P9-AFH-699

# NEUROGENETICS

**CONTEMPORARY NEUROLOGY SERIES AVAILABLE:**

**19** THE DIAGNOSIS OF STUPOR AND COMA, EDITION 3
Fred Plum, M.D., and Jerome B. Posner, M.D.

**26** PRINCIPLES OF BEHAVIORAL NEUROLOGY
M-Marsel Mesulam, M.D., *Editor*

**32** CLINICAL NEUROPHYSIOLOGY OF THE VESTIBULAR SYSTEM, EDITION 2
Robert W. Baloh, M.D., and Vincente Honrubia, M.D.

**36** DISORDERS OF PERIPHERAL NERVES, EDITION 2
Herbert H. Schaumburg, M.D., Alan R. Berger, M.D., and
P.K. Thomas, C.B.E., M.D., D.Sc., F.R.C.P., F.R.C.Path.

**38** PRINCIPLES OF GERIATRIC NEUROLOGY
Robert Katzman, M.D., and John W. Rowe, M.D., *Editors*

**42** MIGRAINE: MANIFESTATIONS, PATHOGENESIS, AND MANAGEMENT
Robert A. Davidoff, M.D.

**43** NEUROLOGY OF CRITICAL ILLNESS
Eelco F.M. Wijdicks, M.D., Ph.D., F.A.C.P.

**44** EVALUATION AND TREATMENT OF MYOPATHIES
Robert C. Griggs, M.D., Jerry R. Mendell, M.D., and Robert G. Miller, M.D.

**45** NEUROLOGIC COMPLICATIONS OF CANCER
Jerome B. Posner, M.D

**46** CLINICAL NEUROPHYSIOLOGY
Jasper R. Daube, M.D., *Editor*

**47** NEUROLOGIC REHABILITATION
Bruce H. Dobkin, M.D.

**48** PAIN MANAGEMENT: THEORY AND PRACTICE
Russell K. Portenoy, M.D., and Ronald M. Kanner, M.D., *Editors*

**49** AMYOTROPHIC LATERAL SCLEROSIS
Hiroshi Mitsumoto, M.D., D.Sc., David A. Chad, M.D., F.R.C.P., and
Eric P. Pioro, M.D., D.Phil., F.R.C.P.

**50** MULTIPLE SCLEROSIS
Donald W. Paty, M.D., F.R.C.P.C., and George C. Ebers, M.D., F.R.C.P.C.

**51** NEUROLOGY AND THE LAW: PRIVATE LITIGATION AND PUBLIC POLICY
H. Richard Beresford, M.D., J.D.

**52** SUBARACHNOID HEMORRHAGE: CAUSES AND CURES
Bryce Weir, M.D.

**53** SLEEP MEDICINE
Michael S. Aldrich, M.D.

**54** BRAIN TUMORS
Harry S. Greenberg, M.D., William F. Chandler, M.D., and Howard M. Sandler, M.D.

**55** THE NEUROLOGY OF EYE MOVEMENTS, Edition 3
R. John Leigh, M.D., and David S. Zee, M.D.
(book and CD-ROM versions available)

**56** MYASTHENIA GRAVIS AND MYASTHENIC DISORDERS
Andrew Engel, M.D., *Editor*

# Neurogenetics

*Edited by*

Stefan-M. Pulst, M.D., Dr. Med.

*Warschaw Chair and Director*
*Division of Neurology*
*Cedars-Sinai Medical Center*
*Professor of Medicine*
*University of California School of Medicine*
*Los Angeles, CA*

New York Oxford
Oxford University Press
2000

Oxford University Press

Oxford New York
Athens Auckland Bangkok Bogotá Buenos Aires Calcutta
Cape Town Chennai Dar es Salaam Delhi Florence Hong Kong Istanbul
Karachi Kuala Lumpur Madrid Melbourne Mexico City Mumbai
Nairobi Paris São Paulo Singapore Taipei Tokyo Toronto Warsaw

and associated companies in
Berlin Ibadan



Published by Oxford University Press, Inc.
198 Madison Avenue, New York, New York 10016



Library of Congress Cataloging-in-Publication Data
Neurogenetics / edited by Stefan-M. Pulst.
p. cm.—(Contemporary neurology series : 57)
Includes bibliographical references and index.
ISBN 0-19-512975-X
1. Nervous system—Diseases—Genetic aspects. 2. Neurogenetics.
I. Pulst, Stefan-M. II. Series.
[DNLM: 1. Genetic Engineering. 2. Genetics, Medical. 3. Nervous System Diseases—genetics.
W1 CO769N v. 57 2000 / WL 140 N4913 2000]
RC346.4.N48 2000 616.8'0442—dc21
DNLM/DLC for Library of Congress 99-22365

The science of medicine is a rapidly changing field. As new research and clinical experience broaden our knowledge, changes in treatment and drug therapy do occur. The author and the publisher of this work have checked with sources believed to be reliable in their efforts to provide information that is accurate and complete, and in accordance with the standards accepted at the time of publication. However, in light of the posibility of human error or changes in the practice of medicine, neither the author, nor the publisher, nor any other party who has been involved in the preparation or publication of this work warrants that the information contained herein is in every respect accurate or complete. Readers are encouraged to confirm the information contained herein with other reliable sources, and are strongly advised to check the product information sheet provided by the pharmaceutical company for each drug they plan to administer.

1 2 3 4 5 6 7 8 9

Printed in the United States of America
on acid-free paper

To my father,
for introducing me to the wonders of
neurology from an early age,
to my wife,
with love and gratitude for
opening my mind to genetics,
and to our children,
Johannes and Alexandra,
for maintaining their interest in
science and medicine despite
many parental absences.

# FOREWORD

The Editor of this book, Stefan Pulst, is a special new type of neurologist, a molecular neurologist. And this important book of his shows the reader how powerful and penetrating his new discipline, molecular neurogenetics, is in its ability to define and characterize the mechanisms of neurological disease.

For over one hundred years, and even until about 20 years ago, neurological texts were descriptive summaries of clinical features, the patient's phenotype, with little information about the biochemical or molecular basis of disease. Recently, there has been a revolution in medical genetics. The methodologies of restriction enzymes, southern, northern, and western blotting, cloning techniques, polymorphisms, knock-out and knock-in and other transgenic animal models, the polymerase chain reaction, and other approaches are now used to define the precise cause of an inherited disease. This approach is now being pioneered by molecular neurologists—as exemplified by the contributors to this book—to provide a clear understanding of the pathogenesis of genetic neurological disease at the molecular level. The progress being made to define gene mutations for neurological diseases is really phenomenal.

There is detailed information about the structure, sequence and regulation of about 3% of the human genome—or about 2100 genes in a human cell expressing about 70,000 genes. There are about 5000 human genetic diseases described in clinical catalogues, and there is detailed information about the gene defect in about 200 human genetic diseases, including neurogenetic diseases. *Neurogenetics* covers this tremendous amount of necessary information in a clear and well-focused manner. The book includes the new and rapidly expanding studies of the molecular basis of Alzheimer's disease, peripheral nerve disease, the epilepsies, the muscular dystrophies, primary tumors of the nervous system, prion diseases, the inherited ataxias, the inherited dementias, hereditary motor neuron diseases, mitochondrial diseases, and genetic issues involved in demyelinating diseases, migraine and cerebrovascular disease. Emphasis on the molecular genotype, rather than the vagaries of the clinical phenotype, is at the core of these chapters. This provides a good foundation to understand the basis of genetic disease, with variable gene expression and penetrance constantly changing within and between families with a constant genotype. Unstable trinucleotide repeat disease mechanisms that are seen in Huntington's disease, the inherited ataxias, myotonic dystrophy, and Kennedy syndrome are hallmarks of new molecular–clinical correlations that the clinician will commonly encounter in a busy practice, and they are wonderfully explained by several contributors. Apoptosis is becoming an important disease-causing mechanism in neurogenetic disease, and it too is well covered.

The Human Genome Project, as of mid-1999, has sequenced about 4% of the human genome, including about 2500–2800 genes. There is about 96% of the genome still to go, representing 65,000 genes being expressed in the human brain, some exclusively in neurons, some exclusively in glia, and many in both. The field of neurogenetics will experience a quantum jump in detailed information by 2003 when the sequencing has been achieved completely. Thousands of new genes, regulatory elements, non-coding regions, repetitive DNA, and polymorphisms will be discovered. Only about 1% of the genome represents coding regions. The remaining 99% contains repetitive DNA, "junk" DNA, regulatory and intronic (non-coding) DNA. This 99% will provide important information about gene regulation and expression and, ultimately, the nuances of neurogenetic disease expression. Many new genetic diseases will be uncovered, and many complex traits due to several genes, possibly interacting with the environment, will be identified

In my view, the next two projects that will require development will be the Human Gene Regulatory Project and, especially for neuroscience, the Human Brain Project. The Human Genome Project is focusing on gene structure. The Human Gene Regulatory Project will emphasize the intricacies of gene expression, including multiple gene interactions with reciprocal inductions, modulations, and inhibitions of genes in a single cell. The Human Brain Project will deal exclusively with coordinate gene expression in multiple neurons or glia that subserve a functional population of neurons and glia to store a unit of information umder normal conditions and an altered pattern of expression in a neurogenetic disease. Gene therapy will be perfected for several neurological diseases including brain tumors, Parkinson's disease, motor neuron diseases and several inherited dementias. We will have to expect the unexpected when following the exponential progress that will ensue in the first two decades of the twenty-first century.

It is apparent that the contributors to this volume are all well aware of the revolution in molecular neurogenetics that is beginning and that will change the face of the practice of neurology. Their insights provide the many clues of what is beginning to take place. It is gratifying to see that neurology as a discipline is finally going to be able to provide the essential data to define complex inherited diseases and lead to effective therapy. The new leadership, as exemplified by Stefan Pulst and his coauthors, represent a synthesis of molecular neurobiology and clinical neurogenetics that will provide far-reaching consequences. *Neurogenetics* represents a new breed of neurology text that provides satisfying answers at last.

Dallas, Tex — Roger N. Rosenberg, M.D.

# PREFACE

Just as our understanding of pathology transformed neurology in the nineteenth century, new genetic knowledge has permeated many aspects of neurology today. Indeed, genetic methods and disease gene identification have changed our basic understanding of neurologic disease processes, and the definition of diseases themselves has undergone changes as DNA based testing is substituted for clinical, morphological or biochemical definitions as a gold standard for diagnosis.

This book is written for neurologists, geneticists, and genetic counsellors. All of the authors are familiar with the differential diagnosis and treatment of the neurogenetic disorders that their chapters cover, and are aware of the issues surrounding DNA-based testing. In addition to covering practical issues, chapters address disease gene function, effects of mutations on phenotype, and animal models that will make this book of interest to the molecular biologist working on fundamental issues of human diseases of the nervous system.

Neurogenetics is a rapidly growing field; new disease genes are identified weekly. Disease groups discussed in this book were selected for their importance to neurologists and geneticists as well as for their illustration of specific mutation or disease mechanisms. The first two chapters provide an introduction to the field of neurogenetics intended for those less familiar with molecular-genetic terminology. The ensuing chapters provide detailed descriptions of inherited diseases covering all aspects of the nervous system. Each chapter begins with descriptions of the clinical phenotypes followed by analysis of disease genes and disease gene function as well as description of cellular and animal models. The correlation of genotype with phenotype is provided to aid the physician in counselling and to provide the basic scientist with a model for the effect of mutant alleles at the organismal level.

It is already apparent that the challenge of the next decade will be the understanding of complex trait genetics. It is likely that single genes responsible for monogenic diseases will emerge as modifiers of more common traits. Reduced penetrance of specific alleles will be traced back to interaction with other alleles or environmental factors that ameliorate or worsen the phenotype. The chapters on migraine, epilepsy, stroke, multiple sclerosis, and Alzheimer disease discuss both rare single gene defects and the presence of more common predisposing alleles in the general population.

Like any other clinical test, DNA-based testing raises the problems of specificity and sensitivity. In a cost-conscious healthcare environment physicians need to be aware of these parameters when testing patients with a positive family history or those patients that appear to be sporadic cases. In contrast to other clinical tests that usually involves only the individual being tested, a positive DNA test has immediate implications for other family members. Testing of presymptomatic individuals raises its own set of specific challenges. These important problems are addressed in the last chapter of the book.

I would like to recognize the major contributions of the chapter authors who did not tire while updating chapters to include the most recently identified disease genes. Lauren Enck provided excellent assistance as medical editor at Oxford University Press, ensuring that the volume maintained clarity and readability throughout. Charles Annis competently served as production editor. Thanks also go to members of my laboratory, past and present, who have provided many stimulating discussions, and to Carmen and Louise Warschaw, whose endowment for neurology has supported many projects in neurogenetics. Finally, in the names of the contributors I wish to thank the patients and families whose participation in genetic studies has made the discovery of disease genes possible.

Los Angeles
July 1999

S.-M.P.

# CONTENTS

# CONTRIBUTORS

CAMERON ADAMS, M.D.
Division of Neurology
Cedars-Sinai Medical Center
Assistant Clinical Professor of Medicine,
UCLA School of Medicine
Los Angeles, CA

ROBERT W. BALOH, M.D.
Professor of Neurology
Department of Neurology
UCLA School of Medicine
Los Angeles, CA

ROBIN L. BENNETT, M.D.
Departments of Neurology and Medicine
University of Washington School of Medicine
VA Puget Sound Health Care System
Seattle, WA

THOMAS D. BIRD, M.D.
Professor, of Neurology and Medical Genetics
University of Washington School of Medicine
VA Puget Sound Medical Center
Seattle, WA

ROBERT H. BROWN, D.PHIL., M.D.
Professor of Neurology
Day Lab for Neuromuscular Research
Harvard Medical School
Massachusetts General Hospital
Charlestown, MA

JEFFREY R. BUCHHALTER, M.D., PH.D.
Associate Professor of Neurology
Mayo Medical School
Mayo Clinic and Foundation
Rochester, MN

PHILLIP F. CHANCE, M.D., F.A.C.M.G.
Chief, Division of Genetics and Development
Children's Hospital and Regional Medical Center
Professor of Pediatrics and Neurology
University of Washington School of Medicine
Seattle, WA

MARIE-PIERRE DUBÉ, PH.D.
Center for Research in Neuroscience
McGill University
Montreal General Hospital Research Institute
Montreal, Quebec, Canada

D. DYMENT, M.SC.
Department of Clinical Neurological Sciences
University of Western Ontario
Vancouver Hospital and Health Sciences Centre-UBC Pavilions
Vancouver, British Columbia, Canada

RICARDO FADIC, M.D.
School of Medicine
Catholic University
Santiago, Chile

THOMAS GASSER, M.D.
Ludwig Maximillians Universitat
Oberarzt der Neurologischen Klinik
München, Germany

ROBERT G. GRIGGS, M.D.
Professor of Neurology
Chair, Department of Neurology
University of Rochester School of Medicine
Rochester, NY

DAVID H. GUTMANN, M.D., PH.D.
Department of Neurology
Washington University School of Medicine
St. Louis, MO

MICHAEL R. HAYDEN, M.D., CH.B., PH.D., F.R.C.P(C), F.R.S.C.
Professor
Director, Center for Molecular Medicine and Therapeutics
University of British Columbia
Vancouver, British Columbia, Canada

DONALD R. JOHNS, M.D.
Associate Professor of Neurology and Ophthalmology
Harvard Medical School
Director, Division of Neuromuscular Disease
Beth Israel Deaconess Medical Center
Boston, MA

H.A. KRETZSCHMAR, M.D.
Professor
Institut fur Neuropathologie
University of Göttingen
Gottingen, Germany

EPHRAT LEVY-LAHAD, M.D.
Department of Medicine
Shaare Zedek Medical Center
Jerusalem, Israel

WOLFGANG H. OERTEL, M.D.
Professor of Neurology
Department of Neurology
Philipps-University
Center for Nervous Diseases
Marburg, Germany

GEORGE W. PADBERG, M.D., PH.D.
University Hospital Nijmegen St. Tadboud
Nijmegen, Netherlands

SUSAN L. PERLMAN, M.D.
Associate Clinical Professor of Neurology
UCLA School of Medicine
Los Angeles, CA

STEFAN-M. PULST, M.D., DR. MED.
Warschaw Chair and Director
Division of Neurology
Cedars-Sinai Medical Center
Professor of Medicine, UCLA School of Medicine
Los Angeles, CA

GUIDO REIFENBERGER, M.D., PH.D.
Institut fur Neuropathologie
Universitaet Bonn
Bonn, Germany

MICHAEL ROSE, M.D.
Department of Neurology
King's Regional Neurosciences Centre
London, England

ALLEN D. ROSES, M.D.
Jefferson Pilot
Professor of Neurobiology and Neurology
Duke University Medical Center
Research Triangle Park, NC

GUY A. ROULEAU, M.D., PH.D.
Center for Research in Neuroscience
Montreal General Hospital
McGill University
Montreal, Quebec, Canada

A. DESSA SADOVNICK, PH.D.
Department of Medical Genetics
University of British Columbia
Vancouver, British Columbia, Canada

JEFFREY SAVER, M.D.
Associate Professor of Neurology
Reed Neurological Research Center
UCLA School of Medicine
Los Angeles, CA

YOSHIHIDE SUNADA, M.D., PH.D.
Professor of Neurology
Division of Neurology
Department of Internal Medicine
Kawasaki Medical School
Okayama, Japan

TITI TAMBURI, M.D.
Consultant in Neurology
University Hospital of Albania
Tirana, Albania

RABI TAWIL, M.D.
Associate Professor of Neurology
Department of Neurology
Rochester University School of Medicine
Rochester, NY

OTTO WINDL, PH.D.
University of Gottingen
Gottingen, Germany

# NEUROGENETICS

Chapter 1

# INTRODUCTION TO MEDICAL GENETICS

Stefan M. Pulst, MD, Dr Med



Gregor Mendel, an Austrian monk, is generally credited with performing the first controlled genetic experiments. By observing the inheritance of specific traits in garden peas, he formulated the fundamental rules of genetics. In contrast to previous animal and plant breeders, Mendel did not stop at the descriptive level, but by analyzing the ratios of observed traits in the offspring he was able to conclude that there must be dominant and recessive traits. Mendel's original publications can now be viewed on the World Wide Web in the original German or an English translation.[1]

When Mendel undertook his seminal controlled breeding experiments in the 1860s, it had already been observed that heredity was transmitted through egg and sperm cells. Soon thereafter, the hereditary material in the nucleus was made visible through special dyes. Subsequently, it was shown that the sex cells contain half the number of chromosomes (*haploid*) than the number found in somatic cells (*diploid*). It took until 1902, however, to advance the hypothesis that half of an individuals chromosomes were contributed by each parent. This year also marked the first description of an "inborn error of metabolism" by Garrod. The term *gene* was coined in 1909 by Johannsen.

The first genetic trait assigned to a chromosome was actually sex itself, when it was discovered that females carry two X chromosomes whereas males carry one X and one Y chromosome. When Bateson rediscovered Mendel's work at the beginning of the twentieth century, the school of biometricians led by Francis Galton regarded mendelian traits as explaining only a small number of largely irrelevant traits. The biometricians followed a statistical study of quantitative traits that they believed was not amenable to mendelian genetics. These opposing theories were finally unified by Fisher, who showed that quantitative traits could be explained by the action of many mendelian genes.

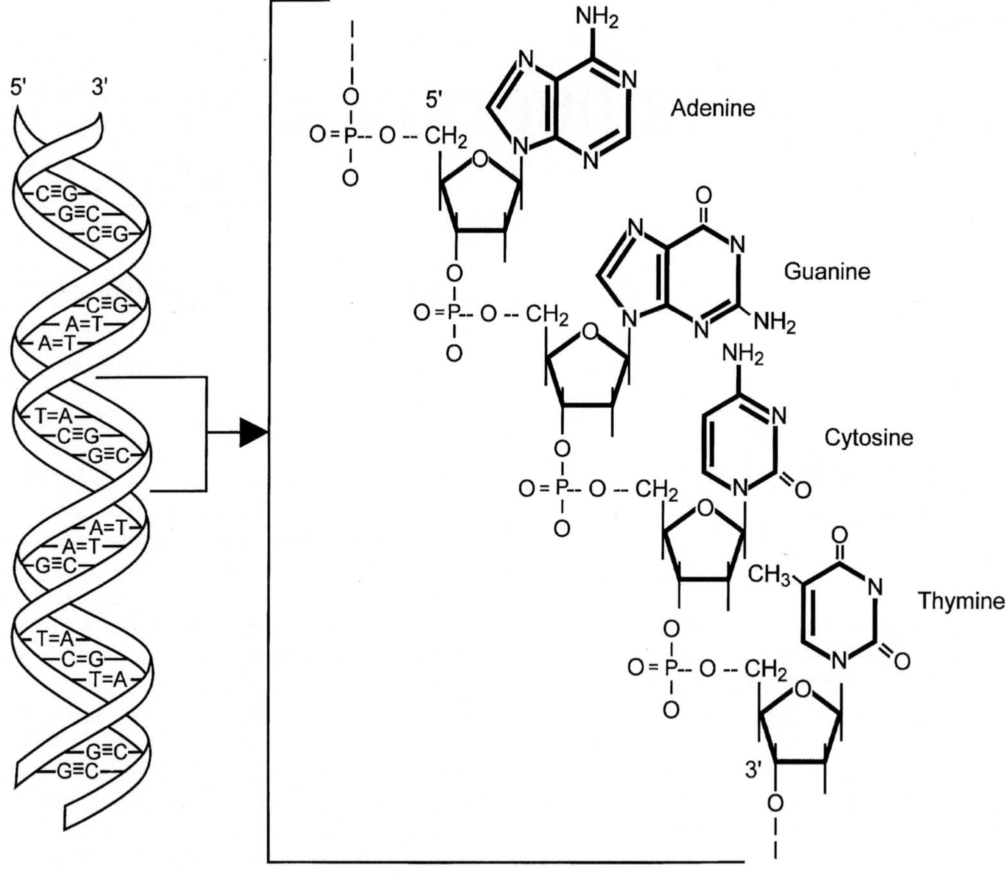


**Figure 1–1.** Structure of DNA. A schematic of the DNA double helix is shown on the left. The chemical structure of four DNA bases connected by phosphodiester bonds is shown on the right.

It was not until the 1940s that Avery and colleagues demonstrated that genetic information is encoded by deoxyribonucleic acid (DNA). Using the detailed x-ray structural DNA studies by Rosalind Franklin, Watson and Crick[2] in 1953 proposed the correct structure for DNA. This structure is now commonly referred to as the DNA *double helix.* In 1956, Tjio and Levan correctly determined the number of chromosomes in a human cell as 46. Three years later it was discovered that Down syndrome was caused by an extra copy of chromosome 21.

The following discussion summarizes some of the basic knowledge concerning molecular and medical genetics. For more detailed descriptions, the reader is referred to specialty textbooks [3,4] and recent reviews.[5–17] For reference citations, preference was given to recent reviews of the subject rather than to original articles. Additional information and figures can be found on the Web.[18,19]

## STRUCTURE OF DNA AND GENES

### DNA Structure

DNA is composed of nucleotide bases, sugar (deoxyribose) groups, and phosphate groups. The nucleotide bases are the two purines A (adenine) and G (guanine) and the two pyrimidines T (thymidine) and C (cytosine).

DNA structurally consists of two unbranched intertwined antiparallel chains, which coil around a common axis (Fig. 1–1). The sugar and phosphate groups form the backbone of each chain. The nucleotide bases pair in a unique fashion so that A always pairs with T and C always pairs with G. Hydrogen bonds stabilize the pairing. Due to the presence of three hydrogen bonds, the G–C pairs have higher thermal stabilities than the A–T pairs, which have only two hydrogen bonds. *Antiparallel* refers to the fact that the 5' end of one strand is aligned with the 3' end of the other strand.

The precise nature of the base-pairing process ensures that the two antiparallel strands are complementary. This provides a means for error correction because one of the strands can serve as a template to repair the other one. In addition, the complementarity of the DNA strands facilitates faithful replication, with each strand serving as the template for a new strand. In 1958, Meselson and Stahl demonstrated this mechanism of DNA replication. It is referred to as *semiconservative replication.*

The complementary nature of DNA has important implications for experimental strategies in molecular research. To identify a DNA fragment with a particular sequence in a complex mixture of DNA molecules, its complementary (or near complimentary) sequence can be used to find this molecule in hybridization-based assays, or complementary oligonucleotide primers can be used in PCR-based assays (see Chapter 2).

## The Structure of a Gene

Genes are the units of heredity. Discrete genes are located linearly at fixed positions along a chromosome. Genes encode information that results in the production of functional end products, either proteins or ribonucleic acid (RNA) molecules. Figures 1–2 and 1–3 graphically depict the structure of a gene and the processes leading from genomic DNA to transcription into messenger RNA (mRNA). After modifications, mRNA is transported out of the nucleus, hence the name messenger RNA, because this type of RNA transports the DNA-encoded information to the cytoplasm. In the cytoplasm, the ribosomal machinery translates this information into an amino acid sequence and synthesizes the protein.

The expressed part of a gene that gives rise to an mRNA transcript is not continuously encoded. Instead, a gene contains interspersed noncoding DNA sequences. These DNA sequences are called *introns* and are present in the primary transcript but are later spliced out when the mature mRNA is formed. Those parts of the gene that remain in the mature transcript and (mostly) code for protein are called *exons.* The processed mRNAs (without introns) exit from the nucleus to the cytoplasm. The following section describes the different steps involved in transcribing the genetic information into mRNA, the processing and modification of the mRNA, and, finally, the translation of mRNA into protein.

## Transcription

Transcription is the process that converts the information contained in the DNA sequence on chromosomes into mRNAs that can leave the nucleus and relay the information to the protein synthesis machinery in the cytoplasm. The amount of mRNA transcribed from a specific gene is regulated and results in cell type–specific transcription patterns.

### PROMOTERS AND ENHANCERS

The primary level of control of gene products is the regulation of gene transcription, the step from DNA to RNA.[10,13,17] The direction of transcription is 5' to 3' and results in a single-stranded RNA molecule. RNA synthesis uses an RNA polymerase with DNA as the template and ATP, CTP, GTP, and UTP (uridinetriphosphate) as RNA precursors. In eukaryotes, three RNA polymerases exist. RNA polymerase II transcribes the genes encoding polypeptides, which represent the vast majority of genes.

The DNA sequences that regulate transcription are located 5', or upstream, of the transcription start site and are referred to as the *promoter.* The sequences are usually clustered within a region not more than 500 base pairs (bp) upstream of the transcription start site. These short sequences bind transcription factors that in turn activate RNA polymerase. Several different sequence motifs influence transcription. In many genes, the promoter is specified by

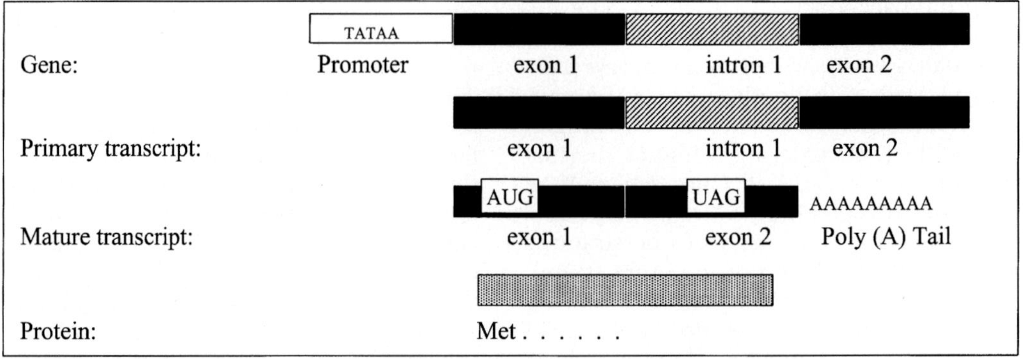


**Figure 1–2.** Simplified representation of the organization of a gene, with its primary and mature transcripts and protein. TATAA box = sequence found in gene promoters; AUG = translation start site (the portion of exon 1 preceding the first AUG codon is not translated; UTR = untranslated region); UAG = stop codon, end of translation.

specific sequences referred to as TATA and CCAAT boxes. The TATA sequence is found around 30 bp 5' to the transcription start site, whereas the CCAAT box may be found 75 to 80 bp upstream of the start site. Promoter sequences are rich in GC pairs (GC box, consensus sequence GGGCGG) that influence transcriptional efficiency and direct tissue-specific expression through the binding of specific transcription factors. One can identify sequences important for the transcriptional control of a gene by linking upstream sequences to reporter genes encoding easily quantifiable gene products and determining their expression after transfer of these constructs into the appropriate cell type.

Other sequences in the vicinity of a gene may influence its transcription. In contrast to promoter sequences, enhancer sequences can exert their effect over greater and variable distances of up to thousands of base pairs and are unaffected by inversion of the enhancer sequences. Enhancers may be located within introns and may act in a tissue-specific fashion.

## RNA PROCESSING

After a protein-encoding gene has been transcribed into an RNA copy in the nucleus, many steps remain to control the readout of information. First, both ends of the single-stranded RNA are modified. At

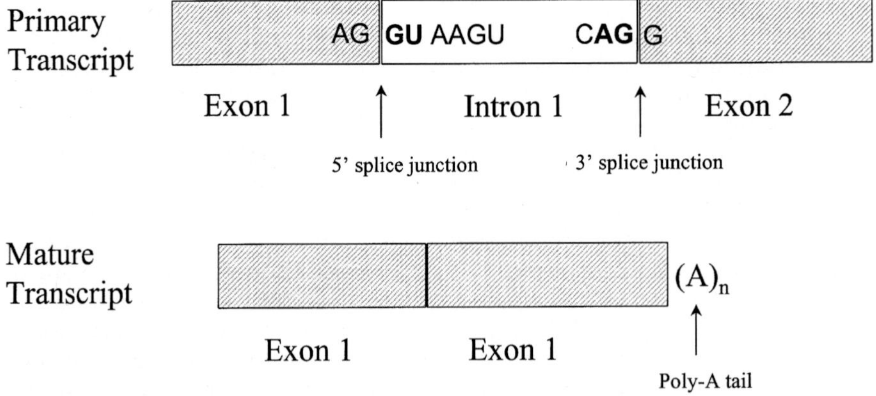


**Figure 1–3.** Splicing of the primary transcript results in the formation of the mature transcript. AG-GUA and CAG-G are splice signals that result in removal of intronic sequences. The bolded intronic sequences (GU-AG) are almost always present. $(A)_n$ = polyA tail added to the primary transcript.

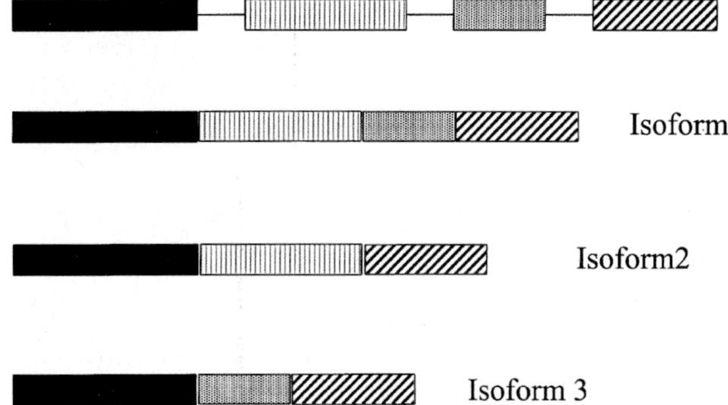


**Figure 1–4.** Different mRNAs are generated by differential splicing of the primary transcript. The genomic organization of a gene is shown at the top, with the transcript isoforms resulting from differential splicing below. These RNA isoforms are translated into different proteins.

the 5' end, a special nucleotide structure, called a *cap*, is added. The function of the cap is to protect the molecule from exonuclease attack to facilitate splicing and transport to the cytoplasm and to help attach the mRNA to cytoplasmic ribosomes, thus increasing efficiency of translation.

At the 3' end of the RNA in the noncoding region lies a sequence (AAUAAA) that acts as a signal for the addition of a stretch of adenine bases to the 3' end of the RNA. About 30 bp downstream of this signal the RNA molecule is cleaved, and approximately 200 adenylate (AMP) residues are added. This polyA tail is important for the stability of the RNA transcript and may facilitate transport to the cytoplasm and translational efficiency.

## SPLICING

As noted earlier, most eukaryotic genes have their coding regions interrupted by introns that must be removed to generate a mature mRNA that in turn can be translated into a protein. This process is referred to as *splicing* and depends on a complex molecular apparatus containing RNA and protein molecules.

The sequences at the 5' and 3' ends of introns show a high degree of sequence similarity. Most introns begin with a GT (the splice donor) and end with an AG (the splice acceptor). This has also been referred to as the GT–AG rule. Extensive sequence analyses of exon–intron boundaries have established that the consensus sequence extends further to adjacent base pairs at the 5' and 3' ends. Not all consensus sequences are utilized, however, indicating that these sequences are necessary but not sufficient for splicing. Mutations at exon–intron boundaries may occasionally activate these "cryptic" splice sites. Although introns do not code for protein sequences, mutations located in introns can affect the protein sequence by altering splicing patterns.

The precise functions of the splicing machinery are only now being understood. The splice sites are bound in a process involving snRNAs (small nuclear RNAs), which contain a sequence complementary to the splice junction donor. Proteins are part of the splicing complex and provide tissue specificity and splicing activity.

Some primary gene transcripts are processed in different ways with or without specific exons. This process is called *alternative splicing* and results in the production of distinct RNA molecules that each encode a slightly different protein (Fig. 1–4). Alternative splicing may occur during development and may be related to differentiation of a tissue, or it may occur in a tissue-specific fashion. Alternative splicing greatly enhances the number of proteins that can be produced by a single gene.

The abbreviation *cDNA* stands for complementary DNA and refers to a specific kind of DNA that is obtained when an mRNA transcript is reverse transcribed (copied) into a complementary DNA strand. To prime (initiate) this reaction, an oligo-dT primer complementary to the polyA tail at the 3' end of the transcript is used, and the cDNA strand is synthesized by the enzyme reverse transcriptase (see later). Alternatively, random primers can be used to prime this reaction. The synthesis of cDNAs is the first step in making a cDNA library and in reverse transcriptase polymerase chain reaction (see Chapter 2).

## Translation

Translation is the process whereby mRNA is decoded on ribosomes to specify the synthesis of a specific protein. After the capped, polyadenylated, and spliced mRNA has been transported from nucleus to cytoplasm, ribosomes scan the mRNA beginning at its 5' end for a sequence specifying the beginning of translation. This *translation start site* is the first AUG codon (in addition to other consensus sequences such as the Kozak sequence) encountered by the ribosomal machinery. A group of three nucleotides (codon) specifies a particular amino acid. Because there are 64 ($4^3$) possible codons, but only 20 amino acids, some amino acids are encoded by more than one codon.

The first AUG is not necessarily close to the 5' end of the mRNA, and several genes have a relatively extended *5' untranslated region* (5'-UTR). The functions of the 5'-UTR are not well defined but may relate to transcript stability as well as to translational efficiency. Similar to the first AUG, there is also a signal that indicates the end of translation. This signal is encoded by three *translation stop codons* that have the sequence UAA, UAG, or UGG.

The first AUG determines the *reading frame* (Fig. 1–5) of the subsequent mRNA sequence. Reading frame refers to the organization of DNA sequence into codons, which in turn determine the amino acid sequence. Figure 1–5 illustrates the effect of changing the reading frame, which may happen with deletions or insertions into the DNA sequence that are not a multiple of 3 bp (or with the normal or abnormal splicing of exons that contain a number of base pairs not divisible by three). Almost immediately after the insertion or deletion, the amino acid sequence is changed and the change in frame produces one of the three stop codons, resulting in premature truncation of translation.

When a genomic DNA sequence of unknown function is examined for the potential of a long open reading frame (ORF), six reading frames need to be examined, three reading the sequence from the "Watson" strand and three reading it from the "Crick" strand.[5] Figure 1–5 shows the three reading frames derived from one strand only.

At the ribosome the mRNA sequence is decoded by tRNAs (transfer RNAs). Each tRNA binds a specific amino acid and has a centrally located specific trinucleotide sequence (anticodon) that binds to the mRNA codon. This mechanism ensures that the information encoded in the mRNA is faithfully transferred to the amino acid sequence. The tRNA transfers the amino acid to the ribosome, where the amino acid is incorporated into the growing polypeptide chain.

## Post-Translational Modifications

Once a protein has been synthesized, it may not yet be functional. Some proteins undergo extensive modifications such as cleavage into smaller polypeptides or addition of functional groups. A common way to regulate the activity of a protein is to add or remove phosphate groups on tyrosine and other amino acid residues (phosphorylation and dephosphorylation). The activity of enzymes (kinases and phosphatases) catalyzing these modifications may be regulated as well, leading to signaling cascades.

Protein modification is important not only for the function of a protein but also for its degradation. The addition of several ubiquitin molecules to a protein (ubiquitination) marks the protein for degradation. Ubiquitinated aggregates have been identified in many neurodegenerative diseases.

# GENOME ORGANIZATION AND CHROMOSOME STRUCTURE

The term *genome* is used to describe the total genetic information in a cell. The human cell actually contains two genomes, a nuclear and a mitochondrial genome. The mitochondrial genome consists of a little more than 16 kilobase pairs (kb) of DNA and is further described in Chapters 2 and 15. The DNA in the haploid human ge-

**ATTTCTGCTAATTATAACGAGTTAATCAGCACCGAGAATATAAATGCA**

**ATT TCT GCT AAT TAT AAC GAG TTA ATC AGC ACC GAG AAT ATA AAT GCA**
***Ile Ser Ala Asn Tyr Asn Glu Leu Ile Ser Thr Glu Asn Ile Asn Glu***

**TTT CTG CTA ATT ATA ACG AGT TAA TCA GCA CCG AGA ATA TAA ATG CA**
***Phe Leu Leu Ile Ile Thr Ser*** **STOP**

**TTC TGC TAA TTA TAA CGA GTT AAT CAG CAC CGA GAA TAT AAA TGC A**
***Phe Cys*** **STOP**

**Figure 1–5.** Different reading frames result in different predicted proteins. A cDNA sequence is on top. The next three lines depict the putative translation products in three different reading frames, each shifted by 1 bp.

nome (one genome equivalent contained in germ cells as opposed to diploid genome in all somatic cells) contains 3 billion bp. The human genome is organized into 22 autosomes and 2 sex chromosomes. Each human somatic cell contains two sets of the autosomes and either two X chromosomes or one X and one Y chromosome, making a total of 46 chromosomes per cell.

## Gene Density and Gene Families

The DNA content of individual chromosomes ranges from 55 million base pairs (Mbp) in chromosome 21 to approximately 250 Mbp in chromosome 1. The human genome is estimated to contain between 60,000 and 90,000 genes. Genes are not evenly distributed in the genome. Gene density can vary significantly between chromosomes and between chromosomal regions. Gene density is high on chromosomes 19 and 22 and in subtelomeric regions.[20]

Although many genes are unique in their sequence composition, others are part of larger gene families with highly conserved DNA sequences. These gene families arise by gene duplication. Members of gene families are occasionally clustered on the same chromosome but are most often found on different chromosomes. Gene duplication often results in nonfunctional (nonprocessed) pseudogenes, when mutations result in premature stop codons. There are also processed pseudogenes that are the result of integration into a chromosome of a natural cDNA sequence that was generated by reverse transcriptase. These genes are nonfunctional due to the lack of an appropriate promoter at the integration site. For molecular diagnosis, highly conserved sequences in gene families may give rise to errors because, instead of the intended gene segment, a related gene sequence or a pseudogene may be analyzed.

The size of genes (exons and introns) ranges from the largest known gene, the dystrophin gene, which covers 2.4 Mbp, to genes that are 20 kb or less such as the insulin or interferon-α genes. There is a similar range in internal organization. The dystrophin gene has 79 exons, whereas the insulin gene has only 3.

## Repetitive DNA

Only about 5% of human DNA codes for expressed sequences that ultimately result in the synthesis of proteins. Of the noncoding DNA, as many as 20% to 30% consist of repetitive DNA sequences. The remainder of DNA is called *single-copy DNA*. As the name implies, single-copy DNA sequences occur only once in the genome and make up approximately 70% to 75% of the genome. Single-copy DNA includes those sequences coding for proteins.

### DISPERSED REPETITIVE DNA

Repetitive DNA can be divided into dispersed repetitive DNA and satellite DNA. The most abundant family of dispersed repeated DNA sequences belongs to the SINES (short interspersed elements) family and is called the *Alu family* because they contain the recognition sequence (AGCT) for the restriction enzyme *Alu*I. These sequences, which are approximately 300 bp long, exist in up to 1 million copies in the genome. An Alu sequence occurs on average every 3000 bp and is specific to human DNA (less than 50% sequence identity between species). The great number of repeats may cause problems in hybridization experiments because a DNA probe containing an Alu sequence will hybridize not only to its single copy target but also to many other fragments containing an Alu sequence. On the other hand, Alu probes can be used to identify clones containing human DNA inserts.

### SATELLITE DNA

α-Satellite DNA is found in the centromeric regions of chromosomes and often extends over several million base pairs. Minisatellites consist of repeating units of 20 to 70 bp and do not extend for more than a few thousand base pairs. Microsatellites (see also Chapter 2) have even smaller repeat units (2 to 6 bp), and their length does not exceed a few hundred base pairs. Both minisatellite and microsatellite DNA is highly variable in length (polymorphic). Due to the ease with which they are amplified by the polymerase chain reaction (PCR), microsatellite markers are a preferred type of genetic marker.

## Variability of the Genome

Human genomic DNA varies about 1 to 2 bp in every 1000 bp between individual chromosomes. This variability is now utilized as a new class of genetic marker, designated as a *single-nucleotide polymorphism* (SNP).[21] The DNA sequence variants are nonrandomly distributed and are much more frequent in noncoding DNA. In coding DNA sequences, DNA variants are commonly encountered in the third position of a codon because they may not change the amino acid sequence. For example, glycine is encoded by the four codons GGA, GGC, GGG, and GGU. Some proteins, however, may be highly polymorphic. Different HLA alleles may differ by more than 10% in their amino acid sequence.

### DNA POLYMORPHISMS AND ALLELES

The variant DNA sequences at a particular chromosomal location (locus) are referred to as *alleles* (Fig. 1–6). When the DNA sequence change causes a disease state, we speak of a mutant allele as compared with the wild-type allele. Thus, a patient with Huntington's disease, an autosomal dominant disease, has one mutant allele (with an expanded CAG repeat) and one normal or wild-type allele. Similar to DNA alleles, we refer to the different forms of a protein due to amino acid substitutions as *protein alleles.* Examples are the different Apolipo-protein E4 alleles.

Allelic sequence variation is conventionally referred to as a *DNA polymorphism* if more than one allele (DNA variant) is found with a frequency of at least 1% in human populations. In other words, if a locus has two or more alleles that occur with a frequency of more than 1%, the locus is referred to as *polymorphic.* The limit of 1% was chosen to exclude chance recurrence of a DNA sequence change, although rare DNA polymorphisms with a frequency of less than 1% exist and allele frequencies may vary greatly between different populations.

■ Wildtype allele 1

ATT TCT GCT AAT TAT AAC GAG TTA ATC AGC ACC GAG AAT ATA AAT
Ile Ser Ala Asn Tyr Asn Glu Leu Ile Ser Thr Glu Asn Ile Asn

■ Wildtype allele 2

ATT TCT GCT AAT TAT AAC GAG TTG ATC AGC ACC GAG AAT ATA AAT
Ile Ser Ala Asn Tyr Asn Glu Leu Ile Ser Thr Glu Asn Ile Asn

■ Mutant allele

ATT TCT GCT AAT TAT AAC GAG TTA ACC AGC ACC GAG AAT ATA AAT
Ile Ser Ala Asn Tyr Asn Glu Leu Thr Ser Thr Glu Asn Ile Asn

**Figure 1–6.** Differences in DNA sequences at a locus create different alleles. Short arrow = an A to G change does *not* alter the protein sequence; long arrow = a T to C change alters the protein sequence.

## GENOTYPES AND HAPLOTYPES

When identical alleles occur on both copies of a chromosome pair, the person is said to be homozygous at this locus. When the alleles differ, the person is heterozygous. If one allele is missing, the person is hemizygous at that locus. For example, all males are hemizygous for alleles on the X chromosome. Some diseases are caused by hemizygosity for a particular gene (e.g., hereditary neuropathy with liability to pressure palsies; see Chapter 4), which is also referred to as *haploinsufficiency.*

DNA polymorphisms are more frequent in noncoding than coding DNA because these DNA changes do not affect the structure or function of a protein. When they occur in a coding sequence, they likely involve the third base of a codon, which does not change the amino acid sequence in many cases. Even if changes in the third base of a codon do not change the amino acid sequence, however, they may introduce cryptic splice sites.

DNA polymorphisms have become indispensable tools for the mapping of genetic traits. In contrast to protein polymorphisms, which are not abundant and are less polymorphic due to the functional constraints on the protein, certain types of DNA sequence variations are highly polymorphic. These are further discussed in Chapter 2.

The alleles at a specific locus define the *genotype.* For example, the genotype for the trinucleotide repeat of a patient with spinocerebellar ataxia type 2 *(SCA2)* may be designated as $(CAG)_{37}/(CAG)_{22}$, referring to the fact that this individual has 37 CAG repeats in the ataxin-2 gene on one chromosome 12 and 22 repeats on the other chromosome 12.[22]

A string of alleles on the *same* chromosome are referred to as a chromosomal *haplotype.* To determine a chromosomal haplotype, one must either separate the two homologous chromosomes, for example, by generating somatic cell hybrid cell lines that contain one of the homologous chromosomes in a rodent cell, or determine the "phase" of alleles by determining the parental genotypes. For example, an individual has the alleles 1 and 2 at locus *A* and alleles 3 and 4 at locus *B.* From this information alone it cannot be determined if the chromosomal haplotypes are 1–3 and 2–4 or 1–4 and 2–3. When we determine parental and grandparental genotypes, however, as shown in Figure 1–7, it is possible to determine the haplotype of the proband's chromosomes. Thus, a haplotype defines a specific chromosomal region and distinguishes it from the same region on the homologous chromosome (see also Chapter 2, Fig. 2–12).

## Chromosome Structure

The DNA in a human diploid cell is organized into 46 chromosomes consisting of

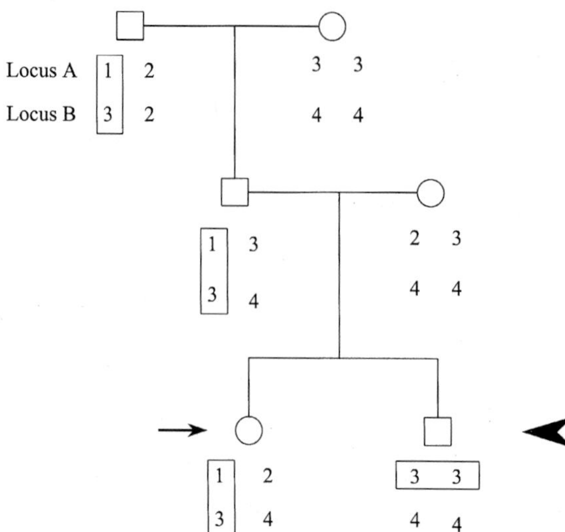


**Figure 1–7.** Three-generation pedigree showing segregated alleles in two adjacent loci. Studying the inheritance of the alleles allows reconstruction of the chromosomal haplotype that is boxed. The haplotypes of the individual marked by an arrow are 1–3 and 2–4. The two alleles at one locus on homologous chromosomes define the genotype. The genotype of the individual marked by an arrowhead is 3/3. Squares = males; circles = females; connecting lines = genetic line of descent.

22 pairs of autosomes (chromosomes 1 through 22), and a twenty-third pair representing the sex chromosomes. One chromosome of each pair is inherited from the father, the other one from the mother. For the sex chromosomes, the Y chromosome is inherited from the father, the X chromosome from the mother or the father.

If the DNA in a cell were stretched out as a straight double helix molecule, it would actually be about 2 m long. To fit DNA into the confines of the cell nucleus, it is coiled several times. This requires an ordered folding of DNA (Fig. 1–8). First, DNA is wrapped in tight turns around a core of histone proteins (nucleosomes). Nucleosomes in turn are coiled into helical solenoids. These are then organized into chromatin loops that attach to a protein scaffold. Each chromatin loop contains about 100 kb of DNA. In the end, the DNA molecules are condensed 10,000-fold compared with their stretched out length.

## FUNCTIONAL ELEMENTS

Chromosomes contain three important functional elements. *Centromeres* ensure proper segregation of chromosomes during mitosis and meiosis. *Telomeres* confer chromosome stability by capping the ends of chromosomes. Both centromeres and telomeres contain long arrays of repeated DNA. DNA replication is initiated at specialized sites on the chromosomes called *origins of replication.* These three sequence elements are sufficient for proper chromosome functioning as has been demonstrated by the creation of artificial chromosomes in yeast and mammalian cells in which large DNA fragments are ligated to these elements.[23]

## CHROMOSOME BANDING

Although chromosomes can be visualized microscopically, it is difficult to distinguish between individual chromosomes. After arrest of cells in metaphase with spindle poisons such as colchicine and the use of staining materials, a characteristic banding pattern is produced that allows one to distinguish individual chromosomes and to detect structural chromosomal abnormalities. Routine banding techniques produce 300 to 400 bands. "High-resolution" banding can increase this number to 800 and allows the detection of subtle chromosome abnormalities.

The short arm of a chromosome is designated p (from French *petite*) and the long arm, q. Major bands are numbered beginning at the centromere. Thus, 12q24 refers to the fourth band in the second region of the long arm of chromosome 12, and 12q24.1 refers to the first subband in this region. The normal male karyotype is de-

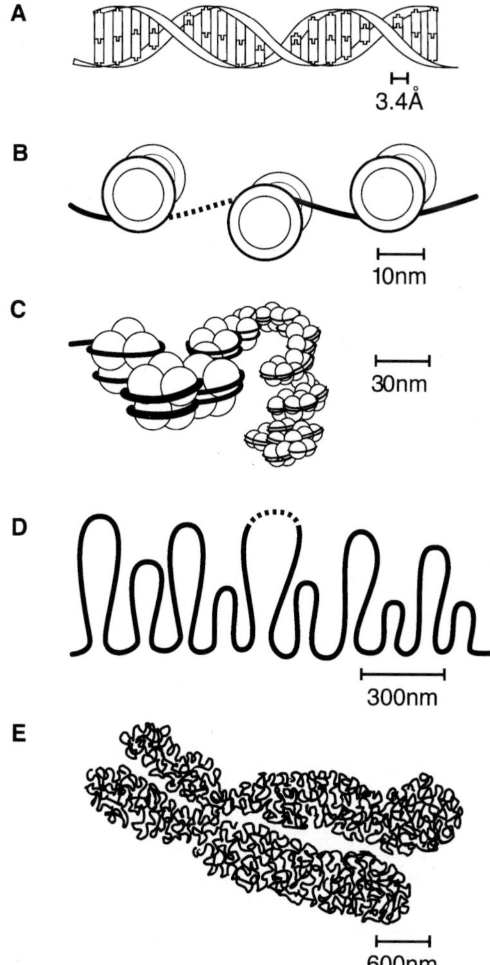


**Figure 1–8.** Progressive compaction of the DNA string leads from a linear double helical molecule to a highly condensed chromosome. *(A)* Double helix, *(B)* nucleosome, *(C)* chromatin fiber, *(D)* Loops of chromatin, and *(E)* metaphase chromosome.

scribed as 46,XY, the normal female karyotype as 46,XX.

## MITOSIS AND MEIOSIS

The human body develops from a single diploid cell, the zygote, to a final number of approximately 100 trillion ($10^{14}$) cells. From the G1 phase of the cell cycle, the cell enters the S phase in which new DNA is synthesized. The S phase is followed by a short G2 phase in which some DNA repair occurs. At the end of G2, the cell contains two complete and identical sets of 46 chromosomes each in which the identical chromosomes are paired (sister chromatids). The process of distributing sister chromatids into the two daughter cells is called *mitosis.* During metaphase (when chromosomes are in their most condensed state), spindle fibers attach to chromosome centromeres and pull the sister chromatids to opposites ends of the cell. At the end of mitosis new nuclear membranes form around each chromosome set, and cytokinesis results in division of the cytoplasm into two parts. Thus, mitosis results in the formation of two identical diploid cells from a single diploid cell.

*Meiosis,* on the other hand, is a specialized form of cell division leading from a diploid cell to a haploid genome, which is contained in sperm or egg cells. Meiosis encompasses two cell divisions. From diploid cells—called *spermatogonia* in males and *oogonia* in females—two haploid cells are formed during meiosis I (reduction division). Meiosis I begins with a duplication of DNA without duplication of the centromeres. After pairing of homologous chromosomes one can see four-stranded chromosomes (tetrads) consisting of two pairs of sister chromatids. Homologous chromosomes are then pulled apart, and two cells with haploid genomes result. In meiosis II, the sister chromatids are separated, resulting in cells containing 23 chromosomes and $3 \times 10^9$ bp.

## INDEPENDENT ASSORTMENT OF PATERNAL AND MATERNAL CHROMOSOMES

Unlike mitosis (or meiosis II), meiosis I is a reductive division because the paternal and maternal homologue of each chromosome are segregated into different cells. This process does not, however, distinguish between maternal and paternal chromosomes, a process referred to as *independent assortment.* On average, in an individual sperm cell, half of the chromosomes are of paternal and half of maternal origin. Even without the effects of recombination (see below), independent assortment results in a tremendous reshuffling of genetic material. For 23 chromosomes, the possibilities of chromosome assortment are $2^{23}$, or a little more than 8 million different ways to assort the chromosomes.

### RECOMBINATION

When the homologous chromosomes closely align in meiosis I, individual chromatids can be seen to cross over one another and form so-called chiasmata. Chiasma formation results in exchange of material between maternal and paternal chromosome homologues (Fig. 1–9). The resulting new "recombined" chromosomes now contain regions derived from the paternal homologue next to regions derived from the maternal homologue. The process of recombination further increases the genetic variation between the gametes of a single individual, which was already enormous just based on the independent assortment of chromosomes.

## PATTERNS OF INHERITANCE

*Mendelian* or *unifactorial inheritance* refers to a pattern of inheritance that can be explained on the basis of mutation in a single gene. Thus, the presence or absence of a genetic character depends on the genotype at a single locus.

Monogenic traits are also referred to as *mendelian* traits because they follow the well-delineated patterns of inheritance first described by Mendel in 1865. Mendelian disorders can be autosomal dominant, autosomal recessive, or X-linked and are caused by mutations in a single gene. In contrast to monogenic disorders, complex genetic traits cannot be explained on the basis of mutations in a single specific gene, and a phenotype is only observed when mutations in several genes have occurred. Examples of complex genetic traits are discussed in the chapters on epilepsies, multiple sclerosis, and stroke.

## Phenotype

Whereas genotype refers to a person's DNA sequence at a specific chromosomal locus, the term *phenotype* describes what can be observed clinically. In addition to the "clinical" phenotype, one can also speak of cellular or biochemical phenotypes that may not be directly observable by physical examination.

There may not be a defined relationship between genotype at a locus and phenotype. Mutations in different genes may produce a similar phenotype. For example, mutations in different genes on different chromosomes may cause familial Alzheimer disease (see Chapter 16). These observations suggest, but do not prove, that the proteins encoded by these genes may be involved in the same cellular pathway.

On the other hand, the same mutation

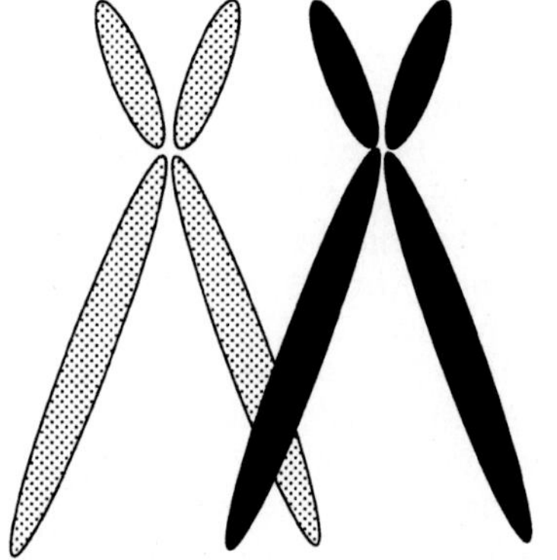

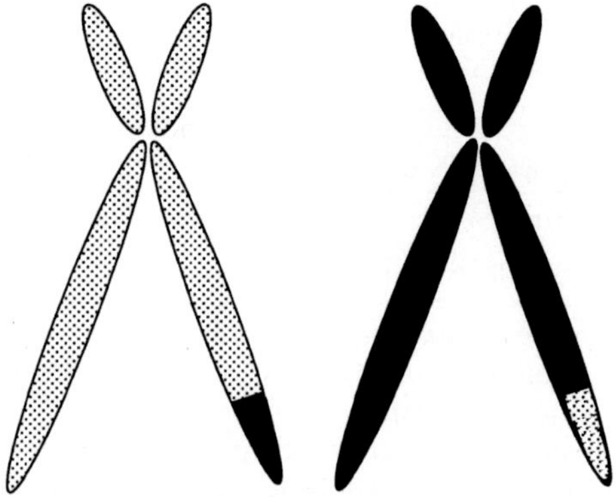

**Figure 1–9.** Chiasma formation results in the exchange of DNA between chromatids of homologous chromosome pairs. Multiple chiasmata are normally formed, but only one is shown for clarity of illustration. The paternal chromosome is shown in black, the maternal chromosome is dotted. The results of recombination are shown on the right with the individual chromatids now containing both paternal and maternal components.

can result in very different phenotypes or in significantly different ages of onset or disease severity. Phenotypic variability associated with a specific mutation may be caused by several genetic and nongenetic factors. The phenotype is determined not only by the genotype at the disease locus, but genotypes at other loci may have an influence as well. These factors are often referred to as modifying loci or modifying alleles. Stochastic events, such as loss of genetic material during mitosis, are important in determining phenotype, especially in patients with tumor suppressor syndromes.[24] This phenomenon is described further in Chapters 8 and 9. In addition, the phenotype may be influenced by the interaction of environmental factors with the genotype. For example, symptoms in patients with certain forms of periodic paralysis may be precipitated by factors such as cold or diet.

## Dominance and Recessiveness

Fundamental to the understanding of mendelian inheritance are the concepts of dominance and recessiveness. Dominance and recessiveness are properties of traits, not of genes, because different mutations in the same gene on the autosomes may show dominant or recessive inheritance. For example, mutations in the same channel protein can lead to dominant as well as recessive traits, depending on the precise location of a missense mutation (see Chapter 3).

Dominance is not a property intrinsic to a particular allele, but describes the relationship between it and the corresponding allele on the homologous chromosome with regard to a particular trait. A trait is dominant if it is manifest in the heterozygote. Dominant alleles exert their phenotypic effect despite the presence of a normal (wild-type) allele on the second homologous chromosome. Thus, if the phenotypes associated with genotypes *AA* and *AB* are identical but are different from the *BB* phenotype, the *A* allele is dominant to allele *B*. Conversely, the *B* allele is recessive to the allele *A*. Recessive mutations lead to phenotypic consequences only when both alleles contain mutations. If the mutations on both alleles are different, this is referred to as *compound heterozygosity*. An example would be a patient with Friedreich's ataxia whose mutation is an expansion of the intronic GAA repeat on one allele while the other allele carries a missense mutation (see Chapter 12).

The same mutation can lead to recessive or dominant traits. Homozygotes for the *HbS* mutation manifest the trait *sickle cell anemia*, and sickle cell anemia is a recessive disease. Sickling, the aggregation of red blood cells at low oxygen tensions, however, is a dominant trait because it is seen in heterozygotes that carry one allele with the *HbS* mutation and one wild-type allele.

Most human dominant syndromes occur only in heterozygotes. Some geneticists refer to dominant mutations that have the same phenotype in heterozygotes and homozygotes as "true" dominant, for example, the rare individuals homozygous for expansion in the Huntington gene. This is distinguished from "semidominant" when the heterozygote *AB* has an intermediate phenotype between the phenotypes of *AA* and *BB*.

If the phenotypes of *AB*, *AA*, and *BB* are identical, alleles *A* and *B* are said to be *codominant*. The human ABO blood system is an example of codominant alleles. Characteristics of different inheritance patterns are summarized in Table 1–1.

### MECHANISMS OF DOMINANCE

The majority of mutations result in an inactive gene product (see later under Types of Mutations). The function of the remaining normal allele, however, is sufficient in most cases to guarantee normal cellular function. Therefore, most mutant alleles are recessive. When the function of the remaining allele is not sufficient to maintain normal function, this is referred to as *haploinsufficiency*.

### GAIN OF FUNCTION

Most dominant mutations lead to a gain of function. This may be due to gene dosage that is a deviation of the normal gene copy number of 2. An example is the duplication of the *PMP22* gene leading to Charcot-

Table 1–1. **Patterns of Inheritance**

| Autosomal Dominant | Autosomal Recessive | X-Linked Recessive | Mitochondrial |
|---|---|---|---|
| 50% risk to offspring | 25% risk to offspring | 50% risk to sons of carrier females | Transmission via females only, all children at risk |
| Males and females equally affected | Males and females equally affected | Only males affected | Males and females at risk |
| Vertical transmission, multiple affected generations, father–son transmission seen | Horizontal transmission, single affected generation | Multiple generations affected, no father–son transmission | Multiple generations affected, maternal transmission only |
| | Consanguinity increased | | Highly variable expression and disease severity |

Marie-Tooth disease type 1 (see Chapter 4). Missense mutations in a gene may lead to proteins with altered or new functions. This may be due to the loss of negative regulatory domains, loss of normal protein degradation, or abnormal protein processing, as has been suggested for the Alzheimer amyloid precursor protein (APP) (see Chapter 16).

Although mutations in most enzymes lead to loss of function and are recessive, certain mutations in the superoxide dismutase gene seen in patients with amyotrophic lateral sclerosis have a dominant effect due to novel functions of the mutant enzyme (see Chapter 14). A toxic gain of function has also been suggested for mutant proteins containing extended polyglutamine stretches (see Chapters 12 and 13).

### LOSS OF FUNCTION MUTATIONS ASSOCIATED WITH DOMINANT TRAITS

Loss of function mutations may be dominant, when they involve a critical rate-limiting step in a metabolic pathway, or involve regulatory genes or structural genes that are sensitive to gene dosage effects. For example, complete loss of one copy of the *PMP22* gene on human chromosome 17p causes hereditary predisposition to pressure palsy (see Chapter 4). *Dominant-negative* mutations result in a mutant protein that interferes with the action of the normal protein. For example, in a homodimeric protein (a protein complex made up of two identical proteins), the mutation of one allele will result in only 25% of the resulting dimers having a normal composition.

Loss of function mutations in certain types of genes are recessive at the level of the cell but dominant at the level of the whole organism. This mechanism is observed in *tumor suppresser gene syndromes.* Germline mutations in these patients (first hit) result in an inactive gene product derived from one allele. When the second allele is lost in specific cell types (second hit), abnormal proliferation of these cells results. Because the second hit occurs with such great frequency over a person's lifetime, the inheritance pattern is that of a dominant disease with high penetrance (Fig. 1–10). Due to the stochastic nature of the second hit, however, tumor formation is age dependent and may be highly variable. Examples of tumors suppressor genes are discussed in Chapters 8 and 9.

## INHERITANCE PATTERNS

The relationship between members of a family are conveniently indicated by a pedigree notation (Fig. 1–11). In addition to their blood relationship, phenotypic and genotypic information can be included in

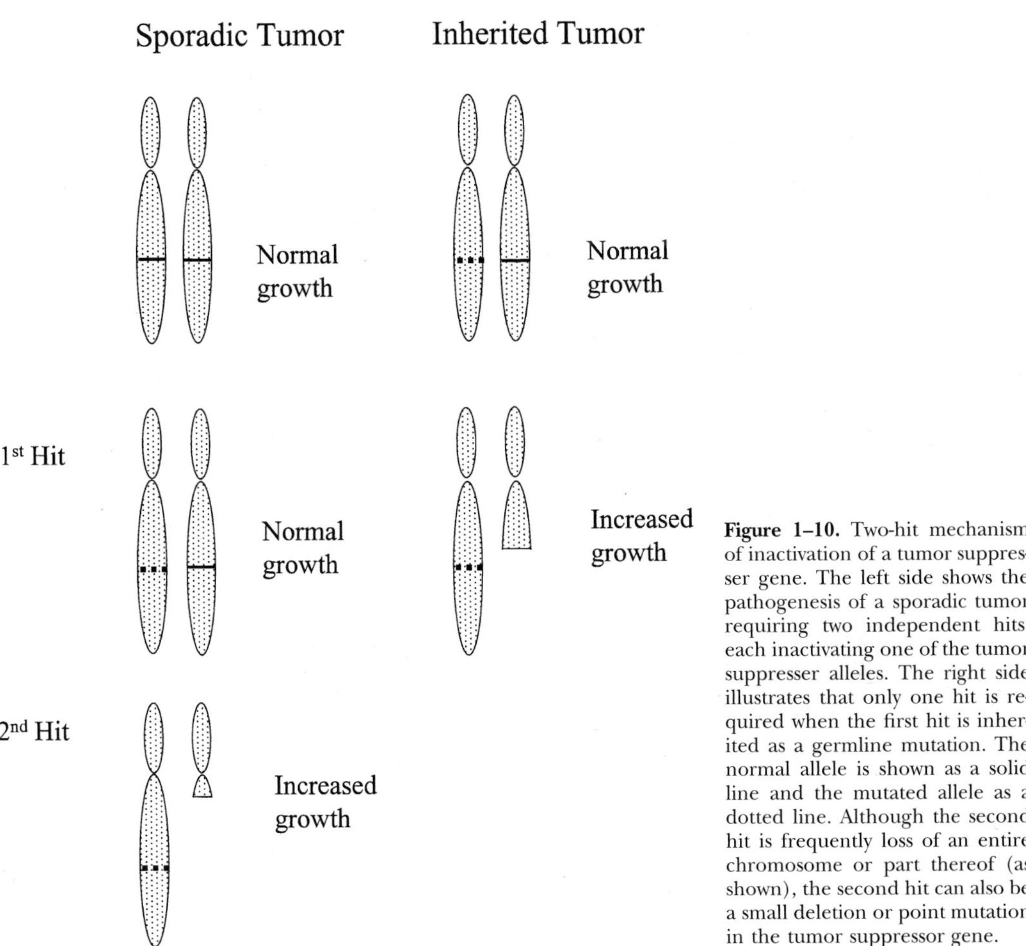


**Figure 1–10.** Two-hit mechanism of inactivation of a tumor suppresser gene. The left side shows the pathogenesis of a sporadic tumor requiring two independent hits, each inactivating one of the tumor suppresser alleles. The right side illustrates that only one hit is required when the first hit is inherited as a germline mutation. The normal allele is shown as a solid line and the mutated allele as a dotted line. Although the second hit is frequently loss of an entire chromosome or part thereof (as shown), the second hit can also be a small deletion or point mutation in the tumor suppressor gene.

one graphic display. The first individual ascertained in a pedigree (the *proband*) is indicated by an arrow.

## Autosomal Dominant

In autosomal dominant disorders, a mutation in a single gene on any of the 22 autosomes produces clinical symptoms or signs. The disease or mutant allele is dominant to the wild-type alleles, and the disease phenotype is seen in heterozygotes.

Offspring are at 50% risk to inherit the disease (Fig. 1–12 *A*). Offspring who inherit the normal allele will not develop the disease or pass it on to their offspring. The disease appears over multiple generations, which appears as *vertical transmission* in the pedigree notation. Males and females are evenly affected, and the disease is passed on from affected fathers or mothers to male and female offspring with equal probabilities. Autosomal dominant disorders may exhibit several important general features: pleiotropism, variable expressivity and delayed age of onset, and variable penetrance.

### PLEIOTROPISM

*Pleiotropism* refers to the phenomenon in which multiple, seemingly unrelated, phenotypic effects are produced by a single mutant gene. The presence of cataracts, insulin intolerance, and muscle weakness in patients with myotonic dystrophy is an example of pleiotropism. Pleiotropism should not be confused with phenotypes seen in

| | Symbol | Comments |
|---|---|---|
| 1. Individual (Male) | | Assign gender by phenotype. |
| 2a. Affected individual (Female) | | Key/legend used to define shading or other fill. (e.g., hatches, dots, etc.) |
| 2b. Affected individual (Male) | | With ≥2 conditions, the individual's symbol should be partitioned accordingly, each segment shaded with a different fill and defined in legend. |
| 3. Multiple individuals (Number known for female) | 5 | Number of siblings written inside symbol. (Affected individuals should not be grouped). |
| 4. Deceased individual (Sex Unknown) | d. 35y | If death is known, write "d." with age at death below symbol. |
| 5a. Proband | | First affected family member coming to medical attention. |
| 5b. Consultand | P | Individual(s) seeking genetic counseling/testing. |
| 6. Spontaneous abortion (SAB) | male | If due to an ectopic pregnancy, write ECT below symbol. Also note sex below symbol. |
| 7. Affected SAB | female | If gestational age known, write below symbol. Key/legend used to define shading. |
| 8. Termination of pregnancy (TOP) | sex unknown | No abbreviations used for sake of consistency. |
| 9. Obligate carrier (will **not** manifest disease) | | Normal phenotype and negative test result. (e.g., Woman with normal physical exam and carrier of a mutation in the frataxin gene) |
| 10. Asymptomatic/ presymptomatic carrier | | Clinically unaffected at this time but could later exhibit symptoms. (e.g., Man age 25 with normal physical exam and positive DNA test) |
| 11. Genetic line of descent (vertical or diagonal) | | Biologic parents shown connected by horizontal line. Offspring are connected to parents by a vertical line. |
| 12. Twins | Monozygotic / Dizygotic | A horizontal line between the symbols implies a relationship line. |
| 13. Consanguinity | | If degree of relationship is not obvious from the pedigree, it should be stated above the relationship line. (e.g., third cousins) |

**Figure 1–11.** Pedigree symbols according to Bennett and associates.[31]

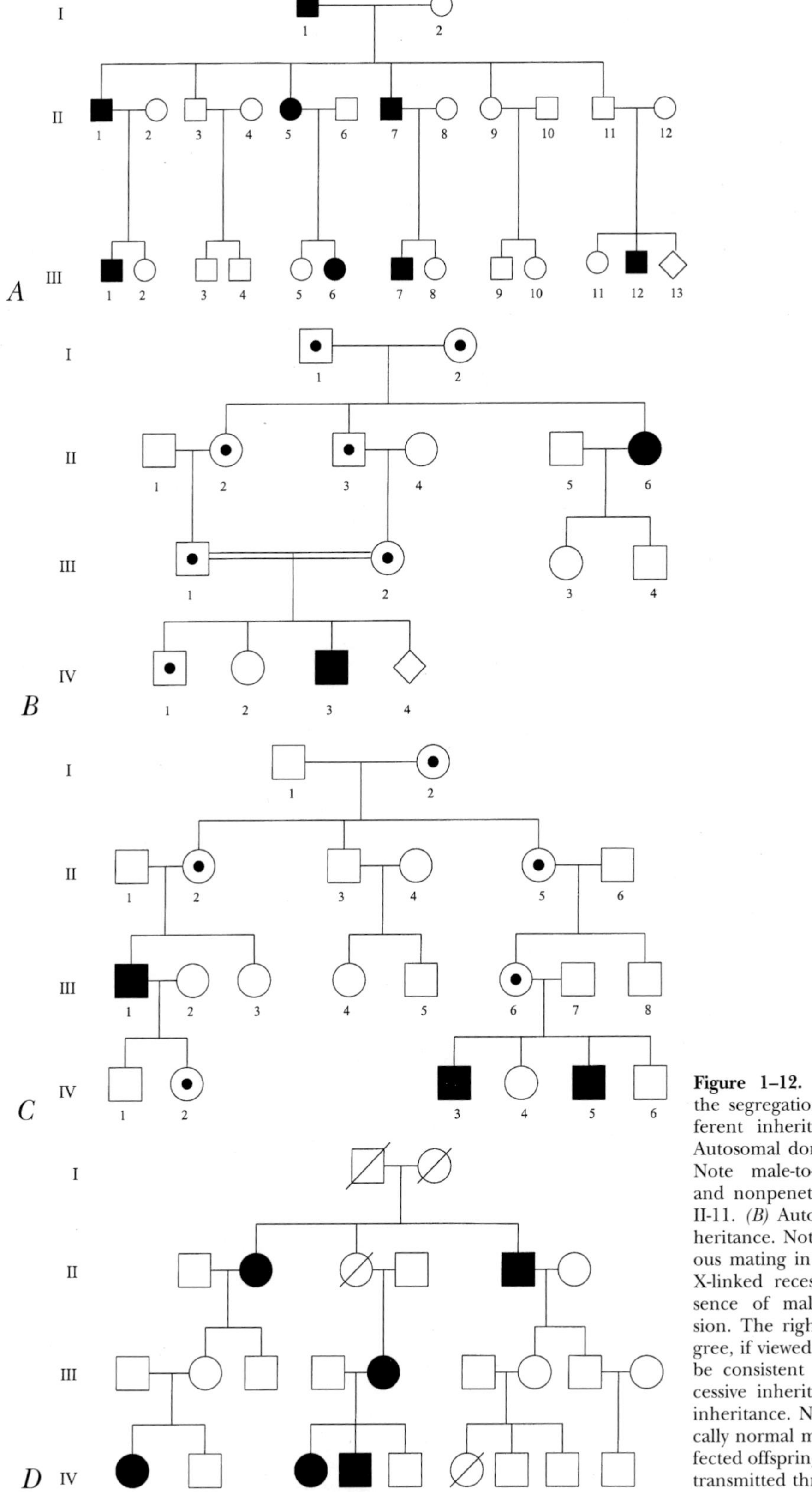


**Figure 1–12.** Pedigrees showing the segregation of traits with different inheritance patterns. *(A)* Autosomal dominant inheritance. Note male-to-male transmission and nonpenetrance in individual II-11. *(B)* Autosomal recessive inheritance. Note the consanguineous mating in generation III. *(C)* X-linked recessive. Note the absence of male-to-male transmission. The right half of the pedigree, if viewed by itself would also be consistent with autosomal recessive inheritance. *(D)* Maternal inheritance. Note that phenotypically normal mothers can have affected offspring. The disease is not transmitted through fathers.

contiguous gene syndromes, where multiple genes that are adjacent to one another are involved in creating a phenotype. This usually occurs through chromosome deletions.

### PENETRANCE

An individual who carries a disease allele may not show any manifestations of the disease phenotype. This individual may, however, transmit the disease to the next generation. Studies have shown that in pedigrees with familial torsion dystonia approximately 30% of individuals who are known to carry the *DYT1* mutation do not show signs of a movement disorder.[25] Thus, the penetrance of mutations in the *DYT1* gene is considered to be 30%. Penetrance is also related to the thoroughness of the clinical examination and to the use of ancillary studies. For example, some individuals carrying a mutation in the *NF1* gene may appear to be nonpenetrant unless a slit-lamp examination is performed and Lisch's nodules (iris hamartomas) are detected (see Chapter 9). Neuroimaging studies can detect the presence of disease in disorders such as tuberous sclerosis or neurofibromatosis 2, when clinical examination does not reveal any abnormalities.

### EXPRESSIVITY

*Variable expressivity* of a mutation can refer to variable severity of disease symptoms or variable age of onset but also to expression of completely different symptoms in carriers of the mutation. Striking examples of variable expressivity can be found in patients with mutations in tumor suppressor genes. For example, in one pedigree, some individuals with *NF1* may show only café-au-lait spots, whereas others have plexiform neurofibromas or optic gliomas. The typical mutation in the *DYT1* gene (i.e., deletion of a GAG codon) causes generalized dystonia in most individuals. In one family, however, individuals with this mutation developed writer's cramp. This is an example of variable expressivity of the mutation.[26]

Variable expressivity may be due to different types of mutations at the disease locus (allelic heterogeneity). Variable expressivity in the same family (where everybody carries the identical mutation) may be due to effects of modifying genes or to stochastic events such as the loss of the second allele in tumor suppresser gene syndromes. Environmental factors may play a role as well.

The terms *penetrance* and *expressivity of a mutation* need to be clearly differentiated. Penetrance is an all-or-none phenomenon. Signs of a given phenotype (e.g., clinical, biochemical, imaging) are either present or not present. Variable expressivity describes the extent and variability of the expression of the phenotype.

## Autosomal Recessive

When both copies of a gene need to be mutated to produce a phenotype, the disorder is inherited as an autosomal recessive trait (Fig. 1–12 *B*). Only individuals homozygous for the disease gene will develop the disease, whereas heterozygous individuals (one normal copy and one mutated copy) are clinically normal. Because heterozygotes may pass on an abnormal gene to their offspring, they are called *carriers*. Parents of affected individuals are usually carriers of the disease gene, and each parent contributes one abnormal copy to the offspring. Disease risk to siblings is 25%, 50% of siblings will be carriers, and 25% will have two normal copies of the gene. In contrast to autosomal dominant inheritance, where vertical transmission is observed, horizontal aggregation is typical for recessive disorders, where multiple individuals in one generation are affected.

The likelihood to encounter recessive disorders is increased in specific populations that have a high frequency of mutant alleles. For example, Tay-Sachs disease is common in Ashkenazi Jews with a heterozygote frequency of 1 in 30, whereas the frequency in Caucasians is only 1 in 3000.

Consanguinity may be present in pedigrees with autosomal recessive inheritance. The probability that a mating was consanguineous increases when the mutant allele is very rare. At a frequency of 0.04 for a mutant gene, the chance of mating with another carrier is 1 in 25. This chance would only be increased to 1 in 8 when mating occurs with a first-degree cousin. Therefore, consanguinity is not a major factor for a disease such as cystic fibrosis. For many of the rare neurologic recessive diseases, consanguinity becomes a factor. For example, at a the low mutant gene frequency of 0.008 for Wilson's disease, half of the cases are the result of consanguineous matings.[27] Consanguinity is seen in many cultures of the Mideast.

## X-Linked Inheritance

In X-linked disorders, the mutation lies on the X chromosome. Because females have two X chromosomes, females with X-linked recessive disorders are usually clinically normal. Sons of carrier females are at 50% risk to inherit the mutation and to develop clinical signs (Fig 1–12 *C*). Affected males carry one copy of the mutated allele, but no normal allele. This state is called *hemizygosity* and differs from heterozygosity in the lack of a second (normal) allele. Daughters of affected males are carriers with 100% risk because all paternal X chromosomes carry the mutated allele.

Although carrier females are usually clinically normal, occasional carrier females are mildly symptomatic or show biochemical signs of the disease. These individuals are called *manifesting heterozygotes*. The basis for this is X-inactivation, a random process that leads to inactivation of one copy of the X chromosome. Inactivation of one X chromosome compensates for the presence of two X chromosomes in females. (Only a small part of the X chromosome escapes inactivation.) Although in most carrier females the normal and abnormal X chromosomes are inactivated approximately half of the time, in occasional individuals the majority of normal chromosomes are inactivated by chance resulting in (usually mild) expression of disease manifestations. Examples of manifesting heterozygotes are seen in Duchenne's dystrophy, most frequently at the biochemical level with increased levels of creatinine phosphokinase.

Because sons inherit their X chromosome from their mother, they cannot pass the disease on when they have a normal phenotype. Thus, X-linked recessive disorders show only affected males, but transmission of the disease occurs through unaffected mothers. Male-to-male transmission excludes X-linked inheritance. Examples of X-linked recessive disorders include the Duchenne and Becker dystrophies, Kennedy's syndrome, and some forms of inherited neuropathies.

X-linked dominant diseases are rare. When a trait is X-linked dominant, females are also affected. The disease, however, is usually more severe in the hemizygous males. Rett's syndrome only occurs in females and may be an example of an X-linked dominant disease that leads to death of male embryos *in utero*. Selective sparing of males in an X-linked dominant disorder has also been described.[28]

## Mitochondrial Inheritance

The mitochondrial genome is distinct from the nuclear genome. A cell contains several hundred mitochondria in its cytoplasm. A single mitochondrion contains up to 10 circular DNA molecules, and each circular DNA molecule in turn contains 16,569 bp. This DNA codes for 13 proteins involved in oxidative phosphorylation, two ribosomal RNAs, and 22 transfer RNAs (see Chapter 15).

The mitochondrial DNA of a fetus is solely contributed by the mother. Although the precise number is not yet known, some evidence suggests that a subset of the oocyte mitochondria contributes all of the embryo's mitochondria. The mitochondria are not all identical so that mutant as well as normal mitochondrial DNAs can be found in the same cell. The presence of normal and mutated mitochondrial DNAs in one cell is called *heteroplasmy*. No mitochondria are contributed by the sperm. This explains why mitochondrial disorders are only transmitted through the mother (Fig.1–12 *D*). The number of mutant mitochondria in each offspring may vary, however, resulting in extremely variable phenotypes. All children are at risk to inherit at least some mutated mitochondria.

## Other Genetic Mechanisms Affecting Phenotype

Issues of nonpenetrance, modifying alleles, and interaction of genotypes with environmental factors are discussed earlier. Two mechanisms that have now been defined at the molecular level are briefly reviewed here.

### ANTICIPATION

In several diseases, a phenomenon of earlier disease onset in successive generations has been observed. This observation, however, was difficult to distinguish from the biased ascertainment of probands or from random variations in the age of onset. With the identification of unstable DNA repeats, this phenomenon now has a molecular basis (see Chapters 7, 12, and 13). Earlier disease onset and increased severity in subsequent generations is correlated with the further expansion of the DNA repeat. It is likely that this mechanism underlies a significant number of neurodegenerative diseases, although anticipation may at times be difficult to recognize.

### IMPRINTING

Most genes are expressed in near equal amounts from the maternal and paternal copies of the gene. Imprinted genes, however, are expressed from only one of the two homologous chromosomes. For mutations in imprinted genes, the parental origin of the mutation matters. For example, if the maternally inherited allele is silenced by imprinting, only mutations of the paternal allele have phenotypic consequences.[29] A well-known example of imprinting is deletion of genes in chromosome 15q12. When the deletion involves the paternal chromosome 15, Prader-Willi syndrome results because the maternal genes are silenced by imprinting. This disease is characterized by moderate mental retardation and obesity. In contrast, a gene in an adjacent region of 15q12 is only expressed from the maternal allele. When this gene is deleted in the maternal chromosome 15, Angelman's syndrome is observed with severe mental retardation, growth retardation, and inappropriate laughter.

At the molecular level, different DNA methylation patterns underlie genomic imprinting. Imprinting should not be confused with sex-specific expression of a phenotype where the sex of the mutation carrier is important, not the sex of the parent from whom the mutation is inherited.

# TYPES OF MUTATIONS

As discussed above, mutations (heritable changes) in DNA are the basis of genetic variation. Types of mutations range from changes of a single base pair in a gene to deletions or duplications of entire exons or even genes. Some mutations involve large alterations of parts or all of a specific chromosome. Chromosome abnormalities cause a significant proportion of genetic disease. They are the leading cause of pregnancy loss and mental retardation.

## Structural Chromosomal Abnormalities

Numerical chromosomal abnormalities can involve either extra copies of the entire set of chromosomes (polyploidy) or loss or gain of a specific chromosome (aneuploidy). Somatic polyploidy is seen in megakaryocytes and regenerating liver cells. Constitutional triploidy or tetraploidy is usually associated with fetal death.

### ANEUPLOIDY

Aneuploidy is frequently observed in cancer cells, but aneuploidy for certain chromosomes is also seen constitutionally. The most common aneuploidy is trisomy 21, which results in Down syndrome, but Down syndrome can also be caused by partial duplication of chromosome 21.[30]

Lack of an entire chromosome is not compatible with live birth. Partial monosomies of some chromosomal regions do not lead to death in utero, usually causing phenotypes with severe mental retardation.

#### DELETIONS AND RING CHROMOSOMES

Two breaks in a single chromosome can lead to loss of the material between the two breaks (interstitial deletion). With the advent of high-resolution chromosome banding, it is now possible to identify small deletions (microdeletions). Examples of microdeletion syndromes are the Prader-Willi syndrome (deletion 15q11–13) and Miller-Dieker lissencephaly (deletion 17p13.3). Smaller deletions involving several 100 kb and only few genes may be detected with molecular methods. They cause diseases as diverse as inherited predisposition to pressure palsies, Duchenne's muscular dystrophy, or neurofibromatosis 1.

Rejoining of the chromosome fragments in a circular fashion results in the formation of a ring chromosome. The chromosomal material between the breaks may also be inverted prior to reintegration. The resulting chromosomal inversion usually does not result in the loss of significant amounts of DNA and may only cause a phenotype if the continuity of a gene is interrupted.

#### TRANSLOCATIONS

Breaks involving two chromosomes and subsequent rejoining of fragments from the two different chromosomes results in chromosome translocations. When the translocation is balanced, the carrier is usually asymptomatic, but the offspring are at risk of partial trisomies or partial monosomies. Occasionally, a balanced translocation may interrupt an important DNA sequence and result in disease.

#### UNIPARENTAL DISOMY

A 46,XX or 46,XY karyotype usually implies a normal karyotype, but it may occasionally represent an abnormal chromosome constitution. This is the case when the chromosomes are not contributed equally by both parents. For example, when one chromosome in a chromosomal trisomy is lost, the two remaining chromosomes may actually be contributed by one parent. Uniparental disomy underlies those cases of Prader-Willi syndrome that do not have a microdeletion because, due to imprinting, the two copies from the father that are silenced by imprinting are present in the offspring.[29]

#### OTHER CHROMOSOMAL ABNORMALITIES

Alterations in chromosome structure, although not necessarily directly disturbing gene structure, can have a profound effect on proper gene function. These position effects are still poorly understood; they are illustrated in Chapter 6 by the effect of shortening of a DNA repeat on an as yet unidentified gene causing facioscapulohumeral dystrophy.

## Single-Gene Mutations

Mutations that affect single genes are most commonly located in the coding region of genes, at intron–exon boundaries, or in regulatory sequences. These changes can be due to changes of single base pairs or to insertions or deletions of one or multiple base pairs. In addition to these changes, gene dosage effects caused by deletion or duplication of the entire gene can be pathogenic (see Chapter 4).

#### SINGLE BASE PAIR SUBSTITUTIONS

Single base pair substitution mutations, also called *point mutations*, result when a single base pair is replaced by another base pair. This may result in a change in the amino acid sequence (missense mutation) or produce a change into one of the three stop codons (nonsense mutation). A third type of mutation may change an existing stop codon into an amino acid–coding codon (stop codon mutation), resulting in the translation of an elongated polypeptide (Fig. 1–13).

Not all amino acid changes are pathogenic. Especially when the amino acid change is conservative (substitution with a similar amino acid), the resulting protein may represent a normal variant and have normal function. At times it may be difficult to distinguish a normal variant from a disease-

**Wildtype**

**ATT TCT GCT AAT TAT AAC GAG TTA A TC AGC ACC GAG TAA ATA AAT GCA**

**Ile Ser Ala Asn Tyr Asn Glu Leu Ile Ser Thr Glu STOP**

**Nonsense**

**ATT TCT GCT AAT TAT AAC GAG T G A ATC AGC ACC GAG TAA ATA AAT GCA**

**Ile Ser Ala Asn Tyr Asn Glu STOP**

**Missense**

**ATT TCT GCT AAT TAT AAC GAG TT C ATC AGC ACC GAG TAA ATA AAT GCA**

**Ile Ser Ala Asn Tyr Asn Glu Phe Ile Ser Thr Glu STOP**

**Stop codon**

**ATT TCT GCT AAT TAT AAC GAG TTA ATC AGC ACC GAG TAC ATA AAT GCA**

**Ile Ser Ala Asn Tyr Asn Glu Leu Ile Ser Thr Glu Tyr Ile Asn Glu**

**Insertion without Frameshift**

**ATT TCT GCT AAT TAT AAC GAG GAG TTA A TC AGC ACC GAG TAA ATA AAT GCA**

**Ile Ser Ala Asn Tyr Asn Glu Glu Leu Ile Ser Thr Glu STOP**

**Deletion with Frameshift**

**ATT TCT GCT AAT T TA ACG AGT TAA TCA GCA CCG AGT AAA TAA ATG CA**

**Ile Ser Ala Asn Leu Thr Ser STOP**

**Figure 1–13.** Different types of mutations and their effects on the gene product: missense, nonsense, stop codon mutation, insertion of a GAG trinucleotide (does not alter the reading frame), and deletion of a T (results in frameshift and premature termination of translation).

causing sequence change, especially when the function of a protein is poorly understood. Many single base pair mutations, even when located in the coding region of a gene, may not change the amino acid sequence due to the redundancy of the genetic code. These are often located in the third position of a codon and are called *silent substitutions.* Although a base pair substitution may not change the amino acid sequence, it may nevertheless be disease causing by introducing cryptic splice signals.

## INSERTIONS AND DELETIONS

The other major type of mutation is deletion or insertion of one or several base pairs of DNA. If the event results in the change of 3 bp or a multiple thereof, amino acids are added or deleted from the protein but the reading frame and the remainder of the protein remain intact. When the reading frame is changed *(frameshift mutations)*, however, deletions and insertions may exert a major effect. Deletions and insertions that are not a multiple of three alter the codons and the resulting amino acid sequence downstream of the deletion or insertion. Often this results in a shortened polypeptide because the frameshift results in the recognition of a premature stop codon. Thus, larger deletions in the dystrophin gene that maintain the reading frame may cause a less severe phenotype than small deletions that change the reading frame (see Chapter 5).

### SPLICE SITE MUTATIONS

Base pair substitutions or insertions or deletions can also interfere with the proper processing of the primary transcript. These *splice site mutations* alter the GT sequence at the 5'-donor site or the AG sequence at the 3'-acceptor site or alter sequences near these sites. These mutations may result in the deletion of an entire exon from the mature transcript or may result in the recognition of normally unused or cryptic splice sites. Depending on the number of bases in the exon, exon deletion by splice site mutations can leave the reading frame intact or change it, often resulting in a truncated protein.

Truncated protein products can thus be generated by nonsense mutations, by deletions or insertions resulting in a frameshift, and by exon deletion due to small interstitial chromosomal deletion. Shortened proteins can also be generated by skipping of exons due to mutations involving exon–intron boundaries.

## SUMMARY

Mendel's postulates have now found a molecular explanation, and the genetics of single gene or mendelian disorders can be extended to complex diseases. This chapter reviews basic terminology and concepts of medical and molecular genetics. Molecular biology has provided detailed insights into DNA structure and the mechanisms of transcription and translation. The molecular basis of clinical phenomena such as anticipation and imprinting is being determined. With the identification of disease genes, phenotypes of human diseases are now correlated with specific types of mutations, leading to new classifications of diseases based on the mutated gene.

## REFERENCES


1. Blumberg RB: Mendel Web Archive: www.netspace.org/MendelWeb/MWtoc.html, 1997 (accessed May 19, 1999)
2. Watson J, Crick FHC: Molecular structure of nucleic acids: A structure for deoxyribose nucleic acid. Nature 171:737–738 1953.
3. Strachan T, Read AP: Human Molecular Genetics. Bios Scientific Publishers, Oxford, England, 1996.
4. Jorde LB, Carey JC, White RL: Medical Genetics. Mosby–Year Book, St. Louis, 1995.
5. Boguski MS: Hunting for genes in computer data bases. N Engl J Med 333:645–647, 1995.
6. Housman D: Human DNA polymorphism. N Engl J Med 332:318–320, 1995.
7. Korf B: Molecular diagnosis (second of two parts). N Engl J Med 332:1499–1502, 1995.
8. Naber S: Molecular pathology—Diagnosis of infectious disease. N Engl J Med 331:1212–1215, 1994.
9. Naber S: Molecular pathology—Detection of neoplasia. N Engl J Med 331:1508–1510, 1994.
10. Papavassiliou AG: Transcription factors. N Engl J Med 332:45–47, 1995.
11. Rosenthal N: Tools of the trade—Recombinant DNA. N Engl J Med 331:315–317, 1994.
12. Rosenthal N: DNA and the genetic code. N Engl J Med 331:39–41, 1994.
13. Rosenthal N: Regulation of gene expression. N Engl J Med 331:931–933, 1994.
14. Rosenthal N: Stalking the gene—DNA libraries. N Engl J Med 331:599–600, 1994
15. Rosenthal N: Recognizing DNA. N Engl J Med 333: 925–927, 1995.
16. Rosenthal N: Fine structure of a gene—DNA sequencing. N Engl J Med 332:589–591, 1995.
17. von Hippel PH: An integrated model of the transcription complex in elongation, termination, and editing. Science 281:660–665, 1998.
18. http://raven.umnh.utah.edu, 1998 (accessed May 18, 1999).
19. http://www.ornl.gov/TechResources/Human_Genome/, 1999 (accessed May 19, 1999).
20. Craig JM, Bickmore WA: The distribution of CpG islands in mammalian chromosomes. Nat Genet 3: 376–382, 1994.
21. Wang DG, Fan JB, Siao CJ, et al.: Large-scale identification, mapping and genotyping of single-nucleotide polymorphisms in the human genome. Science 280:1077–1082, 1998.
22. Adams C, Starkman S, Pulst SM: Phenotype of SCA2 in a large kindred from Southern Italy. Neurology 49:1163–1166, 1997.
23. Harrington JJ, Van Bokkelen G, Mays RW, Gustashaw K, Willard HF: Formation of de novo centromeres and construction of first-generation human artificial microchromosomes. Nat Genet 15:345–355, 1997.
24. Baser ME, Ragge NK, Riccardi VM, Ganz B, Janus T, Pulst SM: Phenotypic variability in monozygotic twins with neurofibromatosis 2. Am J Med Genet 64:563–567, 1996.
25. Pauls DL, Korczyn AD: Complex segregation analysis of dystonia pedigrees suggests autosomal dominant inheritance. Neurology 40(7):1107–1110, 1990.
26. Gasser T, Windgassen K, Bereznai B, Kabus C, Ludolph AC: Phenotypic expression of the DYT1 mutation: A family with writer's cramp of juvenile onset. Ann Neurol 44:126–128, 1998.
27. Saito T: An expected decrease in the incidence of

autosomal recessive disease due to decreasing consanguineous marriages. Genet Epidemiol 5:421–432, 1988.
28. Ryan SG, Chance PF, Zou CH, Spinner NB, Golden JA, Smietana S: Epilepsy and mental retardation limited to females: An X-linked dominant disorder with male sparing. Nat Genet 17:92–95, 1997.
29. Nicholls RD, Saitoh S, Horsthemke B: Imprinting in Prader-Willi and Angelman syndromes. Trends Genet 14:194–200, 1998.
30. Korenberg JR, Chen XN, Schipper R, et al.: Down syndrome phenotypes: The consequences of chromosomal imbalance. Proc Natl Acad Sci USA 91: 4997–5001, 1994.
31. Bennett RL, Steinhaus KA, Uhrich SB, et al.: Recommendations for standardized human pedigree nomenclature. Pedigree Standardization Task Force of the National Society of Genetic Counselors. Am J Hum Genet 56:745–752, 1995.

# Chapter 2

# MOLECULAR GENETIC TOOLS

Stefan-M. Pulst, MD, Dr Med



Before analysis of DNA became possible, two basic hurdles had to be overcome. First, the enormously large, but highly repetitive DNA molecule had to be cleaved into pieces of a specified size in a sequence-specific fashion. Second, technologies had to be generated that allowed the isolation of individual DNA fragments for further analysis and the production of these fragments in large quantities. The first condition was met by the discovery of restriction endonucleases, the second by the ability to propagate and amplify DNA fragments through the creation of recombinant molecules in cloning vectors. Recently, sequence specificity and amplification of DNA molecules were combined in the polymerase chain reaction (PCR). Detailed protocols and more detailed descriptions of various procedures can be found in laboratory manuals and books about molecular biology.[1–3]

## ANALYSIS OF DNA FRAGMENTS

### Restriction Enzymes

Restriction enzymes or restriction endonucleases are enzymes that recognize specific DNA sequences and cleave the DNA in or near a recognition sequence.[4,5] Both DNA strands are cut, and either blunt or overhanging ends are created (Fig. 2–1). These enzymes exist naturally in bacteria, and enzymes are designated according to the organism of origin. For example, *Eco*RI was the first enzyme isolated from *Escherichia coli* strain R. Restriction enzymes serve to pro-

| | | |
|---|---|---|
| **Msp I** | C\|C G G<br>G G C\|C | **overhanging ends**<br>**small fragments** |
| **Hae III** | G G\| C C<br>C C\| G G | **blunt ends**<br>**small fragments** |
| **Not I** | G C\|G G C C G C<br>C G C C G G\|C G | **overhanging ends**<br>**large fragments** |

**Figure 2–1.** Restriction sites of endonucleases. Note that some enzymes produce overhanging ends, and others produce blunt ends. The size of the restriction fragment depends on the base composition and the length of the recognition sequence.

tect bacterial strains from the "invasion" of foreign DNA because their activity is "restricted" or limited to the foreign DNA. They are called *endonucleases* because they cleave DNA within the DNA molecule.

Several hundred restriction enzymes have been isolated, cleaving double-stranded DNA molecules at a large number of sequence permutations. Most enzymes cleave within the recognition sequence, but others cleave outside the sequence. Some enzymes produce staggered ends, where one strand is longer and has an overhang, while others produce blunt ends.

The length and the composition of the recognition sequence determine the average fragment size. For example, *Hae*III and *Msp*I create smaller fragments than *Not*I. Because CpG (C connected to a G by a 3'–5' phosphoclister bond) sequences are rare in the human genome, *Msp*I cleaves DNA less often than *Hae*III, although both have a 4 base pair (bp) recognition sequence. When CpG-rich recognition sequences are combined with a long recognition sequence, very large DNA fragments are created. These "rare cutter" enzymes cleave DNA into fragments from 100 kilo base pairs (kb) up to the million base pair (Mbp) range.

## Electrophoresis

Electrophoresis can resolve DNA fragments according to size. DNA is negatively charged and therefore migrates toward the anode in an electric field. When DNA migrates through a matrix in an electric field, smaller fragments migrate more rapidly through the gel matrix than large fragments (Fig. 2–2).

The type of gel matrix as well as its composition determine which fragment sizes can be resolved. For the resolution of fragments differing by 1 bp, a polyacrylamide gel is used. This type of resolution is required for DNA sequencing or for the resolution of microsatellite marker alleles (see also Fig. 2–11 B). For larger fragments with resolution of differences between ten and several hundred base pairs, agarose gels are used. The concentration of the gel matrix determines the size range of separation. A 1% agarose gel can resolve fragments from

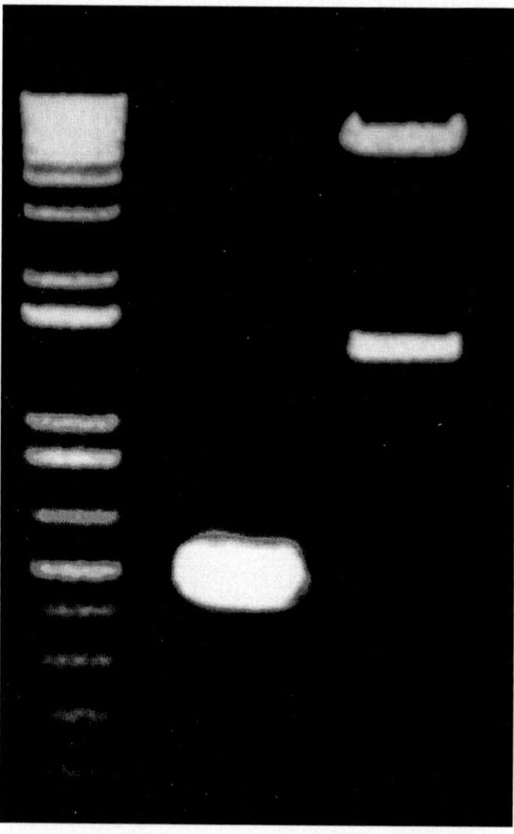

**Figure 2–2.** DNA fragments separated by electrophoresis in a 0.8% agarose gel (10 V/cm, 2 hours). DNA fragments were visualized by staining the gel in 1% ethidium bromide. Left: Molecular weight ladder. Middle: DNA fragment of 700 bp generated by PCR. Right: Recombinant plasmid cleaved with *Bgl* II, showing the vector band of 6 kb and an insert band of 1.2 kb.

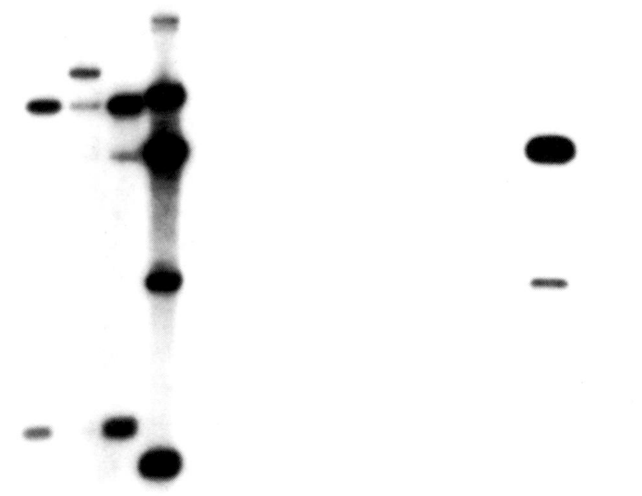


**Figure 2–3.** Effect of hybridization stringency on detection of homologous sequences of a Southern blot of genomic DNA fragments derived from human chromosome 12. After restriction digestion, fragments were separated by gel electrophoresis, transferred to nylon membrane by Southern blotting, and hybridized with a $CAG_{10}$ oligonucleotide probe. On the left is an autoradiograph after low-stringency washes, and on the right the same blot is shown after washes at high stringency. Whereas short CAG repeats and highly interrupted repeats give a signal after low-stringency washes, only long and perfect repeats are able to anneal after washes at high stringency.

approximately 0.5 to 9 kb, whereas a 3% agarose gel is used to separate smaller fragments (i.e., those from about 50 to 1,000 bp).

Even a 0.5% agarose gel cannot resolve fragments of more than 50 kb. A completely different approach to conventional electrophoresis had to be taken for the separation of fragments created by "rare cutter" restriction enzymes such as *Not*I. Fragments up to millions of base pairs in length can be separated when the electrical field is not applied as a continuous field but is changed at specified times. This is called *pulsed-field gel electrophoresis* (PFGE). In its simplest form, PFGE reverses the field every couple of seconds, but the time for the reverse field is shorter than for the forward pulse. Larger DNA molecules cannot "reorient" as rapidly as smaller fragments and therefore migrate more slowly during the forward pulse. PFGE is used in the molecular diagnosis of Charcot-Marie-Tooth disease (see Chapter 4).

## Southern Blotting

The complexity of human genomic DNA is so great that after digestion with a restriction enzyme distinct bands are not visible, but instead a smear is seen reflecting the fact that thousands of fragments of a particular size exist. A specific restriction fragment of interest therefore needs to be identified by its sequence composition. This is achieved by hybridization to a complementary DNA probe. Before this can be done, the DNA is transferred from the agarose gel to a solid support (nylon membrane) by capillary transfer. This procedure is named after its inventor, Ed Southern.[6] By analogy, the transfer of RNA molecules is referred to as *Northern blotting* and the transfer of proteins as *Western blotting*.

## Hybridization

After transfer of the DNA, the nylon membrane is incubated with a complementary DNA probe that has been radioactively labeled. Hybridization is allowed to proceed for 12 to 24 hours. The conditions for hybridization can be varied by adjusting temperature and salt concentration of the hybridization solution and subsequent washes. A rise in temperature and/or a decrease in salt concentration will increase the stringency of hybridization. At high stringency, only DNA sequences with perfect or near perfect matches will stick (anneal) to each other (anneal) to each other (Fig. 2–3).

At lower stringency, hybridization allows the identification of related sequences that are not 100% identical. For example, a hu-

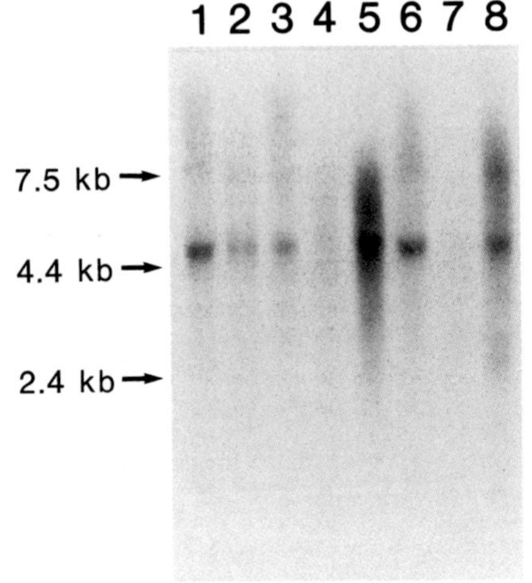


**Figure 2–4.** Autoradiograph of a Northern blot of RNAs extracted from a variety of human tissues. The blot was hybridized with a radioactive cDNA probe for the human ataxin-2 gene. Lane 1, heart; lane 2, brain; lane 3, placenta; lane 4, lung; lane 5, liver; lane 6, skeletal muscle; lane 7, kidney; lane 8, pancreas. (From Pulst and coworkers,[7] with permission.)

man genomic probe can be hybridized to a Southern blot with genomic DNA from several animal species (zoo blot). Because protein coding sequences show a much higher sequence homology across species than other DNA sequences, a zoo blot can be a powerful way to identify genes.

## ANALYSIS OF RNA TRANSCRIPTS AND PROTEINS

### Northern Blotting

Similar to DNA molecules, RNA molecules can be separated by gel electrophoresis according to size. To identify a particular RNA transcript in the mixture of thousands of transcripts in a cell, hybridization with a radioactively labeled probe can be used. Before this can be done, the RNAs are transferred from the polyacrylamide gel to a membrane by application of an electric field. This procedure is called *Northern* blotting in a play of words on *Southern* blotting.

Northern blots can be probed with a variety of fragments, including cDNA or genomic probes. Multiple-tissue Northern blots are often used to provide an initial survey of the expression pattern of a new gene (Fig. 2–4). Surprisingly, many genes causing diseases specific to the nervous system may show widespread tissue expression. When a partial cDNA is used to probe a Northern blot, the observed fragment can provide estimates of the length of the entire transcript. Detection of multiple fragments may point to alternative splicing, the use of alternative promoters, or different lengths of untranslated regions. When Northern blots are hybridized with a probe at lower stringency, transcripts from genes with related sequences may be identified. Quantitative Northern blots assess the change in the expression levels of a particular gene in different tissues or during different stages of development. To control for the loading of different amounts of RNAs in each lane, the expression level is normalized by comparison with the hybridization signal of a gene expressed at constant levels, for example, the β-actin transcript.

### Western Blotting

Similar to DNA and RNA molecules, proteins can be separated by polyacrylamide electrophoresis, although the polyacrylamide concentrations are higher due to the smaller molecular weight of proteins. After transfer of proteins to a membrane, the protein of interest can be recognized after incubation of the membrane with an antibody that binds to specific recognition sites (epitopes) on the protein (Fig. 2–5). Primary antibody binding to the protein is usually visualized by staining with a secondary antibody. The secondary antibody is directed against the immunoglobulin (Ig) of the animal species in which the primary antibody was raised and labeled with a reagent that allows colorimetric detection of the immune complexes. For example, polyclonal primary antibodies are often raised in rabbits. A biotin-labeled goat antirabbit IgG antibody is used as a secondary antibody. Horseradish peroxidase attached to avidin allows visualization of the immune complex. Primary antibodies can be generated to an entire protein or to synthetic peptides (usually 10 to 20 amino acids) representing part of the protein.

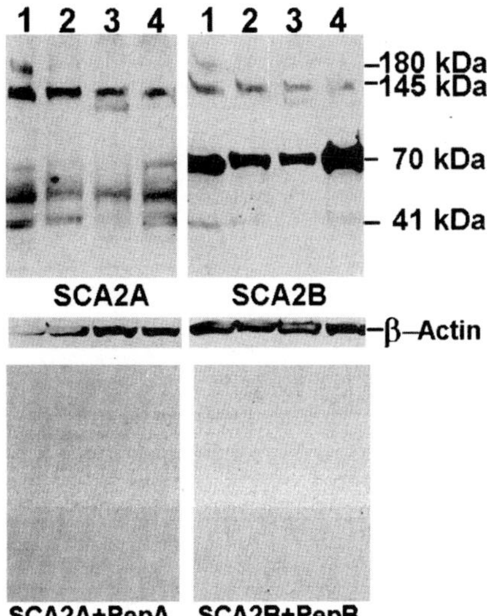


**Figure 2–5.** Expression of ataxin-2 at the protein level. (A): Western blot of brain protein extracts were stained with two antibodies directed to different epitopes of ataxin-2. Note that both antibodies detect the same full-length protein of 145 kDa, but different smaller processed protein fragments. In SCA2 brains, a larger band representing a protein translated from the abnormal allele with an expanded polyglutamine tract can be seen. Lane 1, SCA2 patient; lanes 2 and 3, Alzheimer's disease patients; lane 4, normal individual. (B): Staining of the Western blots with an antibody to β-actin indicates equal loading of the lanes. (C): Preabsorption of the antibodies with their respective peptides abolishes staining. (From Huynh and coworkers,[8] with permission.)

## CREATION OF RECOMBINANT DNA MOLECULES

An important step in DNA analysis was the ability to generate large quantities of specified DNA fragments through the generation of recombinant molecules[9,10] because this was the prerequisite for DNA sequence analysis. This was made possible by the discovery of bacterial minichromosomes called *plasmids*. Plasmids are small circular double-stranded molecules that contain only a few individual genes. Plasmids can be used to function as an *in vivo* machinery to synthesize DNA fragments because they replicate independently of the host genome.

Foreign DNA fragments can be inserted into the plasmid, and the recombinant plasmids can be inserted into a host cell (Fig. 2–6). Both the DNA fragment and the plasmid are cleaved with a restriction enzyme. The restriction enzyme is chosen so that the plasmid is cleaved only once and thus becomes linearized. After the mixture of linearized plasmids and DNA fragments is treated with a DNA ligase, some molecules are generated in which DNA fragments have become ligated in between the two plasmid arms. These plasmids are called *recombinant* because they represent a combination of DNA sequences that did not previously exist in nature. Bacteria serve as host cells in most cases because they replicate rapidly, and the recombinant plasmid can be relatively easily purified. Plasmids are introduced into bacteria by transfection. The plasmid is designated as the *vector* (because it carries the foreign DNA fragment), and the foreign DNA fragment is referred to as the *insert* (see also Fig. 2–2).

### Cloning Vectors

Depending on the size of the insert, different cloning vectors must be used. Smaller inserts are cloned into plasmid or phage vectors. Medium-sized inserts (40 kb) are cloned into cosmid vectors. For genomic mapping it is preferable to insert even larger DNA fragments. Artificial chromosomes with centromeres and telomeres are used for these purposes, and either yeast or bacterial cells can serve as hosts. Yeast artificial chromosomes (YACs) can accept inserts of several hundred to more than 1000 kb, and P1 artificial chromosomes (PACs) or bacterial artificial chromosomes (BACs) can accept inserts of 100 to 300 kb.

### Libraries

A library is a place where material is stored in identifiable units (e.g., books). In molecular biology, a library is a collection of recombinant DNA molecules that can serve as a source of uniquely, identifiable clones. The term *library*, however, is not completely analogous because the clones are not catalogued. An individual clone can only be identified by searching through the whole contents of the library.[11] Thus, searching

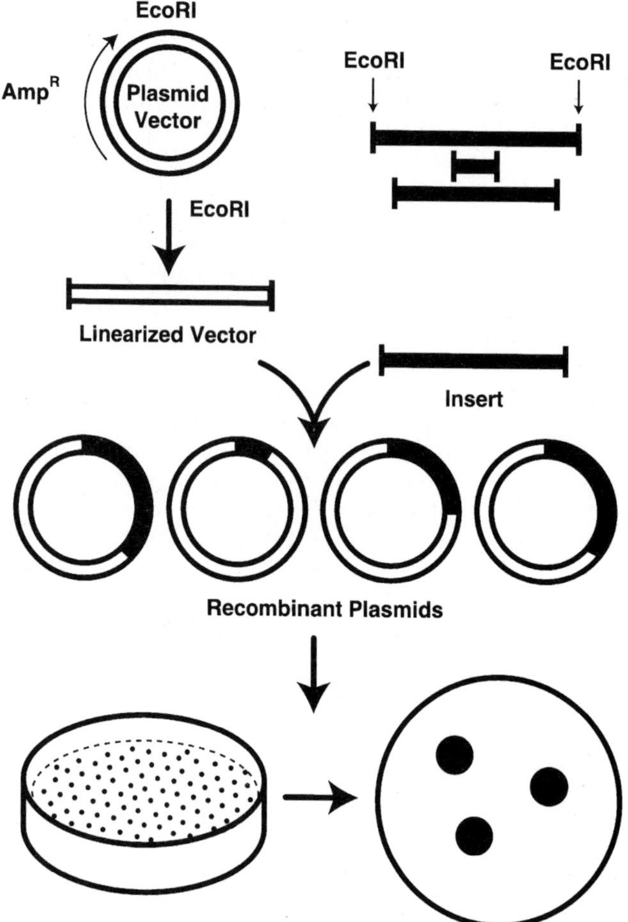


**Figure 2–6.** Generation of a recombinant clone. Plasmid vector (*upper left*) and human genomic DNA (*upper right*) are digested with the same restriction enzyme. Vector and insert DNA are then ligated to create a recombinant plasmid. After transfection of plasmids into bacteria, bacterial clones can be screened by hybridization (*bottom*).

with "To be or not to be" will identify a play by Shakespeare. By analogy, screening of all the clones in a library using a probe with a specific sequence (the sentence) will identify a specific clone (the book).

Libraries can be made from very different starting materials, such as genomic DNA or cDNA (reverse-transcribed mRNA). To make a genomic library, genomic DNA is first digested with a restriction enzyme. The resulting DNA fragments are then linked to vector DNA. Because the vector can self-propagate in bacteria, by linking the insert to the vector we are now able to replicate the insert DNA at will.

After screening of the library, a single clone can be isolated, thus reducing the complexity of the human genome to DNA fragments that can be more easily analyzed (e.g., by DNA sequencing). For library screening, plasmid-bearing bacteria are plated on a growth medium. After transfer of DNA to a nylon membrane, the library can be screened by hybridization with a labeled probe (Fig. 2–6). For example, a cDNA library can be screened with a partial cDNA probe to identify additional cDNA clones containing the entire cDNA (full-length cDNA clones). If screening is performed at lower stringency, related cDNAs can be isolated. In addition to screening by hybridization, screening can also be performed using the PCR to screen pools of library clones.

## POLYMERASE CHAIN REACTION

A novel way to selectively amplify DNA fragments without cloning was the polymerase chain reaction (PCR).[12,13] PCR combines in an ingeniously simple procedure the sequence specificity of restriction enzymes with amplification previously only possible by cloning of restriction fragments. Sequence specificity is provided by the annealing of oligonucleotide probes complementary to the DNA sequence of interest, and amplification is achieved by repeated rounds of oligonucleotide-primed DNA synthesis.

To amplify a fragment of interest, two oligonucleotide primers (usually 20 bp long) are chemically synthesized. One oligonucleotide is complementary to the coding strand 5' of the target sequence, and the second one is complementary to the antisense strand 3' to the target sequence (Fig. 2–7). The oligonucleotides are usually separated by 100 to 1000 bp, but for long-range PCR the distance between them may be much greater. It is important to note that it is not necessary to know the entire sequence of the fragment that is to be amplified as long as sequences at the ends of the fragment are known. An example of the use of PCR in genotyping is shown later in Figure 2–11.

The oligonucleotide primers are used to prime the amplification reaction with DNA polymerase to generate a novel DNA strand. After the oligonucleotide primers have annealed to their target sequences, a heat-resistant DNA polymerase is used to amplify beginning at the 3' end of the primer (extension). After DNA synthesis is completed, the old and newly synthesized DNA strands are separated by denaturation, and the cycle of annealing and DNA synthesis is repeated.

Cycles can be automated due to the development of heat-resistant DNA polymerases that can withstand the high temperatures of denaturation. PCR machines using

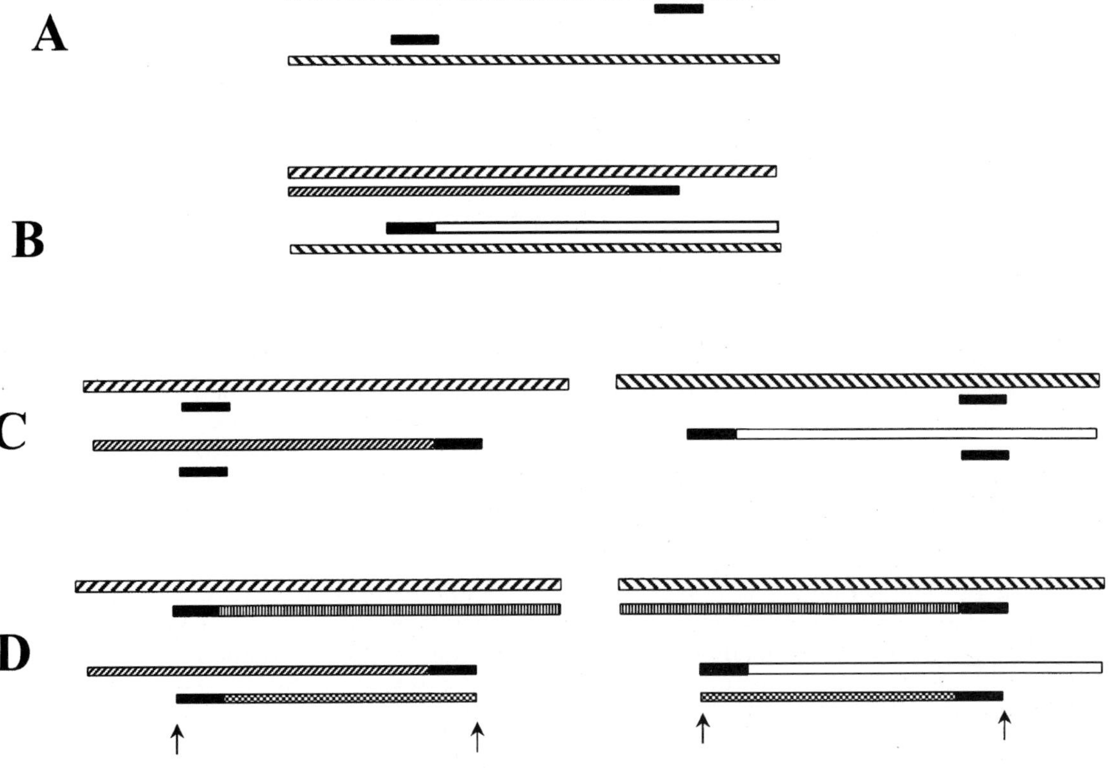


**Figure 2–7.** Schematic of the first two cycles in a PCR amplification (see also Fig. 2–11). (*A*) Annealing of oligonucleotide primers (black boxes) to DNA strands. (*B*) New DNA is synthesized (gray boxes). (*C*) DNA strands are separated by denaturation (not shown), and primers anneal to complementary sequences. (*D*) A second round of DNA synthesis results in doubling of the initial DNA amount. Note that the DNA fragments shown between the arrows have a length defined by the spacing of the oligonucleotide the primers.

heating blocks that hold microtiter plates or Eppendorf tubes can be programmed so that the block can stay at a specific temperature for a specific length of time. A typical PCR cycle is as follows: annealing at 55° C for 1 minute primer extension at 72° C for 1 minute and denaturation at 95° C for 30 seconds.

The specificity of PCR is primarily determined by the annealing temperature. When the annealing temperature is lowered, the primers will anneal to DNA sequences that are not perfectly matched and other fragments will be amplified. This can also be advantageous when the purpose is amplification of related sequences. For molecular diagnosis, however, it is of utmost importance that the amplification occurs in a specific fashion for both normal and mutated alleles.

PCR can also be applied to the study of transcripts. With the enzyme reverse transcriptase and an oligo-dT primer, RNAs are transcribed to create cDNAs. A specific RNA is then amplified with primers derived from the cDNA sequence. Reverse-transcribed PCR is a quick method to analyze tissue samples for the presence of nonabundant transcripts, and it provides an ideal method to detect transcript isoforms generated by alternative splicing (Fig. 2–8).

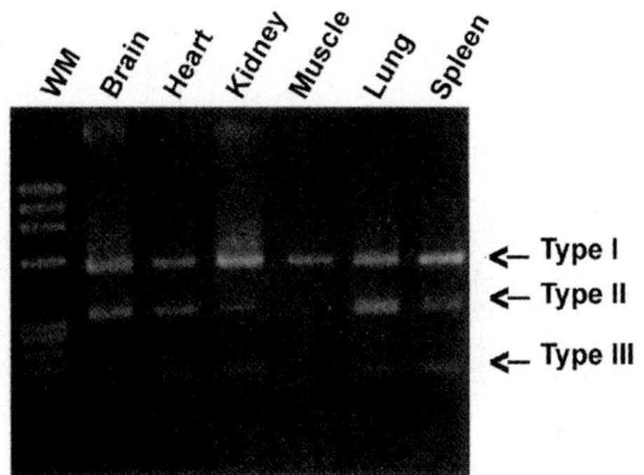


**Figure 2–8.** Transcript analysis of alternative transcripts of the mouse ataxin-2 gene. Ethidium-stained agarose gel with amplicons generated by reverse-transcribed PCR with primers flanking exons 9 and 10. The type II isoform represents a transcript lacking exon 9 and the type III, a transcript lacking exons 9 and 10. Note the absence of type II and III isoforms in muscle. MWM: ϕX174/*Hae* III molecular weight marker. (From Nechiporuk and associates,[14] with permission.)

## DNA SEQUENCING

The ability to decipher the DNA sequence of a fragment has provided the basis for elucidation of the genetic code and is the backbone of the human genome project. Of several sequencing methods, including the enzymatic chain termination method, hybridization-based approaches, and chemical sequencing methods, only the enzymatic chain termination method is described further, because it is the method currently used for automated sequencing. In the chain termination method, a DNA fragment is provided as a template for the synthesis of new DNA strands with a DNA polymerase.[15] The reaction is primed by a sequencing primer usually 17 to 22 bp long that specifically binds to the region being sequenced. In addition to the regular deoxynucleotide triphosphates (dNTPs; *N* stands for any of the four bases), smaller amounts of *dideoxy*nucleotide triphosphates (ddNTPs) are added to the reaction mix. Although the ddNTPs can be incorporated into the growing newly synthesized DNA chain, they cause abrupt termination of the chain because their lack of the 3' hydroxyl group does not permit formation of the phosphodiester bond.

For each nucleotide a separate sequencing reaction is prepared, each containing the four dNTPs but only one of the ddNTPs in much smaller concentration than the dNTPs. For example, one of the four reactions contains ddATP. Chain termination occurs randomly whenever a ddATP is incorporated into the growing chain instead of dATP. Because the number of dATP molecules greatly outnumbers the number of ddATP molecules, many fragments of different lengths are generated that differ by the random integration of ddATP, resulting in chain termination. The length of the fragments can be determined by polyacrylamide gel electrophoresis indicating the presence of an A (adenine) at this position of the DNA chain. Fragments for the remaining three DNA bases are generated in similar reactions. The fragments can be visualized by radioisotope labeling (Fig. 2–9).

Instead of being labeled with a radioac-

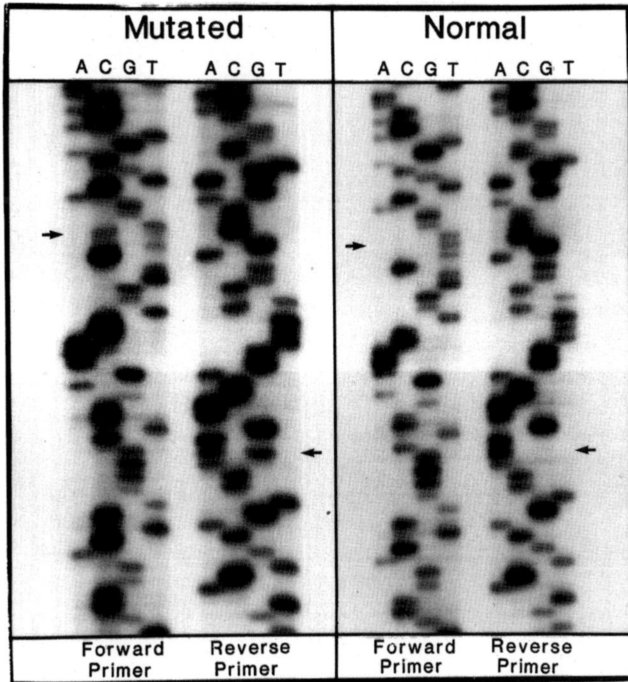


**Figure 2–9.** (*left*) Sequencing gel showing a missense mutation in the *NF2* gene. The T to C transition is marked with an arrow. Note that at the site of the single base pair change, the normal as well as the mutated bases are detected. The mutation is apparent in the forward (sense) and reverse directions. Sequencing in the reverse direction shows the expected A to G change. (*right*) The DNA sequence of a normal individual. (From Scoles and coworkers,[16] with permission.)

tive substance, the sequencing primers or the incorporated dNTPs can be labeled with fluorophores. The use of different fluorophores for each DNA base permits the running of the four sequencing reactions in one lane of the polyacrylamide gel, thus greatly increasing throughput. The DNA sequence is represented as an intensity profile for each fluorescent dye as detected by a fluorescent detector at the bottom of the gel (Fig. 2–10). Automated sequencing with fluorescent dyes provides generally longer sequences than manual sequences and is currently the preferred method for large-scale sequencing.

## DETECTION OF DNA POLYMORPHISMS

In 1980, it was suggested to construct a genetic linkage map of the human genome based on DNA polymorphisms.[17,18] This proposal was feasible because DNA polymorphisms are much more frequent in humans than protein polymorphisms and are more or less randomly distributed throughout the genome. In addition, DNA polymorphisms can be detected more rapidly.

### Restriction Fragment Length Polymorphisms

Before the advent of PCR, the most commonly used procedure to detect differences in DNA sequences involved the use of DNA restriction enzymes. For example, the enzyme *Msp*I cuts DNA between the first and second cytosine bases whenever it encounters the sequence CCGG (see Fig. 2–1). When any base in this recognition sequence is changed, the enzyme will not cut at this site and a larger DNA restriction fragment will be generated. One can thus use the specificity of restriction enzymes to detect DNA polymorphisms by examining changes in the length of restriction fragments, thus the designation RFLP for *r*estriction *f*ragment *l*ength *p*olymorphism.

For the purpose of genetic linkage mapping, RFLPs have been replaced completely by microsatellite markers and recently by single nucleotide polymorphisms (see

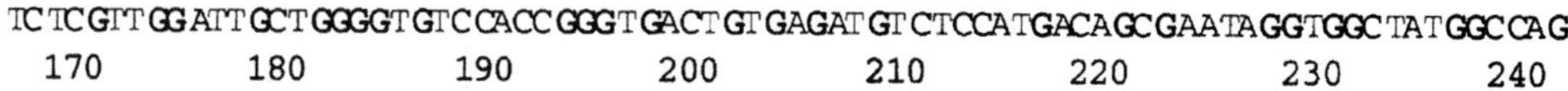


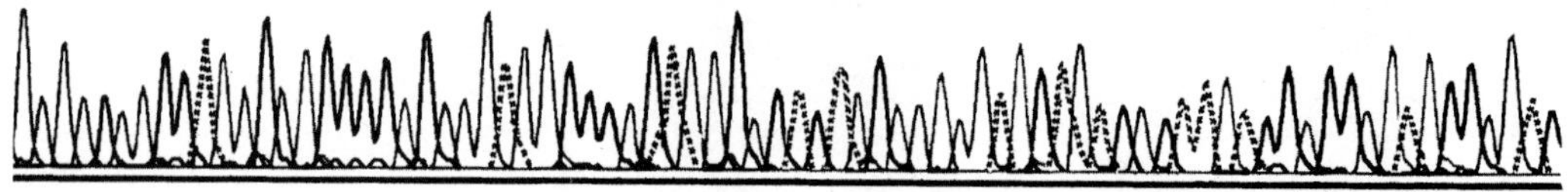

**Figure 2–10.** Automated sequence generated with fluorescently labeled oligonucleotide primers. Instead of representation in color, the different fluorochromes are represented by different shades of gray lines.

later). RFLPs are still used for the detection of mutations in disease genes, however, when a base substitution generates or deletes a restriction site, thus generating a novel restriction fragment. Detection of RFLPs is now combined with PCR-based amplification of the fragment.[19]

## Minisatellite Markers

Markers with a higher degree of polymorphism (greater number of alleles) were developed in the form of minisatellite markers that recognize polymorphic DNA tandem repeats (variable number tandem repeat [VNTR]. Despite the fact that these markers represented an improvement due to their increased heterozygosity, they still required analysis by Southern blotting. Their usefulness was further limited because they were not randomly distributed, but concentrated near the telomeric regions of chromosomes.

## Microsatellite Markers

More recently, RFLP and VNTR markers have been surpassed by microsatellite markers, which are PCR based, highly polymorphic, and well distributed throughout the genome.[20] Microsatellite markers are based on the detection of repeated sequences with a length of two, three, or four nucleotides (e.g., $Ca_n$, $GATA_n$). For this reason, they are also referred to as *short tandem repeat* (STR) markers (Fig. 2–11 *a*).

DNA polymorphisms based on microsatellite repeats can easily be detected. The DNA sequence flanking the repeat is used to synthesize complementary oligonucleotide primers. After PCR amplification, the alleles of different length are resolved by electrophoresis (Fig. 2–11 *b*).

Microsatellite markers have many advantages. They can be relatively easily generated, their use is rapid and inexpensive, and they are often highly polymorphic, sometimes with more than ten alleles. Due to the aforementioned points, genetic maps based on microsatellite markers provide relatively precise genetic distances and now cover the entire genome.[21]

## Single-Nucleotide Polymorphisms

The simplest polymorphisms are those that are generated by substitution of a single base pair and were the basis for most RFLPs. These polymorphisms are almost exclusively bi-allelic and thus not highly polymorphic, but this limitation is overcome by their frequency of one to two polymorphisms per 1000 bp. The ability to probe for these polymorphisms with DNAs arrayed on a chip or glass slide provides the prospect of automated genotyping at extremely high resolution.[23–25] The first genetic maps based on single-nucleotide polymorphisms (SNPs) are being assembled.[26]

# GENETIC LINKAGE ANALYSIS

Genetic linkage analysis is one of the most important tools in the process of identifying disease genes. It is based on the observation that genes that are physically close on a chromosome are inherited together and thus appear genetically linked. With increasing physical distance between two genes, the probability of their separation

5'-CATGGTTA--------------------------------------------
3' AGCGTGGTACCAATATGCTCGACCT**CACACACACACACACACACA**GAACGTCAGTTGCATTACGCGACAGCATGCATCCT- 5'

5' TCGCACCATGGTTATACGAGCTGGA**GTGTGTGTGTGTGTGTGTGT**CTTGCAGTCAACGTAATGCGCTGTCGTACGTAGGA- 3'
------------------------------------------ GCATGCAT-5'

5'-CATGGTTA--------------------------------------------
3' AGCGTGGTACCAATATGCTCGACCT**CACACACACACACACACACACACA**GAACGTCAGTTGCATTACGCGACAGCATGCATCCT- 5'

5' TCGCACCATGGTTATACGAGCTGGA**GTGTGTGTGTGTGTGTGTGTGTGT**CTTGCAGTCAACGTAATGCGCTGTCGTACGTAGGA- 3'
------------------------------------------ GCATGCAT-5'

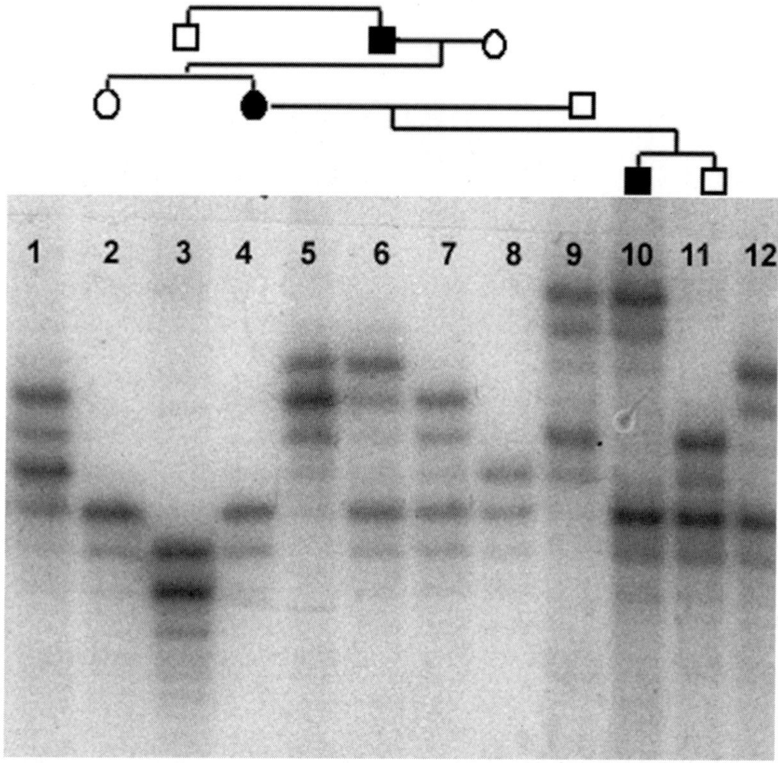


**Figure 2–11.** (*Top*) Schematic of a microsatellite locus. Two alleles containing different $(CA/GT)_n$ tracts, and the location of oligonucleotides used to amplify the polymorphic CA tract, are shown. The oligonucleotides serve as primers for DNA polymerase, and two new templates are synthesized. The dashed lines denote the newly synthesized DNA strand. (*Bottom*) Example of DNA analysis with a microsatellite marker.[32] P-labeled oligonucleotide primers flanking a CA repeat marker (AFM164ze3 in the *D22S275* locus) are used to generate PCR amplicons. These are separated on a polyacrylamide gel and visualized by autoradiography. Note the great heterozygosity of this marker system. Mendelian inheritance of the alleles can be seen by comparison with the pedigree symbols provided above the autoradiograph (From Pulst,[22] with permission.)

during meiotic chiasma formation increases (Fig. 1–9).

Linkage and nonlinkage between an autosomal dominant disease trait and alleles at three marker loci are illustrated in Figure 2–12. Individual II-1 is heterozygous at the three marker loci so that the markers are informative in all meioses and can be used to track the chromosomes. Comparison of haplotypes of individuals I-1 and II-2 indicates that the 1–2–4 haplotype marks the chromosome with the disease mutation or, in other words, that this haplotype is "in phase" with the mutation. The 2 allele of

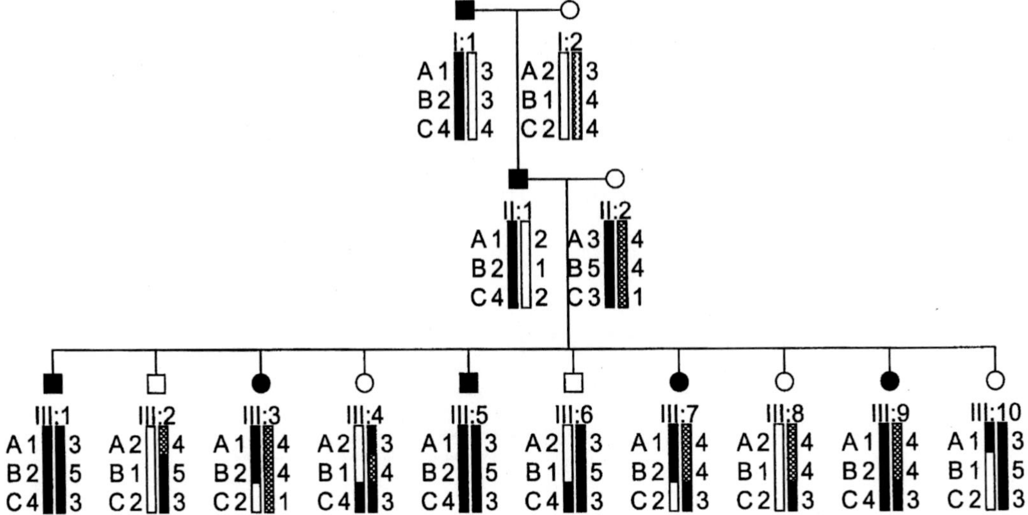


**Figure 2–12.** Three-generation pedigree segregating an autosomal dominant trait. Alleles at three marker loci are shown. Squares, males; circles, females; open symbols, normal phenotype; solid symbols, disease phenotype. (From Pulst,[22] with permission.)

marker B shows perfect cosegregation with the disease trait (i.e., all affected offspring inherited the 2 allele), whereas all unaffected offspring inherited the 1 allele. Thus, the disease locus and the locus for marker B are closely linked. Marker A shows one recombination event in the unaffected individual III-10. If penetrance of the disease is less than 100%, however, this individual may actually carry the disease mutation (and not show a phenotype), which would abolish the recombination event (Table 2–1). Comparison of the disease phenotype with alleles for marker C shows that multiple recombination events occurred. Thus, the disease trait shows linkage to markers A and B but not to marker C.

Just as recombination between a marker and the disease phenotype can be determined, one can also count recombination events between markers. Three recombination events are observed between markers A and B. Two occurred on the maternal chromosome and one on the paternal chromosome. Thus the maternal recombination fraction is 20%, while the paternal recombination fraction is 10%. This gives a sex-averaged recombination fraction of 15%. Eight recombination events are detected between markers B and C, giving a sex-averaged recombination fraction of 40%.

## Lod Score Analysis

The significance of observed linkage depends on the number of meioses in which the two loci remain linked. It is intuitively obvious that the observation of linkage in four meioses is less significant than the observation of linkage in 20 meioses. A measure for the likelihood of linkage is the logarithm of the odds (lod) score. The lod score $z$ is the logarithm of the odds that the loci are linked divided by the odds that the loci are unlinked.[27] Expression of the likelihood as a logarithm allows summation of likelihood observed in different pedigrees. For perfect pedigree structures, lod score calculations can be carried out by hand. For real-life pedigrees with missing family members and reduced penetrance assumptions, however, computer programs such as MLINK and LIPED are necessary.[28]

Because the true genetic distance between two loci is frequently not known, the lod score is calculated for different genetic distances, providing a maximum likelihood

Table 2–1. **Pairwise Lod Scores for Pedigree Shown in Figure 2–12.**

| | | RECOMBINATION FRACTION | | | | | | |
|---|---|---|---|---|---|---|---|---|
| **Locus** | **Penetrance** | **0** | **0.01** | **0.05** | **0.1** | **0.2** | **0.3** | **0.4** |
| *A* | $p = 1.0$ | −INF | 1.0 | 1.5 | 1.6 | 1.4 | 1.1 | 0.6 |
| | $p = 0.5$ | 1.8 | 1.8 | 1.7 | 1.6 | 1.2 | 0.9 | 0.5 |
| *B* | $p = 1.0$ | 3.0 | 2.9 | 2.8 | 2.6 | 2.0 | 1.5 | 0.8 |
| | $p = 0.5$ | 2.1 | 2.1 | 1.9 | 1.8 | 1.4 | 1.0 | 0.5 |
| *C* | $p = 1.0$ | −INF | −5.0 | −2.3 | −1.3 | −0.4 | 0.0 | 0.1 |
| | $p = 0.5$ | −4.9 | −2.5 | −1.1 | −0.6 | −0.1 | 0.0 | 0.1 |

INF: Infinity

estimate for the recombination fraction ($\Theta_{max}$) at which the greatest lod score ($z_{max}$) is observed. Pairwise lod scores for the three markers in Figure 1–12 and the disease trait are shown at fixed recombination fractions (Table 2–1). Because no recombination events occurred between marker locus B and the disease, the $z_{max}$ is observed at $\Theta = 0$. Due to the one recombination event observed in III-10, the most likely distance between marker A and the disease locus is calculated to be at a recombination fraction of 10%.

A lod score of more than 3.0 is generally accepted as evidence for linkage when mendelian traits are examined. Although a lod score of 3 would translate into odds of 1000: 1 favoring linkage, the corresponding significance level is closer to $p = 0.05$ in a genome-wide screen for linkage due to the calculation of linkage for multiple markers with the concomitant increase in observing a positive lod score by chance. A lod score of less than −2 is accepted as evidence against linkage. Between −2 and 3, the analysis is inconclusive, and additional pedigrees need to be examined to accept or reject linkage.

Lod score analysis assumes precise genetic models that include penetrance, disease gene frequency, and the clear classification of individuals as affected or unaffected. Thus, the lod scores in Table 2–1 undergo significant changes when penetrance is reduced to 0.5. Similarly, the lod score and the calculated location of the disease gene can be drastically changed by the misdiagnosis of one individual or by the presence of similar phenotypes (phenocopies) that are not caused by mutations in the gene under study.

Instead of calculating lod scores between two loci at a time, one can calculate maximum likelihood estimates for multiple loci at a time. Thus, it is possible to order loci and to place a disease locus on a map of ordered genetic marker loci. Multipoint analysis also compensates for noninformativeness of markers in specific meioses and will have renewed importance for mapping using SNPs.[28]

## Association

Linkage and association should not be confused with one another. *Linkage* relates to the physical location of genetic loci, whereas *association* refers to the concurrence of a specific allele with another trait at a frequency greater than predicted by chance. Thus, linkage refers to the relationship of *loci*, whereas association refers to the relationship of *alleles* at a frequency greater than predicted by chance. To study association, one has to determine allele frequencies in unrelated cases and compare them with the allele frequencies found in controls. For association studies, it is imperative to repeat the analysis in different patient populations to minimize effects provided by population stratification, particularly when individuals with the disease belong to a genetically distinct subset of the population.

Table 2–2. **Association between Tau Alleles and Progressive Supranuclear Palsy (PSP)***

| Tau Genotype | Young Subject Control ($n$ = 108) | PSP ($n$ = 30) | Alzheimer's Disease ($n$ = 44) |
|---|---|---|---|
| *A0/A0*† | 38 | 87 | 55 |
| *A0/A1* | 4 | 3 | 7 |
| *A0/A3* | 48 | 10 | 34 |
| *A1/A1* | 1 | 0 | 0 |
| *A1/A3* | 3 | 0 | 0 |
| *A3/A3* | 7 | 0 | 1 |

*Modified after Oliva et al., 1998.[29] Only the most prevalent alleles and not all control populations are shown.

†Genotypes are shown as a percentage of the total.

Association studies may point to genetic factors involved in the pathogenesis or susceptibility of a disease. Table 2–2 shows the association between specific alleles of the tau protein and the presence of progressive supranuclear palsy (PSP).[29] There was a significant overrepresentation of the *A0/A0* genotype in PSP patients. Other examples of association studies are given in the chapters on Alzheimer's disease and multiple sclerosis.

## Linkage Disequilibrium

*Linkage disequilibrium* refers to the occurrence of specific alleles at two loci with a frequency greater than expected by chance. It is a powerful tool for genetic mapping. At the population level it can be used to investigate processes such as mutation, recombination, admixture, and selection.

If the alleles at locus *A* are *A1* and *A2* with frequencies of 70% and 30% and the alleles at the locus *B* are *b1* and *b2* with frequencies of 60% and 40%, the expected frequencies of haplotypes would be a1b1 = 0.42, a1b2 = 0.28, a2b1 = 0.18, and a2b2 = 0.12. Even if the two loci were closely linked, unrestricted recombination would result in allelic combinations that are close to the frequencies given above. When a particular combination occurs at a higher frequency, for example, a2b2 at a frequency of 25%, this is called *linkage disequilibrium.* Linkage disequilibrium may result from natural selection, or it may appear by chance. When a disease mutation arises on a founder chromosome and not much time has elapsed since the mutational event, the disease mutation will be in linkage disequilibrium with alleles from loci close to the gene.

The closer a marker is to the mutated gene, the stronger the disequilibrium will be. For example, the CAG repeat that is expanded in Huntington's disease is followed by an adjacent polymorphic CCG/CCT repeat. On normal chromosomes, 50% have the form $(CCG)_7/(CCT)2$, 48% $(CCG)_{10}/(CCT)2$, and 2% $(CCG)_7/(CCT)_2$. On chromosomes with the Huntington's disease mutation, however 85% have the form $(CCG)_7/(CCT)_2$, indicating that there is significant linkage disequilibrium between Huntington's disease and the CCG polymorphism.[30]

## GENETIC AND PHYSICAL MAPS

The development of highly polymorphic markers in conjunction with large insert cloning vectors has led to rapid advances in the completion of genetic and physical maps of the human genome. Physical maps measure distances in base pairs, whereas genetic maps measure distances in recombinational units named after the geneticist Morgan. One centimorgan (1 cM) approximates 1% recombination. Because the chance of recombination increases with increasing physical distance, there is an approximate relationship between distances in genetic and physical maps. On average, when two loci are separated by 1 million base pairs (Mbp), one observes 1% recombination between them; thus 1 Mbp approximates 1 cM.

The total human genome contains close to 3300 cM. Recombination rates are not the same for male and female chromosomes, and there may be significant changes in the rates of recombination along specific chromosomal segments. Chromosomal regions with increased recombination are referred to as *recombination hot spots.*

Current human genetic maps provide an

average marker density of better than one genetic marker per centimorgan. Genetic linkage maps provide the backbone to order physically contiguous clones (contigs) when gaps were shown to exist between contigs. Physical and genetic maps of the human genome can be accessed at several sites on the Internet (Table 2–3).[21] Genetic and physical maps are completed, or are in process, for several model animal organisms, including bacteria, yeast, and the nematode *Caenorhabditis elegans.*

## DETECTION OF MUTATIONS

Methods for mutation detection can be divided into screening methods and direct sequence-based methods. Screening methods are used to evaluate candidate genes before disease gene identification and for disease genes that show extensive allelic heterogeneity (a large number of different mutations). Direct mutation detection is employed for small genes once a disease gene is known and for the detection of common mutations. With the automation offered by novel DNA sequence techniques, it is likely that screening methods will be increasingly replaced by direct sequence analysis.

### Screening Methods

Screening methods have the advantage of speed and lower cost and are usually em-

Table 2–3. **Examples of Sites on the World Wide Web with Molecular Genetic Databases**

| Address | Name |
|---|---|
| http://www.ncbi.nlm.nihgov/Omim/ | Online Mendelian Inheritance in Man |
| http://www.uwcm.ac.uk/uwcm/mg/hgmd0.html | Human Gene Mutation Database |
| http://fruitfly.berkeley.edu | Berkeley Drosophila Genome project |
| http://www.ncbinlm.nih.gov/ncicgap/ | Cancer Genome Anatomy Project (CGAP) |
| http://www.ataxia.org | National Ataxia Foundation |
| http://www.nf.org | National Neurofibromatosis Foundation |
| http://www.turner.syndrome-us.org/ | The Turner's Syndrome society of the US |
| http://www.pwsyndrome.com/index.html | The Prader-Willi Conection |
| http://www.pcnet.cpm/~orphan/ | National Organization for Rare Disorders |
| http://www.downs-syndrome.org.uk/ | Down's Syndrome Association |
| http://www.niaaa.nih.gov/ | National Institute on Alcohol Abuse and Alcoholism |
| http://www.senn.com | Molecular Resources (site sponsored by Nature and Scientific American) |
| http://www.who.ch/ncd/hgn/hgn-home.htm | WHO Human Genetics Programme |
| http://www.wiley.com/genetherapy/ | Gene Therapy |
| http://esg.www.mit.edu:8001/esgbio/7001main.html | Biology Project |
| http://www.biology.arizona.edu/ | The Biology Project (site for basics in biology and genetics) |
| http://www.mblab.gla.ac.uk~julian/Dict.html | A Dictionary of Cell Biological Terms |
| http://morgan.rutgers.edu/ | A well-illustrated genetics tutorial |
| http://wsrv.clas.virginia.edu/~rjh9u/humbiol.html | Human Biology |
| http://cti.itc.Virginia.EDU/~cmg/ | Interactive Biochemistry |
| http://www.kumc.edu/biochemistry/bioc800/start.html | Medical Biochemistry |
| http://www.mc.vanderbilt.edu/gcrc/gene/index.html | Introduction to Gene Therapy Home Page |
| http://www.acs.ucalgary.ca/~browder/dev-biol.html | Dynamic Development |
| http://sdb.bio.purdue.edu/dbcinema/index.html | Developmental Biology Cinema |

ployed to evaluate candidate genes before identification of the actual disease gene. Also, for large disease genes that contain a great number of nonrecurring mutations, screening methods are often employed to prevent having to sequence the entire gene in each individual patient.

Many of these methods are based on detecting confirmational differences of double- or single-stranded DNA fragments with slightly differing base composition. A commonly used method is single-strand conformational polymorphism analysis (SSCP or SSCA). A DNA fragment is amplified by PCR, and single DNA strands are generated by denaturation. A difference in as little as 1 bp may induce a conformational change in the mutant DNA strand, which results in a different migration pattern in a nondenaturing polyacrylamide gel[31] (Fig. 2–13).

Denaturing gradient gel electrophoresis (DGGE) subjects double-stranded DNA fragments to migration through a gel with increasing concentrations of denaturants. A single base pair difference between a normal and a mutant DNA duplex can result in melting of the duplex at different denaturant concentrations. After strand separation, the DNA fragments do not migrate much further, allowing the detection of differences in mutant and normal duplexes. Denaturing gradient gel electrophoresis is highly sensitive, but may be costly due to the necessity to synthesize special PCR primers containing a GC-clamp.[32]

For the detection of truncating mutations, the protein truncation test (PTT) can be used.[33] In this assay, RNA transcripts are converted to cDNA using reverse-transcribed-PCR and a special 5' primer containing the T7 promoter and a translation initiation codon. *In vitro*, this promoter is used to generate RNA, which is then translated into protein. When these *in vitro* generated protein products are run out on a gel, the likely location of the mutation can be predicted from the size of the truncated proteins. When PTT is used for mutation detection, it is imperative that mutations are confirmed at the DNA level.

## Direct Mutation Detection

For diseases caused by a specific mutation, direct detection of the mutation is simple and inexpensive. For example, diseases caused by expansion of a CAG repeat can be detected by amplification of the region containing the repeat and by detection of a larger than normal fragment by gel electrophoresis (see Fig. 12–1). The same is true for other mutations that result in deletion or additions of codons. In the case of heterogeneity of mutant alleles, use of multiplex PCR allows for the simultaneous detection of deletions (see Fig. 5–3).

If single base pair changes alter the recognition sequence of a restriction enzyme, this can be easily recognized by digestion of

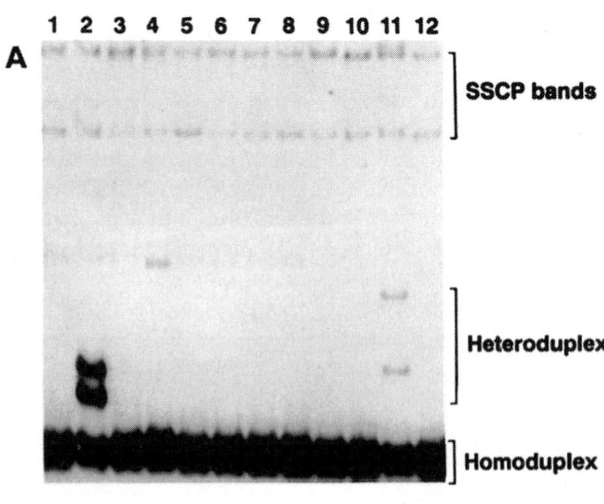


**Figure 2–13.** Single-stranded conformational polymorphism (SSCP) analysis of DNA from vestibular schwannomas. A portion of the NF2 transcript was amplified by reverse-transcribed PCR from tumor RNAs and analyzed by nondenaturing gel electrophoresis. Mutations in DNAs in lanes 2 and 11 result in abnormal heteroduplex bands as well as an abnormal SSCP band at the top of lane 11. (From Sainz and colleagues,[29] with permission.)

a PCR-generated fragment and separation of the fragments on an agarose gel. Single base pair changes can also be recognized with allele-specific hybridization with oligonucleotide probes. These are designed to bind to either the normal or the abnormal allele with high specificity.

Finally, direct sequence analysis is becoming increasingly feasible to analyze genes for point mutations. This approach is particularly useful when several different mutations are clustered in one exon and can be analyzed by sequencing of a single PCR product. The DNA sequence has to be of sufficient quality to recognize the presence of a heterozygous mutation (see Fig. 2–9). The availability of chip technology will undoubtedly broaden the applicability of sequence analysis to larger genes with multiple different mutations.[26]

## MOLECULAR GENETIC TESTING

DNA-based diagnosis falls into two broad categories: direct mutation detection and indirect detection of a mutated gene with segregation (linkage) analysis. When the chromosomal location of a disease gene is known, but the gene itself has not been identified, DNA diagnosis can be performed with polymorphic DNA markers, which are used to track the disease chromosome in a given family. When the disease gene has been identified and the types of mutations are limited, direct mutational analysis is possible. For some diseases, however, the number of disease-causing mutations is greatly variable, and no mutational "hot spots" exist so that indirect testing is technically more feasible than direct mutational analysis. As discussed later, there are many important differences between direct and indirect testing with regard to requirements for DNAs from affected family members and the sensitivity and specificity of the information obtained.

### Indirect Analysis with Linked Genetic Markers

For indirect testing, samples from at least two affected first-degree relatives are required because the phase of the marker alleles and the disease need to be established (see Fig. 2–12). Once phase is established, this information can be used to track the disease chromosome in other family members. Tracking of the disease chromosome (or, more precisely, the chromosomal *region* that contains the gene) can be performed independent of the precise mutation causing the disease. Thus, when a disease is caused by a great number of different mutations in a large gene, indirect testing is at the moment the only feasible modality.

Indirect testing requires that markers flanking the disease gene be identified and that these markers ideally show no recombination with the disease locus. When a marker shows 5% recombination with the disease locus, the accuracy of the prediction in a standard pedigree falls to approximately 95%. When markers are used that closely flank the disease gene, predictive accuracy reaches virtually 100% (with the caveats mentioned later). Given the density of genetic markers, recombination between the disease locus and a genetic marker is usually not a problem, especially because intragenic markers can be used. However, for large genes such as the Duchenne's muscular dystrophy gene, recombination between genetic markers and the disease mutation may be a problem.

In contrast to direct mutational testing, the accuracy of indirect molecular testing is dependent on the correctness of the diagnosis in all individuals used for testing. For example, if the diagnosis of neurofibromatosis 2 (NF2) is missed in the proband and the diagnosis of neurofibromatosis 1 (NF1) is made, indirect testing would employ markers on chromosome 17 flanking the *NF1* gene instead of markers on chromosome 22 flanking the *NF2* gene.

In addition, nonallelic heterogeneity must be absent for the phenotype being examined. In other words, the phenotype must be caused by mutations in only one locus. For example, it has now been well established that all patients with an NF2 phenotype have mutations in the *NF2* gene on chromosome 22. On the other hand, early onset Alzheimer's disease is caused by mutations in at least three distinct genes located on different chromosomes.

Therefore, it would not be possible to use indirect testing for families with early onset Alzheimer's disease unless the pedigree size is sufficiently large to establish linkage to one of the Alzheimer's disease loci before testing of specific individuals.

### Direct Mutational Analysis

In contrast to indirect testing, for which blood samples from at least two affected family members are required, the direct genetic test more closely resembles a conventional laboratory test. A blood sample is taken from a patient, and the test is used to determine whether the individual carries a *specific mutation* in a given gene with a yes/no answer. Barring technical problems resulting in false-positive results, a positive test indicates that the patient has the disease. A positive result is independent of the accuracy of the clinical assessment. Phenotype and mutation analysis, however, still need to be correctly matched. For a patient with dominant spinocerebellar ataxia (SCA), a negative test for *SCA1* or *SCA3* does not mean that he or she does not have a dominant SCA because the mutation could be in one of the several other *SCA* loci.

Examples of direct testing include testing for expansion of trinucleotide repeats and analysis for known recurrent mutations in a gene. An example of direct mutation detection after identification of the mutated exon with SSCP is shown in Figure 2–9. If mutations in a gene do not cluster in hot spots, a greater number of assays need to be performed. If a gene is large, it may be impractical to perform a large number of assays to detect a mutation in an individual patient. In these cases, mutation analysis is only possible with an indirect approach with linked genetic markers. Novel methods for sequence analysis will make direct mutation detection in these diseases possible in the future.[24]

## ANIMAL MODELS

Genetic techniques have provided the tools to create animal models that resemble human diseases even if the diseases do not naturally occur in the animals. At this point, these techniques have been restricted mainly to mice, although in principle they can be applied to other rodents or other mammals. Two main approaches to alter the genetic constitution of animals are utilized. The first involves insertion of a novel, often mutated gene into the mouse germline, and the second involves an alteration of endogenous mouse genes by gene targeting.

### Expression of Foreign Transgenes

Transgenes can be injected into fertilized oocytes, which are then transferred into pseudopregnant mothers. Alternatively, embryonic stem (ES) cells can be used instead of the pseudopregnant mothers. These pluripotent cells are derived from 3.5 day postcoitum embryos and arise from the inner cell mass of the blastocyst. Foreign genes can be introduced into ES cells by electroporation. A selectable marker (such as the *neo* gene) can be joined to the transgene so that only ES cells bearing the transgene survive in culture. These are then added to the blastocyst. The resulting animals are chimeric because they have some wild-type cells and some cells bearing the transgene. In some animals, the transgene-bearing ES cells contribute to the germline so that the transgene can be stably transmitted to the offspring.

The expression of transgenes in mice does not necessarily mirror the expression of a mutated allele in human disease conditions. First, the transgene is expressed in addition to the two endogenous mouse alleles. Often multiple copies of the transgene insert into the mouse genome. Second, unless the endogenous promoter is used, expression may be higher than under physiological conditions or expression may occur in different sets of cell types. Even if the physiological promoter is used, the transgene construct may lack all the appropriate regulatory elements. Finally, by chance, the transgene can integrate into an endogenous mouse gene and disrupt proper functioning of this gene (so-called insertional mutagenesis).

### Gene Targeting (Knock-Out, Knock-In)

With homologous recombination, a cloned gene or gene segment can be exchanged for the endogenous gene.[34,35] With insertion of the mutation into the cloned gene, the mutation can be transferred into the animal cell. When the cloned gene contains a nonsense mutation, the gene will be inactivated after recombination (knock-out). Vectors for homologous recombination contain a marker gene so that successful recombination can be monitored and site-specific integration of the vector construct can be ensured.

Gene targeting can be achieved in somatic cells but has its greatest value when it is performed with ES cells. With backcrossing of chimeric animals, mice can be generated that are heterozygous for the mutation in all tissues. In these animals, the gene is now transcribed only from the one remaining normal allele. Mating of heterozygous animals creates homozygous offspring in which no functional gene product is made. For a gene with the symbol *Gs*, the animals thus produced are designated $Gs^{+/-}$ for the heterozygote and $Gs^{-/-}$ for the homozygote.

Instead of a nonsense mutation, the gene fragment used for homologous recombination can also contain a missense mutation (knock-in). Such animals are potentially closer models of human disease than mice expressing a transgene because the proper endogenous promoter is used and gene dosage is not disturbed.[36]

A problem with homozygous knock-outs for many genes is that embryonic lethality results because the respective genes have a function not only in adult tissues but also during embryogenesis. This can be circumvented by generation of chimeric animals that carry a mixture of wild-type and homozygously deficient cells. For example, with the *Cre–loxP* recombination system, mice containing alleles with inserted *loxP* sites can be mated with mice expressing a *Cre*-recombinase transgene under the control of a tissue-specific promoter so that function of a gene is only abolished in a specific tissue.[37]

## DATABASES FOR MOLECULAR GENETIC RESEARCH

The old adage of "clone by phone" has now in part been replaced by "get it on the Web," also referred to as "data mining." Much information is contained in publicly available databases. These may contain information on testing sites for disease gene mutations and extensive information on the genetic and physical location of DNA markers. More recently, these databases also contain the locations and the expression patterns of genes. Table 2–3 lists different kinds of databases that in turn contain links to other relevant sites.

## SUMMARY

The development of novel molecular tools has greatly enhanced the ability and speed of the analysis of DNA, RNA, and protein molecules. Due to its large size and repetitive composition of only four bases, DNA was difficult to analyze until recombinant molecules could be generated that enabled the production of specific DNA fragments in large quantities. The PCR has further revolutionized DNA analysis and is the basis for many DNA-based diagnostic tests. These techniques have been used to create highly detailed genetic and physical maps of the human genome that constitute the framework for the human genome sequencing project. These maps also provide a foundation from which to identify disease genes by positional cloning or candidate gene approaches once the mutation has been mapped to a specific chromosomal region. DNA-based testing for inherited disease utilizes flanking genetic markers (indirect testing) or can detect specific mutations once a disease gene has been isolated (direct testing).

## REFERENCES

1. Sambrook J, Fritsch EF, Maniatis T: Molecular Cloning: A Laboratory Manual, ed 2. Cold Spring Harbor Press, Cold Spring Harbor, NY, 1989.
2. Watson JD, Gilman M, Witkowski J, Zoller M: Recombinant DNA, 2nd edition. Scientific American Books, New York, 1992.

3. Strachan T, Read AP: Human Molecular Genetics. Bios Scientific Publishers, Ltd., Oxford, 1996.
4. Meselson M, Yuan R: DNA restriction enzyme from *E. coli.* Nature 217:110–1114, 1968.
5. Kelly TJ, Smith HO: A restriction enzyme from *Hemophilus influenzae,* II. Base sequence of the recognition site. J Mol Biol 51:393–409, 1970.
6. Southern EM: Detection of specific sequences among DNA fragments separated by gel electrophoresis. J Mol Biol 98:503–517, 1975.
7. Pulst SM, Nechiporuk A, Nechiporuk T, et al.: Identification of the SCA2 gene: Moderate expansion of a normally biallelic trinucleotide repeat. Nat Genet 40:269–276, 1996.
8. Huynh DH, Del Bigio MR, Sahba S, Ho DH, Pulst SM: Expression of ataxin 2 in brains from normal individuals and patients with Alzheimer disease and spinocerebellar ataxia 2. Ann Neurol 45:232, 1999.
9. Jackson D, Symons R, Berg P: Biochemical method for inserting new genetic information into DNA of simian virus 40: Circular SV40 DNA molecules containing lambda phage genes and the galactose operon of *Escherichia coli.* Proc Natl Acad Sci USA 69: 2904–2909, 1972.
10. Cohen S, Chang A, Boyer H, Helling R: Construction of biologically functional bacterial plasmids *in vitro.* Proc Natl Acad Sci USA 70:3240–3244, 1973.
11. Grunstein M, Hogness DS: Colony hybridization: A method for the isolation of cloned DNAs that contain a specific gene. Proc Natl Acad Sci USA 72: 3961–3965, 1975.
12. Saikai RK, Scharf SJ, Faloona F, et al.: Enzymatic amplification of beta-globin sequences and restriction site analysis for diagnosis of sickle cell anemia. Science 230:1350–1354, 1985.
13. Mullis KB: The unusual origin of the polymerase chain reaction. Sci Am 262:56–65, 1990.
14. Nechiporuk T, Huynh D, Figueroa K, Sahba S, Nechiporuk A, Pulst SM: The mouse SCA gene: cDNA sequence, alternative splicing, and protein expression. Hum Mol Genet 7:1301–1309, 1998.
15. Sanger F, Nicklen S, Coulson AR: DNA sequencing with chain-terminating inhibitors. Proc Natl Acad Sci USA 74:5463–5467, 1977.
16. Scoles D, Baser ME, Pulst SM: A missense mutation in the neurofibromatosis 2 gene occurs in patients with mild and severe phenotypes. Neurology 47: 544–546, 1996.
17. Kan YW, Dozy AM: Polymorphism of DNA sequence adjacent to human beta-globin structural gene: Relationship to sickle mutation. Proc Natl Acad Sci USA 75:5631–5635, 1978.
18. Botstein D, White RL, Skolnick M, Davis RW: Construction of a genetic linkage map in man using restriction fragment length polymorphisms. Am J Hum Genet 32:314–331, 1980.
19. Vaughan J, Durr A, Tassin J, et al.: The alpha-synuclein Ala53Thr mutation is not a common cause of familial Parkinson's disease: A study of 230 European cases. European consortium on genetic susceptibility in Parkinson's disease. Ann Neurol 44:270–273, 1998.
20. Weber JL, May PE: Abundant class of human DNA polymorphisms which can be typed using the polymerase chain reaction. Am J Hum Genet 44:388–396, 1989.
21. http://www.chlc.org/ChlcMaps.html, 1999 (accessed May 17 1999).
22. Pulst SM: Genetic linkage analysis. Arch Neurol (in press).
23. Wang DG, Fan JB, Siao CJ, et al.: Large-scale identification, mapping and genotyping of single-nucleotide polymorphisms in the human genome. Science 280:1077–1082, 1998.
24. Brown PO, Botstein D: Exploring the new world of the genome with DNA microarrays. Nat Genet 21(suppl):33–37, 1999.
25. Hacia JG: Resequencing and mutational analysis using oligonucleotide microarrays. Nat Genet 21(suppl):42–47, 1999.
26. Hacia JG, Brody LC, Chee MS, Fodor SP, Collins FS: Detection of heterozygous mutations in BRCA1 using high density oligonucleotide arrays and two-color fluorescence analysis. Nat Genet 14:441–447, 1996.
27. Morton NE: Sequential tests for the detection of linkage. Am J Hum Genet 7:277–318, 1955.
28. Terwiliger J, Ott J: Handbook for Human Genetic Linkage. John Hopkins University Press, Baltimore, MD, 1994.
29. Oliva R, Tolosa E, Ezquerra M, et al.: Significant changes in the tau A0 and A3 alleles in progressive supranuclear palsy and improved genotyping by silver detection. Arch Neurol 55:1122–1124, 1998.
30. Pecheux C, Mouret JF, Durr A, et al.: Sequence analysis of the CCG polymorphic region adjacent to the CAG triplet repeat of the HD gene in normal and HD chromosomes. J Med Genet 32:399–400, 1995.
31. Sainz J, Huynh D, Figueroa K, et al.: Mutations of the neurofibromatosis type 2 gene and lack of the gene product in vestibular schwannomas. Hum Mol Genet 3:885–891, 1994.
32. Mercel P, Hoang-Xuan K, Sanson M, et al.: Screening for germ-line mutations in the NF2 gene. Genes Chrom Cancer 12:117–127, 1995.
33. Pegoraro E, Marks H, Garcia CA, et al.: Laminin alpha2 muscular dystrophy: Genotype/phenotype studies of 22 patients. Neurology 51:101–110, 1998.
34. Thomas KR, Capecchi MR: Introduction of homologous DNA sequences into mammalian cells induces mutation in the cognate gene. Nature 324: 34–38, 1986.
35. Doetschman T, Gregg RG, Maeda N, et al.: Targetted correction of a mutant HPRT gene in mouse embryonic stem cells. Nature 330:576–578, 1987.
36. Wheeler VC, White JK, Auerbach W, et al.: Huntington's disease knock-in mice. Am J Hum Genet 63:A345, 1998.
37. Sauer B: Inducible gene targeting in mice using the Cre/lox system. Methods 14:381–392, 1998.

Chapter 3

# CHANNELOPATHIES

Rabi Tawil, MD
Robert C. Griggs, MD
Michael Rose, MD



Membrane ion channels serve multiple functions within the central and peripheral nervous system. Channels conduct ions and select specific ions for transmembrane transport. Ion channels open and close in response to specific signals: electrical (voltage gated); chemical (e.g., transmitter gated), and mechanical (pressure or stretch). Despite remarkable similarities in protein structural elements, ion channels are selective both in their discrimination between specific ions and in the activation of their gating function.

The discovery of the structures of various ion channels and the characterization of the protein sequences of many have paved the way for recognition of genetic and acquired disorders of many different channels. Although the focus of this chapter is on genetic voltage-gated channel disorders (Table 3–1), it also acknowledges the large number of acquired disorders, usually autoimmune, that are mediated at least in part by antibodies to specific receptor proteins (Table 3–2).

## STRUCTURAL CONSTITUENTS AND PHYSIOLOGICAL ELEMENTS OF ION CHANNELS

Most membrane ion channels contain *subunits*, usually four, that are designated

Table 3–1. **Channelopathies**

| Disorders | Chromosomal Location |
|---|---|
| Skeletal muscle sodium channel α-subunit | 17q23–25 |
| Hyperkalemic periodic paralysis | |
| With myotonia | |
| Without myotonia | |
| With paramyotonia congenita | |
| Paramyotonia congenita | |
| Sodium channel myotonias | |
| Myotonia fluctuans | |
| Myotonia permanens | |
| Acetazolamide-responsive myotonia | |
| Skeletal muscle calcium channel α-subunit | 1p |
| Hypokalemic periodic paralysis | |
| Skeletal muscle chloride channel | 7q32 |
| Autosomal dominant myotonia congenita (Thomsen's disease) | |
| Autosomal recessive myotonia congenita (Becker's disease) | |
| Potassium channel | 12p13 |
| Episodic ataxia type 1 (EA1) | |
| Brain-specific calcium channel $\alpha_1$-subunit | |
| Episodic ataxia type 2 (EA2) | 19p13 |
| Familial hemiplegic migraine | 19p13 |
| Putative channelopathies | |
| Paroxysmal dyskinesias | |
| Andersen's syndrome | |
| Schwartz-Jampel syndrome | 19q12 |
| Familial hemiplegic migraine | 1q21–q23, q31 |

α-and β-subunits. Subunits in turn consist of large repetitive *domains* composed of smaller *segments* (α-helices) that span the cell membrane. These segments mediate specific channel functions: Typically the $S_4$ segment serves the gating function, and the β-helix between segments 5 and 6 serves as the ion pore. Domains are linked by a *cytoplasmic loop*, and there are often extracellular elements that mediate specialized functions.

## STRATEGIES FOR DEFINING A CHANNELOPATHY

This chapter focuses primarilly on peripheral nervous system channelopathies because the majority of diseases defined in molecular terms involve skeletal muscle and peripheral nerve. It is likely that a larger number of hereditary central nervous system diseases will prove to be the result of mutations of channel genes.

The characterization of the specific molecular defect in a channel has resulted from the convergence of a number of research strategies. Often, physiological data from studies with intact muscle or nerve fibers implicated a specific ion channel. The cloning of specific channels and the study of channel structures in various species provided candidates for linkage to disease and also suggested the most critical, evolutionarily conserved sequences of the channel molecule. The study of carefully defined patient kindreds indicated approximate chromosome locations and suggested candidate loci for the specific disease under study. Study of patient DNA then allowed detection of point mutations in the candidate gene.

Table 3–2. **Examples of Putative Autoimmune Channelopathies**

| |
|---|
| $Na^{+}$ channel: Multiple sclerosis, chronic inflammatory demyelinating polyneuropathy |
| $Ca^{2+}$ channel: Myasthenic syndrome (Lambert-Eaton syndrome) |
| $Cl^{-}$ channel: Focal epilepsy |
| $K^{+}$ channel: Continuous muscle fiber activity syndrome |

## SKELETAL MUSCLE SODIUM CHANNELOPATHY

Several distinct, autosomal dominant disorders of muscle membrane excitability with overlapping features result from mutations of the α-subunit of the skeletal muscle sodium channel. These disorders can be grouped clinically into three major categories: the hyperkalemic periodic paralysis group (HYPP), paramyotonia congenita (PC), and sodium channel myotonias (NaM) (see Table 3–1). The various clinical syndromes are first described and then pathogenesis, genetics, and treatment are discussed.

### Hyperkalemic Periodic Paralysis

Hyperkalemic periodic paralysis can be further subdivided into HYPP with myotonia and HYPP without myotonia. Both conditions are characterized by the occurrence of episodic weakness brought on by rest after physical exertion, by fasting, or by the intake of potassium-rich foods.[1] Myotonic stiffness is variable in HYPP patients with myotonia, at times detectable only with electromyography (EMG). Attacks in HYPP are usually brief, lasting from 1 to several hours. Between attacks, neurologic examination can be normal or show a variable degree of myotonia, predominantly lid lag and eyelid closure. Muscles are sometimes hypertrophied.[1] Older patients often develop a progressive proximal myopathy.

The diagnosis of the HYPP is usually evident by the history and examination and by documentation of a rise in potassium level during attacks. The presence of myotonia detected by EMG or physical examination further supports the diagnosis of HYPP with myotonia. In patients whose history is suggestive of HYPP, but myotonia is not present, an oral potassium challenge may be helpful. This test is potentially hazardous and should not be done in patients with renal disease or diabetes. After an overnight fast, the oral administration of 0.05 g/kg of KCl in a sugar-free solution is followed by serial monitoring of strength and serum potassium levels every 15 minutes. A repeated challenge with 0.10 to 0.15 g/kg of KCl may be indicated if the initial challenge did not precipitate an attack.[1] Secondary forms of HYPP should be ruled out by screens for renal and adrenal disorders as well as a careful history of drug intake.

### Paramyotonia Congenita

In PC, myotonic stiffness is the major symptom. Myotonia in PC is worsened by exposure to cold and paradoxically to exercise.[1] Exercise in cold temperature initially leads to increased myotonic stiffness followed by flaccid paralysis. In some kindreds, the typical PC symptomatology overlaps with HYPP, with affected individuals having episodic weakness unrelated to cold exposure. Physical examination shows prominent musculature, paradoxical myotonia of eye closure, and lid lag myotonia as well as generalized myotonia. Strength remains normal. The diagnosis can be confirmed electrophysiologically by inducing loss of membrane excitability and muscle weakness with the forearm cooling test.[2]

### Sodium Channel Myotonias

Several unusual myotonic disorders without periodic paralysis but clinically different from myotonia congenita have been associated with mutations of the skeletal muscle sodium channel. One is an acetazolamide-responsive myotonia with variable myotonic stiffness worsened by fasting and the intake of potassium-rich foods.[3] Myotonia is also worsened by cold, but at no time is there associated weakness. Another disorder, termed *myotonia fluctuans,* is characterized by fluctuating myotonia, at times worsened by potassium intake but not by exposure to cold.[4] Other myotonic syndromes also occur.[5]

## Genetics and Pathogenesis

After the initial linkage of HYPP to the α-subunit of the human sodium channel,[6] PC and NaM were found to be allelic disorders also linked to the sodium channel.[3,7] To date, about 16 different point mutations causing single amino acid substitutions have been found. Their locations are shown in Figure 3–1.[8] The assignment of a clinical phenotype with a particular mutation is somewhat variable, reflecting a lack of consensus on how the various clinical phenotypes should be defined.[9,10] What were previously classified as distinct disorders may in fact represent a clinical continuum. This is best exemplified by a kindred in which the different affected family members manifested distinct clinical phenotypes (Fig. 3–2).[11]

The α-subunit of the sodium channel has four homologous domains each with six membrane-spanning segments (see Fig. 3–1).[8] *In vitro* electrophysiological studies of mutant sodium channels corresponding to HYPP, PC, and NaM all show lack of normal inactivation of the channel.[8] This lack of inactivation is reflected clinically by muscle cell hyperexcitability as manifested by myotonic stiffness and eventually by inexitability of the fiber, resulting in paralysis. Why adjacent mutations of the sodium channel cause different clinical phenotypes remains unclear. One possible explanation is that the charge and size of the resultant amino acid substitution determines the resultant phenotype.[8] A variety of sodium channel mutations have been introduced into cell lines, the study of their effects on voltage-dependent activation and deactivation.[12,13] In a recent expression study in human embryonic kidney cells, slow channel inactivation, which limits the availability of Na channels from seconds to minutes, was found to be impaired in HYPP but not in PC and NaM.[13a]

## Treatment

Prophylactic treatment for HYPP is aimed at preventing or decreasing the frequency of attacks. This goal is achieved by changes in lifestyle (patients should avoid fasting and strenuous physical activity) as well as by pharmacological interventions. Thiazide diuretics are the first line of treatment, followed by acetazolamide and other carbonic anhydrase inhibitors. Treatment of an acute

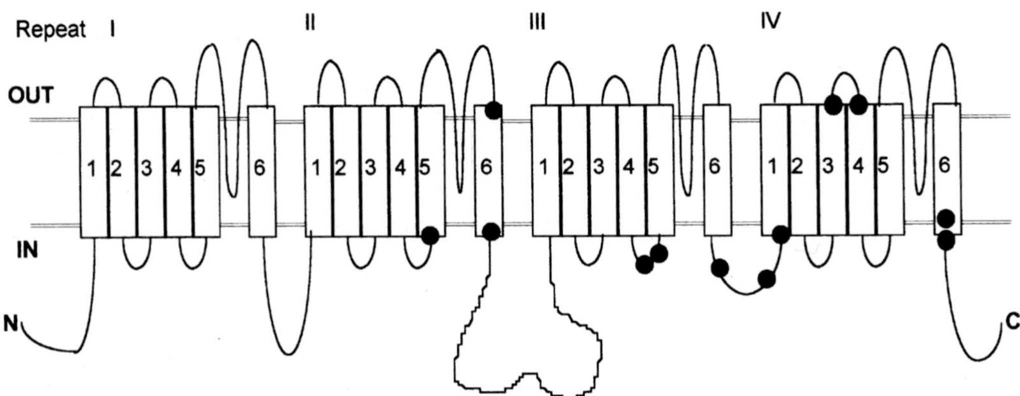


**Figure 3–1.** Skeletal muscle sodium channel showing sites of known point mutations (closed circles).

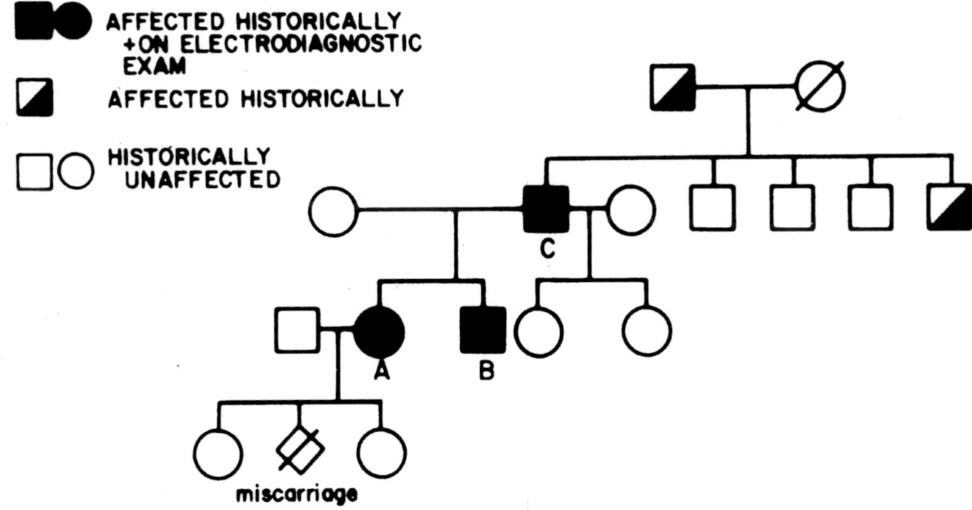


**Figure 3–2.** A kindred with a myotonic disorder and variable phenotype. Patient A: Hyperkalemic periodic paralysis; patient B: hyperkalemic periodic paralysis; patient C: paramyotonia congenita. (Adapted from De Silva et al.[89])

attack is only necessary if the attack is severe or associated with life-threatening hyperkalemia. Interventions aimed at shifting potassium intracellularly have been variably effective for acute attacks of HYPP. Such interventions include intravenous glucose boluses with or without insulin, inhaled β-adrenergic agents, and intravenous calcium gluconate.[11,13]

In PC and some sodium channel myotonias, oral lidocaine congeners (tocainide, mexiletine) are effective in the treatment of severe myotonic stiffness. These agents, however, will not lessen the frequency and severity of weakness in PC associated with HYPP. In such conditions, a combination of a diuretic and an oral lidocaine congener may provide the optimal treatment.[11]

## SKELETAL MUSCLE CALCIUM CHANNELOPATHIES: HYPOKALEMIC PERIODIC PARALYSIS

### Clinical Features

Onset is usually during adolescence, with an age range of 6 to 25 years.[14,15] Only rarely has an age of onset of 60 to 70 years been described.[16] Spontaneous attacks of weakness occur most frequently late at night, and patients often wake up with variable degrees of weakness. Common precipitating factors include large carbohydrate meals and rest following exertion.[14,16] Attacks can also occur with exposure to cold, alcohol ingestion, and emotional stress.[16] Stiffness, heaviness of the limbs, and diaphoresis often precede the attacks.[16] Weakness starts proximally in the lower extremities and can progress to flaccid quadriplegia.[16,17] Ocular, bulbar, and respiratory muscles are rarely involved.[15,16,18] Interattack examination is normal in younger patients with the exception of eyelid myotonia. Older patients frequently have fixed proximal weakness. During the attacks, flaccid weakness with hyporeflexia proportionate to the degree of weakness is noted.[16,19] Single attacks can last from 2 to 72 hours,[14,16] and attack frequencies range from one per day to one or two in a lifetime.[16,19] With increasing age, attack frequency usually diminishes and is often replaced by persistent proximal weakness or a state of fluctuating but persistent weakness.[14,15] Bradycardia and sinus arrhythmia are commonly observed during hypokalemic periodic paralysis (HYOPP) attacks and are directly related to the degree of hypokalemia.[15,16,20,21]

Mortality during paralytic attacks has been reported to be as high as 10%,[22] but

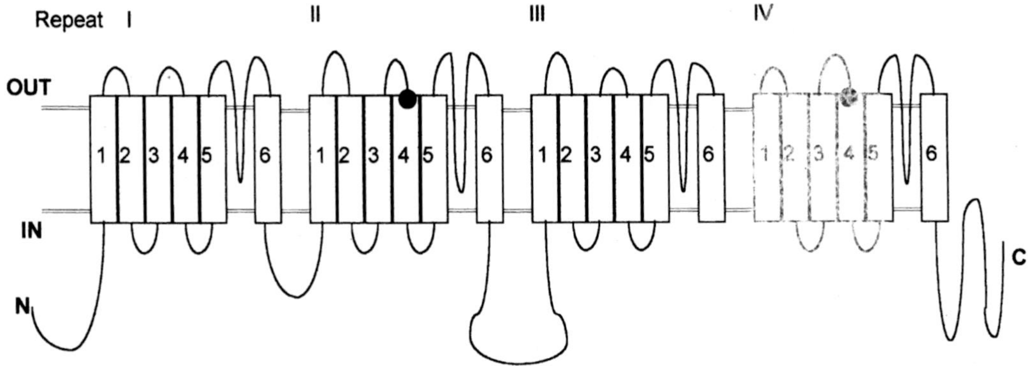


**Figure 3–3.** Skeletal muscle calcium channel showing sites of known point mutations (closed circles).

the report was based on pre-1941 literature and overestimated mortality because of inaccurate diagnoses and less sophisticated medical care.[16] Recent reports of death are rare; when it does occur, it is in the setting of severe, prolonged untreated attacks, mostly as a result of aspiration rather than cardiac complications.[16,18,23]

## Diagnosis

The diagnosis of HYOPP is made by documenting hypokalemia during a spontaneous or induced attack, a consistent clinical profile, and, in two-thirds of cases, a positive family history. Secondary causes of hypokalemic paralysis, such as thyrotoxicosis, toxins, or renal, adrenal, and gastrointestinal potassium-wasting disorders should be excluded in patients with atypical presentations. When spontaneous attacks are infrequent, provocative tests with oral or intravenous glucose combined with insulin may be necessary. Another method, more time consuming, consists of giving hourly oral doses of glucose (50 g/150 mL water) until an attack is precipitated, usually after 8 to 10 doses.[24]

Electrophysiological studies are useful adjunctive tests in the diagnosis of HYOPP. Documentation of electrical myotonia on EMG virtually excludes HYOPP. The exercise nerve conduction test demonstrates a significant and sustained drop in compound muscle action potential amplitudes following isometric exercise.[25] This procedure, with a sensitivity of 71%, is useful to establish the diagnosis of periodic paralysis in questionable cases.[25] However, it does not differentiate between the primary and secondary forms of periodic paralysis or between the various forms of primary periodic paralyses.[25]

## Genetics and Pathogenesis

HYOPP is an autosomal dominant disorder with variable penetrance in women. Sporadic cases, which likely represent new mutations,[26] are relatively common and are clinically indistinguishable from familial cases. Estimates of disease prevalence range from 0.4/100,000 in Finland[15] to 1.25/100,000 in Denmark,[16] but these are likely underestimates of the true prevalence given the disease's variable penetrance. Recently, HYOPP was linked to the skeletal muscle dihydropyridine receptor (CACNL1A3), a calcium channel on chromosome 1q.[26,27] Initially, three mutations within the *CACNL1A3* gene were identified. The most common, initially identified as a *de novo* mutation in a sporadic case, is a histidine to arginine substitution in the $S_4$ segments of receptor domain IV (Fig. 3–3).[26] Two other point mutations have been identified in the $S_4$ segments of domains II and IV.[26,27] Recently, Fouad and associates studied a group of 45 HYOPP patients and identified three mutations in 30 patients.[28] The R528H and R1239G mutations made up the majority of the mutations.

Skeletal muscle weakness in HYOPP results from transient inexcitability of muscle fibers.[29] A normal contractile apparatus[30] and neuromuscular junction[31] in HYOPP implied the presence of a defective muscle membrane as a cause of this inexcitability. *In vitro* studies have consistently demonstrated the presence of lower than normal resting potentials in HYPP muscle.[29,32] The HYOPP muscle fibers, moreover, respond paradoxically to both insulin[32] and decreased extracellular potassium concentrations,[29] becoming depolarized and inexcitable rather than hyperpolarized.[29]

The physiological changes described earlier would not have predicted a causal association between HYPP and the dihydropyridine receptor whose primary role is electrochemical coupling. This voltage-gated channel interacts with the ryanodine receptors, leading to the opening of calcium channels in the sarcoplasmic reticulum, influx of calcium into the cytoplasm, and, finally, contraction of muscle. Preliminary studies on the net effect of the described HYOPP mutations suggest loss of function of the dihydropyridine receptor.[9] It is not clear, however, how the loss of dihydropyridine receptor function explains the paradoxical response of HYOPP muscle fibers to insulin and hypokalemia. To explain the dominant inheritance, it is postulated that the functional channel is composed of multiple subunits where an amino acid substitution results in a dominant negative alteration of channel function.[9]

### Treatment

Acute paralytic attacks are treated with oral potassium replacement. Intravenous replacement should be avoided because usual diluants for potassium, such as glucose and saline, can initially exacerbate hypokalemia.[14] For the prevention of attacks, acetazolamide, a carbonic anhydrase inhibitor, is the drug of choice. It is effective in both reducing attack frequency and improving persistent weakness.[33] Dichlorphenamide, a more potent carbonic anhydrase inhibitor, appears to be beneficial in patients whose response to acetazolamide is waning.[34,35] Acetazolamide may be better tolerated in the periodic paralyses than in other disorders because of the smaller average doses required.[36] Alternatively, potassium-sparing diuretics can be used. Dietary manipulations such as low-carbohydrate and low-sodium diets are variably effective in controlling attack frequency. Given the recent information about pathogenesis, drugs that modulate the function of the dihydropyridine receptor should be considered as potential therapeutic agents. None, however, has thus far been formally tested.

## SKELETAL MUSCLE CHLORIDE CHANNELOPATHIES: MYOTONIA CONGENITA

The congenital myotonias are disorders of muscle membrane whose major symptoms are the result of myotonic muscle stiffness. They occur in two allelic varieties: an autosomal dominant form (ADMC, Thomsen's disease) and an autosomal recessive form (ARMC, Becker's disease).[37]

### Clinical Features

Diffuse painless myotonia is the major symptom of both ADMC and ARMC. Symptom onset is in the first or second decade of life. Myotonia is provoked by muscle contraction, especially with sudden physical exertion following a period of rest. The myotonia resolves with repeated muscle contraction. Myotonia is sometimes followed by a weakness that lasts up to 30 minutes in ARMC.

On examination, muscles are often hypertrophied, especially in the lower extremities. Strength and muscle stretch reflexes are usually normal as are deep tendon reflexes. Grip, percussion, lid lag, and paradoxical eye closure myotonia is easily elicited. To demonstrate generalized myotonia, patients rest supine for 5 to 10 minutes and are then asked to stand up quickly. On electromyography, runs of typical myotonic discharges are evident.[37]

### Diagnosis

The differential diagnosis of myotonia congenita includes a number of distinctive

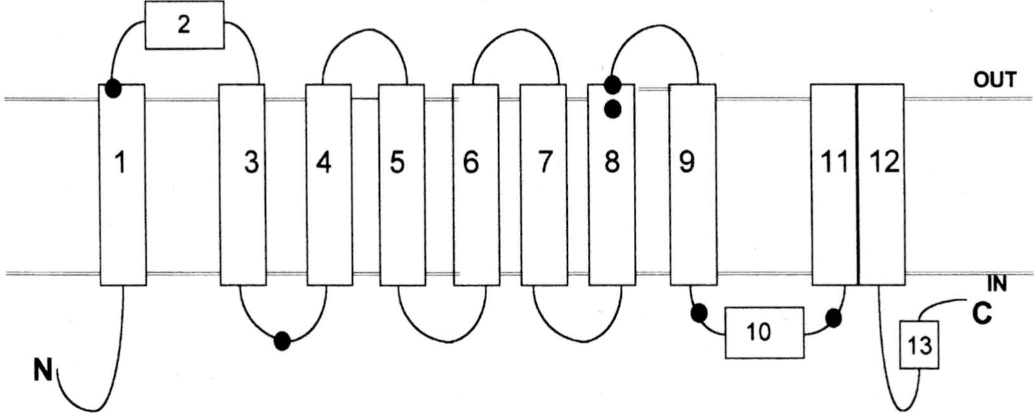


**Figure 3–4.** Skeletal muscle chloride channel showing sites of known point mutations (closed circles).

myotonic syndromes: myotonic dystrophy, proximal myotonic myopathy, paramyotonia congenita, myotonia fluctuans, and chondrodystrophic myotonia. Both myotonic dystrophy and proximal myotonic myopathy have systemic manifestations (such as cataracts, cardiac involvement, glucose intolerance) as well as a progressive myopathy that help distinguish these entities from other myotonic syndromes. Chondrodystrophic myotonia (Schwartz-Jampel syndrome) is a rare myotonic disorder with characteristic muscle stiffness, small stature, and multiple skeletal deformities. Clinical distinction between paramyotonia congenita and myotonia congenita can sometimes be difficult. Symptomatic generalized myotonia is prominent in both conditions, as is muscle hypertrophy. Demonstration of cold-induced weakness can establish the diagnosis of paramyotonia congenita. Alternatively, EMG can be used in problematic cases. Prolonged decrement of the compound muscle action potential in response to cold and exercise is seen in paramyotonia congenita but not in myotonia congenita.[37]

## Genetics and Pathogenesis

Based on the physiological evidence, genetic linkage studies in ADMC were undertaken with a marker on chromosome 7q32 encoding the human muscle chloride channel *(CLCN1)*. Linkage was established to this locus in ADMC[38,39] and a missense (G to A) mutation was identified, resulting in the substitution of a glutamic acid for a highly conserved glycine residue (Fig. 3–4).[40] Interestingly, ARMC has also been linked to the same locus.[39] The presence of an unusual restriction site in two consanguineous ARMC families led to the identification of a missense (T to G) mutation, predicting a phenylalanine to cysteine substitution in the putative transmembrane domain D8 of the channel protein (Fig. 3–5).[39] No locus heterogeneity was found for ARMC with the study of additional families.[41] The T to G mutation, however, was identified in only 15% of cases, suggesting the presence of other disease-causing mutations within the *CLCN1* gene.[41] Therefore, different mutations within the same voltage-gated skeletal muscle chloride channel gene can cause either a dominant or a recessive form of myotonia congenita.[42]

Studies in myotonic goats and in human myotonia congenita have demonstrated the presence of increased chloride conductance across the transverse tubular system.[9] The increased conductance renders the muscle membrane hyperexitable, leading to repetitive firing, which in turn results in clinical myotonia. When the G230E mutation was expressed in mammalian cells, significant changes in channel pore function occurred.[43]

## Treatment

Pharmacological treatment of myotonia traditionally includes procainamide, quinine,

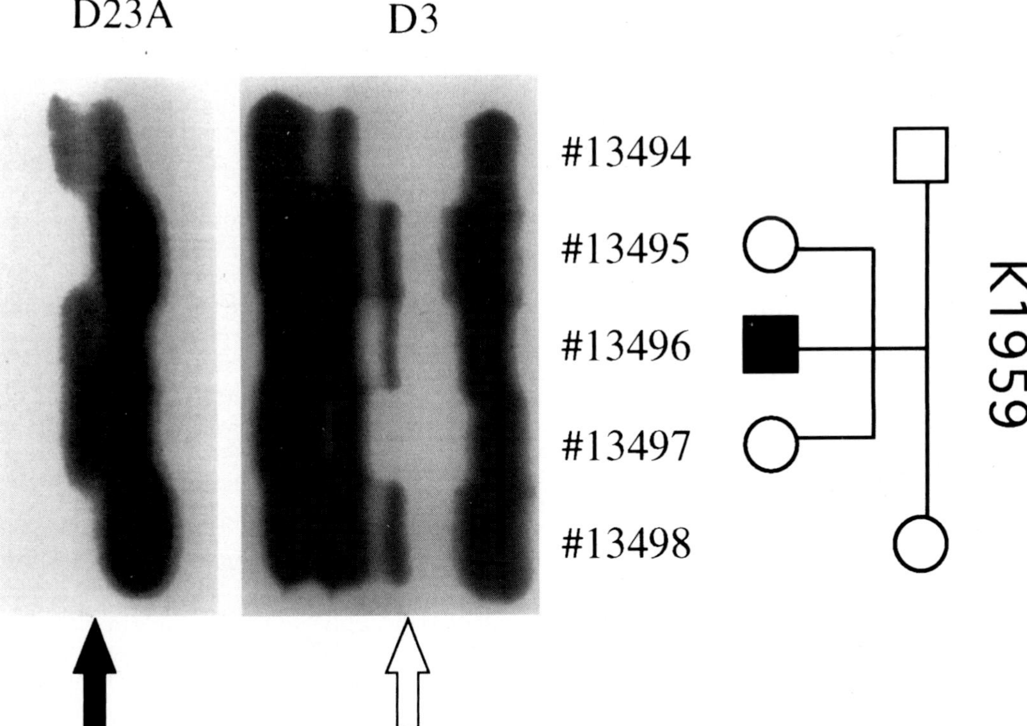


**Figure 3–5.** A recessive myotonia congenita kindred showing an affected sibling (closed square). Single strand confirmation polymorphism analysis shows aberrant band in exon 5 (D3, open arrow) and exon 23 (D23A, closed arrow). Only the affected son inherited both mutations. (Adapted from Zhang et al.[42])

and phenytoin. In severe myotonia, dantrolene has also been reported to be effective.[44] Currently the oral lidocaine congener mexiletine is the drug of choice to treat chloride channel myotonia[44] Tocainide, another lidocaine congener, is also effective but should be avoided because of its potential for bone marrow suppression. The recommended starting dose of mexiletine is 150 mg bid (maximum, 300 mg tid).

## CEREBELLAR/PERIPHERAL NERVE POTASSIUM CHANNELOPATHIES: EPISODIC ATAXIA TYPE 1

In the original 1946 publication on periodic ataxias,[45] 4 of the 11 cases were familial, and the rest were sporadic, secondary to multiple sclerosis. The list of causes for acquired episodic ataxia has since expanded (Table 3–3. Familial episodic ataxia is most often caused by autosomal recessive inherited metabolic diseases (Table 3–3), but also recognized are two distinct, autosomal dominant disorders without enzyme deficiency or other known etiology.[46–50]

### Clinical Features

The clinical features of episodic ataxia type 1 (EA1) have been described in several families.[51–56] Symptoms begin at 2 to 15 years of age, and attack frequency can reach 15 times per day. Attacks occur spontaneously but are more commonly provoked by the initiation of movement, postural change, or exercise, particularly when there is associated emotional excitement or anxiety. Fatigue, startle, intercurrent illness, and menses[53] may also exacerbate the tendency to attacks. Hunger, sleep deprivation, and alcohol, on the other hand, do not seem to influence the likelihood of attacks.[51]

The attacks usually peak within 30 seconds and last up to 15 minutes. Speech may be slurred or completely disrupted. Some

Table 3–3. **Causes of Episodic Ataxia**

| |
|---|
| Sporadic, acquired |
| Multiple sclerosis |
| Arnold-Chiari malformation |
| Intraventricular tumor |
| Basilar migraine |
| Vertebral basillar insufficiency |
| Labyrinthine abnormalities |
| Familial autosomal recessive |
| Hartnup's disease |
| Maple syrup urine disease |
| Refsum's disease |
| Leigh's disease |
| Hyperammonemia type II |
| Pyruvate dehydrogenase deficiency |
| Familial autosomal dominant |
| With myokymia (EA1) |
| Acetazolamide-responsive with interictal nystagmus (EA2) |

patients complain of stiffening of the limbs[53] with cramping of the hands resembling carpopedal spasm.[53,54,56] Shaking, jerking, or tremor of the limbs or head may occur, with clumsiness of the arms and hands. Some reports describe vertigo, diplopia, and oscillopsia,[56] but nausea, vomiting, and headache have not been described. Examination during attacks reveals gait ataxia, limb incoordination with dysdiadokinesis, slurred speech, but no nystagmus.[51]

Interictal examination shows no weakness, reflex abnormalities, or sensory impairment. Fixed cerebellar signs were reported in one family. The most common, but not invariable, interictal finding is that of continuous motor activity, myokymia, which is particularly evident in the face and as a mild tremor of the fingers when the hands are placed in a relaxed prone position. Occasionally myokymia of the limb musculature produces rippling of the skin. Myokymia is generally subtle and in some cases may only be detected on EMG.[51] Myokymia can occur in affected patients in the absence of ataxic episodes (Rose and associates, unpublished data). In some patients, the continuous motor activity results in muscle hypertrophy with bulky calves; opposition of the thumb or Achilles tendon shortening can also occur.[52,56] Congenital fixed postures of the hands and feet have been reported (Rose and associates, unpublished data).

## Diagnosis

Motor and sensory nerve conduction studies are generally normal,[52,53,56] but EMG shows the continuous motor unit activity of myokymia. Discharges are seen most often in doublets or triplets, with occasional singlets or multiplets. This activity is observed most frequently in the hands and the proximal limbs and occasionally in the face.[51,53] The peripheral nerve origin of the discharges was established by their resistance to local nerve block or general anesthesia and by their abolition by regional curare.[52,53,55] Interictal electroencephalograms either are normal or show paroxysmal slowing, which can be lateralized.[51,54–56]

## Genetics and Pathogenesis

The role of potassium channels in maintaining the membrane resting potential as well as in limiting the duration of the action potential and the hyperpolarization afterpotential led to the hypothesis that mutations of potassium channel genes could be responsible for hyperexcitable syndromes such as EA1. In four families with EA1, linkage analysis was performed with markers for regions near known potassium channel genes. Linkage was found to chromosome 12p13, containing a cluster of potassium channel genes (*KCNA5, KCNA6,* and *KCNA1*).[57] A calcium channel gene (*CACNL1A1*) located in the same region was excluded as the site of the defect. There was no evidence for locus heterogeneity in the four families studied. Genetic linkage analysis with microsatellite markers excluded the *KCNA5* and *KCNA6* genes. Each of the four families had a different missense point mutation in the *KCNA1* gene (Fig. 3–6). Because all the mutations were in regions of the gene that are highly conserved across species (from *Drosophila,* mouse, rat, and human) and are also conserved between other members of the potassium channel gene family, it was likely that they were primary pathogenic mutations. This was confirmed when it was found that the mutations were only present in affected family members and not in controls. Similar methods have identified three further point mutations in the *KCNA1* gene (Rose and

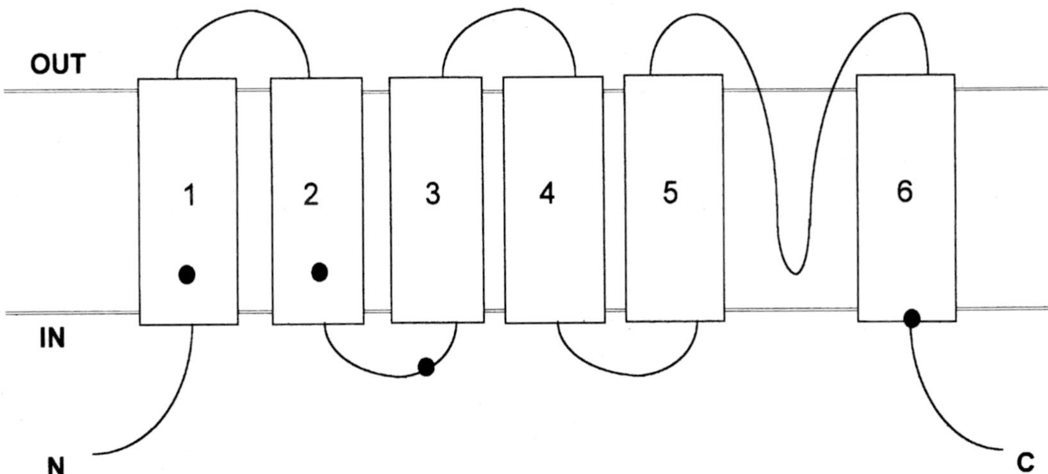


**Figure 3–6.** Schematic representation of the potassium channel polypeptide with putative function of the different regions: voltage sensor, S4; voltage dependence of channel opening, S4 to S5 linker; part of channel pore, S5 to S6 linker. N terminus regulates the rate of inactivation, and the C terminus regulates the rate of recovery from inactivation. Sites of point mutations are shown (closed circles).

colleagues, unpublished data)[52,56,58] (see Fig. 3–6). All affected individuals are heterozygous for the mutation.

The *KCNA1* potassium channel gene is a member of the Shaker group of potassium channel genes. These genes lack introns, and each expresses a single protein subunit that contains six hydrophobic, highly conserved regions (S1 to S6). These form amphipathic helixes spanning the cell membrane (see Fig. 3–6). *In vivo*, a potassium channel consists of four symmetrically grouped protein subunits that may arise from the same gene (homomeric) or from different genes within the same subfamily (heteromeric). This allows for considerable diversity in the properties of potassium channels.

All potassium channel genes appear to be expressed in brain, but the precise expression in other tissues is unknown for humans. The *KCNA1* gene homologue in rats is expressed in cerebellum and peripheral nerve[59]; this would explain why a mutation in this gene gives rise to cerebellar ataxia, and disturbance of peripheral nerve function (i.e., myokymia).

Functionally, the channel produced by the *KCNA1* gene is a fast delayed rectifier potassium channel principally involved in reducing the depolarizing after-potential, thereby limiting re-excitation of the axon. When these channels are blocked with 4-aminopyridine, bursts of action potentials occur after a single short stimulus.[60] Two of the mutations (Val408Ala and Phe184Cys) form functional subunits producing channels with altered kinetics compared with wild-type channels. Four of the mutations result in homomeric nonfunctional channels and cause a reduction in the current amplitude when present as heteromers with wild-type subunits.[61] As all the mutations are heterozygous, the mixture of mutant and wild-type subunits would allow some potassium channel function. The nonfunctional mutant subunits may be causing altered channel function by interfering with the assembly of normal subunits, by altering the stability of the tetramer so that it is rapidly degraded, or by changing the biophysical characteristics of the channels.

## Treatment

Attacks show a variable response to phenytoin[51,53,55] and no response to clomipramine, phenobarbitone, clonazepam, or cinnarizine.[51] Both the frequency and severity of attacks were reduced in one case treated with flunarizine.[55] Poor tolerance of carbonic anhydrase inhibitors such as acetazolamide[51,54,55] and diclorphenamide[51] has limited their use, but sulthiame was better tolerated and appeared to produce a sustained benefit.[51]

## BRAIN-SPECIFIC CALCIUM CHANNELOPATHIES: EPISODIC ATAXIA TYPE 2

Episodic ataxia type 2 (EA2) is an autosomal dominant episodic ataxia with features distinct from EA1. Episodic ataxia type 2 is characterized by the absence of myokymia, the presence of interictal cerebellar signs, and a dramatic response to treatment with acetazolamide. The early literature describes several autosomal dominant episodic ataxias with interictal nystagmus,[47–50,52] but the dramatic cessation of attacks with acetazolamide therapy, a hallmark of EA2, was a serendipitous discovery first reported in 1977.[62] Thus the clinical features of EA2 given here are confined to the literature in which the attacks of episodic ataxia are acetazolamide responsive.

### Clinical Features

Onset is generally in childhood or early adulthood, but onset as early as 7 weeks of age and as late as the fifth decade have been described.[63] Attacks can occur daily,[64] but usually range from three to five per week to one a month. Most attacks have no precipitating factors, but physical or emotional stress, fatigue, and exercise can be provoking factors.[64–66] The attacks are not provoked by startle or movement. Attacks develop gradually over 30 minutes and usually last a few hours, sometimes up to a day. There may be prodromal symptoms of sweating, flushing, heaviness in the head, light headedness, or sensory symptoms.[65] During an attack, patients complain of gait ataxia, dysarthria, and clumsiness, which can be incapacitating. In some patients vertigo is the principal symptom. Nausea, vomiting, and headache can be prominent features.[46] Following an attack, some patients have residual gait difficulties for the rest of the day.

Ataxia, dysdiadokinesis, dysarthria, and nystagmus, but no weakness or sensory abnormalities and normal reflexes, are noted on examination during an attack.[64] Between attacks neurologic examination can be normal, but many patients have nystagmus on lateral or vertical gaze, sometimes with impaired smooth pursuit eye movements or ocular dysmetria. Occasionally there is dysarthria, impaired tandem walking, mild limb ataxia,[9] or dysdiadokinesis.[52] A glove-and-stocking sensory impairment and mild pyramidal signs are infrequent findings. All ten affected members in one family had mild mental retardation, and one of these had a psychosis of unknown origin.[66]

### Diagnosis

Metabolic studies for defects of amino acid metabolism or of pyruvate dehydrogenase activity are normal.[65,67,68] Electroencephalograms can be normal or show slow wave activity, "generalized dysrhythmia," paroxysmal sharp- and slow-wave activity, and spikes and sharp waves.[63,68,69] Brain imaging can also be normal, but in some cases scans have shown cerebellar atrophy, particularly of the vermis.[66,70,71] Brain stem auditory evoked potentials can be unilaterally or asymmetrically abnormal and were reported to normalize with acetazolamide.[67]

### Genetics and Pathogenesis

The clinical similarities between EA2 and familial hemiplegic migraine (FHM) led to the supposition that they might be allelic disorders. Familial hemiplegic migraine is a rare autosomal dominant form of migraine associated with ictal hemiparesis. Nystagmus occurs in cases of FHM,[72,73] and nausea, vomiting, and headache can be prominent features of EA2; cerebellar atrophy occurs in both. The gene for FHM has been mapped to the short arm of chromosome 19.[74,75] Linkage analyses with six markers spanning the FHM interval were performed in two large families with EA2[66,76] and established that the gene for this condition was in the same 30 cM region as the FHM locus. Recently, mutations in a brain-specific calcium channel $\alpha_1$-subunit gene *(CACNL1A4)* were found in both EA2 and FMH.[72] FHM is discussed further in Chapter 20. The *CACNL1A4* gene is also mutated in *SCA6* through expansion of a CAG repeat (see Chapter 12). Moreover, two families with CAG expansion in CACNL1A4 manifest variable phenotypes, ranging from those typical of EA2 to those of a progressive spinocerebellar ataxia (SCA6).[72a]

## Treatment

The response to acetazolamide in doses of 250 mg twice daily is dramatic and sustained in almost all cases. Some patients who do not respond to acetazolamide, or who are unable to tolerate it, respond well to sodium valproate.[65] Phenytoin and phenobarbitone can worsen the attacks in some cases.[77] Some cases of nonfamilial episodic ataxia have responded to acetazolamide; characterization of these will have to await more specific genetic information. The mechanism of action of acetazolamide in this condition is unknown, but magnetic resonance spectroscopy has shown an abnormal elevation of pH in the cerebellum that corrects with acetazolamide.[15] By changing the pH of the cell membrane, acetazolamide may be altering the properties of voltage-gated ion channels. This effect might be important in the mechanism of action of acetazolamide in channelopathies in general.

# PUTATIVE CHANNELOPATHIES

Several disorders have features suggestive of a channelopathy, but the channel in which the mutation has occurred has not yet been identified. In some of these, such as the paroxysmal dyskinesias, the gene defects have been mapped by genetic linkage analysis, but the mutated genes have not yet been identified. The relationship of the paroxysmal dyskinesias to EA1 and EA2 are discussed here; the genetic analysis is discussed further in Chapter 12.

## Paroxysmal Dyskinesias

Mount and Reback[73] first described familial paroxysmal choreoathetosis in 1940. Since then, numerous cases of paroxysmal dyskinesia have been reported, and these have been reviewed recently.[78,79] Several classifications have been proposed for these cases based on combinations of phenomenology, etiology, duration of attacks, and precipitating events.[80–83] The original classification[82] proposed a split between kinesigenic-induced, short-duration (seconds to 5 minutes) choreoathetotic attacks with paroxysmal kinesigenic choreoathetosis (PKC) and prolonged attacks (2 minutes to 4 hours) with dystonic choreoathetosis (PDC). When attacks have not been witnessed, it can be difficult to be sure whether the abnormal movements are dystonic or choreoathetotic. In addition, not all kinesigenic attacks are of short duration, and not all dystonic attacks are prolonged. Therefore, subsequent classifications have added further categories to deal with overlap cases and additional etiologies and precipitants, such as prolonged exercise or sleep.[79,81,82] Nevertheless, the two entities of PKC and PDC have been largely retained.

There are some similarities among familial PKC, PDC, EA1, EA2. All are inherited as autosomal dominant traits with a similar age of onset and decline in attacks with age, more so for PKC than for PDC. All four share similar prodromal features. The attacks in PKC and EA1 have a frequent kinesigenic precipitant, and there is overlap in the symptomatology of the attacks, with dystonic posturing occurring in some cases of EA1.[52,56] Dystonic posturing has also been reported in EA2.[77] Myokymia was seen in one case of PDC, and, in common with EA2, the attacks were aborted by sleep.[84] In one case of PDC there was a background of familial ataxia, with ataxia worsening during attacks of PDC.[85] The response to therapy is more disparate. PKC responds dramatically to anticonvulsants, probably more so than does either EA1 or EA2. The effect of acetazolamide on familial paroxysmal dyskinesia is not known.

## Other Conditions

Andersen's syndrome is a distinct disorder consisting of a triad of periodic paralysis, cardiac dysrhythmias with prolonged QT intervals, and distinct facial and limb anomalies.[13,86,87] It is an intriguing disorder that combines features of a known skeletal muscle channelopathy with features of long-QT syndrome, known to result from a cardiac channel disorder. Linkage to the skeletal muscle sodium channel has been excluded as has linkage to one long-QT syndrome locus on chromosome 11. Schwartz-Jampel syndrome, or chondrodystrophic myotonia, is a rare autosomal recessive disorder with small stature, multiple skeletal deformities, and contractures. The presence of characteristic muscle stiffness and myotonia make it a candidate for a channelopathy.

Familial hyperekplexia, a rare autosomal dominant disorder characterized by hypertonia and an exaggerated startle response, has been found to have point mutations in the $\alpha_1$-subunit of the inhibitory glycine receptor (GLRA1), which is a ligand-gated chloride channel.[88] The responsiveness of some epilepsies to acetazolamide suggests that ion channels may be candidates for the molecular lesion underlying these prototypically episodic disorders.

## SUMMARY

Channelopathies result from dysfunction of specific ion channels. Most channelopathies are characterized by episodic symptomatology. The specific neurologic manifestation of each disorder is dictated by the site of expression of the defective ion channel within the neuraxis. Thus, defective skeletal muscle sodium and calcium channels result in hyperkalemic and hypokalemic periodic paralysis, respectively. Skeletal muscle chloride channel mutations result in dominant and recessive myotonia congenita. Similar myotonic disorders are also caused by sodium channel mutations different than those resulting in hyperkalemic periodic paralysis. The two episodic ataxia syndromes are the result of defective cerebellar- and peripheral nerve-specific potassium channels (type 1) and brain-specific calcium channel (type 2). Different mutations within the same brain-specific calcium channel also cause familial hemiplegic migraine and spinocerebellar ataxia type 6.

## REFERENCES

1. Griggs RC, Mendell JR, Miller RG: Periodic paralysis and myotonia. In Griggs RC, Mendell JR, Miller RG (eds). Evaluation and Treatment of Myopathies. FA Davis, Philadelphia, 1995, pp318–354.
2. Ricker K, Lehmann-Horn F, Moxley RT: Myotonia fluctuans [see comments]. Arch Neurol 47:268–272, 1990.
3. Ptacek, LJ, Tawil R, Griggs RC, Storvick D, Leppert M. Linkage of atypical myotonia congenita to a sodium channel locus. Neurology 42:431–433, 1992.
4. Ricker K, Moxley RT, Heine R, Lehmann-Horn F. Myotonia fluctuans. A third type of muscle sodium channel disease. Arch Neurol 51:1095–1102, 1994.
5. Lerche H, Heine R, Pika U, et al.: Human sodium channel myotonia: Slowed channel inactivation due to substitutions for a glycine within the III–IV linker. J Physiol 470:13–22, 1993.
6. Fontaine B, Khurana TS, Hoffman EP, et al.: Hyperkalemic periodic paralysis and the adult muscle sodium channel alpha-subunit gene. Science 250: 1000–1002, 1990.
7. Ptacek LJ, Trimmer JS, Agnew WS, Roberts JW, Petajan JH, Leppert M. Paramyotonia congenita and hyperkalemic periodic paralysis map to the same sodium-channel gene locus. Am J Hum Genet 49: 851–854, 1991.
8. Hayward LJ, Brown RH, Cannon SC: Inactivation defects caused by myotonia-associated mutation in the sodium channel ui-iv linker (abstract). J Gen Physiol 107:559–576, 1996.
9. McClatchey AI, McKenna-Yasek D, Cros D, et al.: Novel mutations in families with unusual and variable disorders of the skeletal muscle sodium channel. Nat Genet 2:148–152, 1992.
10. Van den Bergh P, Thonnard JL: Genotype–phenotype correlations in human skeletal muscle sodium channel diseases (letter; comment). Arch Neurol 52:1045–1046, 1995.
11. Lehmann-Horn F, Engel AG, Ricker K, Rudel R. The periodic paralysis and paramyotonia. In Engel AG, Franzini-Armstrong C (eds). Myology, ed 2. McGraw Hill International, New York, 1994, pp1303–1334.
12. Featherstone DE, Fujimoto E, Ruben PC: A defect in skeletal muscle sodium channel deactivation exacerbates hyperexcitability in human paramyotonia congenita. J Physiol 506:627–638, 1998.
13. Plassart-Schiess E, Lhuillier L, George AL Jr, et al.: Functional expression of the Ile693 Thr Na+ channel mutation associated with paramyotonia congenita in a human cell line. J Physiol 507:721–727, 1998.
13a. Hayward LJ, Sandoval GM, Cannon SC: Defective slow inactivation of sodium channels contributes to familial periodic paralysis. Neurology 52:1447–1452, 1999.
13b. Hanna MG, Stewart J, Schapira AH, et al.: Salbutamol treatment in a patient with hyperkalemic periodic paralysis due to a mutation in the skeletal muscle sodium channel gene (SCN4A). J Neurol Neurosurg Psychiatry 65:248–250, 1998.
14. Griggs RC: Periodic paralysis (abstract). Semin Neurol 3:285–293, 1983.
15. Kantola IM, Tarssanen LT: Familial hypokalaemic periodic paralysis in Finland. J Neurol Neurosurg Psychiatry 55:322–324, 1992.
16. Johnsen T. Familial periodic paralysis with hypo-

kalaemia. Experimental and clinical investigations (review). Dan Med Bull 28:1–27, 1981.
17. Schipperheyn JJ, Wintzen AR, Buruma OJ: Periodic paralysis. In Rowland LP, DiMauro S (eds). Handbook of Clinical Neurology. Elsevier Science, Holland, 1992, pp457–477.
18. Ionasescu V, Schochet SSJ, Powers JM, Koob K, Conway TW: Hypokalemic periodic paralysis. Low activity of sarcoplasmic reticulum and muscle ribosomes during an induced attack. J Neurol Sci 21: 419–429, 1974.
19. Gamstrop I. Disorders characterized by spontaneous attacks of weakness connected with changes of serium potassium (abstract). Prog Clin Biol Res 306:175–195, 1989.
20. Fukuda K, Ogawa S, Yokozuka H, Handa S, Nakamura Y. Long-standing bidirectional tachycardia in a patient with hypokalemic periodic paralysis. J Electrocardiol 21:71–75, 1988.
21. Kramer LD, Cole JP, Messenger JC, Ellestad MH: Cardiac dysfunction in a patient with familial hypokalemic periodic paralysis. Chest 75:189–192, 1979.
22. Talbot JH: Periodic paralysis (abstract). Medicine 20:85–143, 1940.
23. Links TP, Zwarts MJ, Wilmink JT, Molenaar WM, Oosterhuis HJ: Permanent muscle weakness in familial hypokalaemic periodic paralysis. Clinical, radiological and pathological aspects. Brain 113: 1873–1889, 1990.
24. Johnsen T. A new standardized and effective method of inducing paralysis without administration of exogenous hormone in patients with familial periodic paralysis. Acta Neurol Scand 54:167–172, 1976.
25. McManis PG, Lambert EH, Daube JR: The exercise test in periodic paralysis. Muscle Nerve 9:704–710, 1986.
26. Ptacek LJ, Tawil R, Griggs RC, et al.: Dihydropyridine receptor mutations cause hypokalemic periodic paralysis. Cell 77:863–868, 1994.
27. Jurkat-Rott K, Lehmann-Horn F, Elbaz A, et al.: A calcium channel mutation causing hypokalemic periodic paralysis. Hum Mol Genet 3:1415–1419, 1994.
28. Fouad G, Dalakas M, Servidei S, et al.: Genotype–phenotype correlations of DHP receptor alpha 1-subunit gene mutations causing hypokalemic periodic paralysis. Neuromusc Disord 7:33–38, 1997.
29. Rudel R, Ricker K. The periodic paralysis. Trends Neurosci 8:467–470, 1985.
30. Engel AG, Lambert EH, Resevear JW, Tauxe WN: Clinical and electrophysiologic studies in a patient with primary hypoklemic periodic paralysis (abstract). Am J Med 38:626–640, 1965.
31. Grob D, Johns RJ, Liljestrand A. Potassium movement in patients with familial periodic paralysis (abstract). Am J Med 23:356–375, 1957.
32. Hoffman WW, Adornato BT, Reich H. The relationship of insulin receptors to hypokalemic periodic paralysis (abstract). Muscle Nerve 6:48–51, 1983.
33. Resnick JS, Engel WK, Griggs RC, Stam AC: Acetazolamide prophylaxis in hypokalemic periodic paralysis. N Engl J Med 278:582–586, 1968.
34. Dalakas MC, Engel WK: Treatment of "permanent" muscle weakness in familial hypokalemic periodic paralysis. Muscle Nerve 6:182–186, 1983.
35. Griggs RC, Engel WK, Resnick JS: Acetazolamide treatment of hypokalemic periodic paralysis. Prevention of attacks and improvement of persistent weakness. Ann Intern Med 73:39–48, 1970.
36. Tawil R, Moxley RT, Griggs RC: Acetazolamide-induced nephrolithiasis: Implications for treatment of neuromuscular disorders. Neurology 43:1105–1106, 1993.
37. Streib EW: AAEE minimonograph 27: Differential diagnosis of myotonic syndromes (review). Muscle Nerve 10:603–615, 1987.
38. Abdalla JA, Casley WL, Hudson AJ, et al.: Linkage analysis of candidate loci in autosomal dominant myotonia congenita. Neurology 42:1561–1564, 1992.
39. Koch MC, Steinmeyer K, Lorenz C, et al.: The skeletal muscle chloride channel in dominant and recessive human myotonia. Science 257:797–800, 1992.
40. George AL, Crackower MA, Abdalla JA, et al.: Molecular basis of Thomsen's disease (autosomal) dominant myotonia congenita) (abstract). Nat Genet 3:305–310, 1993.
41. Koch MC, Ricker K, Otto M, et al.: Evidence for genetic homogeneity in autosomal recessive generalised myotonia (Becker). J Med Genet 30:914–917, 1993.
42. Zhang J, George AL, Criggs RC, Fouad GT, et al.: Mutations in the human skeletal muscle chloride channel gene (CLCN1) associated with dominant and recessive myotonia congenita. Neurology 47: 993–998, 1996.
43. Fahlke C, Beck CL, George AL Jr. A mutation in autosomal dominant myotonia congenita affects pore properties of the muscle chloride channel. Proc Natl Acad Sci USA 94:2729–2734, 1997.
44. Kwiecinski H, Ryniewicz B, Ostrzycki A. Treatment of myotonia with antiarrhythmic drugs. Acta Neurol Scand 86:371–375, 1992.
45. Parker HL: Periodic ataxia. In Hewlett RM, Nevling AB, Minor JR, et al. (eds). Collected Papers of the Mayo Clinic. WB Saunders, Philadelphia, 1946, pp642–645.
46. Donat JR, Auger R. Familial periodic ataxia. Arch Neurol 36:568–569, 1979.
47. Farmer TW, Mustian VM: Vestibulocerebellar ataxia (abstract). Arch Neurol 8:471–480, 1963.
48. Hill W, Sherman H. Acute intermittent familial cerebellar ataxia. Arch Neurol 18:350–357, 1968.
49. Sogg RL, Hoyt WF: Intermittent vertical nystagmus in a father and son (abstract). Arch Ophthalmol 68:515–517, 1962.
50. White JC: Familial periodic nystagmus, vertigo, and ataxia. Arch Neurol 20:276–280, 1969.
51. Brunt ER, van Weerden TW: Familial paroxysmal kinesigenic ataxia and continuous myokymia. Brain 113:1361–1382, 1990.
52. Gancher ST, Nutt JG: Autosomal dominant episodic ataxia: A heterogeneous syndrome. Mov Disord 1:239–253, 1986.
53. Hanson PA, Martinez LB, Cassidy R. Contractures, continuous muscle discharges, and titubation. Ann Neurol 1:120–124, 1977.

54. Lubbers WJ, Brunt ER, Scheffer H, et al. Hereditary myokymia and paroxysmal ataxia, linked to chromosome 12 is response to acetazolamide (abstract). J Neurol Neurosurg Psychiatry 59:400–405, 1995.
55. Vaamonde J, Artieda J, Obeso JA: Hereditary paroxysmal ataxia with neuromyotonia. Mov Disord 6: 180–182, 1991.
56. VanDyke DH, Griggs RC, Murphy MJ, Goldstein MN: Hereditary myokymia and periodic ataxia. J Neurol Sci 25:109–118, 1975.
57. Litt M, Kramer P, Browne D, et al.: A gene for episodic ataxia/myokymia maps to chromosome 12p13. Am J Hum Genet 55:702–709, 1994.
58. Browne DL, Brunt ER, Griggs RC, et al.: Identification of two new KCNA1 mutations in episodic ataxia/myokymia families. Hum Mol Genet 4: 1671–1672, 1995.
59. Beckh S, Pongs O: Members of the RCK potassium channel family are differentially expressed in the rat nervous system. EMBO J 9:777–782, 1990.
60. Baker M, Bostock H, Grafe P, Martius P: Function and distribution of three types of rectifying channel in rat spinal root myelinated axons. J Physiol 383:45–67, 1987.
61. Adelman JP, Bond CT, Pessia M, Maylie J: Episodic ataxia results from voltage dependent potassium channels with altered functions (abstract). Neuron 15:1449–1454, 1995.
62. LaFrance R, Griggs R, Moxley R, et al.: Hereditary paroxysmal ataxia responsive to acetazolamide (abstract). Neurology 27:370, 1977.
63. Friedman JH, Hollmann PA: Acetazolamide responsive hereditary paroxysmal ataxia (review). Mov Disord 2:67–72, 1987.
64. Griggs RC, Moxley RT, Lafrance RA, McQuillen J: Hereditary paroxysmal ataxia: Response to acetazolamide. Neurology 28:1259–1264, 1978.
65. Bain PG, O'Brien MD, Keevil SF, Porter DA: Familial periodic cerebellar ataxia: A problem of cerebellar intracellular pH homeostasis. Ann Neurol 31:147–154, 1992.
66. Vahedi K, Joutel A, Van BP, et al.: A gene for hereditary paroxysmal cerebellar ataxia maps to chromosome 19p (abstract). Ann Neurol 37:289–93, 1995.
67. Koller W, Bahamon-Dussan J: Hereditary paroxysmal cerebellopathy: Responsiveness to acetazolamide. Clin Neuropharmacol 10:65–68, 1987.
68. Neufield MY, Nisipeanu P, Chistik V, Korcyn AD: The electroencephalogram in acetazolamide responsive periodic ataxia (abstract). Mov Disord 11: 283–288, 1996.
69. Bogaert VP, Nechel VC, Szliwowski HB: EEG findings in a family with acetazolamide responsive paroxysmal ataxia (abstract). Neurology 43:A378, 1993.
70. Hawkes CH: Familial paroxysmal ataxia: Report of a family. J Neurol Neurosurg Psychiatry 55:212–213, 1992.
71. Vighetto A, Froment JC, Trillet M, Aimard G: Magnetic resonance imaging in familial paroxysmal ataxia. Arch Neurol 45:547–549, 1988.
72. Ophoff RA, Terwindt GM, Vergoume MV, et al.: Familial hemiplegic migraine and episodic ataxia type-2 are caused by mutations in the $CA^{2+}$ channel gene CACNL1A4. Cell 87:543–552, 1996.
72a. Jodice C, Mantuano E, Veneziano L, et al.: Episodic ataxia type 2 (EA2) and spinocerebellar ataxia type 6 (SCA6) due to CAG repeat expansion in the CACNA1A gene on chromosome 19p. Hum Mol Genet 16:1973–1978, 1997.
73. Mount LA, Reback S: Familial paroxysmal choreoathetosis (abstract). Arch Neurol Psychiatry 44: 841–847, 1940.
74. Joutel A, Ducros A, Vahedi K, et al.: Genetic heterogeneity of familial hemiplegic migraine. Am J Hum Genet 55:1166–1172, 1994.
75. Joutel A, Bousser MG, Biousse V, et al.: A gene for familial hemiplegic migraine maps to chromosome 19. Nat Genet 5:40–45, 1993.
76. Kramer PL, Smith E, Carrero-Valenzuela R: A gene for nystagmus associated episodic ataxia maps to chromosome 19p (abstract). Am J Hum Genet 55: A191, 1994.
77. Zasorin NL, Baloh RW, Myers LB: Acetazolamide-responsive episodic ataxia syndrome. Neurology 33:1212–1214, 1983.
78. Fahn S. The paroxysmal dyskinesias. In Marsden CD, Fahn S (eds): Movement Disorders 3. Butterworth-Heinemann, Oxford, 1994, pp310–345.
79. Demirkiran M, Jankovic J: Paroxysmal dyskinesias: Clinical features and classification. Ann Neurol 38: 571–579, 1995.
80. Goodenough DJ, Fariello RG, Annis BL, Chun RW: Familial and acquired paroxysmal dyskinesias. A proposed classification with delineation of clinical features. Arch Neurol 35:827–831, 1978.
81. Lance JW: Familial paroxysmal dystonic choreoathetosis and its differentiation from related syndromes. Ann Neurol 2:285–293, 1977.
82. Byrne E, White O, Cook M: Familial dystonic choreoathetosis with myokymia; a sleep responsive disorder. J Neurol Neurosurg Psychiatry 54:1090–1092, 1991.
83. Mayeux R, Fahn S: Paroxysmal dystonic choreoathetosis in a patient with familial ataxia. Neurology 32:1184–1186, 1982.
84. Codina A, Acarin PN, Miquel F, Noguera M: Familial hemiplegic migraine associated with nystagmus [in French]. Rev Neurol 124:526–530, 1971.
85. Young GF, Leon-Barth CA, Green J: Familial hemiplegic migraine, retinal degeneration, deafness, and nystagmus. Arch Neurol 23:201–209, 1970.
86. Tawil R, Ptacek LJ, Pavlakis SG, et al.: Andersen's syndrome: Potassium-sensitive periodic paralysis, ventricular ectopy, and dysmorphic features (see comments). Ann Neurol 35:326–330, 1994.
87. Sansone V, Griggs RC, Meola G, et al.: Andersen's syndrome: A distinct periodic paralysis. Ann Neurol 42:305–312, 1997.
88. Shiang R, Ryan SG, Zhu YZ, et al.: Mutational analysis of familial and sporadic hyperekplexia. Ann Neurol 38:85–91, 1995.
89. De Silva SM, Kuncl RW, Griffin JW, Cornblath DR, Chavoustie S: Paramyotonia congenita or hyperkalemic periodic paralysis? Clinical and electrophysiologic features of each entity in one family. Muscle Nerve 13:21–26, 1990.

# Chapter 4

# HEREDITARY NEUROPATHY

Phillip F. Chance, MD



## CHARCOT-MARIE-TOOTH NEUROPATHY: BACKGROUND AND CLINICAL SUBTYPES

Charcot-Marie-Tooth (CMT) neuropathy, also called *hereditary motor and sensory neuropathy*, is a heterogeneous group of inherited diseases of peripheral nerve.[1,2] CMT is a common disorder that affects both children and adults and causes significant neuromuscular impairment. An estimated 1 in 2500 persons has a form of CMT, making it one of the largest diagnostic categories of genetic disease.

Motor and sensory nerve function are affected in CMT. The clinical features of these disorders include distal muscle weakness and atrophy, impaired sensation, and absent or diminished deep tendon reflexes. The onset of CMT is usually during the first or second decade of life, although it may be detected by electrophysiological methods in infancy. Ninety-seven percent of individuals who have inherited CMT will manifest clinical symptoms by age 27 years.[3] The variation in clinical presentation is wide, ranging from patients with severe distal atrophy and marked hand and foot deformity to individuals whose only clinical finding is pes cavus and no distal muscle weakness.

With the advent of neurophysiological techniques, heterogeneity with regard to motor and sensory nerve conduction velocities in CMT became apparent. A current classification that is widely used designates this group of disorders as hereditary motor and sensory neuropathies (HMSN).[2] Type I HMSN (HMSNI) includes individuals with a hypertrophic demyelinating neuropathy ("onion bulbs") and reduced nerve conduction velocities, whereas type II HMSN (HMSNII) includes individuals with an axonal neuropathy and normal or near-normal nerve conduction velocities. Other forms of HMSN have also been delineated (e.g., HMSNIII, Dejerine-Sottas disease; HMSNIV, Refsum's disease). CMT1 may be used to refer to HMSNI patients, and CMT2 may be used to refer to HMSNIII patients. CMT1 and CMT2 have evolved as the preferred nomenclature and are used in this chapter.

## MAPPING GENES FOR CMT1

In the majority of CMT1 and CMT2 pedigrees, the mode of inheritance is autosomal dominant; however, pedigrees exhibiting X-linked inheritance and even rarer ones with autosomal recessive inheritance are recognized. Initial genetic linkage studies in three families indicated that CMT1 was linked to the Duffy *(Fy)* blood group locus on the long arm of chromosome 1.[4,5] Further studies, however, identified other pedigrees with CMT1 in which linkage to Duffy could not be demonstrated.[6,7] The discovery of families having CMT1 that is not linked to Duffy suggested that there are at least two clinically indistinguishable disorders within the category of CMT1. Families with CMT1 not linked to Duffy were designated as having CMT1A, while those who showed linkage to Duffy were designated as having CMT1B.[6]

Linkage to two markers on the proximal short arm of chromosome 17 was detected in six non-Duffy–linked CMT1 families.[8] This observation of linkage of CMT1A to chromosome 17 was confirmed by other studies.[9–14] It became apparent from subsequent research that the majority of CMT1 pedigrees demonstrate linkage to chromosome 17p11.2–12 (CMT1A).

Two clinically typical, autosomal dominant CMT1 pedigrees that did not map to the region of the Duffy locus on chromosome 1q (CMT1B) or the proximal chromosome 17p (CMT1A) were reported, extending genetic heterogeneity in CMT.[10] Pedigrees with autosomal dominant CMT1 not mapping to chromosome 1q or to 17p are designated as CMT1C. The CMT1C locus (or perhaps even loci) remains unassigned; however, myelin genes identified in the future are strong candidates. The various chromosomal locations and genetic mechanisms underlying forms of CMT and related disorders are listed in Table 4–1.

## CHROMOSOME 17p11.2–12 DUPLICATION ASSOCIATED WITH CMT1A

Attempts to further refine the localization of CMT1A through positional cloning led to the identification of a tandem DNA duplication in chromosome 17p11.2–12 associated with CMT1A.[15,16] The size of the duplication is approximately 1.5 megabases (Mb) and represents a genetic distance of approximately 6 centimorgans (cM).[17,18] The duplication is completely associated with CMT1A patients and has been detected in many ethnic groups. The region of chromosome 17 involved in CMT1A is depicted in Figure 4–1 should be noted that individuals with CMT1A are trisomic for DNA segments mapping within the duplicated region. Therefore, when molecular probes mapping to the CMT1A duplicated region (e.g., VAW409R3) are used in standard Southern blot analysis of CMT1A patient DNA, they detect a "dosage effect" (an increased relative hybridization signal comparing alleles), as shown in Figure 4–2. Such analysis provides an easy molecular-based test for the CMT1A duplication.

Surprisingly, the duplication can arise as a frequent *de novo* event. Nine of ten patients with sporadic CMT1 had evidence of *de novo* genesis of the 17p11.2–12 duplication.[19] The *de novo* duplication in CMT1A may account for some cases of CMT1 that were thought to occur on the basis of autosomal recessive inheritance. The duplication is also associated with the generation of a novel 500 kilobase pair (kb) *Sac*II junctional fragment, detected by markers mapping within the duplicated region.[15] An example of the novel 500 kb *Sac*II junctional fragment is shown in Figure 4–3. Interestingly, the majority of patients with inherited and *de novo* CMT1A associated with the duplication have a novel fragment of approximately the same size. There are two implications for the apparent uniformity of both size of the novel fragment and extent of the region duplicated in CMT1A: *(1)* molecular-based testing through an assay for the novel fragment may have application to the majority of CMT1A patients; and *(2)* a precise, recurring molecular mechanism may un-

Table 4–1. **Charcot-Marie-Tooth Neuropathy (Hereditary Motor and Sensory Neuropathy) and Related Disorders**

| Disorder | Locus | Gene | Mechanism |
|---|---|---|---|
| Charcot-Marie-Tooth type 1 (HMSNI) | | | |
| CMT1A | 17p11.2–12 | *PMP22* | Duplication/point mutation |
| CMT1B | 1q22–23 | $P_0$ | Point mutation |
| CMT1C | Unknown | Unknown | Unknown |
| CMTX | Xq13.1 | *CX32* | Point mutation |
| CMT4 | 8q | Unknown | Unknown |
| Charcot-Marie-Tooth type 2 (HMSNII) | | | |
| CMT2A | 1p36 | Unknown | Unknown |
| CMT2B | 3q | Unknown | Unknown |
| CMT2C | Unknown | Unknown | Unknown |
| CMT2D | 7p14 | Unknown | Unknown |
| Dejerine-Sottas disease (HMSNIII) | | | |
| DSDA | 17p11.2–12 | *PMP22* | Point mutation |
| DSDB | 1q22–23 | $P_0$ | Point mutation |
| Congenital hypomyelination | | | |
| CH | 1q22–23 | $P_0$ | Point mutation |
| Hereditary neuropathy with pressure palsies | | | |
| HNPPA | 17p11.2–12 | *PMP22* | Deletion/point mutation |
| HNPPB | Unknown | Unknown | Unknown |
| Hereditary neuralgic amyotrophy | | | |
| HNA | 17q24–25 | Unknown | Unknown |

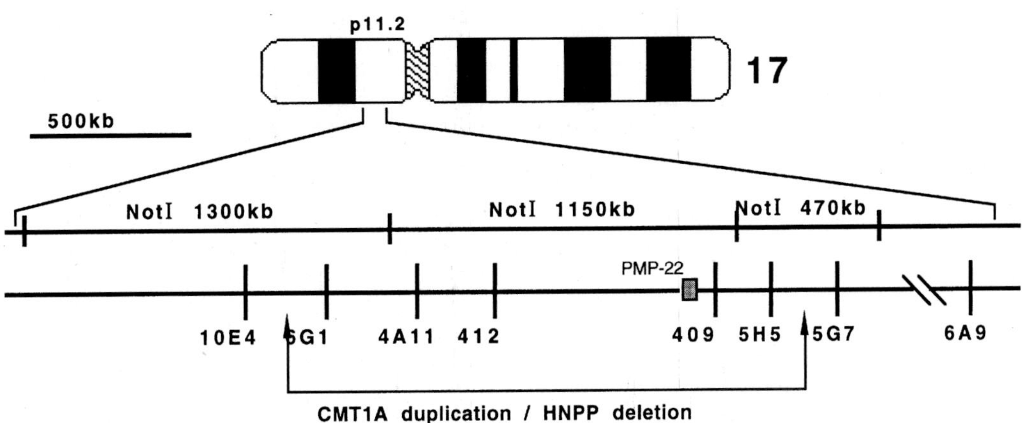


**Figure 4–1.** Map of markers from chromosome 17p11.2. Markers mapping to the CMT1A duplication and the HNPP deletion are shown, as are intervals containing the duplication/deletion breakpoints. Approximate physical distances are represented by *NotI* fragments spanning the CMT1A region. The CMT1A/HNPP region contains the gene for peripheral myelin protein 22 *(PMP22)*.

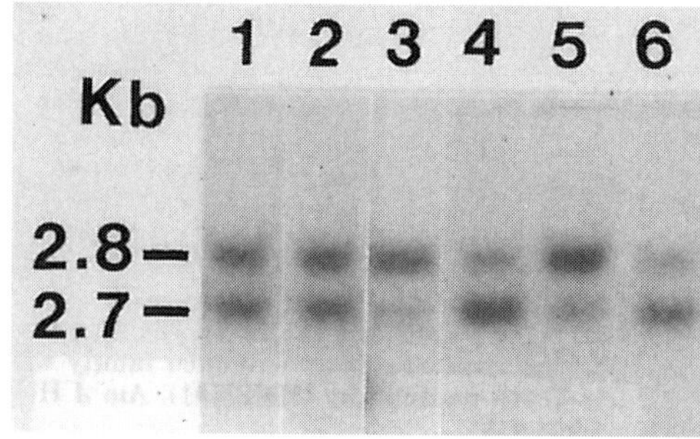


**Figure 4–2.** Genotypes at the VAW409R3 locus (*Msp*I digest) demonstrate a dosage effect in CMT1A patient DNA. Lanes 1 and 2, normal persons; lanes 3–6, affected individuals from each of four CMT1A pedigrees known to map to chromosome 17p11.2 showing differences in dosage intensities at VAW409R3 alleles.

derlay genesis of the duplication. Two reports have suggested that rare patients may have duplications in 17p11.2–12 with different breakpoints.[20,21]

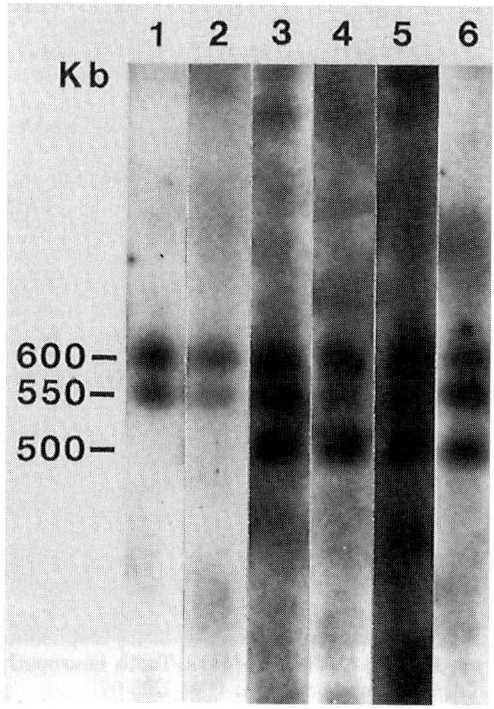


**Figure 4–3.** Presence of a novel 500 kb *Sac*II fragment in CMT1 patient DNAs detected with VAW409R3. Lanes 1 and 2 are from normal persons, showing fragments of 600 and 550 kb. A 500 kb fragment is seen in each of four affected persons (lanes 3–6) from four CMT1A pedigrees, which map to chromosome 17p11.2.

## GENETIC MECHANISMS LEADING TO CMT1A

Identification of the duplication in 17p11.2–12 raised questions regarding the molecular mechanism underlying CMT1A. Two principal models included were gene disruption, whereby a critical gene is altered by a duplication breakpoint, and gene dosage, in which the phenotype results from having an extra copy of the gene (trisomic overexpression). Identification of a critical CMT1A gene affected by duplication remained of great import. Observations in humans and other organisms have helped to explain how the duplication results in the CMT1A phenotype. A small number of patients have been identified who have total or partial trisomy 17p, including bands 17p11.2–12, the region of the DNA duplication in CMT1A patients.[22,23] The consistent phenotypic features of these patients are mental retardation and multiple somatic anomalies, including micrognathia, hypoplastic low-set ears, and foot deformities. Features consistent with CMT1A were detected in three patients with either partial or complete trisomy 17p, supporting the hypothesis that the duplication in CMT1A may have phenotypic consequences through a gene dosage effect.[24–26]

The *trembler* mutation *(Tr)* in the mouse is a dominant disorder that results in a hypomyelinating neuropathy[27,28] and is a proposed murine model for CMT1A. The *Tr* locus maps to mouse chromosome 11,[29] which has conserved synteny with human chromosome 17p, in the region of the CMT1A locus.[30] A gene for the *Tr* locus was identified when a point mutation was found in the peripheral myelin protein-22 *(PMP22)* gene,[31] which is expressed in Schwann cells and is identical to the growth arrest–specific gene *gas3*.[32–34] These observations in *Tr* suggested that the human *PMP22* gene might map to chromosome 17p11.2–12 in the region of the CMT1A gene and might actually be the critical gene for CMT1A. To test this hypothesis and further characterize the DNA duplication associated with CMT1A, several laboratories constructed sets of overlapping yeast artificial chromosomes (YACs) in the region of the CMT1A locus on chromosome 17p11.2–12 and mapped *PMP22* to the CMT1A gene region.[35–38]

The *PMP22* gene encodes a 160 amino acid membrane-associated protein with a predicted molecular weight of 18 kilodaltons (kDa) that is increased to 22 kDa by glycosylation.[32] The PMP22 protein is localized to the compact portions of peripheral nerve myelin,[39] contains four putative transmembrane domains, and is highly conserved in evolution.[36] Two tissue-specific forms (neural and non-neural) of PMP22 arise through different transcripts regulated by two alternatively used promotors.[40] It is postulated that the neuropathy phenotype in patients with the 17p11.2–12 duplication actually results from having three copies of *PMP22*, leading to a speculated 50% increase in expression at this locus. A study of sural nerve biopsy specimens taken from CMT1A patients suggested that mRNA levels for PMP22 are higher than those in normal persons.[41]

CMT1A patients with point mutations in *PMP22* have also been identified. A CMT1 pedigree linked to 17p11.2–12 markers in which the duplication was not present was detected, suggesting that forms of CMT1A may exist in which other mechanisms (e.g., a point mutation) are present.[42] This hypothesis was confirmed when a missense mutation within the *PMP22* gene was found in the same nonduplicated pedigree.[43] Interestingly, the point mutation in this family is identical to that found in the $Tr^J$ mouse, a variant of *Tr*. Furthermore, in another family the CMT1A phenotype was found to result from a *de novo* point mutation in the *PMP22* gene.[44]

It has been found that 70% to 80% of patients with a clinical diagnosis of CMT1 carry the 17p11.2–12 duplication,[45] implying that an assay for the duplication provides a powerful marker for screening suspected patients and at-risk family members. As DNA testing for CMT1A becomes more widely available, it may become an accepted part of the evaluation of any patient with suspected hereditary neuropathy.

## MOLECULAR BASIS OF CMT1B

The human myelin protein zero gene ($P_0$) was isolated and mapped to chromosome 1q22–q23 in the region of the CMT1B locus.[46] $P_0$ became an especially attractive candidate for CMT1B, as it was known to be the major structural component of peripheral nervous system myelin (approximately 50% by weight) and about 7% of Schwann cell message.[47] $P_0$ is a member of the immunoglobulin gene superfamily of cell adhesive molecules and localizes to the compact portion of peripheral nerve myelin. $P_0$ protein is composed of 284 amino acids having both intracelluallar and extracellular domains with a single transmembrane segment. Analysis of $P_0$ as a candidate gene for CMT1B did detect point mutations in pedigrees with this disorder.[48–50] Analysis of $P_0$ as a candidate gene for CMT1B detected different point mutations (Asp90Glu and Lys96Glu) in the two pedigrees with this disorder originally linked to chromosome 1.[48] In an additional pedigree showing linkage to chromosome 1, a deletion of a serine codon at position 34 was documented.[49] The point mutations in these two families fully cosegregated with the CMT1B phenotype, suggesting that abnormalities in the $P_0$ gene are responsible for CMT1B. Thirteen additional mutations in $P_0$ associated with CMT1B pedigrees have been described.[51–54]

## DEJERINE-SOTTAS DISEASE: EXTENSION OF THE CMT1 PHENOTYPIC SPECTRUM

Dejerine-Sottas disease (DSD; also called *hereditary motor and sensory neuropathy type III* [HMSMIII]) is a severe, infantile- and childhood-onset, hypertrophic demyelinating polyneuropathy.[2] Nerve conduction velocities are greatly prolonged, and elevations in cerebrospinal fluid protein may be present. The clinical features of DSD overlap with those of severe CMT1. Many cases of DSD appear to be sporadic and were usually thought to result from an autosomal recessive gene.

Recent molecular genetic studies, however, have revealed that DSD may be associated with dominant point mutations in either the $P_0$ or the *PMP22* gene.[55,56] Analyses in two pedigrees with DSD have identified mutations in *PMP22* (Met 69 Lys and Ser 72 Leu), both located within the second transmembrane segment.[56] On the other hand, mutations in the $P_0$ gene in clinically typical patients with DSD have also been detected.[55] In an analysis of two unrelated patients with DSD, apparent *de novo* mutations were identified in the extracellular domain (Cys 63 Ser) and within the transmembrane portion (Arg 163 Gly) in the $P_0$ gene. A third patient with DSD was found to have a *de novo* insertional mutation in exon 6.[57] Interestingly, in patients with the DSD phenotype studied to date, all mutations have been present in the heterozygous state, suggesting that DSD may actually be caused by dominantly acting genetic defects. Molecular studies have not found evidence for recessive inheritance in DSD. The phenotypic spectrum resulting from mutations in the $P_0$ gene was recently expanded to include patients with a very severe, infantile-onset congenital hypomyelination.[58]

## HEREDITARY NEUROPATHY WITH LIABILITY TO PRESSURE PALSIES

Hereditary neuropathy with liability to recurrent pressure-sensitive palsies (HNPP; also called *tomaculous neuropathy, recurrent pressure-sensitive neuropathy,* and "bulb digger's palsy") is an autosomal dominant disorder that produces an episodic, recurrent demyelinating neuropathy.[59] This condition generally develops during adolescence and may cause attacks of numbness, muscular weakness, and atrophy. Peroneal palsies, carpal-tunnel syndrome, and other entrapment neuropathies are frequent manifestations of this disorder. Motor and sensory nerve conduction velocities may be reduced in clinically affected patients, as well as in asymptomatic gene carriers.[59] Pathological changes observed in peripheral nerves of HNPP patients include segmental demyelination and, in some pedigrees, tomaculous or "sausage-like" formations.[60] Because of mild overlap of clinical features with CMT1, HNPP patients may on occasion be misdiagnosed as having CMT1. HNPP and CMT1 are both demyelinating neuropathies; however, their clinical, pathological, and electrophysiological features are quite distinct.

The *HNPP* locus has been assigned to chromosome 17p11.2–12[61,62] and is associated with a 1.5 Mb deletion.[61,63] All DNA markers known to map to the region in 17p11.2–12 associated with the CMT1A duplication, including the *PMP22* gene, are deleted in *HNPP*. The deletion breakpoints in *HNPP* have been found to map to the same intervals in which the CMT1A duplication breakpoints map. In one pedigree, *de novo* deletion of paternal origin was detected as a basis for sporadic HNPP. It is possible that HNPP results from deletion of the *PMP22* gene and underexpression of this locus. Further support for the hypothesis that HNPP results from reduced expression at the *PMP22* locus was provided by the identification of a nondeleted HNPP kindred in which a 2 bp deletion leading to an early termination codon within exon 1 of PMP22 was present.[64]

The possibility of genetic heterogeneity in HNPP was raised by the identification of an HNPP pedigree that did not demonstrate linkage to the region of 17p11.2–12.[65]

## MEIOTIC UNEQUAL CROSSOVER: GENESIS OF CMT1A AND HEREDITARY NEUROPATHY WITH LIABILITY TO PRESSURE PALSIES

The mechanism underlying generation of the CMT1A DNA duplication and the HNPP deletion deserves careful investigation. It has been proposed that the deleted chromosome in HNPP and the duplicated chromosome in CMT1A are the reciprocal products of unequal crossing over,[61] a likely mechanism for generating the DNA duplication and the deletion. The apparent homogeneity for size of the duplication/deletion in unrelated patients[15,45,61] and detection of *de novo* duplication/deletion events[16,17,61] suggest that a common mechanism may account for the generation of the duplicated CMT1A chromosome and

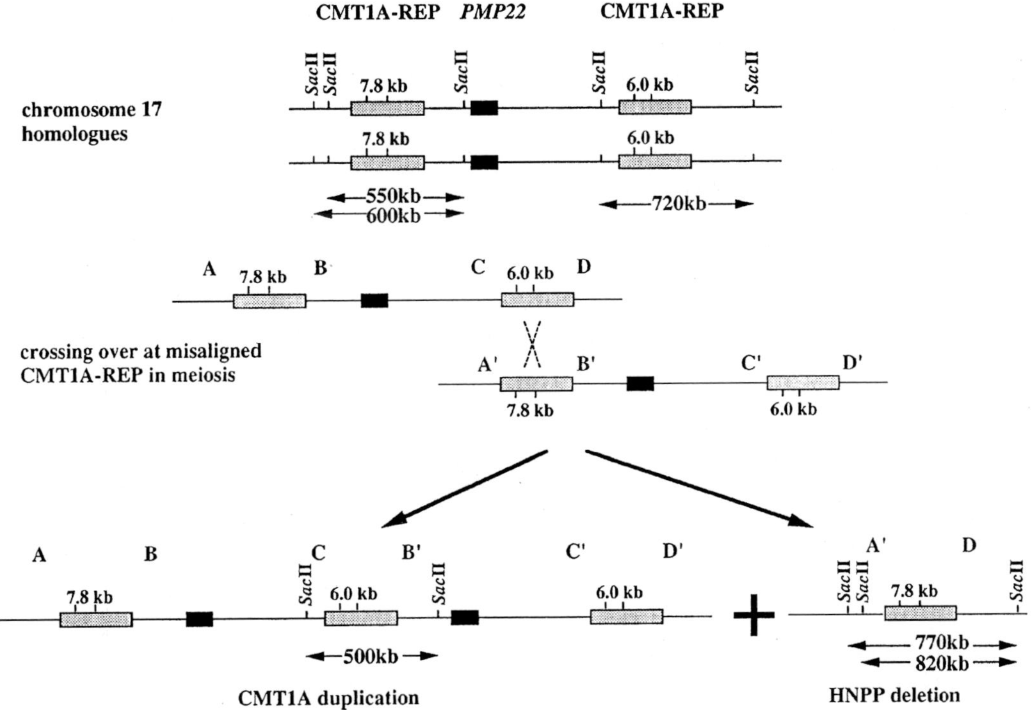


**Figure 4–4.** Model for generation of the CMT1A duplication and the HNPP deletion. Positions of the CMT1A-REP sequences (stippled boxes) are shown relative to the peripheral myelin protein-22 *(PMP22)* gene (black boxes). Approximate distances are shown in kilobases (kb), and *Sac*II sites are depicted. Unequal crossover is postulated to occur through misalignment mediated by the CMT1A-REP sequences to produce a duplicated and deleted recombinant chromosome. These recombinant chromosomes have novel junction fragments, 500 kb for the CMT1A duplication and 770 and 820 kb for the HNPP deletion. (From Chance et al.[67])

the deleted HNPP chromosome. Because the duplicated/deleted segment spans an estimated 1.5 Mb, two homologous regions, widely separated within chromosome 17p11.2–12, are required for unequal crossing over to occur.

As this model predicted, a low-copy-number repeat sequence (CMT1A-REP repeat) that flanks the proximal and distal duplication breakpoint regions on normal (nonduplicated) chromosomes was identified.[66] The CMT1A-REP sequence, which is an intrinsic property of a normal chromosome 17, appears to mediate misalignment of homologous chromosomal segments during meiosis with subsequent crossing over to produce the duplicated CMT1A chromosome. Therefore, the CMT1A-REP repeat sequence specifically flanks the 1.5 Mb segment of chromosome 17p11.2–12, which is duplicated in CMT1A and deleted in HNPP. The CMT1A-REP repeat represents a complex low-copy-number repeat sequence and is present in three copies on the CMT1A duplicated chromosome.[66] Furthermore, the CMT1A-REP repeat was found to be present in only one copy on HNPP deletion chromosomes, strengthening the model that the duplicated chromosome in CMT1A and the deleted chromosome in HNPP are reciprocal products of unequal crossover.[67]

A proposed molecular model for generating the CMT1A duplication and the HNPP deletion is shown in Figure 4–4. Cloned fragments from CMT1A-REP repeat regions have been used to determine the size of the repeats, to assess regions of homology, and to map the crossover breakpoints in a series of unrelated CMT1A and HNPP patients.[68] The CMT1A-REP repeat appears to be continuous and spans approximately 24 kb.[66,68] Approximately 75% percent of CMT1A and HNPP patients have been found to have breakpoints that map to a small interval (2 to 3 kb) within the CMT1A-REP repeat, providing evidence for a recombinational hotspot within the CMT1A-REP repeat.[68–71] DNA sequence analysis of a portion of the interval containing the majority of crossovers revealed over 98% sequence identity between proximal and distal CMT1A-REP repeat sequences.[68–70] The basis for the recombinational hotspot is unknown; however, a *mariner*-like transposon sequence maps within the CMT1A-REP repeat approximately 700 bp centromeric to the hotspot.[69,70] Analysis of this sequence suggests that it does not encode a functional human transposon. It remains possible, however, that specific CMT1A-REP sequences may be a target for an active transposase encoded elsewhere in the genome.

The functional relationship of the *mariner*-like element to the recombinational hotspot remains unknown. The origin of the CMT1A-REP repeat has been investigated through an analysis of homologous sequences in nonhuman primates. Southern blot analysis indicated that the chimpanzee has two copies of a CMT1A-REP–like sequence, whereas gorilla, orangutan, and gibbon have a single copy.[70] These observations suggest that the CMT1A-REP sequence appeared as a repeat before the divergence of chimpanzee and human, but after gorilla and human around 6 to 7 million years ago.

## TRANSGENIC ANIMAL MODELS FOR *PMP22* AND $P_0$

As previously stated, in humans, having only one normal copy of the *PMP22* gene leads to a mildly abnormal phenotype (HNPP); two copies are needed for a normal phenotype, three copies lead to a moderately abnormal phenotype (CMT1A), and four copies cause a severely abnormal phenotype resembling DSD. These observations indicate a direct relationship between gene dosage at the *PMP22* locus and phenotype. One might predict that the total absence of the *PMP22* gene would also cause demyelinating neuropathy, likely more severe than HNPP. Such patients have not yet been found, but a murine model with this genotype has been described.[72] Homozygous deletion ($pmp22^{-/-}$) "knock-out" mice develop a severe demyelinating neuropathy, with very slow conduction velocities (7 m/s) and striking demyelination on pathological examination, including the evolution of demyelinated axons in $pmp22^{-/-}$ mice, as tomaculous myelin sheaths are replaced by thin to absent ones. Heterozygous deletion ($pmp22^{+/-}$) mice are less affected, with minimal slowing of conduction velocities and little evidence of demyelination in biopsy specimens, although numerous tomaculi eventually develop in affected nerves.[72] This data strongly implicates the loss of the *pmp22* gene, and not another gene in the 1.5 Mb deletion, as the cause of HNPP and provides an ideal animal model for further study.

Dosage effects of the $P_0$ gene also cause demyelination, as evidenced by analysis of homozygous deleted ($P_0^{-/-}$) and heterozygous ($P_0^{-/-}$) transgenic mice.[73] $P_0^{-/-}$ mice have severe demyelination, which is evident soon after myelination begins and does not improve over time. Myelination begins normally in $P_0^{+/-}$ mice, but, beginning around age 4 months, there is progressive demyelination so that by 12 months there is mild but significant slowing of nerve conductions, as well as demyelination and remyelination in nerve biopsy specimens. A long delay before the onset of demyelination in ($P_0^{+/-}$ mice indicates that $pmp22^{+/-}$ mice may also develop a more pronounced phenotype.[74] The phenotypes of the $P_0^{+/-}$ and $P_0^{+/-}$ mice suggest that heterozygous deletion of the $P_0$ gene in humans might cause a mild demyelinating neuropathy and that deletion of both $P_0$ genes would lead to a phenotype as severe as (or even worse than) that of DSD.[74]

The actual mechanism of demyelination in $pmp22^{+/-}$ and $P_0^{+/-}$ mice is unknown. It can be speculated that these mice synthesize only one-half as much PMP and $P_0$ protein as their wild-type counterparts, thereby altering the stoichiometry of the proteins in compact myelin, which in turn leads to demyelination.

## HEREDITARY NEURALGIC AMYOTROPHY

Hereditary neuralgic amyotrophy with predilection for the brachial plexus (HNA; also called *familial brachial plexus neuropathy*) is an autosomal dominant disorder that causes attacks of pain, muscle weakness, and sensory disturbances in the brachial region, frequently beginning in childhood.[59] Electrophysiological studies in patients with HNA have found evidence for axonal interruption at the level of the brachial plexus in the affected limb.[75] Distal to the brachial plexus, motor nerve conduction velocities are either normal or mildly prolonged. There is no evidence to suggest that a generalized neuropathy is present in HNA. Pathological studies have demonstrated axonal degeneration in nerves examined distal to the plexus abnormality.[76] In some HNA pedigrees there are mild dysmorphic features of hypotelorism and short stature.[77] The prognosis for recovery of normal function of affected limbs in HNA is good. The underlying pathogenesis of HNA is unknown.

Although HNPP and HNA appear to be distinct disorders on clinical grounds alone, the occurrence of brachial plexopathy in HNPP has lead to the speculation that these disorders may represent the same condition or may be allelic variants of the same locus.[60,75,78,79] Despite the distinctive clinical, electrophysiological, and pathological features of HNPP and HNA, these two disorders are sometimes confused. This is partly because both disorders are episodic in nature and, in the case of HNPP, may affect the brachial plexus.[75,79] Approximately 10% of HNPP patients have had involvement of the brachial plexus, and in some patients a brachial plexopathy is the initial or only expression of HNPP. HNPP is a demyelinating neuropathy involving the altered expression of a myelin gene *(PMP22)*, while evidence suggests that HNA is an axonal process.[76] Painful brachial plexus neuropathy and mildly dysmorphic features are important points of differentiation and likely occur exclusively in HNA.

Two studies have addressed the possible allelic heterogeneity of HNA and have analyzed pedigrees with HNA with gene markers from the HNPP region on chromosome 17p11.2–12.[80–82] These studies in pedigrees with clinically typical HNA found no evidence that abnormalities are present in the *PMP22* gene or that the chromosome 17p11.2–12 deletion seen in many patients with HNPP is present in HNA. It is also evident that HNA is not an allele of CMT1A. In addition to the other clinical, electrophysiological, and pathological features that permit delineation of these two peripheral neuropathies, these studies provide genetic evidence that HNA and HNPP are distinct disorders and are not variant clinical manifestations at the same locus. The HNA gene was mapped to chromosome 17q23–25.[83]

## CMT2

Charcot-Marie-Tooth neuropathy type 2 (CMT2) is a less common disorder than CMT1 (all forms combined). Generally, CMT2 has a later age of onset, has less involvement of the small muscles of the hands, and does not have palpably enlarged nerves. Extensive demyelination with "onion bulb" formation is not present in CMT2. Motor nerve conduction velocities are normal or only slightly prolonged in affected persons.

CMT2 appears to be genetically distinct from all mapped forms of CMT1. Linkage of the neuropathy in three CMT2 pedigrees to the CMT1A region in 17p11.2–12 and the CMT1B region in 1q2 was excluded.[84] A CMT2 locus was assigned by linkage studies to the short arm of chromsome 1 (1p36) and designated as CMT2A.[85] Additional families fulfilling the diagnostic criteria for CMT2 did not have evidence of linkage to this region on chromsome 1, suggesting genetic heterogeneity within CMT2.[85] One CMT2 pedigree was found to link to markers from chromosome 3q and is designated CMT2B.[86] Further genetic heterogeneity within CMT2 is likely as kindreds with the features of axonal neuropathy with diaphragm weakness and vocal cord paralysis have been described and are designated as having CMT2C.[87] The CMT2C locus does not map to the regions of the *CMT2A* or *CMT2B* genes.[88] More recently, an autosomal dominant form of CMT2 was mapped to chromosome 7p14 and designated as CMT2D.[89]

## X-LINKED CHARCOT-MARIE-TOOTH NEUROPATHY

Numerous reports document the existence of X-linked CMT (CMTX).[90] The clinical features of CMTX include demyelinating neuropathy, absence of male-to-male transmission, and a generally earlier onset and faster rate of progression of illness in males.

The initial regional assignment for CMTX was made to the proximal long arm of the X chromosome (Xq) by demonstration of linkage to marker DXYS1.[91] Refinements in the localization of CMTX to the region of Xq13–q21 have been made by many groups.[92–97] The *connexin32 (Cx32)* gene, which encodes a major component of gap junctions, was within the CMTX candidate region and was found to be expressed in peripheral nerve.[98]

An analysis of *Cx32* in unrelated CMTX pedigrees showed multiple point mutations associated with the CMTX phenotype.[98] This observation has been confirmed in other laboratories.[99,100] At least 24 different Cx32 mutations have now been found in 27 CMTX families. *Cx32* has a pattern of expression in peripheral nerve similar to that of other myelin protein genes; however, immunohistochemical studies show a different localization.[98] Unlike PMP22 and $P_0$, which are present in compact myelin, *Cx32* is located at uncompacted folds of Schwann cell cytoplasm around the nodes of Ranvier and at Schmidt-Lanterman incisures.[98] This localization suggests a role for gap junctions composed of Cx32 in providing a pathway for the transfer of ions and nutrients around and across the myelin sheath.

## AUTOSOMAL RECESSIVE NEUROPATHY

Families with rare autosomal recessive motor and sensory neuropathy have been reported, particularly in Tunisian families with parental consanquinity. Both demyelinating and axonal types have been described and given the designation CMT4. One form of autosomal recessive demyelinating neuropathy has been mapped to chromosome 8q (CMT4A).[101] Other families with CMT4 do not show linkage to chromosome 8q; the other chromosomal loci have not yet been determined.

## GENETIC EVALUATION OF PATIENTS WITH CHARCOT-MARIE-TOOTH AND HEREDITARY NEUROPATHY WITH LIABILITY TO PRESSURE PALSIES

Before the application of genetic principles to clinical situations, an accurate diagnosis of neuropathy, consistent with a form of CMT (CMT1 or CMT2), should be established. Other causes of peripheral neuropathies (e.g. heavy metal poisoning, immune neuropathies) should also be considered and, if necessary, ruled out. Environmental exposures may involve multiple family members, thereby potentially mimicking a hereditary illness. CMT is usually a chronic, slowly progressive condition. One should be suspicious of cases that seemingly have a rapid course of deterioration. The neurologic findings show tremendous variability in patients with CMT and possibly even more variability in gene carriers for HNPP. In the cases of CMT, the only physical findings may include mild pes cavus and depressed deep tendon reflexes. Examination of multiple family members for subtle signs of neuropathy may help to establish a diagnosis. It is important for all probands persons at risk, and, if possible parents, to undergo nerve conduction velocity (NCV) and electromyographic studies. For patients who clearly lack sensory impairment and do not show evidence of sensory nerve dysfunction on electrophysiological studies, the diagnosis may include other disorders (e.g., spinal muscle atrophy, juvenile amyotrophic lateral sclerosis).

The pedigree is of paramount import and may assist in making the diagnosis. The genetic counseling given will depend not only on the accuracy of the diagnosis but also on the type of CMT and the mode of inheritance. For example, the occurrence of male-to-male transmission excludes the possibility of CMTX. The sporadic case in a male can be especially difficult to evaluate because the pattern of inheritance can be autosomal dominant, X-linked, or even autosomal recessive. Sporadic cases may also represent *de novo* duplications (CMT1A) or *de novo* deletions (HNPP). False paternity is another explanation for apparent sporadic cases of CMT or HNPP. For this reason, both parents need to be examined clinically and by electrophysiological methods to determine if there is any evidence for neuropathy. If a proband has evidence for CMT1, determination of NCV is a useful screening tool for parents and other at-risk family members. Studies have determined that the CMT1 gene is penetrant in early life, and correct disease status can probably be determined with NCV screening by age 5 years.[102] If a proband's NCV is normal or only mildly prolonged, however, the diagnosis may be CMT2. In this case the screening examination needs to focus on determination of amplitudes and other electrical signs of denervation.

The odds indicate that the overwhelming proportion of CMT1 and CMT2 pedigrees have autosomal dominant inheritance. In pedigrees lacking male-to-male inheritance and/or those in which males are more severely affected than females and have an earlier onset, CMTX should be suspected. Determination of autosomal dominant versus X-linked CMT is important because the counseling for these two modes of inheritance are different. For autosomal CMT, the likelihood of an affected parent (of either sex) having an affected child is 50% for each pregnancy regardless of the sex of the child. For CMTX, all daughters of an affected father will inherit the gene, and none of the sons will be affected. For a woman with CMTX, there is a 50% likelihood of her having affected children regardless of their sex.

It has been estimated that 70% to 80% of patients with a clinical diagnosis of CMT1 carry the 17p11.2–12 duplication.[45,103] The duplication is specific for CMT1A. This implies that an assay for the duplication may provide a powerful marker for screening suspected patients and at-risk family members. DNA testing for the duplication associated with CMT1A is available and should be a part of the evaluation of any patient with suspected hereditary neuropathy. The 1.5 Mb deletion of 17p11.2–12 is highly specific for HNPP, but additional heterogeneity studies are needed to determine if HNPP may also result from other types of molecular abnormalities. Patients with CMT1 phenotypes who lack the duplication may have point mutations in the $P_0$ or *Cx32* genes. The presence of male-to-male transmission of the neuropathy would exclude this possibility for a mutation in Cx32.

## SUMMARY

The inherited disorders of peripheral nerves represent a common group of neurologic diseases. CMT1 is a genetically heterogeneous group of chronic demyelinating polyneuropathies with loci mapping to chromosome 17 (CMT1A), chromosome 1 (CMT1B), the X chromosome (CMTX), and to another unknown autosome (CMT1C). CMT1A is most often associated with a tandem 1.5 Mb duplication in chromosome 17p11.2–12, or, in rare patients, CMT1A may result from a point mutation in the *PMP22* gene. CMT1B is associated with point mutations in the $P_0$ gene.

The molecular defect in CMT1C is unknown. CMTX is associated with mutations in the *Cx32* gene. CMT2 is an axonal neuropathy, also of undetermined cause. One form of CMT2 maps to chromosome 1p36 (CMT2A) and another to chromosome 3p (CMT2B).

Dejerine-Sottas disease, also called *hereditary motor and sensory neuropathy type III* (HMSNIII), is a severe, infantile-onset demyelinating polyneuropathy syndrome that may be associated with point mutations in either the *PMP22* gene or the $P_0$ gene. HNPP is an autosomal dominant disorder that results in a recurrent, episodic demyelinating neuropathy. HNPP is associated with a 1.5 Mb deletion in chromosome

17p11.2–12 and likely results from reduced expression of the *PMP22* gene. CMT1A and HNPP are apparent reciprocal duplication/deletion syndromes originating from unequal crossover during germ cell meiosis. Hereditary neuralgic amyotrophy (familial brachial plexus neuropathy) is an autosomal dominant disorder causing painful, recurrent brachial plexopathies and maps to chromosome 17q23–25.

## ACKNOWLEDGMENTS

This work was supported by the Muscular Dystrophy Association, the March of Dimes Birth Defects Foundation, the National Institutes of Health, and the Myer S. Shandelman Trust.

## REFERENCES

1. Lupski JR, Garcia CA, Parry GJ, Patel PI: Charcot-Marie-Tooth polyneuropathy syndrome: Clinical, electrophysiological and genetic aspects. In Appel S (ed): Current Neurology. Mosby–Yearbook, Chicago, 1991 pp1–25.
2. Dyck PJ, Chance PF, Lebo RV, Carney JA: Hereditary motor and sensory neuropathies. In Dyck PJ, Thomas PJ, Griffin JW, Low PA, Poduslo JF (eds): Peripheral Neuropathy, ed 3. WB Saunders, Philadelphia, 1993 pp1094–1136.
3. Bird TD, Kraft GK: Charcot-Marie-Tooth disease: Data for genetic counselling. Clin Genet 14:43–49, 1978.
4. Bird TD, Ott J, Giblett ER: Evidence for linkage of Charcot-Marie-Tooth neuropathy to the Duffy locus on chromosome 1. Am J Hum Genet 34:388–394, 1982.
5. Stebbins NB, Conneally PM: Linkage of dominantly inherited Charcot-Marie-Tooth neuropathy to the Duffy locus in an Indiana family. Am J Hum Genet 34:195A, 1982.
6. Bird TD, Ott J, Giblett ER, Chance PF, Sumi SM, Kraft GH: Genetic linkage evidence for heterogeneity in Charcot-Marie-Tooth neuropathy (HMSN type I). Ann Neurol 14:679–684, 1983.
7. Dyck PJ, Ott J, Breanndan MS, Moore SB, Swanson CJ, Lambert EH: Linkage evidence for genetic heterogeneity among kinships with hereditary motor and sensory neuropathy, type I. Mayo Clin Proc 58: 430–435, 1983.
8. Vance JM, Nicholson GA, Yamaoka LH, et al.: Linkage of Charcot-Marie-Tooth neuropathy type IA to chromosome 17. Exp Neurol 104:186–189, 1989.
9. Raeymaekers P, Timmerman V, De Jonghe P, Swerts L, Gheuens J, Martin JJ: Localization of the mutation in an extended family with Charcot-Marie-Tooth neuropathy (HMSN I). Am J Hum Genet 45:953–958, 1989.
10. Chance PF, Bird TD, O'Connell, et al.: Linkage and heterogeneity in type I Charcot-Marie-Tooth disease (hereditary motor and sensory neuropathy I). Am J Hum Genet 47:915–925, 1990.
11. McAlpine PJ, Feasby TE, Hahn AF, Komarnicki L, James S, Guy C, et al. Charcot-Marie-Tooth neuropathy type IA (CMT1A) maps to chromosome 17. Genomics 7:408–415, 1990.
12. Middleton-Price HR, Harding AE, Monteiro C, Berciano J, Malcolm S: Linkage of hereditary motor and sensory neuropathy type I to the pericentromeric region of chromosome 17. Am J Hum Genet 46:92–94, 1990.
13. Patel PI, Franco B, Garcia C, et al.: Genetic mapping of autosomal dominant Charcot-Marie-Tooth disease in a large French-Acadian kindred: Identification of new linked markers on chromosome 17. Am J Hum Genet 46:801–809, 1990.
14. Vance JM, Barker D, Yamaoka LH, et al.: Localization of Charcot-Marie-Tooth disease type 1A (CMT 1A) to chromosome 17p11.2. Genomics 9: 623–628, 1991.
15. Lupski JR, de Oca-Luna RM, Slaugenhaupt S, et al.: DNA duplication associated with Charcot-Marie-Tooth disease type 1A. Cell 66:219–232, 1991.
16. Raeymaekers P, Timmerman V, Nelis E, et al.: Duplication in chromosome 17p11.2 in Charcot-Marie-Tooth neuropathy type 1A. Neuromusc Disord 1:93–97, 1991.
17. Raeymaekers P, Timmerman V, Nelis E, et al.: Estimation of the size of the chromosome 17p11.2 duplication in Charcot-Marie-Tooth neuropathy type 1A (CMT1A). J Med Genet 29:5–11, 1992.
18. Wright EC, Goldgar DE, Fain PR, Barker DF, Skolnick MH: A genetic map of human chromosome 17p. Genomics 7:103–109, 1990.
19. Hoogendijk JE, Hensels GW, Gabreels-Festen AA, et al.: *De-novo* mutation in hereditary motor and sensory neuropathy type 1. Lancet 339:1081–1082, 1992.
20. Ionasescu VV, Ionasescu R, Searby C, et al.: Charcot-Marie-Tooth neuropathy type 1A with both duplication and non-duplication. Hum Mol Genet 2:405–410, 1993.
21. Valentijn LJ, Baas F, Zorn I, et al.: Alternatively sized duplication in Charcot-Marie-Tooth disease type 1A. Hum Mol Genet 2:2143–2146, 1993.
22. Feldman GM, Baumer JG, Sparkes RS: Brief clinical report: The dup(17p) syndrome. Am J Med Genet 11:299–304, 1982.
23. Magenis RE, Brown MG, Allen L, et al.: *De novo* partial duplication of 17p (dup(17)(p12–p11.2)): Clinical report. Am J Med Genet 24:415–420, 1986.
24. Chance PF, Bird TD, Matsunami N, et al.: Trisomy 17p associated with Charcot-Marie-Tooth neuropathy I phenotype: Evidence for gene dosage as a mechanism in CMT1A. Neurology 42:2295–2299, 1992.
25. Lupski JR, Wise CA, Kuwano A, et al.: Gene dosage is a mechanism for Charcot-Marie-Tooth disease type 1A. Nat Genet 1:29–33, 1992.
26. Upadhyaya M, Roberts SH, Farnharm, J, et al.: Charcot-Marie-Tooth disease 1A (CMT1A) associated with a maternal duplication of chromosome 17p11.2–12. Hum Genet 91:392–394, 1993.
27. Falconer DS: Two new mutants, "Trembler" and

"Reeler," with neurological actions in the mouse (*Mus musculus L.*). J Genet 50:192–201, 1951.
28. Aguayo JA, Attiwell M, Trecarten J, Perkins S, Bray GM: Abnormal myelination in transplanted Trembler mouse Schwann cells. Nature 265:73–75, 1977.
29. Davisson MT, Roderick TH: Status of the linkage map of the mouse. Cytogenet Cell Genet 22:552–557, 1978.
30. Buchberg AM, Brownell E, Nagata S, Jenkins NA, Copeland NE: A comprehensive genetic map of murine chromosome 11 reveals extensive linkage conservation between mouse and human. Genetics 122:153–161, 1988.
31. Suter U, Welcher AA, Ozcelik T, et al.: Trembler mouse carries a point mutation in a myelin gene. Nature 356:241–244, 1992.
32. Manfioletti G, Ruaro ME, Del Sal G, Philipson L, Schneider C: A growth arrest–specific (*gas*) gene codes for a membrane protein. Mol Cell Biol 10: 2924–2930, 1990.
33. Spreyer P, Kuhn G, Hanemann CO, Gillen C, Schaal H, Lemke G, Muller HW: Axon-regulated expression of a Schwann cell transcript that is homologous to a "growth arrest–specific gene." EMBO 10:3661–3668, 1991.
34. Welcher AA, Suter U, De Leon M, Snipes GJ, Shooter EM: A myelin protein is encoded by the homolog of a growth arrest–specific gene. Proc Natl Acad Sci USA 88:7195–7199, 1991.
35. Matsunami N, Smith B, Ballard L, et al.: Peripheral myelin protein-22 gene maps in the duplication in chromosome 17p11.2 associated with Charcot-Marie-Tooth 1A. Nat Genet 1:176–179, 1992.
36. Patel PI, Roa BB, Welcher AA, et al.: The gene for the peripheral myelin protein PMP-22 is a candidate for Charcot-Marie-Tooth disease type 1A. Nat Genet 1:157–165, 1992.
37. Timmerman V, Nelis E, Van Hul W, et al.: The peripheral myelin protein gene *PMP-22* is contained within the Charcot-Marie-Tooth disease type 1A duplication. Nat Genet 1:171–175, 1992.
38. Valentijn LJ, Bolhuis PA, Zorn I, et al.: The peripheral myelin gene *PMP-22/GAS-3* is duplicated in Charcot-Marie-Tooth disease type 1A. Nat Genet 1:166–170, 1992.
39. Snipes GJ, Suter U, Welcher AA, et al.: Characterization of a novel peripheral nervous system myelin protein (PMP-22/SR13). J Cell Biol 117:225–238, 1992.
40. Suter U, Snipes GJ, Schoener-Scott R, et al.: Regulation of tissue-specific expression of alternative peripheral myelin protein-22 (PMP22) gene transcripts by two promoters. J Biol Chem 26:25795–25808, 1994.
41. Yoshikawa H, Nishimura T, Fujimura H, et al.: Elevated expression of messenger RNA for peripheral myelin protein 22 in biopsied peripheral nerve of patients Charcot-Marie-Tooth disease type 1A. Ann Neurol 35:445–450, 1994.
42. Hoogendijk JE, Janssen EAM, Gabreels-Festen AA, et al.: Allelic heterogeneity in hereditary motor and sensory neuropathy type Ia (Charcot-Marie-Tooth disease type Ia). Neurology 43:1010–1014, 1993
43. Valentijn LJ, Baas F, Wolterman RA, et al.: Identical point mutations of the peripheral myelin protein-22 in Trembler-J mouse and a family with Charcot-Marie-Tooth disease. Nat Genet 2:288–291, 1992.
44. Roa BB, Garcia CA, Suter U, et al.: Charcot-Marie-Tooth disease type 1A: Association with a spontaneous point mutation in the *PMP22* gene. N Engl J Med 329:96–101, 1993.
46. Hayasaka K, Nanao K, Tahara M, et al.: Isolation and sequence determination of cDNA encoding the major structural protein of human peripheral myelin. Biochem Biophys Res Commun 180:515–518, 1991
47. Lemke G: The molecular genetics of myelination: An update. Glia 7:263–271, 1993.
48. Hayasaka K, Himoro M, Sato W, et al.: Charcot-Marie-Tooth neuropathy type 1b associated with mutations in the myelin protein zero gene. Nat Genet 5:31–34, 1993.
49. Kulkens T, Bolhuis PA, Wolterman RA, et al.: Deletion of the serine 34 codon from the major peripheral myelin protein *P0* gene in Charcot-Marie-Tooth disease type 1B. Nat Genet 5:35–39, 1993.
50. Hayasaka K, Takada G, Ionasescu VV: Mutation of the myelin *P0* gene in Charcot-Marie-Tooth neuropathy type 1B. Hum Mol Genet 2:1369–1372, 1993.
51. Hayasaka K, Ohnishi A, Takada G, et al.: Mutation of the myelin *P0* gene in Charcot-Marie-Tooth neuropathy type 1. Biochem Biophys Res Commun 194:1317–1322, 1993.
52. Himoro M, Yoshikawa H, Matsui T, et al.: New mutation of the myelin *P0* gene in a pedigree with Charcot-Marie-Tooth neuropathy type 1. Biochem Mol Biol Int 31:169–173, 1993.
53. Roa BB, Warner LE, Garcia CA, et al.: Myelin protein zero (MPZ) mutations in non duplication type 1 Charcot-Marie-Tooth disease. Hum Mutat 7:35–45, 1996.
54. Nelis E, Timmerman V, De Jonghe P, et al: Rapid screening of myelin genes in CMT1 patients by SSCP analysis: Identification of new mutations and polymorphisms in the $P_0$ gene. Hum Genet 94: 653–657, 1994.
55. Roa BB, Dyck PJ, Marks HG, et al.: Dejerine-Sottas syndrome associated with point mutation in the peripheral myelin protein 22 *(PMP22)* gene. Nat Genet 5:269–273, 1993.
56. Hayasaka K, Himoro M, Sawaishi Y, et al.: *De novo* mutation of the myelin $P_0$ gene in Dejerine-Sottas disease. Nat Genet 5:66–268, 1993.
57. Rautenstrauss B, Nelis E, Grehl H, et al.: Identification of a *de novo* insertional mutation in $P_0$ in a patient with a Dejerine-Sottas phenotype. Hum Mol Genet 3:1701–1702, 1994.
58. Warner LE, Hilz MJ, Appel SH, et al.: Clinical phenotypes of different MPZ ($P_0$) mutations may include Charcot-Marie-Tooth type 1B, Dejerine-Sottas, and congenital hypomyelination. Neuron 17:451–460, 1996.
59. Windebank AJ: Inherited recurrent focal neuropathies. In Dyck PJ, Thomas PJ, Griffin JW, Low PA, Poduslo JF (eds). Peripheral Neuropathy, ed 3. WB Saunders, Philadelphia, 1993, pp1137–1148.
60. Madrid R, Bradley WG: The pathology of neuropathies with focal thickening of the myelin sheath (tomaculous neuropathy): Studies on the forma-

tion of the abnormal myelin sheath. J Neurol Sci 25:415–418, 1975.
61. Chance PF, Alderson MK, Leppig KA, et al.: DNA deletion associated with hereditary neuropathy with liability to pressure palsies. Cell 72:143–151, 1993.
62. Marimann ECM, Gabreels-Festen AAVM, van Beersum SEC, et al.: The gene for hereditary neuropathy with liability to pressure palsies (HNPP) maps to chromosome 17 at or close to the locus for HMSN type I. Hum Genet 93:87–90, 1993.
63. Le Guern E, Sturtz F, Gugenheim M, et al.: Detection of deletion within 17p11.2 in 7 French families with hereditary neuropathy with liability to pressure palsies (HNPP). Cytogenet Cell Genet 65:261, 1994.
64. Nicholson GA, Valentijn LJ, Cherryson AK, et al.: A frame shift mutation in the *PMP22* gene in hereditary neuropathy with liability to pressure palsies. Nat Genet 6:263–266, 1994.
65. Marimann ECM, Gabreels-Festen AAVM, van Beersum SEC, et al.: Evidence for genetic heterogeneity underlying hereditary neuropathy with liability to pressure palsies. Hum Genet 93:151–156, 1994.
66. Pentao L, Wise CA, Chinault AC, et al.: Charcot-Marie-Tooth type 1A duplication appears to arise from recombination at repeat sequences flanking the 1.5 Mb monomer unit. Nat Genet 2:292–300, 1992.
67. Chance PF, Abbas N, Lensch MW, et al.: Two autosomal dominant neuropathies result from reciprocal duplication/deletion of a region of chromosome 17. Hum Mol Genet 3:223–228, 1994.
68. Kiyosawa H, Lensch MW, Chance PF: Analysis of the CMT1A-REP repeat: Mapping crossover breakpoints in CMT1A and HNPP. Hum Mol Genet 4: 2327–2334, 1995.
69. Reiter LT, Murakami T, Koeuth T, et al.: A recombination hotspot responsible for two inherited peripheral neuropathies is located near a mariner transposon-like element. Nat Genet 12:288–297, 1996.
70. Kiyosawa H, Chance PF: Primate origin of the CMT1A-REP repeat and an analysis of a putative transposon-associated recombinational hotspot. Hum Mol Genet 5:745–754, 1996.
71. Lopes J, LeGuern E, Gouider R, et al.: Recombination hot spot in a 3.2 kb region of the Charcot-Marie-Tooth type 1A repeat sequences: New tools for molecular diagnosis of hereditary neuropathy with liability to pressure palsies and of Charcot-Marie-Tooth type 1A. Am J Hum Genet 58:1223–1230, 1996.
72. Martini R, Zielasek J, Toyka KV, et al: $P_0$-deficient mice show myelin degeneration in peripheral nerves characteristic of inherited human neuropathies. Nat Genet 11:281–286, 1995.
73. Adlkofer K, Martini R, Aguzzi A, et al.: Hypermyelination and demyelinating peripheral neuropathy in *pmp22* deficient mice. Nat Genet 11:274–280, 1995.
74. Scherer SS, Chance PF: Myelin genes: Getting the dosage right. Nat Genet 11:226–228, 1995.
75. Bradley WG, Madrid R, Thrush DC, Campbell MJ: Recurrent brachial plexus neuropathy. Brain 98: 381–398, 1975.
76. Tsairis P, Dyck PJ, Mulder DW: Natural history of brachial plexus neuropathy. Arch Neurol 27:109–117, 1972.
77. Jacob JC, Andermann F, Robb JP: Heredofamilial neuritis with brachial predilection. Neurology 11: 1025–1033, 1961.
78. McKusick VA: Mendelian Inheritance in Man, ed 10. The Johns Hopkins University Press, Baltimore, 1992.
79. Martinelli P, Fabbri R, Moretto G, Gabellini AS, D'Alessandro RD, Rizzuto N: Recurrent familial brachial plexus palsies as the only clinical expression of tomaculous neuropathy. Eur Neurol 29:61–66, 1989.
80. Gouider R, Le Guern E, Emile P, et al.: Hereditary neuralgic amyotrophy and hereditary neuropathy with liability to pressure palsies: Two distinct clinical, electrophysiological and genetic entities. Neurology 44:2250–2252, 1994.
81. Chance PF, Lensch MW, Lipe H, Brown RH Sr, Brown RH Jr, Bird TD: Hereditary neuralgic amyotrophy and hereditary neuropathy with liability to pressure palsies: Two distinct genetic disorders. Neurology 44:2253–2257, 1994.
82. Windebank AJ, Schenone A, Dewald G: Hereditary neuropathy with liability to pressure palsies and inherited brachial plexus neuropathy: Two genetically distinct disorders. Mayo Clin Proc 70:743–746, 1995.
83. Pellegrino JE, Rebbeck TR, Brown MJ, et al.: Mapping of hereditary neuralgic amyotrophy (familial brachial plexus neuropathy) to distal chromosome 17q. Neurology 46:1128–1132, 1996.
84. Loprest LJ, Pericak-Vance MA, Stajich J, et al.: Linkage studies in Charcot-Marie-Tooth disease type 2:Evidence that CMT1 and CMT2 are distinct genetic entities. Neurology 42:597–601, 1992.
85. Ben Othmane K, Middleton LT, Loprest LJ, et al.: Localization of a gene for autosomal dominant Charcot-Marie-Tooth type to chromosome 1p and evidence for genetic heterogeneity. Genomics 17: 70–375, 1993.
86. Kwon JM, Elliot JL, Yee W, et al.: Assignment of a second locus for Charcot-Marie-Tooth type II locus to chromosome 3q. Am J Hum Genet 57:853–858, 1995.
87. Dyck PJ, Litchy WJ, Minnerath S, et al.: Hereditary motor and sensory neuropathy with diaphragm and vocal cord paresis. Ann Neurol 35:608–615, 1994.
88. Yoshioka R, Dyck PJ, Chance PF: Genetic heterogeneity in Charcot-Marie-Tooth neuropathy type 2. Neurology 46:658–571, 1995.
89. Ionasescu V, Searby C, Sheffield VC, Roklina T, Nishimura D, Ionasescu R: Autosomal dominant Charcot-Marie-Tooth axonal neuropathy mapped on chromosome 7p (CMT2D). Hum Mol Genet 5: 1373–1375, 1996.
90. Fryns JP, Van den Berghe H: Sex-linked recessive inheritance in Charcot-Marie-Tooth disease with partial manifestations in female carriers. Hum-Genet 55:413–415, 1980.
91. Gal A, Mucke J, Theile H, et al.: X-linked dominant Charcot-Marie-Tooth disease: Suggestion of linkage with a cloned DNA sequence from the proximal Xq. Hum Genet 70:38–42, 1985.

92. Fischbeck KH, ar Rushdi N, Pericak-Vance M, Rozear MP, Roses AD, Fryns JP: X-linked neuropathy: Gene localization with DNA probes. Ann Neurol 20:527–532, 1986.
93. Ionasescu VV, Trofatter JL, Haines JL, Ionasescu R, Searby C: Mapping of the gene for X-linked dominant Charcot-Marie-Tooth neuropathy. Neurology 42:903–908, 1992.
94. Mostacciuolo ML, Muller E, Fardin P, et al.: X-linked Charcot-Marie-Tooth disease: A linkage study in a large family using 12 probes of the pericentric region. Hum Genet 87:23–27, 1991.
95. Ionasescu VV, Trofatter J, Haines, JL, Summers AM, Ionasescu R, Searby C: Heterogeneity in X-linked recessive Charcot-Marie-Tooth neuropathy. Am J Hum Genet 48:1075– 1083, 1991.
96. Bergoffen J, Trofatter J, Pericak-Vance MA, et al.: Linkage localization of X-linked Charcot-Marie-Tooth disease. Am J Hum Genet 52:312–318, 1993.
97. Fain PR, Barker DF, Chance PF: Refined genetic mapping of the X-linked Charcot-Marie-Tooth neuropathy locus. Am J Hum Genet 54:229–235, 1994.
98. Bergoffen J, Scherer SS, Wang S, et al.: Connexin mutations in X-linked Charcot-Marie-Tooth disease. Science 262:2039–2042, 1993.
99. Fairweather N, Bell C, Cochrane S, et al.: Mutations in the connexin32 gene in X-linked dominant Charcot-Marie-Tooth disease (CMTX). Hum Mol Genet 3:29–34, 1994.
100. Ionasescu V, Searby C, Ionasescu R: Point mutations of the connexin32 (GJB1) gene in X-linked dominant Charcot-Marie-Tooth neuropathy. Hum Mol Genet 3:355–358, 1994.
101. Ben Othmane K, Hentati F, Lennon F, et al.: Linkage of a locus (CMT4A) for autosomal recessive Charcot-Marie-Tooth disease to chromosome 8q. Hum Mol Genet 2:1625–1628, 1993.
102. Nicholson GA: Penetrance of the hereditary motor and sensory neuropathy type 1A mutation: Assessment by nerve conduction studies. Neurology 41:547–552, 1991.
103. Ionasescu VV: Charcot-Marie-Tooth neuropathies. From clinical description to molecular genetics. Muscle Nerve 18:267–275, 1995.

Chapter 5

# THE MUSCULAR DYSTROPHIES

Yoshihide Sunada, MD, PhD



Muscular dystrophy is a group of inherited diseases that primarily affect skeletal muscle and are clinically characterized by progressive muscular atrophy and weakness. Dystrophic muscle tissue has both necrotic and regenerating fibers, as well as increased amounts of fatty connective tissue. At the cellular level, there are centrally placed nuclei, and there is a marked variation in fiber size. The clinical diagnosis of muscular dystrophy is mainly based on these clinical features and on the histopathological findings of biopsied skeletal muscle. There are a number of distinct types of muscular dystrophy, which are classified based on clinical phenotype (e.g., age of onset, progression pattern, distribution of affected muscle) and inheritance pattern. Table 5–1 lists common types of muscular dystrophy subgrouped by their genetic traits.

The causative genes and pathogenesis of muscular dystrophies were unknown until the Duchenne's muscular dystrophy (DMD) gene was identified in 1987 with the strategy of positional cloning (see Chapter 2). Subsequent biochemical studies revealed that the DMD gene product, a protein called *dystrophin,* is associated with several novel glycoproteins to form a large oligomeric complex called the *dystrophin–glycoprotein complex* (DGC). Most recently, primary defects in several components of the DGC have been proven to result in limb-girdle muscular dystrophy (LGMD) or congenital muscular dystrophy (CMD). This chapter focuses on the molecular genetics of these DGC-related muscular dystrophies and briefly describes several other muscular dystrophies for which the underlying genetic mutations have been identified.

## THE DYSTROPHIN–GLYCOPROTEIN COMPLEX: AN OVERVIEW

### Positional Cloning of the DMD Gene

In the early 1980s, several DMD or Becker's muscular dystrophy (BMD) patients were identified who had cytogenetic defects in

Table 5–1. **Classification and Genetics of Muscular Dystrophies**

| Muscular Dystrophy | Symbol | Gene Locus | Protein Product |
|---|---|---|---|
| X-linked recessive | | | |
| Duchenne/Becker | DMD/BMD | Xp21 | dystrophin |
| Emery-Dreifuss | EDMD | Xq28 | emerin |
| Autosomal recessive | | | |
| Limb-girdle | LGMD 2A | 15q15.1 | calpain 3 |
| | LGMD 2B | 2p13 | dysferlin |
| | LGMD 2C | 13q12 | γ-sarcoglycan |
| | LGMD 2D | 17q21 | α-sarcoglycan |
| | LGMD 2E | 4q12 | β-sarcoglycan |
| | LGMD 2F | 5q31 | δ-sarcoglycan |
| | LGMD 2G | 17q11–q12 | unknown |
| Congenital | CMD | | |
| Fukuyama type | FCMD | 9q31–33 | fukutin |
| Merosin-deficient | | 6q2 | laminin α2 |
| Miyoshi distal myopathy | | 2p13 | dysferlin |
| Epidermolysis bullosa simplex with muscular dystrophy | MD-EBS | 8q24 | plectin |
| Autosomal dominant | | | |
| Facioscapulohumeral | FSHD | 4q35 | unknown |
| Limb-girdle | LGMD 1A | 5q22–q34 | unknown |
| | LGMD 1B | 1q11–21 | unknown |
| | LGMD 1C | 3p25 | caveolin-3 |
| Scapuloperoneal | SPMD | 12q21 | unknown |
| Oculopharyngeal | OPMD | 14q11.2–q13 | poly(A)binding protein 2 |
| Bethlem myopathy | | 21q22 | α1(VI) collagen |
| | | 21q22 | α2(VI) collagen |
| | | 2q37 | α3(VI) collagen? |

band Xp21 (translocation or deletion).[1,2] In addition, DNA fragments isolated from the Xp21 region identified restriction fragment length polymorphisms (RFLPs) that segregated with the disease phenotype in several DMD families,[3] indicating that patients without cytogenetic abnormalities also had a defect at Xp21. Subsequently, the DMD gene fragments were isolated by two independent approaches.

Using DNA from a female BMD patient with a t(Xp21) translocation, Worton's group[4,5] cloned the junctional fragment bridging the translocation in which the DMD gene had recombined with a block of ribosomal RNA genes on chromosome 21. Kunkel's group[6] isolated DNA fragments that corresponded to the deleted region in a DMD patient with multiple X-linked disease caused by a contiguous gene deletion syndrome involving band Xp21. One of their detected clones, PERT 87, revealed deletions in a subset of DMD patients.[7] Subsequently, Monaco and colleagues[8] were able to isolate the first cDNA clone from a fetal muscle cDNA library, which in turn corresponded to the deleted genomic segment. The cDNA probes identified a 14 kilobase pair (kb) mRNA in skeletal muscle. In 1987, the complete cDNA was isolated in a series of overlapping cDNA clones, which encoded a novel protein of 3685 amino acids.[9] This protein was given the name *dystrophin.*[10]

## The DMD Gene and Dystrophin

The DMD gene at Xp21 is one of the largest genes thus far identified, spanning approximately 2.3 megabase (Mb) or about 1% of the entire X chromosome and containing at least 80 exons.[11] The coding sequence constitutes only 0.6% of the entire gene. Large introns up to 200 kb are common in the 5' third of the gene.

Dystrophin is the protein product of the 14 kb full-length DMD gene transcript in muscle and brain. There are eight different promoters driving their own first exon and producing the cell type–specific expression of distinct dystrophin isoforms. As shown in Figure 5–1, muscle, cortical and Purkinje cell–type promoters give rise to 427 kDa, full-length dystrophins differing only at the first few amino acids. Retinal (R) promoter regulates the expression of 260 kDa retinal dystrophin. Brain/kidney (B/K), Schwann cell (S), and general or glial (G) dystrophin promoters give rise to distal transcripts that encode C-terminal proteins Dp140, Dp116, and Dp71, respectively.[12–14] The primary structure predicts that dystrophin is a rod-shaped cytoskeletal protein consisting of four structurally distinct domains: an N-terminal actin-binding domain, a large spectrin-like rod domain, a cysteine-rich domain, and a unique C-terminal domain.[15] Dystrophin is localized to the inner surface of the sarcolemma in normal skeletal muscle, but is totally missing from skeletal muscle of DMD patients and significantly deficient in BMD patients.[16–18] Neither the exact function nor the precise mechanism of muscle cell degeneration caused by the deficiency of dys-

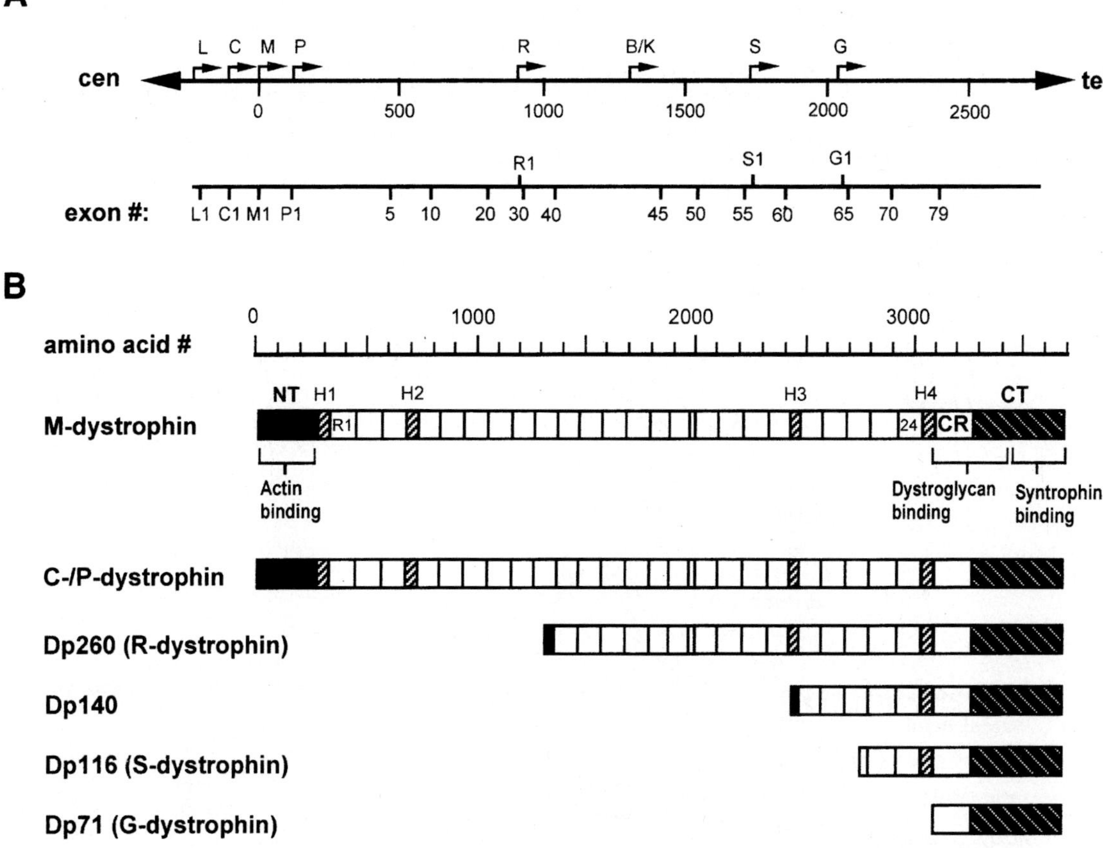


**Figure 5–1.** Schematic diagram of the DMD gene and its protein products. *(A)* Distribution of eight different promoters (upper line) and representative exons (lower line) spanning 2.3 Mb. *(B)* Six different dystrophin isoforms encoded by the DMD gene. Full-length dystrophin consists of four functional domains: NT (N-terminal actin-binding domain), R1–24 (rod domain containing 24 homologous repeats), CR (cysteine-rich domain), and CT (C-terminal domain).

trophin, however, was revealed by its primary structure.

## The DGC

Dystrophin is tightly associated with several sarcolemmal proteins (dystrophin-associated proteins [DAPs]) that form a large oligomeric complex called the *dystrophin-glycoprotein complex.*[19–21] Structural and functional characterizations of dystrophin and DAPs are now providing the clue to the overall molecular organization of the DGC (Fig. 5–2).[22,23] The DAPs constitute three major subcomplexes in the DGC: dystroglycan complex (α- and β-dystroglycans), sarcoglycan complex (α-, β-, γ-, and δ-sarcoglycans), and syntrophin complex (α-, $\beta_1$-, and $\beta_2$-syntrophins, and dystrobrevin).

α-Dystroglycan is a laminin-binding protein, thus mediating the attachment of the sarcolemma to the basement membrane,[24,25] whereas β-dystroglycan directly binds to the C-terminal domains of dystrophin.[26,27] Thus, the dystroglycan complex links the cytoskeletal protein dystrophin to the extracellular matrix. α/β-Dystroglycans are encoded by a single 5.8 kb mRNA,[24] and post-translational modification of a 97 kDa precursor protein results in two mature proteins.[24] The heterotrimeric basement membrane protein merosin (laminin-2) is the extracellular ligand for skeletal muscle α-dystroglycan.

Four transmembrane components, α-, β-, γ-, and δ-sarcoglycans, form a tightly associated subcomplex called the *sarcoglycan complex.* The exact binding site(s) of the sarcoglycan complex to dystrophin and dystroglycan have not been identified. The exact function of the sarcoglycan complex in the DGC remains unknown. The syntrophin complex directly binds to the second half of the C-terminal domain of dystrophin.[28–30] Binding sites for α- and β-syntrophins in the C-terminal domain are tandemly located.[29]

Overall, the DGC provides a link between the subsarcolemmal cytoskeleton and the extracellular matrix. Normal integrity of the DGC is crucial for maintaining normal mus-

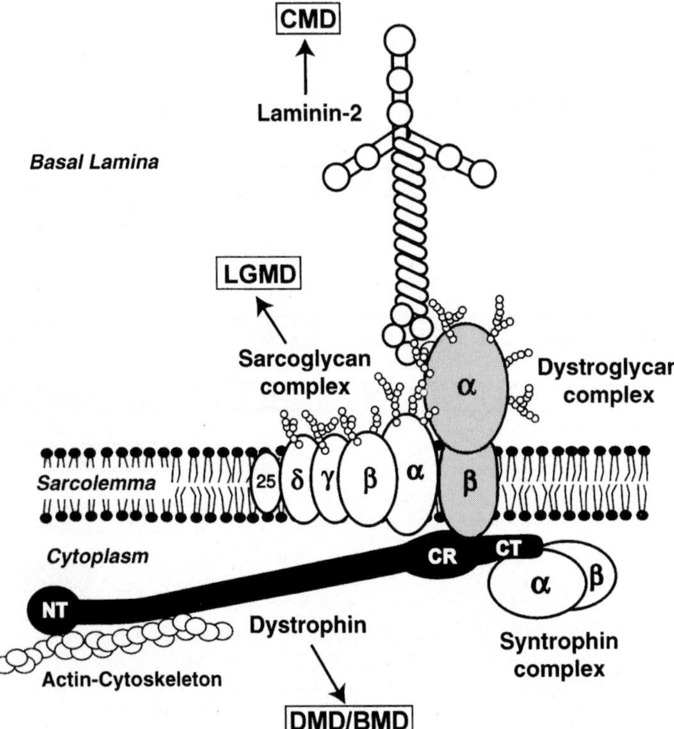


**Figure 5–2.** Schematic model for the DGC presenting the molecular organization and implications in the DGC-related muscular dystrophies. The DGC is comprised of three subcomplexes: the dystroglycan complex, the sarcoglycan complex, and syntrophins. Dystrophin serves as the cytoskeletal linker between the actin-cytoskeleton and dystroglycan. α-Dystroglycan binds laminin-2, a major component of the basal laminae. Precise interaction of the sarcoglycan complex with dystrophin and/or dystroglycan remains unknown. Syntrophins directly bind to the C-terminal domain of dystrophin. CR= cysteine-rich domain; CT = C-terminal domain; NT = N-terminal domain; CMD = congenital muscular dystrophy; LGMD = limb-girdle muscular dystrophy.

cle function, particularly for stability of the sarcolemma. This idea is fully supported by the recent identifications of several distinct types of muscular dystrophy caused by primary defects in the components of this complex.[31]

## DYSTROPHINOPATHIES

### Clinical Phenotype

#### DMD AND BMD

DMD is one of the most severe muscular dystrophies. It was described first by Meryon[32] in 1852 and in more detail by Duchenne[33] in 1868. It begins in early childhood and progresses relatively rapidly. DMD shows an X-linked recessive inheritance pattern and affects 1 in 3300 live male births. However, one-third of patients are estimated to have *de novo* mutations.[34] Infrequently, the disease manifests in females who have abnormalities of X-chromosome structure or function, including Turner's syndrome or abnormal X-chromosome inactivation.

The disease phenotype is usually unremarkable at birth. The initial symptoms indicating muscle weakness are noted when the child starts to walk. The patients are less active than their peers and may fall frequently. At around 2 to 3 years after birth, they have increasing difficulties in walking, running, and climbing stairs. Waddling gait and the tendency of toe walking become more obvious as time passes.

In the early stage of DMD, affected muscles become enlarged but eventually decrease in size, while calf muscle hypertrophy is consistent and a characteristic feature of the disease. Weakness of abdominal and paravertebral muscles accounts for lordosis and protuberant abdomen. When arising from the ground to a standing position, the child first puts his or her hands on the floor to raise the hips and then works each hand alternately up the corresponding thigh (Gowers' maneuver).

The serum creatine kinase (CK) level is increased up to two orders of magnitude in the early stages and then decreases exponentially together with the functioning muscle mass. The clinical course is always progressive, and ambulation is usually lost at around age 10 years. Once the patient is confined to a wheelchair, contractures of hip and knee joints worsen, and severe scoliosis may develop.

Mild degrees of mental retardation, which is nonprogressive, are common. The heart is also commonly involved. Degeneration of cardiac fibers and fibrosis develop, most pronounced in the basal part of the left ventricle. Various types of arrhythmia may appear. Electrocardiography shows tall precordial R waves and deep Q waves in the left precordial and limb leads. Death usually occurs during late adolescence from pulmonary infections and respiratory failure and sometimes from cardiac decompensation.

A small portion of female carriers manifest a moderate degree of myopathy that may mimic LGMD. As discussed later, these manifesting or symptomatic carriers show a unique mosaic immunostaining pattern of dystrophin, which is helpful for genetic counseling.

BMD is an allelic variant of DMD and is characterized by its relatively benign clinical course. The onset is much later (mean age, 12 years; ranging from 5 to 45 years), progression is slower (the average age at the loss of ambulation is 25 to 30 years), and death usually occurs after the fifth decade.

BMD and DMD were distinguished originally on clinical grounds. The most widely accepted differentiating criterion is that BMD patients remain ambulatory beyond the age of 16 years. Its incidence is estimated as 3 to 6 per 100,000 male births,[35,36] which is much less frequent than that of DMD. Overall, the physical picture resembles that of DMD, although cardiac involvement is less frequent and mentation is usually normal.

#### OTHER DYSTROPHINOPATHIES

Extensive DMD gene analysis has revealed that dystrophinopathies do not always take the typical clinical pictures of DMD or BMD. There are several less common clinical forms of dystrophinopathies.

*X-linked dilated cardiomyopathy* (XLDC) is a progressive disorder that presents as congestive heart failure in the second or third decade of life.[37] There is no clinical muscle involvement, however, although the muscle-specific CK isozyme in serum may be elevated mildly or a muscle biopsy may show minimal dystrophic changes. DNA analysis data demonstrated deletions involving the muscle-specific promoter and/or exon 1.[38,39] Analyses of dystrophin mRNA expressed in skeletal muscle suggest that either the brain promoter or Purkinje cell promoter, more than 90 kb upstream of the muscle promoter, drives dystrophin transcription in skeletal muscle.[39a] In contrast, the expression of the full-length dystrophin was undetectable in cardiac muscle.[39b] This data suggests that deletions around exon 1 may lead to compensated expression of brain dystrophins, which rescue dystrophic changes in skeletal muscle but not in cardiac muscle. Reports of XLDC cases with deletions in exons 6 to 13[40] or exons 27 to 30,[41] however, suggest that different mutations outside the 5' region of the DMD gene can underlie this disorder. It remains controversial whether XLDC should be separated from the spectrum of BMD, which sometimes presents with severe cardiomyopathy.

*X-linked familial myalgic-cramp-myoglobinuric syndrome,* described by Gospe and coworkers,[42] shows minimal dystrophic pathology and a relatively nonprogressive clinical course. The patient had a deletion of the first third of the dystrophin gene.

In rarer cases, dystrophin abnormalities were also described in patients clinically diagnosed as having quadriceps myopathy,[43] myopathy with rimmed vacuoles,[44] or congenital muscular dystrophy.[45,46]

## DMD Gene Mutations

In DMD and BMD patients, the underlying DMD gene mutations can be either large rearrangements of genomic DNA (deletions or duplications) or small mutations (point mutations or microdeletions or insertions). Large deletions or duplications in the DMD gene are found in about 70% of DMD cases and in about 85% of BMD cases.[47] Both size and location of deletions are highly heterogeneous. The largest deletions, several thousand kilobases in size, remove neighboring genes and occur in association with glycerol kinase deficiency, McLeod's syndrome (acanthocytosis), chronic granulomatous disease, or retinitis pigmentosa. Smaller deletions remove from one to a few exons. The deletions are usually detected either by Southern blot analysis with dystrophin cDNA probes[48] or by multiplex polymerase chain reaction (PCR) amplification of the deletion-prone exons of the gene.[49,50] In 6% of the mutations, partial gene duplications are detected with quantitative Southern blot analysis[51] or by analysis of large gene fragments by field inversion gel electrophoresis.[52] The large mutations distribute unevenly, with two hot spots: one extending over the first 20 exons, where the introns are particularly large; and the second near the middle of the gene, around exons 45 to 53.[9] Interestingly, large mutations beyond exon 55 are rarely detected.

Mutations in the patients who do not have a large mutation are technically difficult to identify in the huge DMD gene. The frequencies of such small mutations are estimated at about 30% in DMD and 15% in BMD. More than 40 point mutations have been identified in the DMD gene by a systemic analysis of the PCR-amplified message or genomic DNA. Nonsense mutations, in which a single base change produces a stop codon, are most commonly reported. The affected exons are more or less evenly distributed between exons 2 and 76.[53] Point mutations leading to frameshift deletions and insertions and splice site mutations producing exon skipping were also reported. Promoter mutations have also been detected. The deletion of the first muscle exon and the muscle-specific promoter led to reduced expression of dystrophin in two BMD patients[54,55] or severe cardiomyopathy without muscle weakness.[38]

## Genotype–Phenotype Correlation

There is no consistent correlation between the size of a deletion or duplication and the clinical phenotype. The severity can be largely explained as a consequence of the effect of the mutation on the translational reading frame of the transcript (see Chapter 1).[56] Mutations that shift the reading frame result in a premature termination of translation and lead to a synthesis of a truncated dystrophin lacking C-terminal domains that contain interaction sites with dystrophin-associated proteins. Thus, this impairs membrane organization of dystrophin and leads to severe dystrophin deficiency and the DMD phenotype.[57]

In contrast, most nonframeshifting mutations produce internally deleted dystrophins with an intact C-terminus.[58–60] In this situation, phenotype severity is affected by the location and the functional significance of the deleted region. Those deletions involving the rod domain are usually associated with a mild BMD phenotype,[61] whereas those involving the N-terminal or C-terminal domain produce a more severe phenotype.[62] There are exceptions to the frameshift rule; the most commonly reported are in BMD cases with frameshifting deletions of exon 45 and exons 3 to 7. In the former cases, alternative splicing of exon 44 was reported to rescue a continuous reading frame, which would potentially explain the mild phenotype.[63] Although alternative splicing has also been reported in two BMD patients with a deletion of exons 3 to 7,[64] no inframe transcripts were detected in other patients, suggesting that a post-transcriptional mechanism such as ribosomal frameshifting may be involved in restoration of the mRNA reading frame.[65]

## Diagnostic Approaches for DMD and BMD

Before the identification of the DMD gene, the diagnosis of DMD and BMD was mainly based on the clinical features and the histopathological findings in muscle biopsy specimens. Now the diagnosis can be determined by DNA studies or dystrophin protein analysis. This is particularly useful for differentiating BMD from other muscle diseases, including LGMD and spinal muscular atrophy, or for carrier detection and prenatal diagnosis of DMD.

### GENOMIC DNA ANALYSIS

Deletions and duplications in the DMD gene can be detected by either Southern blot analysis with dystrophin cDNA probes[48] or multiplex PCR amplification of deletion-prone exons (Fig. 5–3).[49,50] Because the exon–intron border types on either side of a given deletion can determine its effect on the transcriptional reading frame, identification of deleted exons can predict the severity of the phenotype.[57] Recently, multiplex PCR analysis has replaced Southern blot analysis for routine diagnostic studies. Multiplex PCR analysis of 18 exons in total will detect 98% of all the DMD and BMD deletions detected by Southern blotting.[50] Duplication and carrier detection is more difficult with these methods and require quantitative analysis to distinguish the two copies of the gene segment from the single copy. Direct DNA analysis has the advantage of not requiring a muscle biopsy specimen.

### mRNA ANALYSIS

An alternative approach is to amplify cDNA sequences obtained by reverse transcription of dystrophin mRNA. RNAs isolated from biopsied skeletal muscle, as well as blood cells that contain enough illegitimate transcription, can be used as a starting material. This type of analysis can detect not only deletions and duplications but also the frameshift status of the mutant mRNA by sequencing. Single-strand conformational polymorphism (SSCP) analysis or heteroduplex analysis of PCR products may be helpful for narrowing down the region containing a small mutation. *In vitro* transcription and translation of PCR products, followed by detection of an aberrant size of dystrophin peptides (protein truncation test), offers a useful method for identifying null mutations.[66]

### DYSTROPHIN ANALYSIS

Dystrophin analysis by immunohistochemistry or immunoblotting can detect the defects in the DMD gene product, irrespective of the underlying mutation. Immunostaining of muscle sections with antidystrophin antibodies can examine the normal sarcolemmal localization of dystrophin (Fig. 5–4 *A*), which seems crucial for its biological function. Dystrophin staining is negative, with the exception of rare reverent fibers, in DMD patients (Fig. 5–4 *B*). In BMD muscle, the sarcolemmal staining of dystrophin is de-

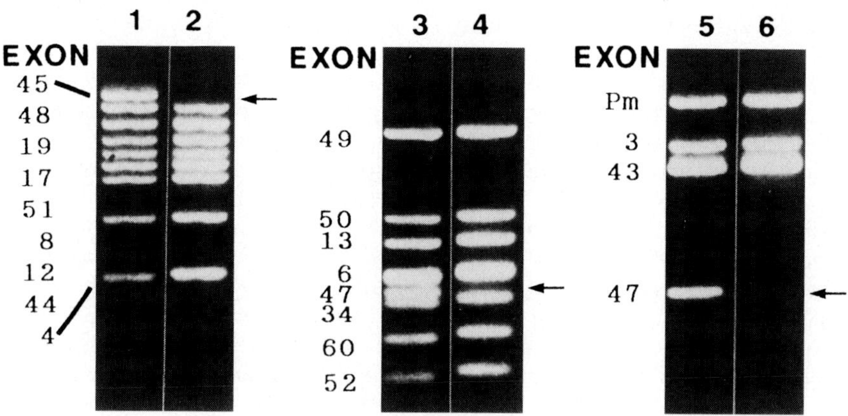


**Figure 5–3.** Multiplex PCR analysis of the DMD gene. Lanes 1, 3, 5, normal control; lanes 2, 4, 6, DMD patient with a deletion of exons 45 to 47. Arrows indicate the missing exons. (Courtesy of Dr. K. Arahata.)

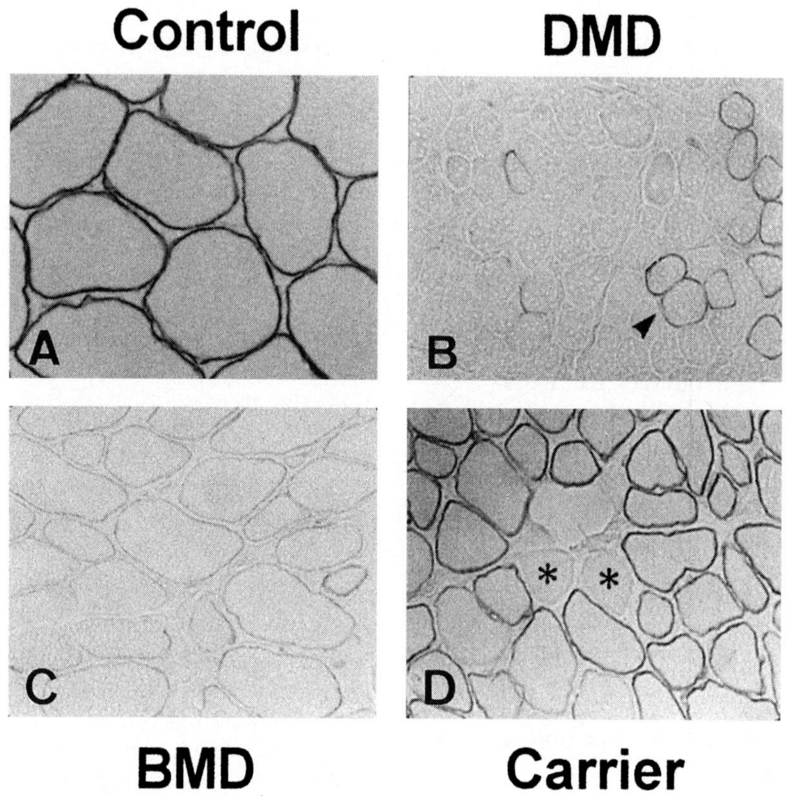


**Figure 5–4.** Immunohistochemistry of skeletal muscle cryosections with an antidystrophin monoclonal antibody. *(A)* Normal control muscle shows homogeneous sarcolemmal localization of dystrophin. *(B)* Negative dystrophin staining in DMD muscle with exceptional revertant fibers (arrowhead). *(C)* Diffuse reduction of dystrophin staining in BMD muscle. *(D)* "Mosaic" pattern of dystrophin staining in a manifesting carrier. Asterisks indicate dystrophin-negative fibers. (Magnifications are variable.)

creased in a diffuse or patchy manner (Fig. 5–4 *C*).[60,67] A patchy staining pattern for BMD diagnosis may be less reliable, however, because it has been observed nonspecifically in other muscle disorders or in poorly stored muscle biopsy materials. Immunoblotting analysis is more informative for the diagnosis of BMD. Manifesting carriers also exhibit a "mosaic" or "patchy" pattern of staining with a mixture of positive and negative fibers (Fig. 5–4 *D*).[67,68] Although asymptomatic carriers may have less abundant dystrophin-negative fibers, the reliability of immunohistochemistry in detecting obligate carriers may not be feasible.

Immunoblot analysis of muscle homogenates with antidystrophin antibodies can provide information on the abundance and size of dystrophin in muscle and the portions of the molecule that are preserved or deleted. Initially immunoblot analysis studies suggested that DMD patients have no detectable dystrophin, whereas most BMD patients have dystrophin of abnormal size (Fig. 5–5).[69] Subsequent extensive studies[59,67,70] with region-specific antibodies and quantitative densitometry demonstrated that

1. In most DMD patients, C-terminal antibodies detect absence of dystrophin, whereas N-terminal or rod domain antibodies detect truncated dystrophin species in a decreased amount.
2. In most cases of BMD, either N- or C-terminal antibodies detect a reduced amount of dystrophin of abnormal size; however, an exception occurs when a given antibody is directed against a deleted epitope.
3. Overall, the abundance of residual dystrophin correlates well with the disease severity.

Ideally, immunoblot analysis should be performed with multiple antibodies directed against different regions of dystrophin (N-terminal, rod domain, and C-terminal). The C-terminal antibody is of particular value in differentiating between DMD and BMD.

**Figure 5–5.** Dystrophin immunoblot analysis with an antidystrophin C-terminal antibody. Normal dystrophin of approximately 400 kDa was detected in normal control lanes, and dystrophin was undetectable in DMD. In a BMD patient, mutant dystrophin with a smaller molecular weight was detectable. The lower panel shows Coomassie blue staining of myosin heavy chain indicating a comparable amount of samples loaded. (Courtesy of Dr. K. Arahata.)

## GUIDELINES FOR DIAGNOSIS

The diagnostic approach for DMD and BMD can vary depending on the cost and availability of the various diagnostic methods. Widely accepted diagnostic guidelines follow:

1. If the patient has a family history of DMD or BMD that is confirmed by gene or protein analysis, the clinical findings alone are sufficient for the diagnosis.
2. For diagnosis of novel cases, multiplex PCR analysis identifies nearly all deletion cases, accounting for at least 65% of the dystrophinopathies. Southern blot analysis is more reliable than PCR for detecting duplications and for determining whether a deletion or duplication is frame shifting. Southern blot is, however, more laborious than PCR.
3. If PCR or Southern analysis fails to detect any deletion or duplication, immunohistochemical analysis of dystrophin in biopsied muscle is valuable for the diagnosis. Immunostaining can identify DMD, BMD, and manifesting heterozygosity based on unique staining patterns.
4. If BMD is suspected by immunohistochemical analysis, the diagnosis can be confirmed by immunoblot analysis.
5. To identify small mutations, mRNA analysis by a reverse-transcribed PCR or protein-truncation test is required, which can be done in selected diagnostic laboratories.

### CARRIER DETECTION

Before the advent of DMD gene cloning, serum CK assay was the most reliable tool for carrier detection. Now various diagnostic methods, including multiplex PCR, Southern blotting, and immunostaining, usually employed to diagnose affected patients, can be used for carrier detection. If these methods are not feasible or fail, carrier detection can be achieved through linkage analysis to determine the presence or absence of a mutant allele by following the inheritance of closely linked markers.

Highly polymorphic CA dinucleotide repeats have been described at the 5' end,[71,72] at the 3' end,[73,74] and in the middle of the gene.[75] These are now the markers of choice for linkage analysis for carrier detection and prenatal diagnosis. Intragenic recombination still prevents accuracy of carrier detection, however, because the recombination rate across the gene has been estimated at 11% based on these markers.[72,76] Even if the above methods fail to detect carriers, protein analysis by immunoblotting or immunostaining may succeed, but this approach requires invasive muscle biopsy.

In addition, germline mosaicism greatly complicates the determination of carrier status because up to 20% of sporadic DMD cases are estimated to be caused by germline mosaicism,[77] in which no mutation can be identified in somatic cells. The risk of having a second affected son or a carrier daughter depends on the proportion of the mother's germ cells carrying the mutation. Thus, all mothers of an affected boy have a significant recurrence risk even when the mutation is not present in their blood cell DNA, and for this reason prenatal diagnosis is recommended for all such women.

### PRENATAL DIAGNOSIS

For the 65% of DMD families carrying a detectable deletion or duplication, prenatal diagnostic procedure in a subsequent pregnancy is to look for the mutation in fetal cells obtained by chorionic villus sampling or by amniocentesis. If the dystrophin mutation in the family is not identified, linkage analysis of fetal cells is often the only recourse. Otherwise, a sonographically guided fetal muscle biopsy specimens, obtained after 19 weeks of gestation, can provide tissue for dystrophin analysis.[78] The risks of this procedure are still undetermined.

## Animal Models

### THE *MDX* MOUSE.

The *mdx* mutant mouse, reported in 1984, has been proven to carry a nonsense mutation in the dystrophin gene on the X chromosome.[79] The mutation abolishes the production of full-length dystrophin but not the distal transcripts such as Dp71. Despite very high serum CK levels and dystrophic muscle pathology, the affected mice show little if any disability and are able to breed. Muscle fiber necrosis increases abruptly at 20 days after birth and then decreases after 60 days and reaches a stable low frequency during the adult life. The diaphragm shows the most severe dystrophic changes, but there is no respiratory impairment.[80] The relatively mild phenotype of dystrophin deficiency in the *mdx* mouse is still not understood.

The *mdx*$^{3CV}$ is another *mdx* mutation produced by chemical mutagenesis and expresses neither full-length dystrophin nor Dp71.[81] The *mdx*$^{3CV}$ mouse differs from the *mdx* mouse only in that fewer offspring survive per litter. These murine models have been useful in the study of mechanisms of muscle degeneration and the evaluation of therapeutic approaches to dystrophin deficiency.

### CANINE X-LINKED MUSCULAR DYSTROPHY

Dystrophin deficiency has been also demonstrated in dystrophic dogs, which is best characterized in golden retrievers.[82] Dystrophic dogs have a severe muscle wasting disease comparable with DMD in humans. The disease is caused by a splice acceptor site mutation of intron 6, resulting in skipping of exons 6 to 8, which results in frameshifting.[83]

## Gene Therapy

There is as yet no effective treatment that can arrest the progression of DMD. The discovery of the dystrophin gene, however, has raised the hope that the progressive course of the disease might be mitigated by introduction of the normal dystrophin gene into a patient's muscle. Myoblast transfer and gene therapy are the two potential approaches.

### MYOBLAST TRANSFER

Injected normal myoblasts carrying an intact DMD gene into dystrophin-deficient muscle are expected to fuse with the existing myofibers; dystrophin encoded by the normal nuclei might rescue the dystrophic process. Initial experimental studies with *mdx* mice demonstrated that the donor cells fuse with the existing muscle and produce dystrophin.[84,85] Based on the limited studies in mice, clinical trials of human myoblast transfer have been started. Four groups of investigators have reported the feasibility, safety, and efficiency of myoblast transfer in DMD.[86–89] All trials showed no serious adverse reaction to the injection of myoblasts, suggesting the safety of this method. Double-blind trials, however, have shown little or no clinical improvement, indicating difficulties in the establishment of myoblast transfer as a valuable approach to the treatment of DMD.

The overall inefficiency of myoblast transfer may be attributed to *(1)* poor mobility of the injected myoblasts through connective tissue barriers, *(2)* failure of myoblasts to fuse with nonregenerating myofibers, *(3)* poor replicative capacity of the donor myoblasts, and *(4)* possible silent immunorejection. Even if these problems could be cleared, the repeated injections of multiple muscles and the inaccessibility of many muscles, including diaphragm, would limit the usefulness of myoblast transfer in the treatment of DMD. As an alternative to direct intramuscular injection, intra-arterial injection was shown to deliver myoblasts to muscle.[90]

### GENE THERAPY

The introduction of short or full-length dystrophin cDNA in a form of plasmid DNA into the germline of *mdx* mice to produce transgenic mice has shown the correction of the muscle pathology and recovery of force generation.[91] Experiments also indicated no deleterious effect of overexpressed dystrophin in skeletal muscle. Although plasmids may be adequate for delivering genes to transgenic mice, they may be quite inefficient at delivering genes to muscle for gene therapy. A promising approach utilizes viral vectors for gene therapy. Viral vectors must be replication defective, be able to carry long DNA inserts, and be able to enter postmitotic cells. With direct injection of recombinant retrovirus vectors, up to 6% of adult *mdx* fibers of the injected muscle expressed dystrophin.[92]

Greater efficiency has been reported for recombinant adenovirus constructs containing minidystrophin cDNA due to a limited capacity for foreign DNA, when injected into young *mdx* muscle.[93,94] This produced dystrophin expression in up to 50% of the muscle fibers 15 days after the injection, which was maintained up to 6 months. Limitations of this approach are *(1)* inability to accommodate the 14 kb full-length dystrophin cDNA, *(2)* inflammatory reactions induced in the recipient, and *(3)* limited longevity because the adenoviral constructs are not integrated into the host's genome. A third-generation adenoviral vector has been developed that contains no viral genes and encodes approximately 28 kb of foreign DNA, including the full-length dystrophin cDNA, with the muscle CK promotor.[95] Intramuscular injection of this construct showed efficient delivery and regional expression of the full-length dystrophin, resulting in the restoration of skeletal muscle membrane stability.[96] Further studies are required to develop a systemic method of adenoviral delivery to skeletal muscle.

Another option for potential DMD therapy came from an exciting recent report that overexpressed utrophin, an autosomal homologue of dystrophin, can functionally replace dystrophin and rescue the dystrophic phenotype in *mdx* mice.[97a] The identification of regulatory elements that can upregulate utrophin expression in dystrophin-deficient muscle could provide a novel therapeutic strategy to fight DMD. Altogether, these experiments demonstrate the potential for gene therapy for DMD, but many hurdles remain to be cleared before human gene therapy will be ready for clinical trials.

## CONGENITAL MUSCULAR DYSTROPHY

Congenital muscular dystrophy (CMD) is a group of clinically and genetically heterogeneous disorders characterized by muscle weakness and hypotonia at birth, or in the first few months of life, and delayed motor development. Contractures are a common clinical feature, and the serum CK levels are high, particularly in the early stages of the disease. The most noticeable features of muscle histopathology are a wide variation in fiber size and a marked increase in endomysial connective tissue. Degenerating or regenerating fibers are less abundant than in other muscular dystrophies such as DMD and BMD.

Several forms of CMD have been described. In the classic or occidental form of CMD, clinical manifestations are limited to skeletal muscle with no clinical involvement of the central nervous system. Two groups of classic-type CMD cases can be distinguished according to the status of merosin (laminin $\alpha_2$-chain); about half of the cases are merosin-negative CMD. There is another major group of CMD that is associated with severe brain anomalies, including Fukuyama-type CMD (FCMD), Walker-Warburg syndrome, and muscle-eye-brain disease.

### Merosin-negative CMD (merosinopathy)

#### MEROSIN: STRUCTURE AND FUNCTION

Laminins are major components of the extracellular matrix and are heterotrimeric molecules consisting of three distinct laminin chains ($\alpha$, $\beta$, and $\gamma$) (Fig. 5–6).[98] Each chain has multiple isoforms and is assembled into different types of laminins with different combinations of isoforms.[99] In skeletal muscle and peripheral nerve, $\alpha$-dystroglycan mainly binds the $\alpha_2$-chain of laminin-2 (formerly called *merosin*).[100,101] Laminin $\alpha_2$-chain was first isolated from human placenta as a laminin $\alpha_1$-chain homologue and is predominantly expressed in striated muscle, peripheral nerve, and placenta.[102–104] Laminin-2 ($\alpha_2$, $\beta_1$, $\gamma_1$) has been indicated to have various biological functions. These include cell attachment, neurite outgrowth promotion,[105] Schwann cell migration,[106] and formation of supramolecular structures by either self-aggregation or interaction with other components (collagen type IV and entactin) of the basal lamina.[107]

The complete primary structure of the laminin $\alpha_2$-chain has been determined in

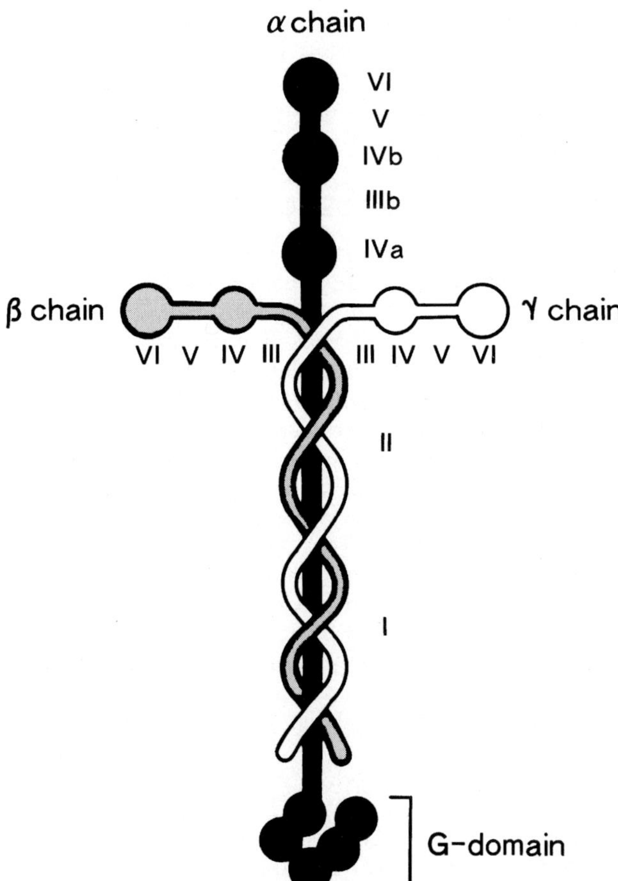


**Figure 5–6.** A schematic model for a laminin heterotrimer. Laminins consist of one longer α2-chain and two shorter β and γ-chains. Laminin $\alpha_2$-chain is a native ligand for dystroglycan in skeletal muscle and peripheral nerve and deficient in merosin-negative CMD.

human[108] and mouse[109] by cDNA cloning. The laminin α2-chain has a domain structure similar to that of the $\alpha_1$-chain (Fig. 5–6); domains VI, IVb, and IVa are predicted to form globular structures. Domains V, IIIb, and IIIa contain cysteine-rich epidermal growth factor–like repeats and are predicted to form rigid rod-like structures. Domains I and II are involved in the formation of a triple-stranded coiled-coil structure that forms the long arm of the laminin heterotrimer together with β and γ-chains. The C-terminal region contains five internal homologous repeats to form a large globular domain (G domain). Laminin heterotrimers self-aggregate in the presence of $Ca^{2+}$ ions and in an entropy-driven manner.[107] In this process, the N-terminal short domains of each chain, including domain VI, interact together and eventually form an independent network in the basal lamina.[110,111] In addition, the laminin network crosslinks to the type IV collagen network via entactin and forms a rigid meshwork in the mature basal lamina. The human α2-chain gene has been mapped to chromosome 6q2[108] and mouse $\alpha_2$-chain gene to a proximal portion of chromosome 10.[100]

## CLINICAL PHENOTYPE

Tomè and colleagues[112] first reported selective laminin $\alpha_2$-chain deficiency in the skeletal muscle in 13 cases of classic-type CMD. They reported the expression of β-and γ-chain comparable with that in controls and upregulated expression of the $\alpha_1$-chain. In some cases of classic-type CMD, expression of the $\alpha_2$-chain was quite normal (merosin-positive CMD), suggestive of genetic heterogeneity of classic-type CMD. Subsequently, homozygosity mapping demonstrated that merosin-negative CMD is linked to chromosome 6q2 in the region containing the $\alpha_2$-chain *(LAMA2)* gene, whereas this linkage was excluded in patients with merosin-positive CMD.[113] Thus, merosin-negative CMD is now considered an established disease entity separate from heterogeneous classic-type CMD.

When compared with merosin-positive CMD, patients with merosin-negative CMD usually show a more severe phenotype; these patients do not achieve independent ambulation, and the serum CK levels are high (>1000 IU/l).[114] A recent histological study of muscle revealed that a transient inflammatory process may occur in the early stages, which leads to the clinical diagnosis of inflammatory myopathy.[115] The clinical phenotype of merosin-negative CMD is most specifically characterized by abnormal high-intensity signals in the brain white matter detected by $T_2$-weighted magnetic resonance imaging (MRI).[113,114] Delayed motor nerve conduction velocity studies suggest the presence of dysmyelination of peripheral nerve.[116] Genetic and biochemical approaches in the diagnosis of merosin-negative CMD, however revealed that the clinical term CMD does not include all merosin-deficient patients. Case reports of merosin-deficient patients with late onset of clinical symptoms illustrate the broad spectrum of disease severity.[117]

## LAMININ $\alpha_2$-CHAIN GENE MUTATIONS

The initial mutation study showed a splice site and a nonsense mutation in two CMD families exhibiting complete deficiency of merosin in muscle biopsies.[118] In one family, a homozygous splice site mutation caused skipping of exon 31 and resulted in a frameshift leading to premature termination in domain II. In the other family, a homozygous nonsense mutation at nucleotide 3767 was identified, which results in premature termination in domain IVa. A large deletion spanning at least 50% of the $\alpha_2$-chain coding sequence was reported in combination with a single base deletion in a compound heterozygous patient with complete merosin deficiency.[115] In partial merosin deficiency, the homozygous missense mutation Cys996Arg[119] and a splice site mutation leading to an inframe deletion of exon 25[120] were identified in a consanguineous Turkish and Saudi family, respectively.

## DIAGNOSTIC APPROACHES

An important clue to the clinical diagnosis of merosin-negative CMD is a high-intensity signal of the brain white matter by $T_2$-weighted MRI. The diagnosis is usually confirmed by immunofluorescence analysis of either skeletal muscle or skin biopsy material.[121] The diagnosis of partial deficiency is less reliable based on the merosin immunostaining alone, however, because secondary deficiency was reported in patients with FCMD.[122] In the diagnosis of partial deficiency, immunoblotting sometimes may be valuable if it detects the expression of the truncated protein.[120]

For identification of the *LAMA2* gene mutation, a practical approach is a systematic analysis of overlapping reverse-transcribed PCR fragments spanning the entire coding region because of the huge size of the gene. SSCP analysis of PCR fragments that can detect aberrant conformers may facilitate the mutation screening. Because the genomic structure of the *LAMA2* gene has been published,[123] one can start with genomic DNA samples for mutation analysis.

Prenatal diagnosis is possible by investigation of the expression of laminin $\alpha_2$-chain in fetal trophoblast tissue from chorionic villus sampling[124] or by haplotype studies for linkage analysis. Normal expression of merosin in fetal trophoblast tissue is taken as an indication for a healthy fetus in affected families.

## ANIMAL MODELS: DYSTROPHIA MUSCULARIS AND *DY$^{2J}$* MICE

An animal model for laminin $\alpha_2$-deficient CMD is the dystrophia muscularis *(dy)* mouse, which is characterized by muscle degeneration and developmental dysmyelination. The mouse $\alpha_2$-chain gene maps to the same region of mouse chromosome 10 to which the *dy* locus has been assigned.[100] Analysis of $\alpha_2$-chain expression in *dy/dy* mice revealed a specific deficiency of the $\alpha_2$-chain in skeletal and cardiac muscles and peripheral nerve.[100,125,126] This data suggests that $\alpha_2$-chain deficiency may be a primary cause of the *dy* phenotype.

The allelic strain $dy^{2J}$ mouse shows a less severe phenotype. Immunofluorescence demonstrated less severe reduction of $\alpha_2$-chain staining. Interestingly, $dy^{2J}$ mice expressed a truncated $\alpha_2$-chain.[127,128] A splice donor site mutation and resulting mutant transcripts have been identified.[127,128] A major variant encoding the truncated $\alpha_2$-chain has a 57 amino acid deletion in the N-terminal domain VI that is critical for self-aggregation of laminin-2 heterotrimers.[128] Thus, this mutation may disrupt the formation of the laminin network in the basal lamina.

### Merosin-Positive CMD

Merosin-positive CMD still encompasses genetically and clinically heterogeneous diseases. Recently, a deficiency of α-actinin 3, a type 2 fiber–specific isoform of α-actinin, one of the actin-binding proteins, was demonstrated in skeletal muscle of merosin-positive CMD patients.[129] Mutation analysis in affected patients has to confirm the specificity of this finding.

### Fukuyama-Type CMD

FCMD is a unique type of congenital muscular dystrophy that, in combination with a developmental defect of the central nervous system,[130] has been almost completely confined to Japan, where it is the second most common form of muscular dystrophy. Clinically all patients show a severe delay in intellectual development in addition to skeletal muscle symptoms such as hypotonia, weakness, atrophy, and joint contractures. Epileptic seizures are common. Motor development is greatly retarded. Although many children are able to sit and crawl, only a few can stand at 4 years of age. The average age of death is 16 years. Brain malformation commonly seen in this disease is cerebral and cerebellar cortical dysplasia (polymicrogyria) probably due to a defect in neuronal migration.

By linkage disequilibrium mapping, the gene locus of FCMD was initially mapped to chromosome 9q31–33.[131] And then narrowed down to within 100 kb of D9S2107.[132] Haplotype analysis with three satellite markers in this region revealed a founder haplotype that is now valuable for prenatal and carrier diagnosis.[132] Most Japanese cases are caused by a retrotransposal insertion into the 3' untranslated region of a novel gene. The encoded protein, termed *fukutin,* is a 461 amino acid protein that may be secreted.[133]

## LIMB-GIRDLE MUSCULAR DYSTROPHY

### Genetic Heterogeneity of LGMD

The limb-girdle muscular dystrophies (LGMD), named by Walton and Nattrass,[134] represent a heterogeneous group of diseases that are characterized by progressive weakness of the pelvic and shoulder girdle muscles. These diseases may be inherited as an autosomal dominant or recessive trait, the latter being more common, with an estimated prevalence of 1 in 100,000 individuals.[135] The existence of this group as a separate disease entity had been questioned for a long time because clinical symptoms overlap with those of BMD patients, manifesting carriers of DMD, patients with spinal muscular atrophy, and patients with metabolic myopathies. Mutations in the six different genes implicated in autosomal recessive LGMD have been identified, however, and one gene locus for an autosomal recessive form determined.

Because of difficulties in classifying LGMD based on the clinical pictures, the European Neuromuscular Center recommended a new classification based on the chromosomal localization of the morbid genes.[136] To date, several genes have been implicated in the etiology of these disorders. The autosomal dominant form, LGMD 1A, was mapped to 5q22–34, whereas seven genes involved in the autosomal recessive forms were mapped to chromosomes 15q15.1 (LGMD 2A), 2p13–16

(LGMD 2B), 13q12 (LGMD 2C), 17q12–21.33 (LGMD 2D), 4q12 (LGMD 2E), 5q33 (LGMD 2F), and 17q11–12 (LGMD 2G). The gene involved in LGMD 2B has recently been identified and the gene product designated *dysferlin.*[137] Mutations in the same gene also cause Miyoshi distal myopathy.[137,137a]

## Sarcoglycanopathies

Extensive analysis of dystrophin-associated proteins in various types of muscular dystrophy revealed a deficiency of α-sarcoglycan (adhalin) in severe childhood autosomal recessive muscular dystrophy (SCARMD) patients in North Africa.[138] SCARMD resembles the DMD phenotype but affects both males and females at equal rates.[137] SCARMD was originally described in Tunisia[139] and then reported from other North African[140] and Middle Eastern countries,[141] Western Europe,[142] and Japan.[143] In several North African families, SCARMD has been linked to chromosome 13q (LGMD 2C)[140,144]; however, this linkage was excluded in other families, including North African families[145–147] suggesting genetic heterogeneity of SCARMD. As discussed later, because of genetic and phenotypic heterogeneity, SCARMD is considered now as a term describing the severity of the phenotype rather than a discrete disease entity.

Primary defects involving four distinct genes were recently shown to cause the SCARMD phenotype. *(1)* the α-sarcoglycan gene at the LGMD 2D locus (17q12–21.33),[148,149] *(2)* the β-sarcoglycan gene at the LGMD 2E locus (4q12),[150,151] *(3)* the γ-sarcoglycan gene at the LGMD 2C locus (13q12),[152] and *(4)* the δ-sarcoglycan gene at the LGMD 2F locus (5q33).[153] These four transmembrane glycoproteins tightly associate and form the sarcoglycan complex in the DGC. A primary deficiency of one component leads to the concomitant reduction of the other three components and results in loss of the whole sarcoglycan complex. Thus, the term *sarcoglycanopathy* has been proposed to represent the muscular dystrophy that is caused by a primary defect in one of four sarcoglycans.[152]

### LGMD 2D: α-SARCOGLYCAN MUTATIONS

In 1995, the human α-sarcoglycan (formerly called *adhalin*) gene (cDNA) was cloned, and the gene locus was mapped to chromosome 17q12–21.33,[148,149] excluding the gene from involvement in 13q-linked SCARMD (LGMD 2C). An intragenic polymorphic marker of the α-sarcoglycan gene, however, was linked to autosomal recessive LGMD in one large French family and missense mutations (compound heterozygotes for Arg98His and Val175Ala) were identified in this family.[148] Since then, an increasing number of α-sarcoglycan gene mutations have been reported in LGMD patients of different ethnic origins with various levels of severity.[154–156] Now, autosomal recessive muscular dystrophy caused by mutations in the α-sarcoglycan gene is classified as LGMD 2D.

The primary structure of α-sarcoglycan predicts a 387 amino acid protein having a single transmembrane domain, two potential N-linked glycosylation sites in the putative extracellular domain, and one consensus site for phosphorylation by $Ca^{2+}$/calmodulin-dependent protein kinase. The N-terminal extracellular domain comprises four closely spaced Cys residues with limited homology to entactin and nerve growth factor receptor, suggesting that α-sarcoglycan may serve as a receptor for an extracellular matrix protein. The expression of α-sarcoglycan is restricted to skeletal, cardiac, and selected smooth muscles. This tissue distribution pattern is consistent with the clinical feature of SCARMD but lacking mental retardation, which is often observed in DMD and BMD.

To date, 25 different mutations have been reported.[157] Interestingly, all the missense mutations occur in the extracellular domain. Among mutations thus far identified, Arg77Cys is the most frequent mutation, which is carried by unrelated subjects on different haplotype backgrounds. Such missense mutations that introduce an additional Cys in the extracellular domain may alter the secondary structure of the protein by rearrangement of the disulfide bond formation. The severity of the phenotype varies greatly from case to case. Patients with null mutations have a SCARMD phenotype. Missense mutations produce a broad range of severity, including a very mild phenotype of exercise intolerance with elevated serum CK levels.

## LGMD 2E: β-SARCOGLYCAN MUTATIONS

Autosomal recessive LGMD among the Amish population of northern and southern Indiana were described by Jackson and colleagues.[158,159] Most of the families in these communities are interrelated by multiple consanguineous links and can be traced back to a common ancestry from Switzerland in the eighteenth and nineteenth centuries.[158] LGMD families from northern Indiana were shown to carry the same Arg769GIn calpain 3 mutation[160] (LGMD 2A) as described later, whereas involvement of this locus was excluded in southern Indiana LGMD families. This genetic heterogeneity of LGMD within this community was quite unexpected. Furthermore, the other known LGMD loci were all excluded, suggesting the existence of yet another locus, LGMD 2E, involved in autosomal recessive LGMD.[161]

β-Sarcoglycan is a 43 kDa transmembrane component of the DGC. In 1995, cloning of the β-sarcoglycan gene (cDNA) was achieved independently by two groups.[150,151] A single open reading frame encodes a 318 amino acid protein with a deduced molecular mass of approximately 35 kDa. The primary structure predicts a single transmembrane domain and no functional signal sequence at the N terminus, indicating that β-sarcoglycan is a type II transmembrane protein that has N-terminal cytoplasmic and C-terminal extracellular segments. This membrane topology is consistent with the location of three putative N-linked glycosylation sites, all of which are C-terminal to the transmembrane domain. β-Sarcoglycan mRNA is expressed in various tissues, including brain, and is particularly enriched in skeletal and. cardiac muscle. The β-sarcoglycan gene was assigned to chromosome 4q12 by fluorescence *in situ* hybridization (FISH) with cosmid clones as probes.

Lim and colleagues[150] mapped LGMD 2E to chromosome 4q12 and identified a missense mutation (Thr151Arg) in the β-sarcoglycan gene, which is present in a homozygous state in all affected Amish patients from southern Indiana. In parallel, Bönnemann and colleagues[151] also identified a sporadic case of Duchenne-like LGMD with a frameshifting and a nonsense mutation in a compound heterozygous state. Genomic screening for a β-sarcoglycan gene mutation in 15 Brazilian LGMD patients identified one frameshifting 2 bp deletion at nucleotide 164 and three missense mutations: Arg91Pro, Met100Lys, and Leu108Arg.[162] Patients with these missense mutations showed a severe DMD-like phenotype in contrast to the milder phenotype in the Amish patients.[162]

## LGMD 2C: γ-SARCOGLYCAN MUTATIONS

γ-Sarcoglycan is a 35 kDa transmembrane glycoprotein. Noguchi and colleagues[152] obtained the cDNA clones encoding human and rabbit γ-sarcoglycan. The predicted protein contains 291 amino acids with a deduced molecular mass of 32.3 kDa. Like β-sarcoglycan, γ-sarcoglycan is considered a type II transmembrane protein with an extracellular C terminus. γ-Sarcoglycan has no significant homologies with other known proteins and is expressed exclusively in skeletal and cardiac muscle. The γ-sarcoglycan gene maps to chromosome 13q12, the same region implicated in Tunisian 13q-linked SCARMD families by linkage analysis.[152] Linkage disequilibrium was demonstrated with the marker D13S232, suggesting that both alleles of the responsible gene should carry an identical mutation in 13q-linked SCARMD families in North Africa.[163] A deletion of a single thymidine base from the span of nucleotides 521 to 525 was identified in three Tunisian SCARMD families and was linked to 13q12.[152] This single base deletion alters the reading frame and produces a stop codon at amino acid 193.

In addition, a 73 bp deletion in the γ-sarcoglycan transcript, producing a premature stop codon at 170, was identified in a sporadic case in Japan.[152] Recent reports described four additional homozygous microdeletions or microinsertions at nucleotide positions 87, 521, 793, and 801 in patients from the United States and Italy[164] and a founder homozygous missense mutation Cys283Tyr in Gypsy families.[165] These results suggest that LGMD 2C is not confined to the North African population, but could affect various ethnic populations. LGMD 2C in the North African population generally presents a severe DMD-like phenotype; however, the identical mutation has been shown to cause much milder symptoms in a Brazilian family, suggesting the presence of other factors that may modify the clinical course.[166]

#### LGMD 2F: δ-SARCOGLYCAN MUTATIONS

The δ-sarcoglycan is a second 35 kDa sarcolemmal glycoprotein that shares high homology with γ-sarcoglycan and is expressed mainly in skeletal and cardiac muscle.[167,168] Despite their similar molecular weights and amino acid sequences, γ- and δ-sarcoglycans are separate entities within the sarcoglycan complex.[166] The δ-sarcoglycan gene was mapped to chromosome 5q33[167,168] within the disease interval for LGMD 2F, which was originally reported in a Brazilian family.[169] Meanwhile, a mutation in the δ-sarcoglycan gene was identified in this family, which indicates that the δ-sarcoglycan gene is the causative gene for LGMD 2F.[153]

#### DIAGNOSIS OF SARCOGLYCANOPATHY

The diagnosis of sarcoglycanopathy can be achieved by immunofluorescence or immunoblotting analysis of sarcoglycans. These methods, however, do not allow a reliable diagnosis to distinguish the four different sarcoglycanopathies because primary defects in a single sarcoglycan usually result in the reduced expression of all sarcoglycans. Thus far there does not seem to be a phenotypic difference between the disorders, and the clinical severity in the patients is highly variable. Unless linkage analysis data is available, mutation assays of genomic DNA recently established for the sarcoglycan genes are required.[154,162,168] Denaturing gradient gel electrophoresis or SSCP analysis may be helpful to narrow down the region to be sequenced for identifying mutations.

#### GENOTYPE–PHENOTYPE CORRELATION

A genotype–phenotype correlation for distinct mutations is not yet applicable. Patients with the same mutation had different phenotypes, and a missense mutation can be as severe as null mutations. In general, autosomal recessive LGMD 2A and 2B present a milder phenotype than sarcoglycanopathies.

### LGMD 2A: Calpain 3 Mutations

Beckman and coworkers[170] mapped a form of autosomal recessive LGMD that in the La Reunion island and the northern Indiana Amish community is present on chromosome 15q15.1–q21.1.[168] This form of LGMD is designated as LGMD 2A based on the European Neuromuscular Center classification. The clinical phenotype is characterized by onset in late childhood (usually between ages 8 and 15 years) and a moderate progression (loss of ambulation around age 30 years). Both the shoulder and pelvic girdles are affected. The muscle weakness varies considerably in severity. The gene encoding the muscle-specific proteolytic enzyme calpain 3 was one of several candidate genes that showed muscle-specific expression in this region. The systematic screening of this gene in LGMD families linked to the 15q locus led to the identification of 15 different mutations that showed complete segregation with the disease phenotype, establishing that mutations in calpain 3 are responsible for LGMD 2A.[160]

This is the first demonstration that an enzymatic rather than a structural protein defect causes muscular dystrophy. For mutation screening, PCR primers were used to amplify the exons, splice junctions, and regions containing putative promoter and polyadenylation signals. Heteroduplex analyses on PCR products followed by DNA sequencing can detect mutations.[160]

## OTHER MUSCULAR DYSTROPHIES

### Emery-Dreifuss Muscular Dystrophy

#### CLINICAL PHENOTYPE

Emery-Dreifuss muscular dystrophy (EDMD) is a relatively mild muscular dystrophy mimicking BMD but has distinct clinical features, most notably early joint contractures and a cardiac conduction defect.[171,172] Onset occurs in the first decade with toe walking and flexion contracture of the elbows. Recognition of this distinct pattern of early contractures and scapulohumeroperoneal distribution of weakness is a clinical clue to diagnosis. In the early stage, the biceps, triceps, and anterior tibial and peroneal muscles are predominantly affected, giving a humeroperoneal distribution. Later the pectoral girdle and pelvic girdle muscles become affected. Another consistent feature is a cardiac conduction defect that may lead to sudden death. There are no reports of significant intellectual impairment as occurs in DMD. Serum CK level is usually elevated in mild degrees (3- to 10-fold over normal levels), considerably lower than that in DMD and BMD. Electromyographic examination shows both myopathic changes and evidence of denervation.

#### GENETICS

EDMD is usually inherited as an X-linked recessive trait, although rare families with a similar clinical picture show autosomal dominant inheritance.[173] The disease has been mapped to distal Xq28, between the DXS52/DXS15 loci and the clotting factor eight (FVIII) gene.[174] Among several candidate genes in this region, unique mutations in EDMD patients were identified in the *STA* gene, encoding a serine-rich protein of 254 amino acids, now called *emerin*.[175] The *STA* gene comprises six exons spanning 2.1 kb of genomic DNA. It encodes a 1218 nucleotide mRNA that is expressed ubiquitously. The primary structure of emerin predicts type II integral membrane protein. Antisera against emerin synthetic peptides detect a 34 kDa protein that is expressed in the nuclear membrane of muscle cells.[176] The specific deficiency of emerin was demonstrated in skeletal muscle from EDMD patients.[176]

A total of 45 different mutations in the *STA* gene from 50 families had been reported by the time of the second international workshop on EDMD in 1996.[177] These mutations are scattered throughout the gene without mutation hot spots, and most are nonsense, frameshift, or putative splice site mutations. For mutation analysis, several different primers to amplify the *STA* gene from patient DNA samples were published.[178,179] Screening of the emerin coding region by SSCP, heteroduplex analysis, or direct sequencing has identified mutations in almost all X-linked EDMD families, as opposed to sporadic cases of EDMD in which only 14 mutations have been found in over 100 patients studied.[177] The molecular pathogenesis regarding how emerin deficiency leads to muscle degeneration remains unknown.

### Bethlem's Myopathy

Bethlem's myopathy is a rare, benign autosomal dominant myopathy that was first described by Bethlem and van Wijingaarden in 1976.[180] The clinical onset is in early childhood, but progression is slow without significant disability or decrease in life expectancy. Most of the patients have early flexion contractures of the elbows, ankles, and fingers. Mild muscle weakness and atrophy occur more predominantly in the proximal muscles than distal muscles. Cardiac muscle is not involved. The serum CK levels range from normal to four times normal. Muscle histology exhibits nonspecific myopathic changes without significant dystrophic features.

Linkage analyses in Dutch families localized the gene locus to 21q22.3 containing the cluster of the $\alpha_1$- and $\alpha_2$-subunits of type VI collagen genes (*COL6A1* and *COL6A2*), suggestive of candidate genes.[181] One French Canadian family showed genetic linkage to chromosome 2q37 close to the

$\alpha_3$-subunit of the type VI collagen gene *(COL6A3)*, providing evidence for genetic heterogeneity in Bethlem's myopathy.[182] Sequence analysis in four families revealed missense mutations in *COL6A1* (G286V) or in *COL6A2* (G250S).[183] Both mutations disrupt the Gly-X-Y motif of the triple helical domain by substitution of Gly for either Val or Ser. Because microfibrillar type VI collagen may play a role in bridging cells with the extracellular matrix, the disruption of cell attachment to the extracellular matrix could be involved in the pathogenesis of the disease.

## Muscular Dystrophy with Epidermolysis Bullosa

In a rare, autosomal recessive variant of epidermolysis bullosa (EB), a group of heritable blistering disorders, a form associated with late-onset muscular dystrophy (EB-MD), has been described.[184–186] The blistering tendency usually occurs at birth and affects the epithelia of various mucous membranes, including the cornea and skin. Careful electron microscopic examination revealed that the tissue separation occurs at the level of the hemidesmosomal inner plaque consisting of plectin, an intermediate filament-associated protein, also expressed in the sarcolemma.[187] Demonstration of plectin deficiency in patients with EB-MD led to the identification of homozygous deletion mutations in the plectin gene *(PLEC1)* on chromosome 8q24.[188] Plectin deficiency presumably leads to defective anchorage of the cytoskeleton to transmembrane complexes in an way analogous to that proposed for dystrophin in the DGC.

## Oculopharyngeal Muscular Dystrophy

Oculopharyngeal muscular dystrophy has a worldwide distribution, with a particularly high prevalence among French Canadians.[189] In most cases of oculopharyngeal muscular dystrophy, the disease begins with ptosis, but occasionally dysphagia is the first symptom. Onset is usually in late adult life. As the disease progresses, eye movements may be impaired with occasional diplopia. The shoulder girdle and, less commonly, the pelvic girdle may be involved with weakness and atrophy. A variant with distal weakness has been described in the Japanese.

In French Canadians, the mutation has been mapped to chromosome 14q11 and a mutation identified in the poly A-binding protein 2 gene *(PABP2)*.[190] A $(GCG)_6$ repeat in the 5' coding region of the gene is expanded to 8 to 13 repeats in patients with oculopharyngeal muscular dystrophy. Homozygosity for a rare $(GCG)_7$ allele causes recessive oculopharyngeal muscular dystrophy. In members of dominant pedigrees more severe phenotypes were seen when the second allele contained seven repeats, establishing this allele also as a modifier of a dominant phenotype. Future studies are needed to determine whether the nuclear filamentous inclusions typical for oculopharyngeal muscular dystrophy are caused by aggregation of proteins containing expanded polyalanine tracts.

## SUMMARY

The identification of the DMD gene and its product dystrophin was a great breakthrough in the history of muscular dystrophy research. The subsequent identification of the dystrophin–glycoprotein complex has given substantial new insights into the basic defects in various types of muscular dystrophy, including DMD and BMD, sarcoglycanopathy (LGMD 2C–E), and merosinopathy (CMD). This indicates the importance of intact molecular links between the cytoskeleton and the extracellular matrix for maintenance of muscle fiber integrity. This idea has been supported by the identification of other molecules implicated in muscular dystrophies: type VI collagen in Bethlem's myopathy and plectin in EB-MD. In LGMD 2A and EDMD, the function of defective proteins still remains elusive. Although our knowledge of the molecular genetic basis of muscular dystrophies is expanding, our detailed understanding of the molecular pathogenesis of the diseases is not yet in hand. Understanding physiological functions and the pathophysiology of the causative proteins will certainly give us insights that will facilitate rational design of treatments for these diseases.

## ACKNOWLEDGMENTS

The author gratefully acknowledges Dr. Kiichi Arahata (NINPT, Tokyo) for providing figures and Drs. Teruo Shimizu and Kiichiro Matsumura for their critical reading of the manuscript.

## REFERENCES


1. Verellen-Dumoulin C, Freund M, Demyer R, et al.: Expression of an X-linked muscular dystrophy in a female due to translocation involving Xp21 and non-random inactivation of the normal X chromosome. Hum Genet 67:115–119, 1984.
2. Franke U, Ochs HD, de Martinville B, et al.: Minor Xp21 chromosome deletion in a male associated with expression of Duchenne muscular dystrophy, chronic granulomatous disease, retinitis pigmentosa, and McLeod syndrome. Am J Hum Genet 37: 250–267, 1985.
3. Davies KE, Pearson PL, Harper PS, et al.: Linkage analysis of two cloned DNA sequences flanking the Duchenne muscular dystrophy locus on the short arm of the human X chromosome. Nucleic Acids Res 11:2303–2312, 1983.
4. Worton RG, Duff C, Sylvester J, Schmickel RD, Willard HF: Duchenne muscular dystrophy involving translocation of the DMD gene next to ribosomal RNA genes. Science 224:1447–1449, 1984.
5. Ray PN, Belfall B, Duff C, et al.: Cloning of the breakpoint of an X;21 translocation associated with Duchenne muscular dystrophy. Nature 318:672–675, 1985.
6. Kunkel LM, Monaco AP, Middlesworth W, Ochs HD, Latt SA: Specific cloning of DNA fragments absent from the DNA of a male patient with an X-chromosome deletion. Proc Natl Acad Sci USA 82: 4778–4782, 1985.
7. Monaco AP, Bertelson CJ, Middlesworth W, et al.: Detection of deletions spanning the Duchenne muscular dystrophy locus using a tightly linked DNA segment. Nature 316:842–845, 1985.
8. Monaco AP, Neve RL, Colletti-Feener C, et al.: Isolation of candidate cDNAs for portions of the Duchenne muscular dystrophy gene. Nature 323: 646–650, 1986.
9. Koenig M, Hoffman EP, Bertelson CJ, Monaco AP, Feener C, Kunkel LM: Complete cloning of the Duchenne muscular dystrophy (DMD) cDNA and preliminary genomic organization of the DMD gene in normal and affected individuals. Cell 50: 509–517, 1987.
10. Hoffman EP, Brown RH, Kunkel LM: Dystrophin: The protein product of the Duchenne muscular dystrophy locus. Cell 51:919–928, 1987.
11. Roberts RG, Coffey AJ, Bobrow M, Bentley DR: Exon structure of the human dystrophin gene. Genomics 16:536–538, 1993.
12. Ahn AH, Kunkel LM: The structural and functional diversity of dystrophin. Nat Genet 3:283–291, 1993.
13. D'Souza VN, Man NT, Morris GE, Karges W, Pillers DAM, Ray PN: A novel dystrophin isoform is required for normal retinal electrophysiology. Hum Mol Genet 4:837–842, 1995.
14. Lidov HGW, Selig S, Kunkel LM: Dp 140: A novel 140 kDa CNS transcript from the dystrophin locus. Hum Mol Genet 4:329–335, 1995.
15. Koenig M, Monaco AP, Kunkel LM: The complete sequence of dystrophin predicts a rod-shaped cytoskeletal protein. Cell 53:219–228, 1988.
16. Arahata K, Ishiura S, Ishiguro T, et al.: Immunostaining of skeletal and cardiac muscle surface membrane with antibodies against Duchenne muscular dystrophy peptide. Nature 333:861–866, 1988.
17. Bonilla E, Samitt CE, Miranda AF, et al.: Duchenne muscular dystrophy: Deficiency of dystrophin at the muscle cell surface. Cell 54:447–452, 1988.
18. Zubrzycka-Gaarn EE, Bulman DE, Karpati G, et al.: The Duchenne muscular dystrophy gene product is localized in sarcolemma of human skeletal muscle. Nature 333:466–469, 1988.
19. Campbell KP, Kahl SD: Association of dystrophin and integral membrane glycoprotein. Nature 338: 259–262, 1989.
20. Ervasti JM, Ohlendieck K, Kahl SD, Gaver MG, Campbell KP: Deficiency of a glycoprotein component of the dystrophin complex in dystrophic muscle. Nature 345:315–319, 1990.
21. Yoshida M, Ozawa E: Glycoprotein complex anchoring dystrophin to sarcolemma. J Biochem 114: 634–639, 1990.
22. Sunada Y, Campbell KP: Dystrophin–glycoprotein complex: Molecular organization and critical roles in skeletal muscle. Curr Opin Neurol 8:379–384, 1995.
23. Ozawa E, Yoshida M, Suzuki A, Mizuno Y, Hagiwara Y, Noguchi S: Dystrophin-associated proteins in muscular dystrophy. Hum Mol Genet 4:1711–1716, 1995.
24. Ibraghimov-Beskrovnaya O, Ervasti JM, Leveille CJ, et al.: Primary structure of the 43K and 156K dystrophin-associated glycoproteins linking dystrophin to the extracellular matrix. Nature 355:696–702, 1992.
25. Ervasti JM, Campbell KP: A role for the dystrophin–glycoprotein complex as a transmembrane linker between laminin and actin. J Cell Biol 122: 809–823, 1993.
26. Suzuki A, Yoshida M, Hayashi K, Mizuno Y, Ozawa E: Molecular organization at the glycoprotein–complex-binding site of dystrophin: Three dystrophin-associated proteins bind directly to the carboxyl terminal portion of dystrophin. Eur J Biochem 220:283–292, 1994.
27. Jung D, Yang B, Meyer J, Chamberlain JS, Campbell KP: Identification and characterization of the dystrophin anchoring site on β-dystroglycan. J Biol Chem 270:27305–27310, 1995.
28. Ahn AH, Kunkel LM: Syntrophin binds to an al-

ternatively spliced exon of dystrophin. J Cell Biol 128:363–371, 1995.
29. Suzuki A, Yoshida M, Ozawa E: Mammalian $\alpha_1$- and $\beta_1$-syntrophin bind to the alternative splice-prone region of the dystrophin COOH terminus. J Cell Biol 128:373–381, 1995.
30. Yang B, Jung D, Rafael JA, Chamberlain JS, Campbell KP: Identification of syntrophin binding to syntrophin triplet, dystrophin, and utrophin. J Biol Chem 270:4975–4978, 1995.
31. Campbell KP: Three muscular dystrophies: Loss of cytoskeletal–extracellular matrix linkage. Cell 80: 675–679, 1995.
32. Meryon E: On granular and fatty degeneration of the voluntary muscles. Med Chir Trans 35:73–84, 1852.
33. Duchenne GB: Recherches sur la paralysie musculaire pseudohypertrophique ou paralysie myosclerosique. Arch Gen Med 11:5–25, 179–209, 305–321, 421–423, 552–588, 1868.
34. Emery AEH: Duchenne Muscular Dystrophy, ed 2. Oxford University Press, New York, 1993.
35. Mostacciuolo ML, Lombardi A, Cambissa V, Danieli GA, Angelini C: Population data on benign and severe forms of X-linked muscular dystrophy. Hum Genet 75:217–220, 1987.
36. Bushby KM, Thambyayah M, Gardner Medwin D: Prevalence and incidence of Becker muscular dystrophy. Lancet 337:1022–1024, 1991.
37. Towbin JA, Hejtmancik JF, Brink P, et al.: X-linked dilated cardiomyopathy: Molecular genetic evidence of linkage to Duchenne muscular dystrophy (dystrophin) gene at the Xp21 locus. Circulation 87:1854–1865, 1993.
38. Muntoni F, Cau M, Ganau A, et al.: Deletion of the dystrophin muscle-promoter region associated with X-linked dilated cardiomyopathy. N Engl J Med 329:921–925, 1993.
39. Yoshida K, Ikeda S, Nakamura A, et al.: Molecular analysis of the Duchenne muscular dystrophy gene in patients with Becker muscular dystrophy presenting with dilated cardiomyopathy. Muscle Nerve 16:1161–1166, 1993.
39a. Muntoni F, Melis MA, Ganau A, et al.: Transcription of the dystrophin gene in normal tissues and in skeletal muscle of a family with X-linked dilated cardiomyopathy. Am J Hum Genet 56:151–157, 1995.
39b. Muntoni F, Wilson L, Marrosu G, et al.: A mutation in the dystrophin gene selectively affecting dystrophin expression in the heart. J Clin Invest 96: 693–699, 1995.
40. Oldfors A, Eriksson BO, Kyllerman M, et al.: Dilated cardiomyopathy and the dystrophin gene: An illustrated review. Br Heart J 72:344–348, 1994.
41. Franz WM, Cremer M, Herrmann R, et al.: X-linked dilated cardiomyopathy. Ann NY Acad Sci 752:470–491, 1995.
42. Gospe SM Jr, Lazaro RP, Lava NS, et al.: Familial X-linked myalgia and cramps: A nonprogressive myopathy associated with a deletion in the dystrophin gene. Neurology 39:1277–1280, 1989.
43. Sunohara N, Arahata K, Hoffman EP, et al.: Quadriceps myopathy: Forme fruste of Becker muscular dystrophy. Ann Neurol 28:634–639, 1990.
44. de Visser M, Bakker E, Defesche JC, et al.: An unusual variant of Becker muscular dystrophy. Ann Neurol 27:578–581, 1990.
45. Prelle A, Medri R, Moggio M, et al.: Dystrophin deficiency in a case of congenital myopathy. J Neurol 239:76–78, 1992.
46. Kyriakides T, Gabriel G, Drousiotou A, et al.: Dystrophinopathy presenting as congenital muscular dystrophy. Neuromusc Disord 4:387–392, 1994.
47. Engel AG, Yamamoto M, Fischbeck KH: Dystrophinopathies. In Engel AG, Franzini-Armstrong C (eds): Myology, ed 2. McGraw-Hill, New York, 1994, pp1130–1187.
48. Baumbach LL, Chamberlain JS, Ward PA, Farwell NJ, Caskey CT: Molecular and clinical correlations of deletions leading to Duchenne and Becker muscular dystrophies. Neurology 39:465–474, 1989.
49. Chamberlain JS, Gibbs RA, Ranier JE, Nguyen PN, Caskey CT: Deletion screening of the Duchenne muscular dystrophy locus via multiplex DNA amplification. Nucleic Acids Res 16:11141–11156, 1988.
50. Beggs AH, Koenig M, Boyce FM, Kunkel LM: Detection of 98% of DMD/BMD gene deletions by polymerase chain reaction. Hum Genet 86:45–48, 1990.
51. Hu X, Ray PN, Murphy EG, Thompson MW, Worton RG: Duplicational mutations at the Duchenne muscular dystrophy locus: Its frequency, distribution, origin, and phenotype/genotype correlation. Am J Hum Genet 46:682–695, 1990.
52. den Dunnen TJ, Grootscholten PM, Bakker E, et al.: Topography of the Duchenne muscular dystrophy (DMD) gene: FIGE and cDNA analysis of 194 cases reveals 115 deletions and 13 duplications. Am J Hum Genet 45:835–847, 1989.
53. Prior TW, Bartolo C, Pearl DK, et al.: Spectrum of small mutations in the dystrophin coding region. Am J Hum Genet 57:22–33, 1995.
54. Boyce FM, Beggs AH, Feener C, Kunkel LM: Dystrophin is transcribed in brain from a distant upstream promoter. Proc Natl Acad Sci USA 88:1276–1280, 1991.
55. Bushby KMD, Cleghorn MJ, Curtis A, et al.: Identification of a mutation in the promoter region of the dystrophin gene in a patient with atypical Becker muscular dystrophy. Hum Genet 88:185, 1991.
56. Monaco AP, Bertelson CJ, Liechti-Gallati S, et al.: An explanation for the phenotypic differences between patients bearing partial deletions of the DMD locus. Genomics 2:90–95, 1988.
57. Koenig M, Beggs AH, Moyer M, et al.: The molecular basis of Duchenne versus Becker muscular dystrophy: Correlation of severity with type of deletion. Am J Hum Genet 45:498–506, 1989.
58. Beggs AH, Hoffman EP, Snyder JR, et al.: Exploring the molecular basis for variability among patients with Becker muscular dystrophy: Dystrophin gene and protein studies. Am J Hum Genet 49:54–67, 1991.
59. Arahata K, Beggs AH, Honda H, et al.: Preservation of the C-terminus of the dystrophin molecule in the skeletal muscle from Becker muscular dystrophy. J Neurol Sci 101:148–156, 1991.
60. Arahata K, Hoffman EP, Kunkel LM, et al.: Dystrophin diagnosis: Comparison of dystrophin abnor-

malities by immunofluorescence and immunoblot analyses. Proc Natl Acad Sci USA 86:7154–7158, 1989.

61. Love DR, Flint TJ, Marsden RF, et al.: Characterization of deletions in the dystrophin gene giving mild phenotypes. Am J Med Genet 37:136–142, 1990.
62. Bies RD, Caskey CT, Fenwick R: An intact cysteinrich domain is required for dystrophin function. J Clin Invest 90:666–672, 1992.
63. Roberts RG, Barby TF, Manners E, Bobrow M, Bentley DR: Direct detection of dystrophin gene rearrangements by analysis of dystrophin mRNA in peripheral blood lymphocytes. Am J Hum Genet 49:298–310, 1991.
64. Chelly J, Gilgenkrantz H, Lambert M, et al.: Effect of dystrophin gene deletions on mRNA levels and processing in Duchenne and Becker muscular dystrophies. Cell 63:1239–1248, 1990.
65. Malhotra SB, Hart KA, Klamut HJ, et al.: Frameshift deletions in patients with Duchenne and Becker muscular dystrophy. Science 242:755–759, 1988.
66. Roest PAM, Roberts RG, Sugino S, van Ommen G-JB, den Dunnen JT: Protein truncation test (PTT) for rapid detection of translation-terminating mutations. Hum Mol Genet 2:1719–1721, 1993.
67. Nicholson LV, Johnson MA, Gardner Medwin D, Bhattacharya S, Harris JB: Heterogeneity of dystrophin expression in patients with Duchenne and Becker muscular dystrophy. Acta Neuropathol 80: 239–250, 1990.
68. Arahata K, Ishiura T, Kamakura K, et al.: Mosaic expression of dystrophin in symptomatic carriers of Duchenne's muscular dystrophy. N Engl J Med 320:138–142, 1989.
69. Hoffman EP, Fischbeck KH, Brown RH, et al.: Characterization of dystrophin in muscle-biopsy specimens from patients with Duchenne's or Becker's muscular dystrophy. N Engl J Med 318: 1363–1368, 1988.
70. Bulman DE, Murphy EG, Zubrzycka Gaarn EE, Worton RG, Ray PN: Differentiation of Duchenne and Becker muscular dystrophy phenotypes with amino-and carboxy-terminal antisera specific for dystrophin. Am J Hum Genet 48:295–304, 1991.
71. Feener CA, Boyce FM, Kunkel LM: Rapid detection of CA polymorphisms in cloned DNA. application to the 5' region of the dystrophin gene. Am J Hum Genet 48:621–627, 1991.
72. Oudet C, Heilig R, Hanauer A, Mandel JL: Nonradioactive assay for new microsatellite polymorphisms at the 5' end of the dystrophin gene, and estimation of intragenic recombination. Am J Hum Genet 49:311–319, 1991.
73. Oudet C, Heilig R, Mandel JL: An informative polymorphism detectable by polymerase chain reaction at the 3' end of dystrophin gene. Hum Genet 84:283–285, 1990.
74. Beggs AH, Kunkel LM: A polymorphic CACA repeat in the 3' untranslated region of dystrophin. Nucleic Acids Res 18 :1931, 1990.
75. Clemens PR, Fenwick RG, Chamberlain JS, et al.: Carrier detection and prenatal diagnosis in Duchenne and Becker muscular dystrophy families, using dinucleotide repeat polymorphisms. Am J Hum Genet 49:951–960, 1991.
76. Abbs S, Roberts RG, Mathew CG, Bentley DR, Bobrow M: Accurate assessment of intragenic recombination frequency within the Duchenne muscular dystrophy gene. Genomics 7:602–606, 1990.
77. van Essen AJ, Abbs S, Baiget M, et al.: Parental and germline mosaicism of deletions and duplications of the dystrophin gene: A European study. Hum Genet 88:249–257, 1992.
78. Kuller JA, Hoffman EP, Fries MH, et al.: Prenatal diagnosis of Duchenne muscular dystrophy by fetal muscle biopsy. Hum Genet 90:34–40, 1992.
79. Sicinski P, Geng Y, Ryder-Cook AS, et al.: The molecular basis of muscular dystrophy in the *mdx* mouse: A point mutation. Science 244:1578–1580, 1989.
80. Stedman HH, Sweeney HL, Shrager JB, et al.: The *mdx* mouse diaphragm reproduces the degenerative changes of Duchenne muscular dystrophy. Nature 352:536–539, 1991.
81. Cox GA, Phelps SF, Chapman VM, Chainberlain JS: New *mdx* mutation disrupts expression of muscle and nonmuscle isoforms of dystrophin. Nat. Genet 4:87–93, 1993.
82. Valentine BA, Winand NJ, Pradhan D, et al.: Canine X-linked muscular dystrophy as an animal model of Duchenne muscular dystrophy: A review. Am J Med Genet 42:352–356, 1992.
83. Sharp NJH, Kornegay JN, Van Camp SD, et al.: An error in dystrophin mRNA processing in golden retriever muscular dystrophy, an animal homologue of Duchenne muscular dystrophy. Genomics 13:115–121, 1992.
84. Partridge TA, Morgan JE, Coulton GR, Hoffman EP, Kunkel LM: Conversion of *mdx* myofibers from dystrophin-negative to-positive by injection of normal myoblasts. Nature 337:176–179, 1989.
85. Karpati G, Pouliot Y, Zubrzycka-Gaarn E, et al.: Dystrophin is expressed in *mdx* skeletal muscle fibers after normal myoblast implantation. Am J Pathol 135:27–32, 1989.
86. Huard J, Bouchard JP, Roy R, et al.: Human myoblast transplantation: Preliminary results of 4 cases. Muscle Nerve 15:550–560, 1992.
87. Gussoni E, Pavlath GK, Lanctot AM, et al.: Normal dystrophin transcripts detected in Duchenne muscular dystrophy patients after myoblast transplantation. Nature 356:435–438, 1992.
88. Karpati G, Ajdukovic D, Arnold D, et al.: Myoblast transfer in Duchenne muscular dystrophy. Ann Neurol 34:8–17, 1992.
89. Law PK, Goodwin TG, Fang Q, et al.: Feasibility, safety and efficacy of myoblast transfer therapy on Duchenne muscular dystrophy boys. Cell Transplant 1:235–244, 1992.
90. Neumeyer AM, DiGregorio DM, Brown RH, Jr: Arterial delivery of myoblasts to skeletal muscle. Neurology 42:2258–2262, 1992.
91. Cox GA, Cole NM, Matsumura K, et al.: Overexpression of dystrophin in transgenic *mdx* mice eliminates dystrophic symptoms without toxicity. Nature 364:725–729, 1993.
92. Dunckley MG, Wells JD, Walsh FS, Dickson G: Direct retroviral-mediated transfer of a dystrophin

minigene into *mdx* mouse *in vivo.* Hum Mol Genet 2:717–723, 1993.
93. Ragot T, Vincent N, Chafey P, et al.: Efficient adenovirus-mediated transfer of a human mini-dystrophin gene to skeletal muscle of *mdx* mice. Nature 361:647–650, 1993.
94. Vincent N, Rogot T, Gilgenkrantz H, et al.: Long-term correction of mouse dystrophic degeneration by adenovirus-mediated transfer of a mini-dystrophin gene. Nat Genet 5:130–134, 1993.
95. Kockanek S, Clemens PR, Mitani K, et al.: A new adenoviral Vector. Replacement of all viral coding sequences with 28 kb of DNA independently expressing both full-length dystrophin and β-galactosidase. Proc Natl Acad Sci USA 93:5731–5736, 1996.
96. Clemens PR, Kochanek S, Sunada Y, et al.: *In vivo* muscle gene transfer of full-length dystrophin with an adenoviral vector that lacks all viral genes. Gene Ther 3:965–972, 1996.
97. Tinsley JM, Potter AC, Phelps SR, et al. Amelioration of the dystrophic phenotype of *mdx* mice using a truncated utrophin transgene. Nature 384:349–353, 1996.
97a. Tinsley J, Deconinck N, Fisher R., et al.- Expression of full-length utophin prevents muscular dystrophy in mdx mice. Nat Med 4:1441–1444, 1998.
98. Beck K, Hunter I, Engel J: Structure and function of of laminin: Anatomy of a multidomain glycoprotein. FASEB J 4:148–160, 1990.
99. Burgeson RE, Chiquet M, Deutzmann R, et al.: A new nomenclature for the laminins. Matirx Biol 14:209–211, 1994.
100. Sunada Y, Bernier SM, Kozak CA, Yamada Y, Campbell KP: Deficiency of merosin in dystrophic *dy* mice and genetic linkage of the laminin M chain gene to the *dy* locus. J Biol Chem 269: 13729–13732, 1994.
101. Yamada H, Chiba A, Endo T, et al.: Characterization of dystroglycan-laminin interaction in peripheral nerve. J Neurochem 66:1518–1524, 1996.
102. Leivo I, Engvall E: Merosin, a protein specific for basement membranes of Schwann cells, striated muscle, and trophoblast, is expressed late in nerve and muscle development. Proc Natl Acad Sci USA 85:1544–1548, 1988.
103. Ehrig K, Leivo I, Argraves WS, Ruoslahti E, Engvall E: Merosin, a tissue-specific basement membrane protein, is a laminin-like protein. Proc Natl Acad Sci USA 87:3264–3268, 1990.
104. Engvall E, Earwicker D, Haaparanta T, Ruoslahti E, Sanes JR: Distribution and isolation of four laminin variants: Tissue restricted distribution of heterotrimers assembled from five different subunits. Cell Regul 1:731–740, 1992.
105. Engvall E, Earwicker D, Day A, Muir D, Manthorpe M, Paulsson M: Merosin promotes cell attachment and neurite outgrowth and is a component of the neurite-promoting factor of RN22 schwannoma cells. Exp Cell Res 198:115–123, 1992.
106. Anton ES, Sandrock AW Jr, Matthew WD: Merosin promotes neurite growth and Schwann cell migration *in vitro* and nerve regeneration *in vivo*: Evidence using an antibody to merosin, ARM-1. Dev Biol 164:133–146, 1994.
107. Yurchenco PD, Cheng YS, Colognato H: Laminin forms an independent network in basement membranes. J Cell Biol 117:1119–1133, 1992.
108. Vuolteenaho R, Nissinen M, Sainio K, et al: Human laminin M chain (merosin): Complete primary structure, chromosomal assignment, and expressiopn of the M and A chain in human fetal tissue. J Cell Biol 124:381–394, 1994.
109. Bernier SM, Utani A, Sugiyama S, Doi T, Polistina C, Yamada Y: Cloning and expression of laminin $\alpha_2$ chain (M-chain) in the mouse. Matrix Biol 14: 447–455, 1994.
110. Schittny JC, Yurchenco PD: Terminal short arm domains of basement membrane laminin are critical for its self-assembly. J Cell Biol 110:825–832, 1990.
111. Yurchenco PD, Cheng Y-S: Self-assembly and calcium-binding sites in laminin: A three-arm interaction model. J Biol Chem 268:17286–17299, 1993.
112. Tomè FMS, Evangelista T, Leclerc A, et al.: Congenital muscular dystrophy with merosin deficiency. C R Acad Sci Ser III Sci Vie 317:351–357, 1994.
113. Hillaire D, Leclerc A, Faure S, et al.: Localization of merosin-negative congenital muscular dystrophy to chromosome 6q2 by homozygosity mapping. Hum Mol Genet 9:1657–1661, 1994.
114. Philpot J, Sewry C, Pennock J, Dubowitz V: Clinical phenotype in congenital muscular dystrophy: Correlation with expression with expression of merosin in skeletal muscle. Neuromusc Disord 5: 301–305, 1994.
115. Pegoraro E, Mancias P, Swedlow SH, et al.: Congenital muscular dystrophy with primary laminin $\alpha_2$ (merosin) deficiency presenting as inflammatory myopathy. Ann Neurol 40:782–791, 1996.
116. Shorer Z, Philpot J, Muntoni F, Sewry C, Dubowitz V: Demyelinating peripheral neuropathy in merosin-deficient congenital muscular dystrophy. J Child Neurol 10:472–475, 1995.
117. Dubowitz V: Workshop report. 41st ENMC international workshop on congenital muscular dystrophy. Neuromusc Disord 4:295–306, 1996.
118. Helbling-Leclerc A, Zhang X, Topaloglu H, et al.: Mutations in the laminin $\alpha_2$-chain gene (LAMA2) cause merosin-deficient congenital muscular dystrophy. Nat Genet 11:216–218, 1995.
119. Nissinen M, Helbling-Leclerc A, Zhang X, et al.: Substitution of a conserved cysteine-996 in a cysteine-rich motif of the laminin $\alpha_2$-chain in congenital muscular dystrophy with partial deficiency of the protein. Am J Hum Genet 58:1177–1184, 1996.
120. Allamand V, Sunada Y, Salih MAM, et al.: Mild congenital muscular dystrophy in two patients with an internally deleted laminin $\alpha_2$-chain. Hum Mol Genet 6:747–752, 1997.
121. Sewry CA, Philpot J, Sorokin LM, et al.: Diagnosis of merosin (laminin-2) deficient congenital muscular dystrophy by skin biopsy. Lancet 347:582–584, 1996.
122. Hayashi YK, Engvall E, Arikawa-Hirasawa E, et al.:

Abnormal localization of laminin subunits in muscular dystrophies. J Neurol Sci 119:53–64, 1993.
123. Zhang X, Vuolteenaho R, Tryggvason K: Structure of the human laminin $\alpha_2$-chain gene (*LAMA2*), which is affected in congenital muscular dystrophy. J Biol Chem 271:27664–27669, 1996.
124. Voit T, Fardeau M, Tome FMS: Prenatal detection of merosin expression in human placenta. Neuropediatrics 25:332–333, 1994.
125. Arahata K, Hayashi YK, Koga R, et al.: Laminin in animal models for muscular dystrophy: Defect of laminin M in skeletal and cardiac muscles and peripheral nerve of the homozygous dystrophic *dy/dy* mice. Proc Jpn Acad 69B:259–264, 1993.
126. Xu H, Chrismas P, Wu XR, Wewer UM, Engvall E: Defective muscle basement membrane and lack of M-laminin in the dystrophic *dy/dy* mouse. Proc Natl Acad Sci USA 91:5572–5576, 1994.
127. Xu H, Wu XR, Wewer UM, Engvall E: Murine muscular dystrophy caused by a mutation in the laminin $\alpha_2$ (Lama2) gene. Nat Genet 8:297–302, 1994.
128. Sunada Y, Bernier SM, Utani A, Yamada Y, Campbell KP: Identification of a novel mutant transcript of lamin $\alpha_2$ chain gene responsible for muscular dystrophy and dysmyelination in $dy^{2J}$ mice. Hum Mol Genet 4:1055–1061, 1995.
129. North KN, Beggs AH: Deficiency of skeletal muscle isoform of α-actinin (α-actinin 3) in merosin-positive congenital muscular dystrophy. Neuromusc Disord 4:229–235, 1996.
130. Fukuyama Y, Osawa M, Suzuki H: Congenital muscular dystrophy of the Fukuyama type. clinical, genetic, and pathological considerations. Brain Dev 3:1–30, 1981.
131. Toda T, Segawa M, Nomura Y, et al.: Localization of a gene for Fukuyama type congenital muscular dystrophy to chromosome 9q31–33. Nat Genet 5: 283–286, 1993.
132. Toda T, Miyake M, Kobayashi K, et al.: Linkage-dysequilibrium mapping narrows the Fukuyama-type congenital muscular dystrophy (FCMD) candidate region to $<$100 kb. Am J Hum Genet 59: 1313–1320, 1996.
133. Kobayashi K, Nakahori Y, Miyake M, et al.: An ancient retrotransposal insertion causes Fukuyama-type congenital muscular dystrophy. Nature 394: 388–392, 1998.
134. Walton JN, Nattrass FS: On the classification, natural history and treatment of myopathies. Brain 77:169–231, 1954.
135. Emery AEH: Population frequencies of inherited neuromuscular diseases: A world survey. Neuromusc Disord 1:19–29, 1991.
136. Bushby KMD, Beckmann JS: The limb-girdle muscular dystrophies: Proposal for a new nomenclature. Neuromusc Disord 5:337–343, 1995.
137. Liu J, Aoki M, Illa I, et al.: Dysferlin, a novel skeletal muscle gene, is mutated in Miyoshi myopathy and limb girdle muscular dystrophy. Nat Genet 20:31–36, 1998.
137a. Bashir R, Britton S, Strachan T, et al.: A gene related to Caenorhabditis elegans spermatogenesis factor *fer-1* is mutated in limb-girdle muscular dystrophy type 2B. Nat Genet 20:37–42, 1998.
138. Matsumura K, Tomé FMS, Collin H, et al.: Deficiency of 50K dystrophin-associated glycoprotein in severe childhood autosomal recessive muscular dystrophy. Nature 359:320–322, 1992.
139. Ben Hamida M, Fardeau M, Attia N: Severe childhood muscular dystrophy affecting both sexes and frequent in Tunisia. Muscle Nerve 6:469–480, 1983.
140. Azibi K, Bachner L, Beckmann JS, et al.: Severe childhood autosomal recessive muscular dystrophy with the deficiency of the 50 kDa dystrophin-associated glycoprotein maps to chromosome 13q12. Hum Mol Genet 2:1423–1428, 1993.
141. Salih MAM, Omer MIA, Bayoumi RA, et al.: Severe autosomal recessive muscular dystrophy in an extended Sudanese kindred. Dev Med Child Neurol 25:43–52, 1983.
142. Fardeau M, Matsumura K, Tomé FMS, et al.: Deficiency of the 50 kDa dystrophin-associated glycoprotein (adhalin) in severe autosomal recessive muscular dystrophies in children native from European countries. C R Acad Sci Paris 316:799–804, 1993.
143. Higuchi I, Yamada H, Fukunaga H, et al.: Abnormal expression of laminin suggests disturbance of sarcolemma–extracellular matrix interaction in Japanese patients with autosomal recessive muscular dystrophy deficient in adhalin. J Clin Invest 94:601–606, 1994.
144. Ben Othmane K, Ben hamida M, Pericak-Vance MA, et al.: Linkage of Tunisian autosomal recessive Duchenne-like muscular dystrophy to the pericentromeric region of chromosome 13q. Nat Genet 2:315–317, 1992.
145. El Kerch F, Sefiani A, Azibi K, et al.: Linkage analysis of families with severe childhood autosomal recessive muscular dystrophy (SCARMD) in Morocco indicates genetic heterogeneity of the disease in North Africa. J Med Genet 31:342–343, 1994.
146. Passos-Bueno MR, Oliveira JR, Bakker E, et al.: Genetic heterogeneity for Duchenne-like muscular dystrophy (DLMD) based on linkage and 50 DAG analysis. Hum Mol Genet 2:1945–1947, 1993.
147. Romero NB, Tomè FMS, Leturcq F, et al.: Genetic heterogeneity of severe childhood autosomal recessive muscular dystrophy with adhalin (50 kDa dystrophin-associated glycoprotein) deficiency. C R Acad Sci Paris 317:70–76, 1994.
148. Roberds SL, Leturcq F, Allamand V, et al.: Missense mutations in the adhalin gene linked to autosomal recessive muscular dystrophy. Cell 78: 625–633, 1994.
149. McNally EM, Yoshida M, Mizuno Y, Ozawa E, Kunkel LM: Human adhalin is alternatively spliced and the gene is located on chromosome 17q21. Proc Natl Acad Sci USA 91:9690–9694, 1994.
150. Lim LE, Duclos F, Broux O, et al.: β-Sarcoglycan: Characterization and role in limb-girdle muscular dystrophy linked to 4q12. Nat Genet 11:257–265, 1995.
151. Bönnemann CG, Modi R, Noguchi S, et al.: β-Sarcoglycan (A3b) mutations cause autosomal recessive muscular dystrophy with loss of the sarcoglycan complex. Nat Genet 11:266–273, 1995.

152. Noguchi S, McNally E, Ben Othmane K, et al.: Mutations in the dystrophin-associated protein γ-sarcoglycan in chromosome 13 muscular dystrophy. Science 270:819–822, 1995.
153. Nigro V, deSa Moreira E, Piluso G, et al.: Autosomal recessive limb-girdle muscular dystrophy, LGMD2F, is caused by a mutation in the δ-sarcoglycan gene. Nat Genet 14:195–198, 1996.
154. Piccolo F, Roberds SL, Jeanpierre M, et al.: Primary adhalinopathy: A common cause of autosomal recessive muscular dystrophy of varieble severity. Nat Genet 10:243–245, 1995.
155. Ljunggren A, Duggan D, McNally E, et al.: Primary adhalin deficiency as a cause of muscular dystrophy in patients with normal dystrophin. Ann Neurol 38:367–372, 1995.
156. Kawai H, Akaike M, Endo T, et al.: Adhalin gene mutations in patients with autosomal recessive childhood onset muscular dystrophy with adhalin deficiency. J Clin Invest 96:1202–1207, 1995.
157. Carrié A, Piccolo F, Leturcq F, et al.: Mutational diversity and hot spots in the α-sarcoglycan gene in autosomal recessive muscular dystrophy (LGND2D). J Med Genet 34:470–475, 1997.
158. Jackson CE, Carey JH: Progressive muscular dystrophy: Autosomal recessive type. Pediatrics 28: 77–84, 1961.
159. Jackson CE, Strehler DA: Limb-girdle muscular dystrophy: Clinical manifestations and detection of preclinical disease. Pediatrics 41:495–502, 1968.
160. Richard I, Broux O, Allamand V, et al.: Mutations in the proteolytic enzyme calpain 3 cause limb-girdle muscular dystrophy type 2A. Cell 81:27–40, 1995.
161. Allamand V, Broux O, Bourg N, et al.: Genetic heterogeneity of autosomal recessive limb-girdle muscular dystrophy in a genetic isolate (Amish) and evidence for a new locus. Hum Mol Genet 4: 459–464, 1995.
162. Bönnemann CG, Passos-Bueno MR, McNally EM, et al.: Genomic screening for β-sarcoglycan gene mutations: Missense mutations may cause severe limb-girdle muscular dystrophy type 2E (LGMD2E). Hum Mol Genet 5:1953–1961, 1996.
163. Ben Othmane K, Speer MC, Stauffer J, et al.: Evidence for linkage disequilibrium in chromosome 13-linked Duchenne-like muscular dystrophy (LGMD2C). Am J Hum Genet 57:732–734, 1995.
164. McNally EM, Duggan D, Gorospe JR, et al.: Mutations that disrupt the carboxyl-terminus of γ-sarcoglycan cause muscular dystrophy. Hum Mol Genet 5:1841–1847, 1996.
165. Piccolo F, Jeanpierre M, Leturcq F, et al.: A founder mutation in the γ-sarcoglycan gene of Gypsies possibly predating their migration out of India. Hum Mol Genet 5:2019–2022, 1996.
166. McNally EM, Passos-Bueno MR, et al.: Mild and severe muscular dystrophy caused by a single γ-sarcoglycan mutation. Am J Hum Genet 59:1040–1047, 1996.
167. Nigro V, Piluso G, Belsito A, et al.: Identification of a novel sarcoglycan gene at 5q33 encoding a sarcolemmal 35 kDa glycoprotein Hum Mol Genet 5:1179–1186, 1996.
168. Jung D, Duclos F, Apostol B, et al.: Characterization of δ-sarcoglycan, a novel component of the oligomeric sarcoglycan complex involved in limb-girdle muscular dystrophy. J Biol Chem 271: 32321–32329, 1996.
169. Passos-Bueno MR, Moreira ES, Vanizof M, Marie SK, Zatz M: Linkage analysis in autosomal recessive limb-girdle muscular dystrophy (AR LGMD) maps a sixth form to 5q33–34 (LGMD2F) and indicates that there is at least one more subtype of AR LGMD. Hum Mol Genet 5:815–820, 1996.
170. Beckmann JS, Richard I, Hillaire D, et al.: A gene for limb-girdle muscular dystrophy maps to chromosome 15 by linkage. CR Acad Sci Paris 312: 141–148, 1991.
171. Emery AEH, Dreifuss FE: Unusual type of benign X-linked muscular dystrophy. J Neurol Neurosurg Psychiatr 29:338–342, 1966.
172. Merlini L, Granata C, Dominici P, Bonfiglioli S: Emery-Dreifuss muscular dystrophy: Report of five cases in a family and review of the literature. Muscle Nerve 9:481–485, 1986.
173. Becker PE: Dominant autosomal muscular dystrophy with early contractures and cardiomyopathy (Hauptmann-Thannhauser). Hum Genet 74:184–1986.
174. Yates JRW, Warner JP, Smith JA, et al.: Emery-Dreifuss muscular dystrophy: Linkage to markers in distal Xq28. J Med Genet 30:108–111, 1993.
175. Bione S, Maestrini E, Rivella S, et al.: Identification of a novel X-linked gene responsible for Emery-Dreifuss muscular dystrophy. Nat Genet 8: 323–327, 1994.
176. Nagano A, Koga R, Ogawa M, et al.: Emerin deficiency at the nuclear membrane in patients with Emery-Dreifuss muscular dystrophy. Nat Genet 12:254–259, 1996.
177. Yates JRW: Workshop report. 43rd ENMC internatinal workshop on Emery-Dreifuss muscular dystrophy. Neuromusc Disord 7:67–69, 1997.
178. Yamada T, Kobayashi T: A novel emerin mutation in a Japanese patient with Emery-Dreifuss muscular dystrophy. Hum Genet 97:693–694, 1996.
179. Bione S, Small K, Aksmanovic VMA, et al.: identification of new mutations in the Emery-Dreifuss muscular dystrophy gene and evidence for genetic heterogeneity of the disease. Hum Mol Genet 4:1859–1863, 1995.
180. Bethlem J, van Wijingaarden GK: Benign myopathy, with autosomal dominant inheritance. Brain 99:91–100, 1976.
181. Jobsis GJ, Barth PG, Boers JM, et al.: Bethlem myopathy: Clinical and genetic aspects. Neurology 46:779–782, 1996.
182. Speer MC, Tandan R, Rao PN, et al.: Evidence for locus heterogeneity in the Bethlem myopathy and linkage to 2q37. Hum Mol Genet 5:1043–1046, 1996.
183. Jobsis GJ, Keizers H, Vreijling JP, et al.: Type VI collagen mutations in Bethlem myopathy, an autosomal dominant myopathy with contractures. Nat Genet 14:113–115, 1996.
184. Niemi K-M, Somer H, Kero M, Kanerva L, Haltia M: Epidermolysis bullosa simplex associated with muscular dystrophy with recessive inheritance. Arch Dermatol 124:551–554, 1988.
185. Kletter G, Evans OB, Lee JA, et al.: Congenital

muscular dystrophy and epidermolysis bullosa simplex. J Pediatr 114:104–107, 1989.
186. Fine J-D, Stenn J, Johnson L, et al.: Autosomal recessive epodermolysis bullosa simplex: Generalized phenotypic features suggestive for junctional or dystrophic epidermolysis bullosa, and association with neuromuscular diseases. Arch Dermatol 125:931–938, 1989.
187. Gache Y, Chavanas S, Lacour JP, et al.: Defective expression of plectin in epidermolysis bullosa simplex with muscular dystrophy. J Clin Invest 97: 2289–2292, 1996.
188. Pulkkinen L, Smith FJD, Shimizu H, et al.: Homozygous deletion mutations in the plectin gene (PLEC1) in patients with epidermolysis bullosa simplex associated with late-onset muscular dystrophy. Hum Mol Genet 5:1539– 1546, 1996.
189. Tome FMS, Fardeau M: Oculopharyngeal dystrophy. In Engel AG, Franzini-Armstrong C (eds): Myology. McGraw-Hill, New York, 1994, pp1233–1245.
190. Brais B, Bouchard JP, Xie YG, et al.: Short GCG expansions in the *PABP2* gene cause oculopharyngeal muscular dystrophy. Nat Genet 18:164–167, 1998.

Chapter 6

# FACIOSCAPULOHUMERAL MUSCULAR DYSTROPHY

George W. Padberg, MD, PhD
Cameron Adams, MD



Recent research to define the molecular genetics of facioscapulohumeral muscular dystrophy (FSHD) has clarified the classification of this and related disorders. The majority of cases are caused by a deletion of an integral number of 3.3 kb tandem repeats at the subtelomere of chromosome 4 (specifically, at 4q35). This inheritance model justifies that the condition be called a *disease,* and the D in the abbreviation FSHD can be read as "disease" or "dystrophy" according to one's liking. When the disorder in a particular family is known to be linked to 4q35 (or when the diagnostic deletion at 4q35 is identified in any given individual) it is referred to as FSHD 1A; if it is known to be not linked there, it is called FSHD 1B. The term "FSHD" without a number implies that the individual has the syndrome described in this chapter, but that the actual linkage or mutation has not yet been defined.

In 1884, patient L died of tuberculosis at the age of 24 years, enabling Landouzy and Déjerine to perform the first postmortem studies on the neuromuscular condition from which L had suffered since the age of 3 years.[1] They established that the condition was a primary myopathy and named it *facioscapulohumeral* to summarize its most remarkable clinical features. Although upper arm weakness rarely is an early sign of the disease, "humeral' was included in the name to contrast this disease with the only established myopathy at the time, described by Duchenne, with onset in the pelvic and lower limb muscles. In a second paper in 1886, Landouzy and Déjerine included sporadic cases with facial involvement, further emphasizing that facial weakness and upper limb onset were hallmarks of the condition, but at the same time this made their work vulnerable to those who hesitated to accept the various forms of progressive muscular dystrophies as separate diseases.

When hereditary mechanisms were first applied to human biology and human diseases, several attempts were made to define the muscular dystrophies based on their patterns of inheritance. Because not all autosomal dominant cases included facial weakness and upper limb involvement, no simple picture for FSHD emerged. It became clear, however, that involvement of the facial muscles was an important discriminatory feature of FSHD. A landmark paper by Walton and Nattrass[2] in 1954 clarified the nosology and described FSHD as an independent entity with either autosomal dominant or autosomal recessive inheritance and also sporadic occurrence.

In the meantime, a different clinical concept had arisen that contributed to semantic and nosological discussion and confusion. In 1929, Oransky (as reported by Davidenkov[3]) described a Russian family with muscular dystrophy that he did not recognize as FSHD because of minimal involvement of facial and upper arm muscles. On the other hand, the term *facioscapulohumeral* had obscured the recognition of early involvement of the foot extensor muscles in FSHD. Because periscapular and foot extensor weaknesses were the major signs in many of Oransky's cases, this family was included in the studies of Davidenkov, who had coined the terms *scapuloperoneal syndrome* and *scapuloperoneal myopathy*.[4] Without the benefit of molecular analysis, it would be quite difficult to determine whether Oransky's cases did in fact have FSHD or a genetically distinct condition, as was implied by him. The term *scapuloperoneal* has proved its usefulness to summarize a clinical syndrome similar to FSHD but in which peroneal involvement is more prominent and facial weakness is minimal at most. Now, since the debate about the extent of the clinical picture of FSHD has died out, the only remaining puzzle is the possible genetic heterogeneity of FSHD, as is suggested by a few familial cases apparently not linked to chromosome 4q35.[5]

## CLINICAL PICTURE

### Age at Onset and Penetrance

Defining age of onset in FSHD patients usually initiates a long discussion. We have seen toddlers with obicularis oculi weakness who remained asymptomatic for 20 years and know of patients with reported congenital facial asymmetry. We usually suggest that age of onset is the age at which a person becomes aware of muscle weakness. With awareness of facial muscle weakness as the onset of the disease, the mean age of onset is in the second decade (on average, 17 years) with variation from 2 to 50 years. These variations occur between families and probably to a lesser extent within families, but the latter has not been studied thoroughly.

Penetrance has been estimated to be less than 5% for ages 0 to 4 years, 21% for ages 5 to 9, 58% for ages 10 to 14, 86% for ages 15 to 19, and 95% for age 20 years and older. The manifestations of myopathy are usually visible to the experienced clinician by the time the patient reaches age 20 years in more than 95% of the cases. Nonpenetrance was observed and estimated by regression analysis in a large study to be less than 2% to 5% at the age of 60 years.[6] The age at onset roughly correlates with the size of the deletion in the 4q35 *Eco*RI fragment detectable by p13E-11 (see later). The relationship is most evident in sporadic cases (new mutations) and is less clear when entire families are considered.[7,8]

### Initial Symptoms

Facial weakness rarely leads to complaints early in the disease, yet family studies have suggested that it is the earliest *sign* of the disease and that it is occasionally present at birth. In a large series of patients, facial weakness was almost invariably present, although it can be minimal.[6] Symptoms of facial weakness become apparent with advanced weakness only; answers to questions about difficulty whistling (as a measure of buccinator weakness) appear unreliable, culturally dependent, and not helpful in making the diagnosis in most cases. Shoulder girdle weakness most often leads to awareness of the disease by the patient. In particular, weakness of the scapula fixators (i.e., the serratus anterior, the rhomboid muscles, and the lower part of the trapezius) are most affected. Often the patient already shows the characteristic high rise of the scapula on attempts to raise the arms above shoulder level, being caused by the relatively strong deltoid muscle pulling at an unrestrained shoulder blade. In the rare patient presenting with foot extensor weakness, shoulder girdle weakness is found on physical examination. Infantile onset might present with pelvic girdle weakness, as most attention by parents is paid to walking and running in this age group; these patients are usually found to have extensive facial weakness when examined by the physician. Muscle pains are reported frequently, often in relation to exercise and occasionally lasting weeks or even longer. Apart from pain, some patients mention chronic excessive fatigue.

## Clinical Course

In patients who develop an advanced clinical picture, the sequence of muscle involvement is generally uniform in the majority of cases. Six stages of progression can be discerned (Table 6–1). A subdivision in two subtypes of progression (i.e., foot extensors first followed by pelvic girdle muscles and the reverse sequence) is impractical. The latter is a rare occurrence, and both types occur in the same families and do not constitute separate genetic entities.

Involvement of the scapular fixators is almost invariably present early in the course of the disease, as is involvement of the pectoralis, distinguishing FSHD from other dystrophies. When the deltoid does become atrophic, the atrophy is often partial, affecting frequently only a proximal part of the muscle by hitherto unexplained mechanisms.

Foot extensor weakness usually heralds a more advanced degree of muscle involvement in FSHD. When examined at that time, weakness of the abdominal muscles and upper arm muscles can be detected. In the rare instances where early signs of pelvic girdle weakness are present, a compensating hypertrophy of the extensor digitorum brevis muscle and a mild foot extensor weakness is often found. As the disease progresses further, the pelvic girdle, upper leg muscles, and wrist extensors become involved. Asymmetry of muscle involvement is much less common and less pronounced in the lower limbs than in the shoulder girdle. The early abdominal weakness, the gluteus maximus paresis, and involvement of the long muscles of the back all contribute at this stage to the development of the steep hyperlordosis that Landouzy and Déjerine considered characteristic of this disease. Neck extensor weakness is an uncommon and late sign. The extraocular, masticatory, and pharyngeal muscles remain unaffected, and ptosis is not part of FSHD. Rare lingual involvement in severe cases has been reported.[9]

The proportion of gene carriers with signs of shoulder girdle weakness with or without facial weakness but without more advanced symptoms is rather high. In studies of completely examined families, at least 30% of all gene carriers were asymptomatic.[6]

Patients develop pelvic girdle weakness at a widely variable age, mostly between 30 and 55 years (average around 40 years). In a large family study, we found that after the age of 50 years approximately 20% of the

Table 6–1. **Clinical Course of FSHD in Stages**

| Stage | Description |
|---|---|
| 0 | Facial weakness only |
| 1 | Shoulder girdle weakness |
| 2 | Abdominal, foot extensor, and upper arm muscle weakness |
| 3 | Pelvic girdle, upper leg, and lower arm weakness |
| 4 | Rise from a chair and climb stairs with support |
| 5 | Ambulatory indoors, unable to climb stairs, wheelchair outside |
| 6 | Wheelchair indoors |

gene carriers were wheelchair dependent, but also that 30% were still asymptomatic.[6] The former reflects a fast progressive course of FSHD and the latter an extremely slow, progressive course. Long periods of apparent arrest as well as periods of rapid progression have been reported, but both are rare.

## Asymmetry of Muscle Involvement

Asymmetry of muscle involvement is a frequent finding in patient with FSHD[10] and some authors consider it to be highly characteristic of the disease. Asymmetry of facial muscle weakness occurs in at least half of the patients and suggests a developmental factor rather than environmental factors. Similarly, partial involvement of the deltoid muscle suggests genetic factors rather than selective (dis)use. Asymmetry of shoulder girdle muscle involvement is often striking, judged by the lateral and anterior displacement of the scapulae. The right shoulder clearly seems to be involved more often than the left. Yet, when strength was measured, only marginally significant differences were observed for several muscle groups on both sides, and relationship to handedness could not be proved.[11] Moreover, these right–left differences were not confirmed by others. Asymmetry of muscle involvement in the lower extremities is less striking and also appears not to be related to one side.

## Unusual Signs of FSHD

Unusual signs are by definition those that differ from the usual descending course of muscle involvement. Although 85% of patients with progression to the lower extremities report foot extensor weakness before pelvic girdle weakness, the reverse pattern is not considered unusual. A truly unusual sign is severe neck extensor weakness leading to a dropping head. Occasionally, finger extensor weakness, particularly index finger weakness, can be observed early in the course.

We saw two patients with early gastrocnemius weakness and atrophy. Ptosis, extraocular weakness, and masseter and pharyngeal weakness are not part of FSHD. Contractures can be seen in FSHD, although they are rare with the exception of ankle contractures, which occur in approximately 10% of cases and occasionally require operation, particularly in early onset cases. Skeletal deformation occurs infrequently. A mild scoliosis may be present, particularly if the disease is of early onset. Both pectus excavatum and pectus carinatum have been mentioned repeatedly but have not been studied systematically.

## Cardiac Muscle Involvement

Overt clinical cardiac involvement is not typically part of the clinical picture in FSHD. Claims in the past likely involved cases with unsatisfactory neuromuscular diagnoses, Emery-Dreifuss muscular dystrophy, autosomal dominant scapuloperoneal syndromes with contractures and cardiomyopathy, or patients with FSHD and incidental cardiovascular disease. A carefully conducted study in a large group of well-defined FSHD patients revealed no significant cardiac involvement.[12] Stevenson and colleagues,[13] however, reported minor and subclinical conduction abnormalities in up to 60% of their patients. Also, the results of a single-photon emission computed tomography study suggest subclinical cardiac involvement in FSHD.[14]

## Hearing Loss

Sensorineural hearing loss is not an infrequent sign of early onset FSHD.[15] In adolescent and adult onset cases, hearing problems are rarely a complaint and, at more advanced ages, high tone hearing loss might be taken for a traumatic effect or presbyacusis. Audiometry in affected and nonaffected siblings in ten kindreds, however, showed that a high tone hearing loss is in fact a subtle part of FSHD in two-third of the patients, with a wide range of involvement within families. There was a poor correlation with severity of the muscle disorder, but there was a tendency toward increased hearing deficit with age.[16] Brainstem auditory evoked potentials are generally normal.[17]

## Ocular Changes

Retinal vascular changes in FSHD patients have been described occasionally since 1968, usually as Coats' disease in severely affected early onset cases, which had led to the suggestion that these patients suffer from a different disease. In more recent reports, it has been established that a retinal vasculopathy is part of all forms of FSHD, but that it remains asymptomatic in the majority of patients.[18] Less than 1% of all gene carriers develop visual loss due to retinal exudates and hemorrhages. Microaneurysms, capillary telangiectasis, and small exudates can be demonstrated in approximately two-third of all patients by fluorescent angiography. These changes, however, cannot be seen by routine ophthalmoscopy. Because of such a low risk, a regular ophthalmological check-up is probably not warranted. Nonetheless, photocoagulation can be quite successful, especially if done early in the disease process.

# LABORATORY TESTS

## Biochemical Analysis

Of the routine biochemical tests, serum creatinine kinase measurements are most useful and probably correlate best with severity of the ongoing myopathic process. Creatinine kinase levels rarely exceed five times the upper limit of normal, and they decline significantly with age and duration of the disease. Other serum enzyme tests do not contribute to the diagnosis or prognosis of the disease.

## Imaging Studies

Because the muscles that are involved early in FSHD are all rather thin, imaging is of little use for early diagnosis. Computed tomography studies, however, reveal a pattern of muscle involvement somewhat distinct from that based on clinical signs because in the lower extremity the hamstrings are involved early in the course of the disease.[19]

## Electrophysiology

Electromyographic studies usually show a widespread pattern of low-amplitude, brief, and polyphasic motor units, especially in clinically affected muscles. Fibrillation potentials are rare.[20] Occasionally, denervation potentials can be found, but neurogenic features never dominate the electromyogram.

## Histology

The morphological changes in FSHD muscles can be variable. A biopsy specimen may be entirely normal when taken from a clinically nonaffected muscle. Variation in fiber diameter, fibrosis, necrosis and regeneration fibrosis, and patchy infiltration are the common features; moth-eaten fibers and whorled fibers are frequently seen, as are small angulated fetal myosin-expressing fibers (Fig. 6–1).[21] Groups of atrophic fibers exclude the diagnosis of FSHD.

Cellular infiltrates are present in more than 30% of biopsy specimens and can be extensive, occasionally leading to the incorrect diagnosis of polymyositis. Therefore, polymyositis with facial weakness warrants DNA analysis for 4q35 deletions. The immune mechanisms responsible for the inflammatory reaction in FSHD muscles are different from those in Duchenne's dystrophy and polymyositis.[22] Electron microscopy has not revealed characteristic changes for FSHD. Freeze-fracture studies showed decreased orthogonal arrays, but unfortunately the molecular correlate of these arrays are unknown.[23] In recent immunohistochemical studies, FSHD biopsy specimens were often examined as controls, revealing a normal presence of dystrophin, dystroglycans, merosin, and emerin.

We showed in three patients that mitochondrial respiratory chain function was reduced in all complexes, similar to findings in Duchenne's muscular dystrophy patients. Others have demonstrated increased incorporation of amino acids in muscle polyri-

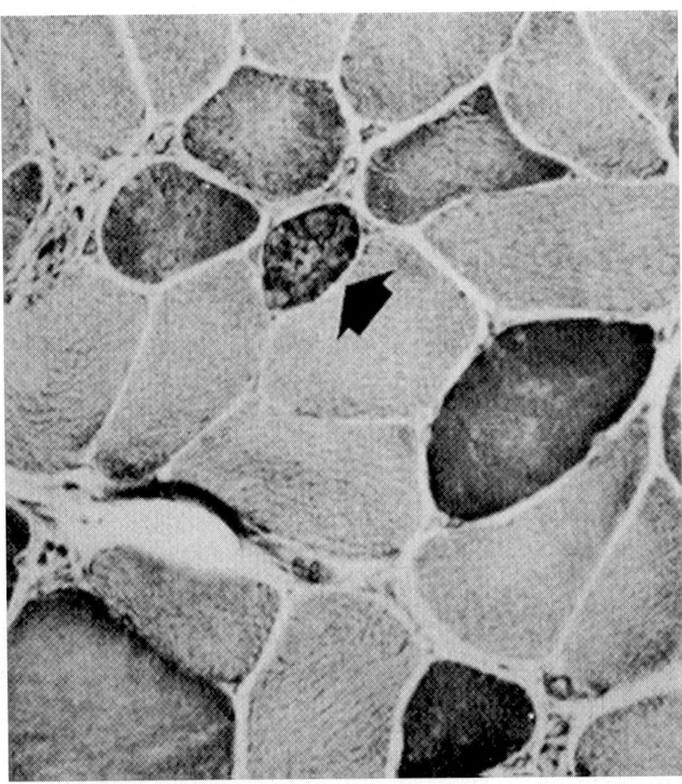

**Figure 6–1.** Histologic findings in FSHD. Biopsy specimen (NADH stain) from a patient with fairly severe weakness showing numerous small, moth-eaten whorled fibers (arrow).

bosomes of patients in early stages of the disease, suggestive of increased protein synthesis.[24]

## GENETIC STUDIES

### Linkage Analysis

In 1990, linkage of FSHD 1A to chromosome 4q35 markers was demonstrated.[25] FSHD 1A was the first disease linked when a member of the now established class of microsatellite markers was used. Soon thereafter other markers were found, and by 1992 the genetic map of 4q35 was as follows: 4 cen-D4S171-D4S163-D4S139-D4S810-FSHD1A-qter.[26] The use of linkage analysis in FSHD has been largely replaced by molecular diagnosis via the p13E-11 probe (see later). Nonetheless, linkage and haplotype analyses still remain useful when the clinical suspicion of FSHD remains high despite the inability to detect a deletion with this molecular probe. An international collaborative study showed that most families were 4q35 linked,[27] and only a very small number of large families are not linked to 4q35 (these pedigrees are referred to as FSHD 1B).[5] The recombination frequency in males appeared slightly higher than in females. Thus far a second locus has not been established.

### p13E-11 and 4q35 Deletions

In the search for potential candidate genes, a cosmid clone was found that mapped to 4q35. From this clone, the probe p13E-11 was obtained that revealed a polymorphism after *Eco*RI digestion. The probe was found not only to be tightly linked but also to show a deletion in the *Eco*RI fragment causally related to the presence of the disease in families. Contained within each of these *Eco*RI restriction fragments is the site bound by the p13E-11 probe and region called the *D4Z4* locus, which is composed of 12 to 85 nearly identical tandem repeats of approximately 3.3 kb each (Fig. 6–2). Each repeat is flanked by a *Kpn*I restriction site, contains two homeobox motives, and has regions showing sequence homology to LSau (a GC-rich region) and hhspm3 (a low-copy human repeat).[28]

The *Eco*RI restriction fragments in controls are 35 to 300 kb. In FSHD 1A patients, the *Eco*RI fragment is smaller than 35 kb, containing up to 9 of the 3.3 kb tandem repeats in the *D4Z4* locus. After a long search, it was determined that these 3.3 kb repeats do not contain any functional genes. The deletion most likely exerts a position effect variegation, silencing a gene or genes more centromerically.[29] Thus far, two genes have been identified. FSHD-related gene 1 (*FRG1*)[30] was found to be transcribed in patients and controls, and therefore is not the FSHD 1A gene. The second gene, the β-tubulin gene,[31] appears to be a pseudogene.

Myopathy, high tone hearing loss, and retinal vasculopathy are at present considered pleiotropic effects of the same gene because all three conditions occur in all multiple families examined. This renders the possibility of a contiguous gene defect less likely. Because position effect variegation is presently considered the mechanism at work in FSHD 1A, however, it might be possible that the auditory disorder and the

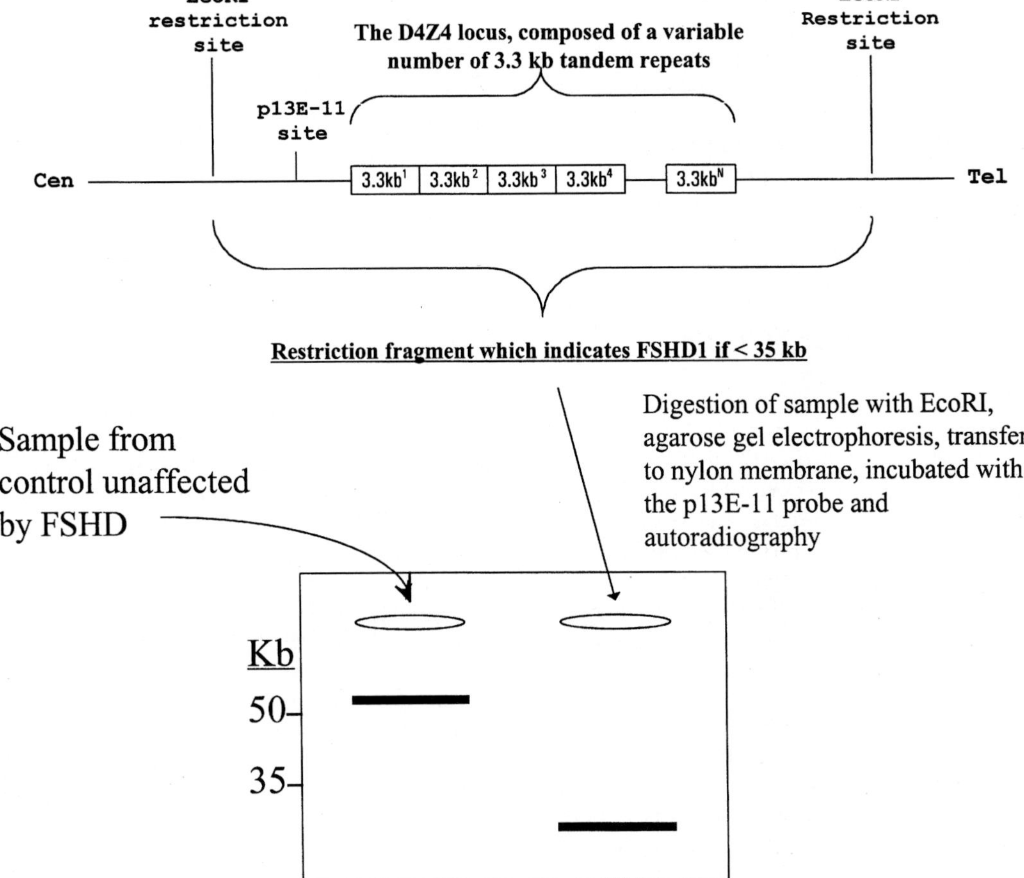


**Figure 6–2.** Simplified restriction map showing the linked region on chromosome 4q35. The locus is much closer to the telomere (Tel) than to the centromere (Cen). Two *Eco*RI restriction sites surround a fragment that is 35 to 300 kb long in controls. The fragment contains the site that is bound by the p13E-11 probe and the D4Z4 locus, which is composed of a variable number of nearly identical 3.3 kb tandem repeats. In FSHD1A, a deletion involving the D4Z4 locus causes the *Eco*RI restriction fragment to be less than 35 kb.

retinal vasculopathy, which did not occur in all FSHD patients, are caused by different genes, less influenced by the position effect.

p13E-11 hybridization of *Eco*RI-digested DNA not only shows two 4q35-associated fragments, but also a constant chromosome Y–related fragment of 9.2 kb and two fragments that map to chromosome 10q26. Chromosome 10 fragments also contain a number of 3.3 kb repeats almost identical to the 4q35 repeats.[32] The 10q homologue and problems with interchromosomal exchange pose challenges to accurate molecular diagnosis, as discussed later under DNA Diagnosis.

With p13E-11, germlike somatic mosaicism has been demonstrated.[33,34] These cases are a strong argument that multiple *de novo* cases in the same sibship are the result of germline mosaicism. In these situations, it is speculated that the spontaneous mutation occurs in a germ cell progenitor cell, leading to mature germ cells carrying either the wild type or mutated gene, but the somatic cells do not contain the mutation. The interesting case of one affected twin in an identical twin set was demonstrated to be caused by an early zygotic mutation.[35]

## GENOTYPE–PHENOTYPE CORRELATIONS

### Sporadic Cases

The demonstration of deletions in FSHD 1A (FSHD with linkage to 4q35 demonstrated) helped to identify new mutations of the disease. The percentage of new mutations in the Dutch FSHD population was found to be at least 9.6%.[36] This is likely to be a conservative figure as it is estimated that not all new mutations are ascertained at present. On the other hand, the 30% new mutations reported from Brazil might equally be too high of a percentage.[37]

Sporadic cases tend to be more severely affected, as patients with greater disability probably have a smaller chance of generating offspring. Patients with new mutations of a mild phenotype have a good chance of being diagnosed late and of having offspring, rendering them familial cases. Several authors found a significant correlation between the age at onset of the disease and the size of the deleted fragment.[7,8] This anticipation is similar to that seen in the DNA trinucleotide repeat syndromes. The question of whether the deletion is meiotically unstable has not yet been entirely addressed, however, so the molecular mechanism for the generation effect in FSHD is yet to be determined.

### Familial Cases

In families, a mild gender difference has been observed by several authors. Among asymptomatic cases there are more women, and there is a tendency for women to have later onset of the disease. In families, the mean age at onset correlated less, but the age of onset of the disease in the proband correlated somewhat more with the size of the deleted fragment. When large families are considered entirely, most authors are more impressed by the large variation in age at onset and severity of the disease in patients having the same deleted fragment.

### Infantile Onset

Symptoms other than facial weakness before the age of 10 years are required to diagnose infantile onset of FSHD. A large number of these children have a severe course of the disease, and many of them have clinically significant hearing loss and retinal vascular changes. Mental retardation has been suggested to occur in these cases, but a relation with FSHD 1A has not been proven sufficiently. In general, these patients show a large 4q35 deletion. We found a minimally affected parent of such a patient to be a somatic mosaic with a small fragment, explaining the peculiar hereditary pattern. On the other hand, in a family with a severely affected boy, both he and his minimally affected parent had a 15 kb fragment. Our present genetic knowledge cannot explain the entire phenotype. Proper genotype–phenotype correlations must await the cloning of the gene.

## COUNSELING

### Mutation Frequency, Incidence, and Prevalence

Based on the previously described data from the Dutch FSHD 1A[36] population, the incidence of FSHD 1A is estimated to be about 1 FSHD mutation in 320,000 live births. The *prevalence* of FSHD 1A in a particular Dutch province is estimated to be a least 1 in 21,000 inhabitants, suggesting that Holland probably contains 750 FSHD 1A gene carriers. These figures might be on the low side because ascertainment is likely to remain incomplete. Reported prevalence figures vary from 2.3 to 66.9 per $10^6$ in the literature, similar to incidence estimates, which vary from 3.8 to 26.0 per 10.[6] Both germline mosaicism and a high mutation rate explain all historic observations of a possible autosomal recessive inheritance.

### DNA Diagnosis

Now that the complexities of the p13E-11 polymorphism have been clarified, it is possible to make a reliable DNA diagnosis with approximately 86% to 95% sensitivity and 98% specificity.[38] As mentioned earlier, one of the challenges in correctly identifying the FSHD 1A mutation is to discern the origin of the *Eco*RI fragment identified by the p13E-11 probe, which can arise from either 4q35 or 10q26. In controls, the 10q26 fragments vary in size from 15 to 300 kb. Approximately 10% of the fragments are smaller than 35 kb and pose a significant diagnostic uncertainty for DNA testing. Demonstrating that the chromosome 10q repeat contains a *Bln* restriction site helped to develop a double-digestion method to cleave chromosome 10–related fragments so that they do not appear on a Southern blot. This restriction analysis turned out to be 95% specific and 95% sensitive.[39] A few patients and families with FSHD were found to have small *Bln*-sensitive fragments. These situations are best explained by postulating an interchromosomal exchange of repeats, which was found in the normal population in approximately 20% of individuals. When a *Bln*-sensitive chromosome 10q26 fragment exchanges with a 4q35 fragment and subsequently gets deleted, a position effect on chromosome 4q35 is created. Such a situation can only be proved by haplotype analysis in familial cases.

Experience with presymptomatic testing has been limited. DNA testing is usually performed to confirm or exclude a diagnosis. Both situations suggest that clinicians are occasionally in doubt about the diagnosis of FSHD. If a small 4q35-related p13E-11 fragment cannot be demonstrated, it is recommended to have the clinical diagnosis confirmed and scapuloperoneal syndrome ruled out by a second physician, examine the parents and children if present, perform 4q35 haplotype analysis with several markers, and obtain a muscle biopsy specimen (to help rule out spinal muscular atrophy, acid maltase deficiency, congenital myopathies, mitochondrial myopathies, or a rare case of polymyositis). Those few incidents when a patient with FSHD does not have a detectable 4q35 deletion may occur due to technical difficulties in preparing the DNA, the translocation of homologous regions between 4q35 and 10q, or locus heterogeneity.[38] Haplotype analysis is useful in this context because it would establish linkage versus nonlinkage to the 4q35 region despite those factors.

## TREATMENT

The management of FSHD remains primarily supportive. As this is one of the more mild forms of muscular dystrophy, many patients go through their entire lives without the disorder significantly interfering with any form of activity. Physical therapy offers a simple benefit for diminishing early contractures. Ankle–foot orthoses may be of benefit for those patients with significant peroneal involvement.

In some FSHD patients, an improvement in upper extremity function, especially elevation of the shoulder past 90 degrees, can result when the examiner manually fixates the scapula. In carefully selected patients such as these, surgical immobilization of the scapula may provide significant functional benefit.[40]

Treatment of FSHD with corticosteroids has had very limited success. In light of the proven temporary benefit of prednisone for Duchenne's muscular dystrophy, may clinicians offer a trial of oral steroids to patients with FSHD, especially those who have significant inflammatory reactions demonstrated by muscle biopsy. Despite earlier isolated reports of benefit from this treatment,[41] the most recent trial found no significant improvement in strength from prednisone 1.5 mg/kg/day for 12 weeks, although the sample size of eight was not large enough to detect a possible deceleration of progression.[42]

Finally, a recent pilot trial of sustained release albuterol 16 mg/day for 3 months in FSHD patients demonstrated a statistically significant increase in the skeletal muscle compartment of lean body mass and an overall 12% improvement in maximal voluntary isometric contraction testing.[43] Albuterol may benefit these patients through $\beta_2$-recepter–induced satellite cell proliferation, increased protein production, and inhibition of muscle proteolysis. Although the results are encouraging, recommendations for the routine use of albuterol for FSHD patients awaits a larger, randomized, double-blind placebo-controlled trial, now in progress.

## SUMMARY

A fundamental change in our view of the clinical picture of FSHD has occurred. The concept of FSHD now encompasses a broad clinical spectrum, ranging from very mild cases to severely affected young patients, and includes extramuscular features such as auditory and retinal pathology. The genetic advances have been enormous, revealing each time another level of complexity. In the vast majority of FSHD patients, deletions of integral numbers of 3.3 kb subtelomeric repeats appear causative for the disease by a position effect variegation. At the same time, interchromosomal exchange of these repeats constitutes an unprecedented mechanism complicating DNA diagnosis. The diagnosis of FSHD is also complicated by genetic heterogeneity. The gene or genes involved in FSHD have not yet been identified.

## REFERENCES

1. Landouzy L, Déjerine J: De la myopathie atrophique progressive (myopathie hereditaire debutant dans l'enfance, par la face sans alteration du systeme nerveux). C R Seances Acad Sci 98:53, 1884.
2. Walton JN, Nattrass FJ: On the classification, natural history and treatment of the myopathies. Brain 77:169, 1954.
3. Davidenkov S: Uber die scapuloperoneale Amyotrophie. (Die Familie "Z"). Z Ges Neurol Psychiatr 122:625, 1929.
4. Davidenkov S: Scapulo-peroneal type of progressive muscular atrophy. J Clin Med (Moscow) 6:337–343, 1926.
5. Gilbert JR, Stajich JM, Wall S, et al.: Evidence for heterogeneity in facioscapulohumeral muscular dystrophy (FSHD). Am J Hum Genet 53:401–408, 1993.
6. Padberg G: Facioscapulohumeral Disease. Doctoral thesis, University of Leiden, Intercontinental Graphics, 1982.
7. Tawil R, Forrester J, Griggs RC, et al.: Evidence for anticipation and association of deletion size with severity in facioscapulohumeral muscular dystrophy. The FSH-DY Group. Ann Neurol 39(6):744–748, 1996.
8. Goto K, Lee JH, Matsuda C, et al.: DNA rearrangements in Japanese facioscapulohumeral muscular dystrophy patients: Clinical correlations. Neuromusc Disord 5(3):201–208, 1995.
9. Shimizu T, Miyamoto K, Hayashi H, Nagashima T, Hirose K, Tanabe H: [Congenital facioscapulohumeral muscular dystrophy associated with tongue atrophy and sensorineural hearing disturbance]. Rinsho Shinkeigaku Clin Neurol 31(4):433–438, 1991.
10. Padberg GW, Lunt PW, Koch M, Fardeau M: Diagnostic criteria for facioscapulohumeral muscular dystrophy—Workshop Report. Neuromuscular Disorders 1(4):231–234, 1991.
11. Brouwer OF, Padberg GW, van der Ploeg RJ, Rugs CJ, Brand R: The influence of handedness on the distribution of muscular weakness of the arm in facioscapulohumeral muscular dystrophy. Brain 115:1587–1598, 1992.
12. de Visser M, de Voogt WG, la Riviere GV: The heart in Becker muscular dystrophy, facioscapulohumeral dystrophy, and Bethlem myopathy. Muscle Nerve 15(5):591–596, 1992.
13. Stevenson WG, Perloff JK, Weiss JN, Anderson TL: Facioscapulohumeral muscular dystrophy: Evidence for selective genetic electrophysiologic cardiac involvement. J Am Coll Cardiol 15:292–299, 1990.
14. Yamamoto S, Matsushima H, Suzuki A, Sotobata IIndo T, Matsuoka Y: A comparative study of

thallium-201 single-photon emission computed tomography and electrocardiography in Duchenne and other types of muscular dystrophy. Am J Cardiol 61(10):836–843, 1988.

15. Brouwer OF, Padberg GW, Wijmenga C, Frants RR: Facioscapulohumeral muscular dystrophy in early childhood. Arch Neurol 51(4):387–394, 1994.
16. Brouwer OF, Padberg WG, Ruys CJ, Brand R, de Latt JA, Grote JJ: Hearing loss in facioscapulohumeral muscular dystrophy. Neurology 41(12):1878–1881, 1991.
17. Verhagen WI, Huygen PL, Padberg GW: The auditory, vestibular, and oculomotor system in facioscapulohumeral dystrophy. Acta Oto-Laryngol Suppl 520(1):140–142, 1995.
18. Fitzsimons RB, Gurwin EB, Bird AC: Retinal vascular abnormalities in facioscapulohumeral muscular dystrophy. Brain 110:631–648, 1987.
19. Horikawa H, Takahashi K, Nishioi H, Mano Y, Takayanagi T: [X-ray computed tomographic scans of lower limb and trunk muscles in facioscapulohumeral muscular dystroohy]. Rinsho Shinkeigaku Clin Neurol 32(10):1061–1066, 1992.
20. Brown WF, Bolton CF: Clinical Electromyography. Butterworth-Heinemann, Boston, 1993, p61.
21. Dubowitz V, Brooke MH: Muscle Biopsy: A Modern Approach. WB Saunders, London, 1973, p212.
22. Arahata K, Ishihara T, Fukunaga H, et al.: Inflammatory response in facioscapulohumeral muscular dystrophy (FSHD): Immunocytochemical and genetic analyses. Muscle Nerve 2:S56–66, 1995.
23. Schotland DL, Bonilla E, Wakayama Y: Freeze facture studies of muscle plasma membrane in human muscular dystrophy. Acta Neuropathol 54(3): 189–197, 1981.
24. Ionasescu V: Distinction between Duchenne and other muscular dystrophies by ribosomal protein synthesis. Medical Genetics 12(1):49–54, 1975.
25. Wijmenga C, Frants RR, Brouwer OF, Moerer P, Wever JL, Padberg GW: Location of facioscapulohumeral muscular dystrophy gene on chromosome 4. Lancet 336(8716):651–653, 1990.
26. Cacurri S, Deidda G, Piazzo N, et al.: Chromosome 4q35 haplotypes and DNA rearrangements segregating in affected subjects of 19 Italian families with facioscapulohumeral muscular dystrophy (FSHD). Hum Genet 94(4):367–374, 1994.
27. Sarfarazi M, Wijmenga C, Upadhyaya M, et al.: Regional mapping of facioscapulohumeral muscular dystrophy gene on 4q35: Combined analysis of an international consortium. Am J Hum Genet 51(2): 396–4032, 1992.
28. Fisher J, Upadhyaya M: Molecular genetics of facioscapulohumeral muscular dystrophy. Neuromusc Disord 7:55–62, 1997.
29. Winokur ST, Bengtsson U, Feddersen J, et al.: The DNA rearrangement associated with facioscapulohumeral muscular dystrophy involves a heterochromatin-associated repetitive element: Implications for a role of chromatin structure in the pathogenesis of the disease. Chromosome Res 2: 225–234, 1994.
30. van Deutekom JCT, Lemmers R, Grewal KP, et al.: Identification of the first gene *(FRG1)* from the FSHD region on human chromosome 4q35. Hum Mol Genet 5:581–590, 1996.
31. Van Deutekom JCT, van Geel M, van Staalduinen A, et al.: A novel β-tubulin gene *(TUBrq)* in the chromosome 4q35 region: A candidate gene for FSHD1. In press.
32. Bakker E, Wijmenga C, Vossen RHAM, Padberg GW, et al.: The FSHD-linked locus D4F104S1 (p13E-11) on 4q35 has a homologue on 10qter. Muscle Nerve 2:S39–44, 1995.
33. Kohler J, Rupilius B, Otto M, Bathke K, Koch MC: Germline mosaicism in 4q35 facioscapulohumeral muscular dystrophy (FSHD1A) occurring predominantly in oogenesis. Hum Genet 98(4):485–490, 1996.
34. Upadhyaya M, Maynard J, Osborn M, Fardine P, Harper PS, Lunt P: Germline mosaicism in facioscapulohumeral muscular dystrophy (FSHD). Muscle Nerve 2:S45–49, 1995.
35. Griggs RC, Tawil R, McDermott M, Forrester J, Figlewicz D, Weiffenfach B: Monozygotic twins with facioscapulohumeral dystrophy (FSHD): Implications for genotype/phenotype correlation. FSH-DY Group. Muscle Nerve 2:S50–55, 1995.
36. Padberg GW, Frants RR, Brouwer OF, Wijmenga C, Bakker E, Sandkuijl LA: Facioscapulohumeral muscular dystrophy in the Dutch population. Muscle Nerve 2:S81–84, 1995.
37. Zatz M, Marie SK, Passos-Bueno MR, et al.: High proportion of new mutations and possible anticipation in Brazilian facioscapulohumeral muscular dystrophy families. Am J Hum Genet 56:99–105, 1995.
38. Tawil R, Figlewicz, Griggs RC, Weiffenbach B, and the FSH Consortium: Facioscapulohumeral dystrophy: A distinct regional myopathy with a novel molecular pathogenesis. Ann Neurol 43(3):279–282, 1998.
39. Deidda G, Cacurri S, Piazzo N, Felicetti L: Direct detection of 4q35 rearrangements implicated in facioscapulohumeral muscular dystrophy (FSHD). J Med Genet 33:361–365, 1996.
40. Ketenjian AY: Scapulocostal stabilization for scapular winging in facioscapulohumeral muscular dystrophy J. Bone Joint Surg 60:476, 1978.
41. Munsat TL, Piper D, Cancilla P, et al.: Inflammatory myopathy with facioscapulohumeral distribution. Neurology 22:335–347, 1972.
42. Tawil R, McDermott MP, Pandya S, et al.: A pilot trial of prednisone in facioscapulohumeral muscular dystrophy. Neurology 48:46–49, 1997.
43. Kissel JT, McDermott MP, Natarajan, MA, et al.: Pilot trial of albuterol in facioscapulohumeral muscular dystrophy. Neurology 50:1402–1406, 1998.

Chapter 7

# MYOTONIC DYSTROPHY

Allen D. Roses, MD
Cameron Adams, MD



Myotonic dystrophy, or dystrophia myotonica (DM), is an autosomal dominant disease that is characterized by the most highly variable expressivity and age-dependent penetrance of any known disease affecting humans. Clinical signs and symptoms that are characteristic of DM appear in virtually every organ system, but the disease can be so variable that a person carrying the DM genetic mutation may also show no signs or symptoms.[1–3] Myotonic dystrophy is named for the sustained depolarization, referred to as *myotonia,* that occurs when skeletal muscle is stimulated. The pattern of progressive muscle weakness presents a characteristic distribution of clinically affected muscles, involving distal small muscles as well as muscles of the trunk, face, eye, and tongue. Myotonic dystrophy also affects cardiac and smooth muscle, cataract formation, endocrine responses, bowel function, and the central nervous system. A severe form of the disease, congenital myotonic dystrophy (CDM), appears in some children born to affected mothers and rarely to affected fathers. The involvement of skeletal muscle in CDM patients is distinct from that observed in adults.[1–3] Congenital myotonic dystrophy is characterized by skeletal muscle hypotonia with decreased electrical activity compared with adult DM in which myotonia develops and is then followed by progressive dystrophy with a course extending over decades. Patients with CDM who survive into early childhood and the teenage years develop an adult DM pattern of muscle involvement.[3]

In the early 1970s, biochemical and physiological evidence led some investigators to propose that the multisystem clinical involvement of DM was due to surface membrane abnormalities common to many cell membranes.[4–6] The proposal was developed from findings of the reduced resting membrane potential of skeletal muscle, the slow development of characteristic cataracts, and the continued presence of myotonia after neuromuscular blockade. Cataracts suggest a disruption of membrane function because few other prominent cellular components are contained within this tissue besides the cell membrane. In myotonia congenita, a less severe muscle disease with more symptomatic clinical myotonia but no dystrophy, an alteration of chloride conductance in the muscle membrane was found to be responsible for the repetitive muscle fiber discharges.[7,8] These repetitive discharges are the electrophysiological equivalent of the clinical myotonia. Although chloride conductance was normal in DM, the implication of an ion channel added support to the suggestions of an alteration of a transmembrane protein, as these types of proteins serve as a conduit for ions between the intracellular and extracellular spaces.[2,4–6,9] Red cell membrane preparations were used as model biochemical membranes, as were skin fibroblasts and occasional muscle biopsy specimens. These experiments suggested an abnormality of the phosphorylated state of intrinsic membrane proteins related to endogenous membrane protein kinase activity.[5,6,10] In particular, abnormal phosphorylation of a component of erythrocyte band 3, once thought to be an anion channel (now known to be multiple proteins and glycoproteins), was implicated. These experiments took place before introns and exons were described, however, and before most of the currently familiar membrane channel families were imagined. Recent molecular experiments have reinforced the concept that abnormal phosphorylation of an intrinsic membrane protein, one of the sodium channels, may be related to the function of myotonin protein kinase (DMPK) and the possible pathophysiology of the myotonia seen in DM patients (see later under Skeletal Muscle).[11] The destruction of muscle fibers responsible for the dystrophy element of the disease likely involves more complex cellular mechanisms (see later under Potential Pathogenic Molecular Events Causing Myotonic Dystrophy).

The inheritance of a highly variable trinucleotide repeat located on the long arm of chromosome 19, $(CTG)_n$, accounts for DM's autosomal dominant mode of inheritance.[12–15] Figure 7–1 shows a Southern blot illustrating variable $(CTG)_n$ repeats in a DM family. This dynamic mutation has been implicated in *anticipation*, the term applied to the increase in severity and earlier age of onset of the disease in subsequent generations.[16] The region can expand from a normal range of less than 50 repeats to several thousand repeats.[17–19] The $(CTG)_n$ repeat is located in the 3' untranslated region of the gene for DMPK, a putative protein kinase.[14,15,20] Initial molecular studies after the identification of the gene examined purely genetic explanations (particularly decreased expression of DMPK mRNA and protein) for the variation of clinical manifestations of DM. As these studies have evolved, the more obvious explanations concerning gene expression and protein translation have yielded few clues to the mechanism of disease pathogenesis.[21,22] Some studies have focused on a neighboring gene at the 3' end of *DMPK*, whose transcription may also be affected by the CTG expansion.[23,24] Other recent studies have expanded genetic analogies to more primitive genes identified in lower organisms, but still there is little insight into the nature of the fascinating diversity of clinical expression seen in DM patients. This chapter summarizes the most important clinical aspects of DM, presents the genetic data emphasizing the role of genetic testing in disease diagnosis, and briefly summarizes the flood of recent hypotheses with respect to possible mechanisms of disease pathogenesis.

## CLINICAL SIGNS AND SYMPTOMS

### Skeletal Muscle

Myotonia is characterized by the sustained contraction of skeletal muscle, usually in response to voluntary contraction, percussion, or electrical stimulation. It is usually a minor clinical symptom in DM, the most common problem being the patient's inability to quickly release a hand grip or jaw clench. Myotonia frequently elicits no complaints from the patient. As a diagnostic sign, the distribution of myotonia that can be elicited in DM often involves small muscles, particularly in the hand, jaw, and tongue. Lingual myotonia may be useful as a very early diagnostic sign in mildly affected patients, but it is rarely symptomatic. The patient's tongue is placed on a tongue depressor, and percussion is applied to the tongue's edge with the side edge of a second depressor that is tapped lightly by a percussion hammer. This produces a contraction, seen as transient notching of the tongue's rounded contour, indicating a sustained contraction of that portion of the tongue muscle.

In patients who have had no weakness, myotonia generally appears or can be detected before the dystrophic process becomes symptomatic.[2] Electromyography is often used to search for repetitive (myo-

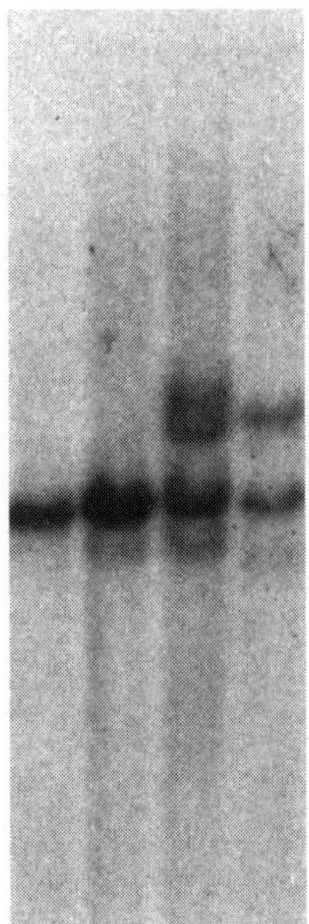


**Figure 7–1.** Southern blot illustrating variable $(CTG)_n$ repeat in a family with dystrophia myotonica (DM). Blood DNA was extracted from each individual in this DM family, cut with *Hin*dIII, subjected to electrophoresis on agarose, and blotted for analysis. The blot was probed with a 1.5 kb *Bam*HI probe that contains the $(CTG)_n$ repeat region and surrounding sequences. The two normal alleles detected by autoradiography are 8.3 and 7.4 kb in length in this analysis. The father has an enlarged $(CTG)_n$ repeat that can be detected by PCR analysis, but is too small to be observed on Southern blot. Both twin sons were patients with CDM and both demonstrated enlarged *Hin*dIII fragments containing very large $(CTG)_n$ repeats. Note that the identical twin sons are not identical with respect to the enlarged $(CTG)_n$ repeats, with differences in the size and pattern of the enlarged repeats.

tonic) discharges in skeletal muscle. These discharges sound like a World War II vintage "dive bomber" when monitored with audio. Electrophysiologically, they are long trains of single fiber discharges that wax and wane in amplitude and frequency. It is possible that the mechanism that leads from the molecular defect to myotonia might also trigger or enhance the dystrophic process. The clinical progression from myotonia to dystrophic changes may be important to understand the pathogenesis of DM in muscle.

The diversity of DM muscle pathology is characterized by variations in fiber size, proliferation of nuclei, fibrosis, hypertrophied and atrophic muscle fibers, fiber splitting, increased numbers of internal nuclei in long rows, sarcoplasmic pads, and ringbinden ("ring fibers").[1,2] Ringbinden, together with sarcoplasmic pads and long rows of internal nuclei, are most characteristic of DM in comparison with other muscular dystrophies. Another early and characteristic change is the atrophy of type 1 fibers (rich in oxidative enzymes and weak in myosin adenosine triphosphate [ATPase] activity). Pathological findings vary in frequency and severity from muscle to muscle and may be mild or absent in some muscle biopsy specimens (Fig. 7–2). Muscle biopsies and extensive electromyographic examinations are no longer necessary for diagnosis with the advent of specific genetic testing, an obvious example of the beneficial effect of modern molecular genetic diagnosis on cost and patient discomfort.

A distinct set of muscle changes in CDM may precede characteristic adult muscle findings. Abnormalities in the peripheral distribution and arrangement of myofibrils have been reported. Also, myofilaments with marked proliferation of the sarcotubular system and high electron dense I-bands (interpreted as a lattice-like network of tubules or infolding of proliferating sarcolemma) have been noted.[24–26] These findings are consistent with the evidence that *DMPK* with an expanded $(CTG)_n$ affects the function of the sodium channel, located in the sarcotubular system.[11] The sarcotubular system is an internal membrane system that is responsible for spreading electrical discharges (ion fluxes) rapidly throughout the muscle cell. If, in muscle, the initial effect of the expanded repeat mutation is on sodium channel phosphorylation, the subsequent changes observed over years in DM muscle could result from secondary cascade mechanisms.

Other ultrastructural studies contribute evidence of immaturity and possible abnormalities of proliferating sarcotubular membranes. Proliferation of the sarcotubular system may be a mechanism to compensate for alterations in sodium fluxes due to the effects of DM-mutated *DMPK*.[11] The sarco-

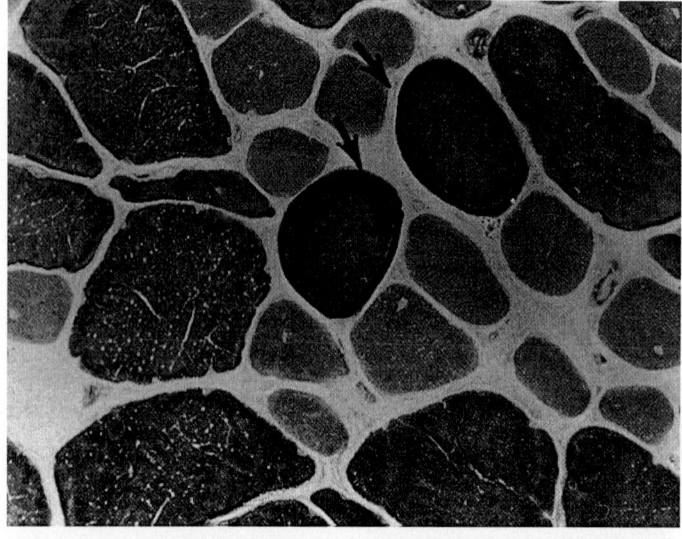

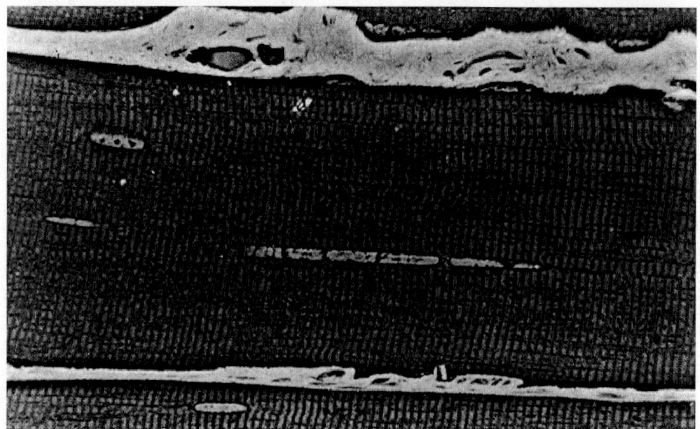


**Figure 7–2.** Typical pathological features in DM. *(A)* Two ring fibers (arrows) with surrounding type I fiber atrophy (myofibrillar ATPase, pH 9.4 staining). *(B)* A longitudinal section showing a chain of four central nuclei (resin section). (From Carpenter S, Karpati G: Pathology of Skeletal Muscle. Churchill Livingstone, New York, 1984.)

plasmic pads or masses located at the periphery of the muscle fiber have been shown to consist of groups of disorganized myofibrils, Z-band material, elements of triads and sarcoplasmic reticulum, and sarcoplasmic components, including glycogen, lipid droplets, and lysosomes.[25–27]

The discovery that the mutation causing DM may disrupt the function of a protein kinase led to recent experiments in which an abnormal phosphorylation state of the sodium channel was induced in frog oocytes when a DM-sized $(CTG)_n$ repeat *DMPK* gene was cotransfected with a skeletal muscle sodium channel instead of a normal-sized *DMPK* gene.[11,13,15] Reduced amplitude of the sodium current and accelerated current decay resulted from normal phosphorylation, but with a DM gene sodium current amplitudes were reduced to an even greater extent and exhibited slower decay kinetics. These effects were dependent on a phosphorylation site in the inactivation mechanism of the channel. Figure 7–3 illustrates the patch current averages observed in oocytes expressing skeletal muscle sodium channels together with normal or DM mutant *DMPK*.[11] These experiments suggest that one of the early effects of the *DMPK* containing an enlarged $(CTG)_n$ repeat may be phosphorylation of cation transport proteins, leading to myotonia and eventually to dystrophic changes.

Recombinant DMPK has also been shown *in vitro* to phosphorylate the β-subunit of the dihydropyridine receptor, a voltage-gated calcium channel.[28] Therefore, calcium in addition to sodium channels

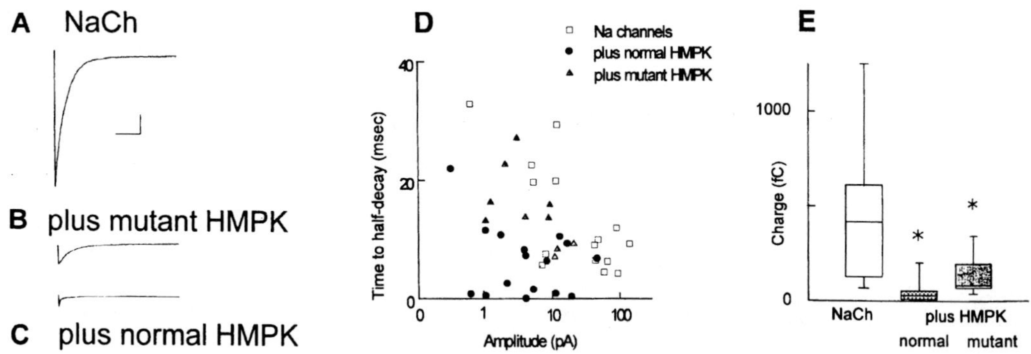


**Figure 7–3.** The patch current averages observed in oocytes expressing skeletal muscle Na channels together with normal or DM mutant myotonin protein kinase. *(A–C)* Patch currents. Average 50 to 100 traces in oocytes expressing skeletal muscle Na channels by themselves *(A)*, with the DM mutant HMPK *(B)*, or with the normal HMPK *(C)*. Bar = 20 ms and 10 pA. *(D)* Time to half-decay as a function of peak amplitude for patch currents in oocytes expressing only Na channels (open squares, n = 15), in oocytes coexpressing normal (closed circles, n = 16), and in DM mutant (open triangles, n = 10). *(E)* Box plots of transmembrane charge movement, calculated as the integral of current waveforms. (*$p < 0.005$ for any pair of groups; Mann-Whitney U test.)

may be involved in this potential channelopathy.

## Heart

Cardiac manifestations of DM can be fatal. In fact, sudden death may be the first and only manifestation of DM.[29,30] With the advent of continuous monitoring and longitudinal studies, there has been increased documentation of progressive cardiac signs.[31–33] Cardiac involvement has been documented in approximately 80% of those patients whose diagnosis of DM was based on skeletal muscle myotonia.[34] Bradycardia, arrhythmias, and other serious cardiac manifestations have been found in "normal" family members who can now be identified as carriers of the DM-expanded *DMPK* $(CTG)_n$ repeat.[3]

Conduction abnormalities are frequent.[30,34] In younger patients, these may be serious and precede other symptoms of the disease. Atrioventricular and intraventricular conduction defects occur in virtually all cases of CDM. Bradycardia and first-degree heart block are common, frequently not associated with any symptoms. Sudden death or syncope during athletic activities in teenagers or young adults in DM families are not uncommon. Myotonic dystrophy patients should have periodic electrocardiograms to detect progressive heart block. Periodic cardiac monitoring of *DMPK* mutation carriers may provide evidence of increasing heart block and suggest the need for further cardiac studies. When the PR interval reaches 0.20 second, more detailed studies are indicated.[30] His bundle-ventricular (HV) electrophysiological studies have demonstrated that conduction defects progress over several years.[31,33] Several patients who were followed up longitudinally activated prophylactic demand pacemakers when complete heart block occurred.

The most common histopathological findings in the cardiovascular system are fibrosis, fatty infiltration, and atrophy.[35] The myocardial metabolic rate for glucose and the phosphorylation rate constant were measured in DM patients with parametric images generated from dynamic cardiac positron emission tomography.[36] A reduction in glucose metabolism and myocardial hexokinase activation appeared to be correlated with the sizes of the $(CTG)_n$ repeat measured in leukocyte DNA. Thus, the DM mutant *DMPK* may affect not only the phosphorylation state of sodium channels but also the phosphorylation of other proteins, contributing to the pleiotropic manifestations of DM mutations.[36–38]

## Eye

Cataracts characteristic of DM are located in the posterior capsular area. They typically appear dust-like, scintillating, and iridescent.[39] Commonly found in adult DM patients, they usually do not impair vision, but frequently hasten the development of mature cataracts. They are best viewed by slit-lamp examination.[40] over several years of observation (frequently longer than a decade,) slit-lamp changes become easier to visualize as cortical spokes and a reticulated appearance of the lens develop Further changes include the coalescence of opacities throughout the lens and the development of star-shaped changes. By this time, the early opalescence disappears, and impairment of vision occurs. Patients with DM present rather late with complaints of clouded vision partly because of the gradual progression of the cataract and partly because of their general reluctance to seek medical consultation.[41]

Other ophthalmological abnormalities include pigmentary retinal degeneration as well as abnormal electroretinograms.[41,42] Perhaps the most obvious ophthalmological signs of DM involve the external ocular muscles. Ptosis is common. Weakness of eye movement can be demonstrated, although complaints of diplopia are surprisingly uncommon. On ophthalmological examination, intraocular pressure is low, resulting in asymptomatic enophthalmos. Although this may be advantageous as a protection against glaucoma, the phenomenon may reflect another manifestation of an underlying abnormality in membrane ion transport affecting the blood–ocular barrier.

## Gastrointestinal System

Pharyngeal weakness with occasional myotonia can cause dysphagia. Dilation and hypomotility of the esophagus or bowel can also be clinically troublesome.[1] This is particularly true in the neonatal period or in old age. Megacolon can cause constipation, colic-like abdominal pain, and diarrhea in adults as well as in children with CDM. In adults, a chronic constipation may gradually change to intermittent diarrhea that is unresponsive to most usual medications. Severe diarrhea can be a debilitating problem during the terminal phase of a patient's illness.

## Endocrine System

Hyperinsulinemia in response to a glucose bolus is characteristic of many DM patients.[43] In fact, insulin levels can be quite elevated, but hypoglycemia does not occur. Peripheral resistance to insulin may also be related to generalized membrane defect. Testicular and ovarian atrophy are also common in DM. Although this factor might limit reproductive fitness, gonadal atrophy generally appears late, usually after the prime reproductive years.[3] Hyperplasia of Leydig cells with degeneration of tubular cells are common findings. Ovarian changes are less well characterized owing to the difficulty in obtaining ovarian biopsy material. There has been considerable interest in endocrine abnormalities associated with calcium metabolism, but there is no general agreement on abnormal mechanisms. Again, abnormal responses by or abnormal transport through a membrane-associated protein may explain the highly varied manifestations of DM.

## Brain

Increased incidences of mild mental retardation and socialization difficulties in patients with DM has been observed. Hypersomnolence is another clinically significant problem. Adult patients may sleep up to 20 hours per day, exacerbating the situation for patients who may already be characteristically apathetic.[44] In fact, hypersomnolence is frequently not a complaint of the DM patient but rather of the primary caretaker. For individuals with preserved intellectual abilities, increasing sleepiness and frank hypersomnolence can interfere with daily functions and be quite refractory to treatment.[3]

Neuropathologically, intracytoplasmic inclusions and Marinesco bodies have been found in the thalamus and the substantia nigra.[45] The pathological significance of these findings and of the focal white matter lesions and anterior temporal lobe abnormalities seen with magnetic resonance imaging are unknown.[46,47]

## GENETIC STUDIES

### The Molecular Lesion

As a result of genetic linkage studies, the genetic mutation in DM was initially localized to the long arm of chromosome 19 and then identified through the efforts of many contributing laboratories organized by the Muscular Dystrophy Association as a Myotonic Dystrophy Task Force. The sharing of clinical and linkage data led to the discovery of a unique mutation on a region of chromosome 19.[13–15] This initial flurry of excitement suggested the rapid delineation of disease mechanisms but, like many other gene searches, knowledge of the molecular mutation did not quickly yield clear insights regarding disease pathogenesis.[3,18,48]

The heritable element responsible for the transmission of DM as an autosomal dominant trait is a variable-length $(CTG)_n$ repeat that does not interrupt the coding region of the gene within which it is found. The $(CTG)_n$ repeat is located in the 3'-untranslated region of a gene originally identified as a protein kinase, named *myotonin protein kinase* (DMPK). Thus, although the trinucleotide repeat expansion in DM patients undoubtedly underlies the clinical manifestations of the disease, the mechanisms involved with pathogenesis in each tissue remain essentially unknown.[3,49–51]

### Relationship of $(CTG)_n$ Repeat Expansion to Inheritance

Every normal human has a $(CTG)_n$ repeat sequence at the identical site. The size of the repeat is variable, but usually less than $(CTG)_{20}$, and is transmitted without an increase in size as a codominant genetic trait. The repeat number ranges from 5 to 37 in the normal population. Thus a normal father with a $(CAG)_5$ and a $(CAG)_{12}$ can transmit either to an offspring, the size of which will remain stable. In DM carriers (who are usually also patients), the size of the repeat ranges from 50 to several thousand. When repeats of this length are transmitted, they usually increase in size. The $(CTG)_n$ repeat size of 38 to 50 is considered a range of instability, or premutation, not associated with a phenotype, but provides a potential source of new disease mutations in subsequent generations.[18,52]

The size of the increased repeat that a patient inherits is roughly correlated with the severity of clinical involvement of DM. In general, a smaller $(CTG)_n$ expansion is associated with milder disease and later onset of signs and symptoms. Large $(CTG)_n$ repeat sizes (in the thousands) are commonly found in CDM patients who have prenatal and neonatal onset and the most severe and penetrant clinical manifestations. Thus, the size of the $(CTG)_n$ repeat may be viewed as a variable rheostat, with larger sizes associated with earlier and more penetrant clinical manifestations. This contributes to the variability in severity between members of the same family and the repetitive nature of this highly variable disease that can be observed in multiple members of different families.[3] The range of observable clinical disease in individuals makes DM the most clinically variable autosomal dominant disease in humans, and the variability between individuals is a recurrent characteristic of large DM pedigrees.

Another $(CTG)_n$ repeat syndrome, spinocerebellar ataxia type 8 (SCA8), has recently been shown to have similar molecular features to those of DM. The $(CTG)_n$ expansion in SCA8 is also in the 3'-untranslated region of the transcript. The range of repeat sizes in individuals affected by SCA8 is 70 to 170, similar to the range seen in adult onset DM. The *SCA8* alleles are highly unstable. Also, like DM, there is a female bias for $(CTG)_n$ repeat expansion.[53]

### Potential Pathogenic Molecular Events

#### ALTERATION IN DMPK EXPRESSION

A series of studies that attempted to quantitate the expression of *DMPK* in DM muscle led to variable results. Several groups documented an increased, abnormally large

*DMPK* transcript, while others reported decreased expression of a normal-sized *DMPK* mRNA.[21, 54–58] All studies found that the normal (wild-type) *DMPK* transcript was expressed, so the rationale for a relationship between the decreased expression of the mutant gene allele to clinical pathogenesis remains obscure. The usual explanation has been a "positive gain of function," but in this case, as opposed to the $(CAG)_n$ repeat diseases, the transcript coded by the allele with the $(CTG)_n$ repeat (noncoding region) is normal. In fact, the hypothesis that the variably increased $(CTG)_n$ repeat may be expressed in CDM and leads to the abnormal gain-of-function characteristic of the CDM syndrome, but not the adult DM syndrome, has gained credibility. Figure 7–4 illustrates mRNA extracted from skeletal muscle of five adult DM patients and one with CDM. This data confirms the initial data describing an enlarged species in CDM.[54,55] The data also confirms that most adult onset DM muscle preparations described in the literature do not demonstrate an enlarged species. In fact, the difference is that the enlarged species (?hn-RNA) is present in muscle and other tissues from CDM patients, whereas adult onset DM patients have only the normal-sized *DMPK* transcript.[21,58] The confusion and controversy in the literature resulted from assuming that the expressions of CDM and DM were the same. In fact, the available data is consistent with a different type of *DMPK* expression in CDM and in adult DM, with the adult pattern appearing in CDM patients as they get older and develop adult DM clinical characteristics.

## GAIN OF FUNCTION OF THE EXPANDED TRINUCLEOTIDE REPEAT AT THE DNA–RNA LEVEL

Several investigators have suggested that the effect of the enlarged $(CTG)_n$ repeat is via abnormal DNA nucleosomes or RNA transcript processing. Wang and coworkers[59] have suggested that the expansion of $(CTG)_n$ repeats increases the efficiency of

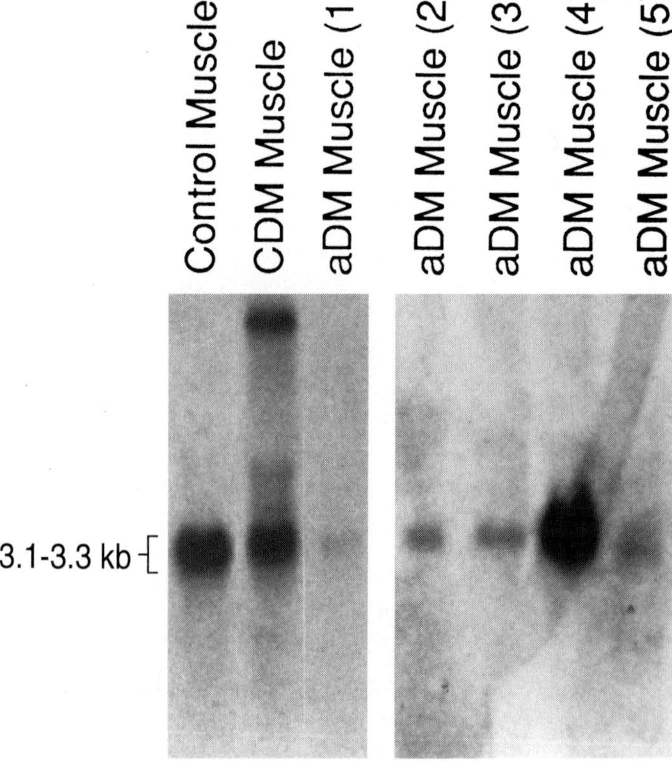


**Figure 7–4.** Northern blots of skeletal muscle biopsys specimens from five adult DM patients and one CDM patient. Two northern blots containing total mRNA extracted from skeletal muscle biopsies from five adult DM (aDM) patients and one CDM patient. These blots were probed with probe 971, a partial coding sequence of myotonin protein kinase that does not contain the $(CTG)_n$ repeat. The 3.1 to 3.3 kb band corresponding to the normal myotonin protein kinase is visualized in each tissue. Larger molecular weight bands are visualized in the CDM patient, but not in adult or control samples. The CDM sample was overloaded compared with the adult DM samples so that coding sequence hybridization at the higher molecular weight could be visualized. The same band can be hybridized with probes to the $(CTG)_n$ repeat sequences

nucleosome formation, which could decrease the efficiency of mRNA transcription. Nucleosomes are the basic structural elements of chromosomes that are constructed by 146 base pairs of DNA coiled about an octomer of histone proteins. These structures mediate general transcription repression. Two homologous RNA CUG-binding proteins (CUG-BP and ETR-3) have been identified and proposed to be sequestered by the expanded CUG repeats in DMPK mRNA, consequently leading to abnormal RNA processing of several RNAs containing CUG repeat sequences in regulatory regions.[60,61]

Using fluorochrome-conjugated $(CAG)_{10}$ probes that hybridized specifically to the expanded $(CTG)_n$ repeats, Taneja[62] could detect $(CTG)_n$ repeats containing transcripts as bright foci in the nuclei of DM fibroblasts and muscle. By simultaneously using a sense-strand probe with a different fluorochrome, Taneja determined that the focal concentrations were post-transcriptional RNA, separated from the DNA in the nuclei and concluded that this "concentration of nuclear transcripts . . . may represent aberrant processing of the RNA." The realization that DMPK RNA is increased in the nucleus, but decreased in the cytoplasm, may clarify earlier, conflicting studies reporting *total* cellular DMPK RNA being either increased or decreased.

### A FIELD EFFECT ON THE ADJACENT GENE FOR MYOTONIC DYSTROPHY–ASSOCIATED HOMEODOMAIN PROTEIN

The region surrounding the *DMPK* gene has been cloned and studied, and two flanking genes have been identified (Fig. 7–5). A growing hypothesis is that the variable clinical expressivity seen in DM patients is probably due to the abnormal effect of the increased triplet repeat on several genes and is not strictly limited to *DMPK*. Although this idea was proposed in 1994,[63] the hypothesis has since received the most experimental study from Johnson and colleagues.[49] These investigators mapped the nearby genes and suggested that a "field effect model . . . could affect gene activity in the region differently. . . . The genes affected in this way could be *DMPK, DMAHP,* 59 or other as yet uncharacterized genes."[49,64]

A possible "field effect" on the gene for DM-associated homeodomain protein *(DMAHP)* is of particular interest because the promoter for this gene overlaps with the mutated $(CTG)_n$ repeat. Consequently, it is quite possible that transcription of *DMAHP* is disrupted along with *DMPK* in this disease. Thornton, and colleagues[23] demonstrated significantly reduced transcription of the *DMAHP* gene tandem to the expanded repeat compared with the allele on the other chromosome in myoblasts, muscle, and myocardium from DM patients. DMAHP belongs to the homeodomain class of proteins that normally are involved in regulating gene expression during development as well as homeostasis in the adult state. This may help to explain why a mutation at the same locus could result in a congenital disorder (CDM) when severe, but also why at other times a less severe mutation creates an adult onset disease.

Although the exact function of DMAHP may not be clear, one clue comes from its homology to another homeodomain protein, AREC3, which binds to the sodium–potassium ATPase $\alpha$ 1-subunit gene regulatory element (ARE) found in myoblasts. Recombinant DMAHP has also been shown to bind to ARE.[24] This connection is intriguing with regards to the myotonia in DM. Disruption of this channel could lead to muscle membrane instability, resulting in the sustained contractions and trains of spontaneous electrical discharges characteristic of this disease. Further work is underway to determine whether disruption of the *DMAHP* gene product is in fact responsible for producing the myotonia as well as other manifestations of the phenotype.

## Animal Models

Reddy and associates[65] reported the results of removing ("knock-out") the *DMPK* gene in mice. The findings are interesting but not congruent with the clinical signs of DM. These mice developed a distal myopathy with variation in fiber size, increased fiber degeneration, and fibrosis. Ultrastructural

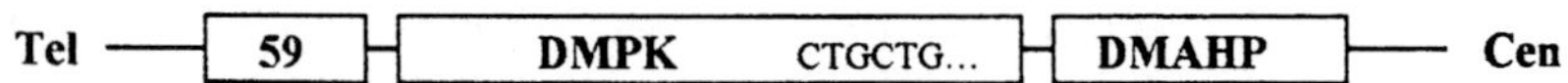


**Figure 7–5.** The DM locus at 19q13. DMPK is flanked by two genes, 59 and DMAHP. The CTG repeat that is expanded in DM is located in the 3' untranslated region of the gene, and this expansion overlaps with the promoter site for DMAHP.

changes included Z-line loss and mitochondrial and sarcoplasmic reticulum abnormalities; sternocleidomastoid muscles from animals without a *DMPK* gene on either chromosome 19 showed a 50% decrease in isometric twitch and tetanic force generation. The findings suggested that "a decrease in DMPK levels may contribute to DM pathology." The model fell short of many of the other characteristic signs, again suggesting involvement of other DM-specific mechanisms.

A valid animal model of DM would recapitulate the variable heritability of the $(CTG)_n$ repeat and also demonstrate variability in characteristic clinical expression. It is now possible to consider constructing transgenic mice with so-called knock-in technology in which the abnormal gene is inserted into the mouse at the correct homologous location (on chromosome 7 of the mouse). Different transgenic strategies have recently been reported. Only very mild myopathic changes in mice were produced by the insertion of multiple tandem copies of the *DMPK* gene into mice.[66] Later, Monckton and coworkers[67] introduced an expansion segment of CTG repeats into transgenic mice and demonstrated some intergenerational repeat length instability, but no detectable myopathic features were produced. The rather unimpressive pathological abnormalities produced in these transgenic models once again underscore the point that multiple molecular mechanisms may be responsible for generating the vast pleiotropic manifestations in DM.

## Current Clinical Applications of Genetic Testing

Within DM pedigrees there are two distinct applications for genetic testing. When DM is known to be in a family, relatives may seek genetic information. This is the more common circumstance in academic situations in which DM families have been studied and many individuals in extended pedigrees were contacted as part of the search for the DM gene. Another situation occurs when a patient presents to a physician with symptoms, physical features, or signs of DM with no known family history. In this case genetic testing is performed as a diagnostic procedure.

The diagnosis of suspected DM has changed radically over the past 5 years and represents a situation in which genetic testing has virtually replaced many less specific, more expensive, and sometimes painful diagnostic procedures. A suspected DM patient with minimal phenotypic symptoms and signs would, at a minimum, undergo electromyography, which could consist of testing muscles in multiple limbs. Unless myotonia was demonstrated, patients would undergo a more extensive examination. Other studies included slit-lamp examination for characteristic cataracts, glucose tolerance test with measurement of glucose and growth hormone, radiographic examination of long bones and skulls, and other endocrine studies. These studies are generally more expensive and less specific than genetic testing. In the United States, commercial laboratories offer DM diagnosis with both Southern blotting and polymerase chain reaction (PCR) analyses. For practical reasons, PCR analyses are usually performed first; if two normal-sized $(CGT)_n$ repeats are detected, no other testing is necessary (Fig. 7–6). DM patients may have a repeat too large to be amplified by standard PCR protocols; in these cases, the patients' PCR test may give the appearance of a single normal allele with the absence of a second allele. Because this can also be the case when a nonaffected individual has two identical normal alleles, Southern blotting (Fig. 7–1) is then performed to identify an enlarged genomic fragment. Southern blotting is a longer procedure that is less automated and more expensive, but is better at delineating very large repeats.

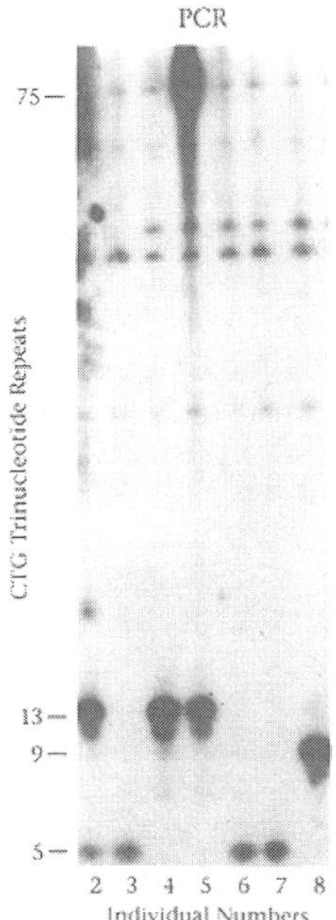


**Figure 7–6.** PCR analysis of a family with dystrophia myotonica (DM). Individual number 2 is unaffected by the disease and has two alleles with repeat lengths within the normal range. Individual 5 is an asymptomatic carrier with a repeat length clearly larger than normal. Individuals 3, 6, 7, and 8 are all DM patients. Only one band is present because the CTG lengths on their other allele was so long that the PCR reaction could not effectively amplify the sequence. Individual 4 does not carry the mutation. However, she only has one visualized band because both her alleles contain 13 CTG repeats. (Printed with permission by Vincent Bertolino, Athena Diagnostics, Inc., a division of Elan Pharmaceuticals.)

There are patients with myotonia who do not have DM. In practice, physical examination of the family is very useful for diagnosis, but this requires access to and willingness among family members. Unless the studies are part of a clinical research project, the costs of family studies are usually prohibitive because insurance carriers may only cover the index patient. Genetic testing of the patient provides the necessary information to either diagnose or rule out DM. The most confusing clinical situations arise in patients with proximal myotonic myopathy (PROMM)[68,69] and in extremely rare DM patients who are in DM pedigrees but do not demonstrate the increased repeat.[70] The discovery of the CTG repeat expansions in DM made it possible to appreciate families who were diagnosed or suspected as DM but in whom the DM repeat size was in the normal range. This familial disorder has become known as PROMM.[69] The 19q13 DM and the loci for the sodium and chloride channels associated with hyperkalemic periodic paralysis (with a form of myotonia) and myotonia congenita, respectively, have been excluded in PROMM families. The PROMM patients usually have proximal, but not distal, weakness of the legs, myotonia that may be intermittent, peculiar muscle pain, occasional cardiac arrhythmias, and cataracts that may appear identical to those in DM. Significant muscle atrophy is unusual, but myopathic muscle pathology (on biopsy) similar to what may be observed in early DM can be found. The genetic mutation for PROMM is unknown, and, although the DM triplet repeat and certain ion channel mutations have been ruled out as loci, the region of chromosome 19 surrounding the DM triplet repeat has not.

Rare families in whom the phenotype is even more similar to that of DM than that of PROMM, but in whom the typical CTG expansion cannot be demonstrated, raise the possibility of locus heterogeneity. Ranum and coworkers[70] described a pedigree with a condition (referred to by them as DM2) that is virtually indistinguishable from classic DM. This disorder maps to chromosome 3q. In affected members of this family, weakness was either equally proximal and distal, or exclusively distal, making PROMM a less appropriate diagnosis. Even more recently, Ricker and coworkers[71] established linkage between nine PROMM families and markers from the region of the DM2 locus on chromosome 3q. Further linkage and mutational analyses will help to determine whether DM2 and these pedigrees of PROMM are allelic disorders or rather caused by closely linked genes.

Is there a medical rationale for aggressive diagnosis of DM? Certainly the ability to provide both counseling and an explanation for many nonspecific troubling symptoms such as intermittent belly pain and aggressive social behaviors provides support for accurate diagnosis. In DM, however, cardiac arrhythmias are potentially fatal complications that can be monitored and prevented. The arrhythmias that are frequently associated with DM can be progressive, related to fibrosis of the conduction system.[30,33,35,72] Complete heart block in DM patients is associated with a bradycardia frequently incompatible with life, and, in a number of patients, pacemakers have avoided a potentially fatal complete heart block.[3] The progression of heart block has usually been encountered in adults, but can be observed to begin at any time. Therefore, a preventive rationale exists for the accurate diagnosis of DM patients.

Because of the characteristic mental status in many DM patients, the demands for medical care in general and genetic testing in particular are usually made by the normal individuals in the families. The unaffected sisters and brothers of DM patients are usually very concerned about ruling out disease, yet the DM patients are often less concerned about the disease or its genetic transmission. Although most DM genetic testing is performed for concerned family members or by new diagnoses when family history is unavailable or reported as negative, prenatal diagnosis is available and occasionally performed. The implications of genetic susceptibility are based on the same ranges as for carrier testing. Either amniotic fluid is taken after 15 weeks gestation or chorionic villus sampling is performed as early as 9 weeks gestation. Testing of maternal blood is usually required to rule out contamination. Field studies of initial negative family histories from DM patients have virtually always led to additional cases.

## SUMMARY

Of all human diseases, DM is characterized by the most variable expressivity of clinical symptoms that appear in virtually every organ system. The inherited DM mutation is an expanded trinucleotide repeat, $(CTG)_n$, located in the 3'-untranslated region of the *DMPK* gene on chromosome 19. The mutation allows rapid and inexpensive DNA testing for the presence of a DM mutation in symptomatic individuals. The protein product of the *DMPK* gene is normally expressed without additional repeated amino acid insertions such as the polyglutamine repeats in $(CAG)_n$ diseases so that a dominant gain of function at the protein level seems unlikely. The effect of the enlarged $(CTG)_n$ repeat on the expression of other genes in the region, or on other regulatory events in chromatin metabolism, are unknown. With the new molecular genetic technology for "knock-in" mutations, it is now possible to attempt to construct a mouse DM model. Myotonic dystrophy is genetically distinct from PROMM and DM2, which map to 3q.

## REFERENCES

1. Harper PS: Myotonic Dystrophy, ed 2. WB Saunders, London, 1989.
2. Roses AD, Harper P, Bossen E: Myotonic Muscular Dystrophy (Dystrophia Myotonica, Myotonia Atrophy). In Vinken PJ, Bruyn CW (eds), Handbook of Clinical Neurology. John Wiley and Sons, New York, 1979.
3. Roses AD: Myotonic Dystrophy, In Rosenberg RN, Prusiner SB, Dimauro S, Barchi RL (eds): The Molecular and Genetic Basis of Neurological Disease, ed 2. Butterworth-Heinemann, Stoneham, MA, 1997, pp. 913–930.
4. Roses AD, Appel SH: Muscle membrane protein kinase in myotonic muscular dystrophy. Nature 250:245–247, 1974.
5. Roses AD, Appel SH: Phosphorylation of component "a" of the human erythrocyte membrane in myotonic dystrophy J Membr Biol 20:51–58, 1977.
6. Hull KLJ, Roses AD: Stoichiometry of sodium and potassium transport in erythrocytes from patients with myotonic muscular dystrophy. J Physiol 254: 169–181, 1976.
7. Lipicky RJ, Bryant SN, Salmon JD: Cable parameters, sodium, potassium, chloride and water content, and potassium efflux in isolated external intercostal muscle of normal volunteers and patients with myotonia congenita. J Clin Invest 50:2091–2103, 1971.
8. Lipicky RJ: Studies in human myotonic dystrophy. In Rowland LP (ed): Pathogenesis of Human Muscular Dystrophies. Excerpta Medica, Amsterdam, 1978, pp.792–738.
9. McComas AJ, Mrozek K: The electrical properties of muscle fibre membranes in dystrophia myotonica and myotonia congenita. J Neurol Neurosurg Psychiatry 31:441–447, 1968.
10. Wong P, Roses AD: Altered component "A" phosphorylation in erythrocyte membrane in myotonic muscular dystrophy. J Membr Biol 45:145–166, 1977.
11. Mounsey JP, Xu P, John JE, et al.: Modulation of skeletal muscle sodium channels by human myotonin protein kinase. J Clin Invest 95:2379–2384, 1995.
12. Jansen G, de Jong PK, Amemiya C, et al.: Physical and genetic characterization of the distal segment

of the myotonic dystrophy area on 19q. Genomics 13:509–517, 1992.
13. Brook JD, McCurrach ME, Harley HG, et al.: Molecular basis of myotonic dystrophy: Expansion of a trinucleotide (CTG) repeat at the 3' end of a transcript encoding a protein kinase family member [published erratum appears in Cell 69:385, 1992]. Cell 68:799–808, 1992.
14. Mahadevan M, Tsilfidis C, Sabourin L, et al.: Myotonic dystrophy mutation: An unstable CTG repeat in the 3' untranslated region of the gene. Science 255:1253–1255, 1992.
15. Fu YH, Pizzuti A, Fenwick RG Jr, et al.: An unstable triplet repeat in a gene related to myotonic muscular dystrophy Science 255:1256–1258, 1992.
16. Ashizawa T, Dunne CJ, Dubel JR, et al.: Anticipation in myotonic dystrophy. I. Statistical verification based on clinical and haplotype findings [see comments]. Neurology 42:1871–1877, 1992.
17. Richards RI, Sutherland GR: Dynamic mutations: A new class of mutations causing human disease. Cell 70:709–712, 1992.
18. Caskey CT, Pizzuti A, Fu YH, Fenwick RG Jr, Nelson DL: Triplet repeat mutations in human disease. Science 256:784–789, 1992.
19. Roses AD: Molecular genetics of neurodegenerative diseases. Curr Opin Neurol Neurosurg 6:34–39, 1993.
20. Brook JD, Zemelman BV, Hadingham K, et al.: Radiation-reduced hybrids for the myotonic dystrophy locus. Genomics 13:243–250, 1992.
21. Fu YH, Friedman DL, Richards S, et al.: Decreased expression of myotonin-protein kinase messenger RNA and protein in adult form of myotonic dystrophy [see comments]. Science 260:235–238, 1993.
22. Roses AD: Muscle biochemistry and a genetic study of myotonic dystrophy. Science 260:235–238, 1993.
23. Thornton CA, Wymer JP, Simmons Z, McClain C, Moxley III RT: Expansion of the myotonic dystrophy CTG repeat reduces expression of the flanking DMAHP gene. Nat Genet 16:407–409, 1997.
24. Winchester CL, Johnson KJ: Is myotonic dystrophy (DM) the result of a contiguous gene defect? In Welsh, Warren (eds): Genetic Instabilities and Hereditary Neurologic Diseases. Academic Press, San Diego, 1998.
25. Fardeau M, Lapresle J, Milhaud M: Contribution a l'etude ultrastructurale des plaques motrices du muscle squelettique: ultrastructure des masses sarcoplasmiques laterales. C R Soc Biol (Paris) 159: 15–17, 1994.
26. Mussini I, Di Mauro S, Angelini C: Early ultrastructural and biochemical changes in muscle in dystrophia myotonic. J Neurol Sci 10:585–604, 1970.
27. Engel WK: Chemocytology of striated annulets and sarcoplasmic masses in myotonic dystrophy. J Histochem Cytochem 10:229–230, 1962.
28. Timchenko L, Nastaincyk W, Schneider T, Pate B, Hofmann F, Caskey CT: Full-length myotonin protein kinase (72 kDa) displays serine kinase activity. Proc Natl Acad Sci USA 92:5366–5370, 1995.
29. Spillane JD: The heart in myotonia atrophica. Br Heart J 13:343–347, 1951.
30. Moorman JR, Coleman RE, Packer DL, et al.: Cardiac involvement in myotonic muscular dystrophy. Medicine 64(6):371–387, 1985.
31. Prystowsky EN, Pritchett EL, Roses AD, Gallagher J: The natural history of conduction system disease in myotonic muscular dystrophy as determined by serial electrophysiologic studies. Circulation 60: 1360–1364, 1979.
32. Melacini P, Villanova C, Menegazzo E, et al.: Correlation between cardiac involvement and CTG trinucleotide repeat length in myotonic dystrophy. J Am Coll Cardiol 25:239–245.
33. Melacini P, Buja G, Fasoli G, et al.: The natural history of cardiac involvement in myotonic dystrophy: An eight year follow-up in 17 patients. Clin Cardiol 11:231–238, 1988.
34. Church SC: The heart in myotonia atrophica. Arch Intern Med 119:176–181, 1967.
35. Nguyen HH, Wolfe JT, Homes DR, Edwards WD: Pathology of the cardiac conduction system in myotonic dystrophy: A study of 12 cases. J Am Coll Cardiol 11:662–671, 1988.
36. Annane D, Duboc D, Mazoyer B, et al.: Correlation between decreased myocardial glucose phosphorylation and the DNA mutation size in myotonic dystrophy. Circulation 90:2629–2634, 1994.
37. Rudel R, Ricker K, Lehmann-Horn F: Genotype–phenotype correlations in human skeletal muscle sodium channel diseases [see comments] Arch Neurol 50:1241–1248, 1993.
38. Rudel R, Ruppersberg JP, Spittelmeister W.: Abnormalities of the fast sodium current in myotonic dystrophy, recessive generalized myotonia, and adynamia episodica. Muscle Nerve 12:281–287, 1989.
39. Vogt A: Die Cataract bei Myotonische Dystrophie. Schweiz Med Wochenschr 29:669–674, 1921.
40. Thomasen E: Myotonia. Universitetsforlaget, Aarbus, 1948.
41. Junge J: Ocular changes in dystrophia myotonica, paramyotonia and myotonia congenita. Doc Ophthalmol 21:1–115, 1996.
42. Burian NM, Burns CA: Ocular changes in myotonic dystrophy. Am J Ophthalmol 63:22–34, 1967.
43. Huff TA, Horton ES, Lebowitz NE: Abnormal insulin secretion in myotonic dystrophy. N Engl J Med 277:837–841, 1967.
44. Culebras A, Feldman RG, Merk FB: Cytoplasmic inclusion bodies within neurons of the thalamus in myotonic dystrophy. J Neurol Sci 19:319–321, 1973.
45. Ono S, Kanda F, Takahashi K, et al.: Neuronal cell loss in the dorsal raphe nucleus and the superior central nucleus in myotonic dystrophy: A clinicopathological correlation. Acta Neuropathol (Berl) 89:122–125, 1995
46. Hashimoto T, Tayama M, Miyazaki M, et al.: Neuroimaging study of myotonic dystrophy. I. Magnetic resonance imaging of the brain. Brain Dev 17:24–27, 1995.
47. Censori B, Provinciali L, Danni M, et al.: Brain involvement in myotonic dystrophy: MRI features and their relationship to clinical and cognitive conditions. Acta Neurol Scand 90:211–217, 1994.
48. Roses AD: Muscle biochemistry and a genetic study of myotonic dystrophy [letter; comment]. Science 264:587–588, 1994.
49. Johnson KJ, Boucher CA, King SK, et al.: Is myotonic dystrophy a single-gene disorder? Biochem Soc Trans 24:510–513, 1996.

50. Johnson K, Siciliano MJ: Report on MDA workshop on myotonic dystrophy, 10 Octobeer, 1994, Montreal, Quebec, Canada. J Med Genet 32:662–665, 1995.
51. Wieringa B: Myotonic dystrophy reviewed: Back to the future? Hum Mol Genet 3:1–7, 1994.
52. Mahadevan MS, Amemiya C, Jansen G, et al.: Structure and genomic sequence of the myotonic dystrophy (DM jubase) gene. Hum Mol Genet 2:229–304, 1993.
53. Koob MD, Moseley ML, Schut LJ, et al: Untranslated CTG expansion causes a novel form of spinocerebellar ataxia (SCA8). Nat Genet 21:379–384, 1999.
54. Roses AD: Myotonic dystrophy. Trends Genet 8: 254–255, 1992.
55. Sabouri LA, Mahadevan MS, Narang M, Lee DS, Surh LC, Korneluk RG: Effect of the myotonic dystrophy (DM) mutation on mRNA levels of the DM gene. Nat Genet 4:233–238, 1993.
56. Hofmann-Radvani H, Junien C: Myotonic dystrophy: Over-expression or/and under-expression? A critical review on a controversial point. Neuromusc Disord 3:497–501, 1993.
57. Novelli G, Gennarelli M, Zelano G, et al.: Failure in detecting mRNA transcripts from the mutated allele in myotonic dystrophy muscle. Biochem Mol Biol 29:291–297, 1993.
58. Krahe R, Ashizawa T, Abbruzzese C, et al.: Effect of myotonic dystrophy trinucleotide repeat expansion on DMPK transcription and processing. Genomics 28:1–14, 1995.
59. Wang Y, Schnegelsberg PN, Dausman J, Jaenisch R: Functional redundancy of the muscle specific transcription factors Myf5f and myogenin. Nature 379:823–825, 1996.
60. Philips AV, Timchenko LT, Cooper TA: Disruption of splicing regulated by a CUG-binding protein in myotonic dystrophy. Science 280:737–741, 1998.
61. Timchenko LT, Lu X, Roberts R, Timchenko NA: Myotonic dystrophy: Gain of function of RNA (CUG) triplet repeat bindings proteins. Am J Hum Genet (in press).
62. Taneja KL: Localization of trinucleotide repeat sequences in myotonic dystrophy cells using a single fluorochrome-labeled PNA probe. Biotechniques 24(3):472–476, 1998.
63. Roses AD, Taylor H, Schwartzbach C, et al.: The mechanisms of disease expression may not be directly related to MPK gene expression in myotonic dystrophy (DM): Alternative interactions of the triplet repeat locus. MDA Symposium on Molecular Mechanisms of Neuromuscular Disease, Tucson, AZ, 1994.
64. Boucher CA, King SK, Carey N, et al.: A novel homeodomain-encoding gene is associated with a large CPG island interrupted by the myotonic dystrophy unstable $(CTG)_n$ repeat. Hum Mol Genet 4:1919–1925, 1995.
65. Reddy S, Smith DB, Rich MM, et al.: Mice lacking the myotonic dystrophy protein kinase develop a late onset progressive myopathy. Nat Genet 325–335, 1996.
66. Jansen G, Groenen PJTA, Bachner D, et al.: Abnormal myotonic dystrophy protein kinase levels produce only mild myopathy in mice. Nat Genet 6: 136–145, 1996.
67. Monckton DG, Coolbaugh MI, Ashizawa KT, Siciliano MJ, Caskey CT: Hypermutable myotonic dystrophy CTG repeats in transgenic mice. Nat Genet 15:193–196, 1997.
68. Taylor HP, Schwartzbach CJ, Gilbert JR, et al.: Myotonic dystrophy in an affected family member inheriting affected parent's normal chromsome. Am J Hum Genet 53:1238, 1993.
69. Ricker K, Koch MC, Lehmann-Horn, et al.: Proximal myotonic myopathy. Clinical features of multisystem disorder similar to myotonic dystrophy. Arch Neurol 52:25–31, 1995.
70. Ranum LPW, Rasmussen PF, Benzow KA, Koob MD, Day JW: Genetic mapping of a second myotonic dystrophy locus. Nat Genet 19:196–198, 1998.
71. Ricker K, Brimm T, Koch MC, et al.: Linkage of proximal myotonic myopathy to chromosome 3q. Neurology 52:170–171, 1999.
72. Morgenlander JC, Nohria V, Saba Z: EKG abnormalities in pediatric patients with myotonic dystrophy. Pediatr Neurol 9:124–126, 1993.

# Chapter 8

# PRIMARY TUMORS OF THE NERVOUS SYSTEM

Stefan-M. Pulst, MD, Dr Med
Guido Reifenberger, MD, PhD



The current knowledge about the molecular genetic alterations associated with the initiation and progression of the most common forms of primary nervous system tumors, which are gliomas, primitive neuroectodermal tumors (PNETs), meningiomas, and schwannomas is reviewed in this chapter. Before that, we briefly review recent epidemiological data and the present histopathological classification of primary nervous system tumors. In addition, we outline the current concepts of the molecular basis of cancer and discuss the hereditary syndromes predisposing to the development of tumors of the nervous system.

## EPIDEMIOLOGY

Estimates of the incidences of the various tumors of the nervous system vary considerably depending on the source of data.[1] According to the first annual report of the Central Brain Tumor Registry of the United States (CBTRUS), the overall annual incidence rate for primary benign and malignant brain tumors in the United States is 10.9 cases per 100,000 population. An estimated 12,600 deaths were attributed to primary malignant brain tumors in 1994. Thus, primary central nervous system (CNS) tumors account for about 2% of all cancer-related deaths. The relative incidence of CNS tumors is age dependent. In children below the age of 15 years, primary tumors of the nervous system comprise close to 20% of all cancers, making them the second most common form of childhood cancer after the leukemias.[2] Interestingly, epidemiological studies have reported evidence of an increasing incidence of primary CNS tumors, particularly gliomas, in the elderly population.[3,4] This increase appears to be independent of the improvements in diagnostic facilities.[5]

## CLASSIFICATION

The most widely used classification system of tumors of the CNS is the World Health Organization (WHO) classification.[6] Although in certain aspects a compromise solution, it is presently the standard classification. The general use of this classification provides a common morphological baseline in neuro-oncology and greatly facilitates comparisons of clinical and laboratory results from different institutions around the world. The WHO classification is based on histopathological tumor typing and on an optional WHO grading scheme ranging from WHO grade I (benign) to WHO grade IV (malignant).

WHO grade I lesions generally include tumors with a minimal proliferative potential and the possibility of cure after surgical resection alone. Typical examples are pilocytic astrocytomas, subependymomas, myxopapillary ependymomas of the cauda equina, a variety of neuronal and mixed neuronal–glial tumors, schwannomas, and most meningiomas. Tumors of WHO grade II are those with low mitotic activity but a tendency for recurrence. The well-differentiated astrocytomas, oligodendrogliomas, mixed gliomas, and ependymomas are classic examples of WHO grade II tumors. WHO grade III is reserved for neoplasms with histological evidence of anaplasia, generally in the form of increased mitotic activity, increased cellularity, nuclear pleomorphism, and cellular anaplasia. WHO grade IV is assigned to mitotically active and necrosis-prone highly malignant neoplasms that are usually associated with a rapid preoperative and postoperative evolution of the disease. These include the glioblastoma and the various forms of PNETs.[6]

## MOLECULAR BASIS OF TUMOR GROWTH IN THE NERVOUS SYSTEM

The etiology of human brain tumors is still largely unknown. Although certain types of CNS and peripheral nervous system (PNS) tumors have been successfully induced in laboratory animals with a number of viral and chemical carcinogens,[7,8] the etiologic relationship of these agents to human tumors is uncertain. Epidemiological studies have suggested an increased incidence of brain tumors in association with certain occupations, but thus far no specific environmental agent has been convincingly shown to be responsible for the development of brain tumors in humans. The development of secondary CNS tumors (mostly gliomas, meningiomas, and sarcomas) in patients previously irradiated for other reasons has been documented in a number of case reports.[1,9,10] Furthermore, children with acute lymphoblastic leukemia who have received prophylatic craniospinal irradiation have been shown to carry an increased risk for the development of a glioma as a second neoplasia.[11] Nevertheless, radiation-induced tumors account for only a minute fraction of nervous system tumors.

In contrast to the little-known significance of environmental factors, certain genetic factors are well known to predispose for the development of CNS tumors. Bondy and coworkers[12] have shown that genetically determined sensitivity to gamma radiation may be associated with an increased risk for the development of a glioma. In addition, a number of familial tumor syndromes, including neurofibromatosis type 1 and type 2, tuberous sclerosis, von Hippel-Lindau syndrome, Li-Fraumeni syndrome, and Turcot's syndrome, are associated with a high risk for certain types of neural tumors. These syndromes are relatively rare disorders, however, and the vast majority of primary nervous system tumors are sporadic neoplasms of unknown etiology.

Recent progress in the understanding of the genetic basis of primary nervous system tumors has come from molecular biological studies showing that the formation of these tumors, similar to many other types of cancer, appears to be related to two fundamental alterations: inactivation of tumor suppressor gene products and activation of proto-oncogene products. These alterations may subvert the normal growth regulatory mechanisms and confer an *in vivo* growth advantage to the affected cell. According to the clonal evolution model of Nowell,[13,14] the development of a tumor is thought to be initiated by the clonal expansion of a single cell carrying a growth-advantageous mutation. Subsequently, any cell of this original clone may acquire additional genetic alterations, giving rise to more rapidly growing subclones. Tumors thus develop in a multistep process by the cumulative acquisition of genetic changes. The best evidence in support of this assumption comes from studies on colorectal tumors for which it has been possible to correlate progression from benign precursor lesions to metastatic carcinomas with the accumulation of alterations of distinct tumor suppressor genes.[15]

In the case of nervous system tumors, there are no known premalignant lesions, but gliomas, especially the diffusely infiltrating variants, frequently progress from relatively benign to more malignant forms. In line with the findings in colorectal tumors, the available data on gliomas also suggests that such progression is caused by progressive accumulation of genetic alterations.

## Tumor Suppressor Genes

The tumor suppressor genes, or antioncogenes, are cellular genes whose products under physiological conditions have a negative growth-regulatory function.[16] Tumor suppressor genes usually function as recessive genes, which means that both alleles need to be altered to cause the loss of function necessary for neoplastic transformation. In some situations, however, alteration of only one allele may be efficient enough for functional inactivation of a tumor suppressor gene product. This so-called dominant negative effect is exemplified by the *p53* tumor suppressor gene. Certain types of *p53* mutations result in the expression of mutant proteins that can inactivate wild-type p53 protein by the formation of functionally inactive oligomeric complexes.[17]

Inactivation of both copies of a tumor suppressor gene can be achieved by different genetic and chromosomal mechanisms, including mutation of both alleles, homozygous deletion, and, most frequently, mutation of one allele combined with loss of the other. In addition, transcriptional silencing by regional hypermethylation of CpG islands at the 5'-end of a gene has been shown to be a further mechanism of tumor suppressor gene inactivation in human tumors.[18–20]

It is important to know that alterations of recessive tumor suppressor genes are not only involved in the formation of sporadic tumors but also cause hereditary tumor syndromes of the nervous system. Most of these syndromes present clinically as dominant disorders even though the responsible mutations in tumor suppressor genes are recessive at the level of the cell. This phenomenon is due to the fact that patients with a hereditary tumor syndrome carry a germline mutation in one allele of a tumor suppressor gene. The second hit, resulting in inactivation of the second allele, occurs in somatic cells of a specific tissue, which then may develop a tumor. This two-hit mechanism (germline alteration followed by somatic alteration), originally proposed by Knudson[21] on the basis of statistical considerations for familial retinoblastoma, is now established for a number of other hereditary cancer syndromes such as neurofibromatosis type 1 and 2 and von Hippel-Lindau syndrome. Because the likelihood of a second hit over a person's lifetime approaches 1.0 for most tumor suppressor genes, the inheritance pattern is that of a dominant disease. If the likelihood of a second hit is less than 1.0, reduced penetrance results. Although sporadic tumors and tumors seen in patients with inherited tumor syndromes have similar pathologies, certain features point to the presence of a germline mutation (Table 8–1).

From a scientific point of view, the existence of families with a hereditary tumor predisposition has greatly facilitated the identification and cloning of tumor sup-

Table 8–1. **Characteristic Features of Hereditary Diseases Caused by Germline Mutations in Tumor Suppressor Genes**

| |
|---|
| Early onset of tumors |
| Bilateral occurrence of tumors |
| Presence of multiple tumor types |
| Positive family history of tumors |
| Non-tumor features for some diseases |
| Skin or eye involvement |
| Developmental abnormalities with or without hamartomatous lesions of other organ systems |

pressor genes by linkage analysis and positional cloning. In fact, most presently known tumor suppressor genes have been discovered by this approach (Table 8–2). Another commonly employed approach to determine the chromosomal location of tumor suppressor genes is the analysis of tumors for loss of heterozygosity (LOH) at well-mapped polymorphic loci, either by the analysis of restriction fragment length polymorphisms (RFLPs) or by the study of microsatellite polymorphisms. The rationale for the LOH approach is that inactivation of tumor suppressor genes in tumors is commonly achieved either by mutation of one allele combined with loss of the other or by deletion of both alleles.[22] Thus, the finding of a high incidence of LOH at a particular chromosomal region in a particular tumor type is indicative of a tumor suppressor gene being located within the lost area. To date, many different candidate tumor suppressor gene loci have been identified in the various forms of cancer with the LOH strategy. In gliomas, for example, this approach has led to the identification of a number of chromosomal regions. For some, the relevant tumor suppressor genes have already been found (e.g., 9p, *CDKN2A;* 10q, *PTEN;* 13q, *RB1;* and 17p, *p53*). For others

Table 8–2. **Inherited Tumor Syndromes Involving the Nervous System**

| Syndrome | Gene | Location | Associated Tumors |
|---|---|---|---|
| Neurofibromatosis type 1 | *NF1* | 17q11.2 | Neurofibroma, malignant peripheral nerve sheath tumor, optic glioma |
| Neurofibromatosis type 2 | *NF2* | 22q12 | Schwannoma, meningioma, ependymoma |
| von Hippel-Lindau syndrome | *VHL* | 3p25 | Capillary hemangioblastoma, renal cell carcinoma, pheochromocytoma |
| Tuberous sclerosis | *TSC1*<br>*TSC2* | 9q34<br>16p13.3 | Subependymal giant cell astrocytoma |
| Li-Fraumeni syndrome | *p53* | 17p13.1 | Soft tissue and bone sarcomas, breast carcinoma, glioma, leukemia, PNET |
| Turcot's syndrome | *APC*<br>*hPMS2*<br>*hMLH1* | 5q21<br>7p22<br>3p21.3–p23 | Colon carcinoma, glioblastoma, PNET |
| Gorlin's syndrome | *PTCH* | 9q22 | Basal cell carcinoma, PNET, meningioma |
| Cowden's syndrome | *PTEN* | 10q23 | Dysplastic gangliocytoma of the cerebellum, meningioma |
| Werner syndrome | *WRN* | 8p12 | Meningioma, astrocytoma |

(e.g., 1p, 6q, 10p, and 19q), they have not been identified.

## Proto-oncogenes

Evidence for the role of dominantly acting transforming genes (so-called oncogenes) in human tumors was originally provided by two independent lines of inquiry converging on the same genes. First, studies investigating the role of retrovirus-encoded genes in tumorigenesis revealed that the transforming retroviral genes (viral oncogenes) were actually mutated forms of normal cellular genes (cellular oncogenes or proto-oncogenes) that the virus had picked up during replication and integrated into its genome. Second, transfection of tumor DNA into immortalized NIH3T3 fibroblasts resulted in the identification of transforming genes that turned out to be mutant forms of the same genes that had been identified by the retroviral approach.[23]

More than 100 proto-oncogenes have been discovered thus far, each of which may become an activated oncogene in one or more of the various forms of cancer. Most of these genes code for proteins involved in the transduction of growth stimulatory signals from the extracellular space to the cell nucleus. That is, they encode growth factors, growth factor receptors, GTP-coupled proteins, protein kinases, or nuclear regulatory proteins.[23,24] Activation of proto-oncogenes to transforming oncogenes may be accomplished by a variety of genetic and chromosomal mechanisms. In human tumors, the most important mechanisms of oncogene activation include mutation, chromosomal translocations, and the increase in gene copy number by gene amplification. Gene amplification represents the most common mechanism of oncogene activation in human malignant gliomas.[25]

Cytogenetic studies have revealed that about 50% of glioblastomas show homogeneously staining regions and/or double minutes as karyotypic hallmarks of gene amplification.[26,27] The resulting gain in gene copy number is usually accompanied by a strong increase in the expression of the respective gene product. This overexpression may provide the affected cell with a selective growth advantage and thus promotes their clonal growth. Interestingly, gene amplifications have been predominantly found in tumors of an advanced grade of malignancy, indicating that this alteration is a major mechanism of tumor progression rather than of tumor initiation.[28]

# HEREDITARY TUMOR SYNDROMES PREDISPOSING TO NERVOUS SYSTEM TUMORS

As stated, nearly all primary nervous system tumors occur in a sporadic fashion, but some brain tumors may also develop as part of certain hereditary tumor syndromes. The germline mutations in such patients usually manifest themselves by the development of other symptoms in addition to nervous system malignancy. Occasionally, however, brain tumors may be the presenting manifestation in such cancer-prone patients. In the following text, we briefly discuss some of the most important hereditary tumor syndromes predisposing for the development of nervous system tumors. For further details, the reader is referred to Chapter 9.

## Neurofibromatosis Type 1 (Von Recklinghausen's Disease)

Neurofibromatosis type 1 (NF1) is transmitted in an autosomal dominant fashion with 50% of patients representing *de novo* mutations. The *NF1* gene is located on the long arm of chromosome 17 and was cloned in 1990.[29] Patients with NF1 typically develop multiple neurofibromas of the peripheral nervous system. Most neurofibromas, including the plexiform variant, are benign tumors, but a small fraction may turn into malignant peripheral nerve sheath tumors, which are life-threatening, highly malignant tumors associated with a poor prognosis. In addition to tumors of the peripheral nervous system, patients with NF1 have a predisposition for the development of gliomas.[30] These most frequently involve the optic nerves or optic chiasm and may be found in up to 15% of patients if detailed neuroimaging is used. The histology is typically that of a benign pilocytic astrocytoma. Less frequently, NF1 patients present with pilocytic astrocytomas in the brain stem, hypothalamus, cerebellum, or spinal cord. Reports of meningiomas in NF1 most likely represent the chance association of a common brain tumor with a common genetic disease.

## Neurofibromatosis Type 2

Neurofibromatosis type 2 (NF2) is much rarer than NF1 and affects approximately 1 in 40,000 individuals.[31] NF2 is caused by a germline mutation in the *NF2* gene, which is located at 22q12 and was cloned in 1993.[32,33] The principal tumor types associated with NF2 are schwannomas of cranial and spinal nerves (typical for NF2 are bilateral vestibular schwannomas) and meningiomas.[34] In addition, patients with NF2 have a predisposition for the development of gliomas. About 80% of gliomas in NF2 patients are intramedullary spinal or cauda equina tumors, and the vast majority of these are ependymomas.[35,36]

## Von Hippel-Lindau Syndrome

The combination of retinal angiomata (angiomatosis retinae) and cerebellar capillary hemangioblastoma represents the classic manifestation of von Hippel-Lindau syndrome (see also Chapter 9). In addition, other organ systems such as the kidneys, the pancreas, the adrenal gland and paraganglia, and the epididymis are frequently affected by either neoplastic or hamartomatous lesions. Capillary hemangioblastomas in von Hippel-Lindau patients tend to manifest in younger patients than do sporadic capillary hemangioblastomas and are more often multifocal.[37] The *VHL* gene maps to chromosome 3p25–p26 and was cloned in 1993.[38]

## Tuberous Sclerosis

Tuberous sclerosis (TS) is the second most frequent hereditary tumor syndrome of the nervous system after NF1.[39] The typical CNS lesions in patients with TS are either hamartomas such as cortical tubers and subependymal nodules or a characteristic type of benign astrocytic tumor called *subependymal giant cell astrocytoma*.[39] Molecular genetic studies have implicated two different genes, located at 9q34 (*TSC1*) and 16p13.3 (*TSC2*), in the genesis of TS.[40] Both genes have been cloned.[41,42] There appear to be no major differences in the phenotypes associated with mutations in either *TSC1* or *TSC2*. A recent study, however, has suggested that mental retardation is significantly less frequent among carriers of *TSC1* than *TSC2* mutations.[43]

## Li-Fraumeni Syndrome

Li-Fraumeni syndrome is a rare, dominantly inherited disorder typically caused by germline mutations in the *p53* tumor suppressor gene.[44] The most common types of tumors occurring in Li-Fraumeni patients are breast carcinomas and sarcomas of bone and soft tissue. Brain tumors account for about 13% of all neoplasms associated with *p53* germline mutations.[45] Histologically, most are astrocytic gliomas (including glioblastoma multiforme), followed by PNETs. This corresponds remarkably well with the findings in sporadic brain tumors, among which somatic *p53* mutations also show a preference for astrocytomas.[45]

An exceptionally high frequency of *p53* germline mutations has been reported in patients with multifocal glioma, glioma with secondary malignancies, glioma with a familial history of cancer, or all three risk factors.[46] This data is debatable, however, because it is not quite clear whether some of these cases may actually represent formes fruste of Li-Fraumeni syndrome. In addition, another study did not identify germline mutations in exons 5 through 9 of the *p53* gene in 26 members of 16 families with glioma.[47]

## Turcot's Syndrome

Turcot's syndrome is a rare disorder characterized by the association of colonic polyposis and primary neuroepithelial tumors of the CNS such as malignant gliomas and PNETs. A subset of patients with Turcot's syndrome carry germline mutations in the gene for familial adenomatous polyposis coli (*APC*).[48,49] In addition, a patient with Turcot's syndrome and congenital hypertrophy of the pigment epithelium, an abnormality also seen in familial APC, has been reported.[50] On the other hand, somatic *APC* mutations are not a major cause of sporadic brain tumors. Mori and colleagues[49] did not detect any *APC* gene mutations in 47 medulloblastomas, 8 glioblastomas, 22 astrocytomas, and 2 oligodendrogliomas.

Tops and coworkers[51] found recombination events between markers linked to *APC* and the Turcot's syndrome phenotype, indicating the involvement of further genes in this disease. This hypothesis has been confirmed by identification of germline mutations in the mismatch repair genes *hPMS2* (human postmeiotic segregation 2) and *hMLH1* (human mutL homologue 1).[52] Of 14 families with Turcot's syndrome, 10 had germline mutations in the *APC* gene, and 2 had mutations in mismatch repair genes. The predominant CNS tumors in the families with *APC* mutations were medulloblastomas, whereas in the other four families glioblastomas predominated.[52] Interestingly, patients with glioblastomas and Turcot's syndrome caused by mutations in mismatch repair genes appear to survive longer on average than patients with sporadic glioblastomas.[52]

## Gorlin's Syndrome

Gorlin's syndrome, also known as *nevoid basal cell carcinoma syndrome,* is an autosomal dominant disorder leading to the development of multiple basal cell carcinomas of the skin, palmar and plantar pits, odontogenic keratocysts, and skeletal anomalies.[53] Intracranial calcifications, especially of the falx, are common, and defects of neuronal migration have also been observed.[54] Childhood medulloblastoma, meningioma, craniopharyngioma, and neurofibroma have been described in patients with Gorlin's syndrome.[55–57] The Gorlin's syndrome gene maps to 9q22 and has been identified as the human homologue of the *Drosophila patched* gene (*PTCH*).[58,59] *PTCH* codes for a transmembrane protein (Ptch) that serves as a receptor for the secreted Sonic hedgehog (Shh) signaling protein.[60] Somatic mutations in *PTCH* have been detected in sporadic basal cell carcinomas, PNETs, and certain other types of sporadic tumors.[61,62]

## Cowden's Syndrome

Cowden's syndrome, also known as *multiple hamartoma syndrome,* is an autosomal dominant cancer syndrome that predisposes to a variety of hamartomas and neoplasms. The major CNS lesion associated with the disease is dysplastic gangliocytoma of the cerebellum (Lhermitte-Duclos disease).[63] Further associated CNS lesions include megalencephaly and gray matter heterotopias. Occasional cases of meningiomas in patients with Cowden's disease have also been documented.[64]

Peripheral manifestations include multiple trichilemmomas of the skin, cutaneous keratoses, oral papillomatosis, gastrointestinal polyps, hamartomas of soft tissues, thyroid tumors, as well as benign and malignant breast tumors.[65,66] Germline mutations in the *PTEN* tumor suppressor gene at 10q23 have been identified as the genetic lesion causing Cowden's disease.[67]

## Werner's Syndrome

Werner's syndrome is a recessive trait with clinical symptoms resembling premature aging. The responsible gene maps to the short arm of chromosome 8 and has been identified by positional cloning.[68] In addition to premature aging, some individuals with Werner's syndrome may develop tumors, including CNS tumors such as meningiomas and, less frequently, astrocytomas.[69–71]

# RELATIVE RISK OF BRAIN TUMORS IN FIRST-DEGREE RELATIVES

Epidemiological studies have detected only a small increase in the risk of nervous system tumors for relatives of patients with brain tumors. Choi and associates[72] found a ninefold increase in the incidence of brain tumors among relatives of glioma patients compared with controls. Even this increased relative risk, however, translated into a small absolute risk of 0.6% in this study. In another study, the increased relative risk was less significant.[73] Gold and associates[74] compared several risk factors in 361 children with brain tumors with 1083 matched controls. In this study, a family history of tumors did not contribute to an increased risk of brain tumors in children, although a modest increase in risk of childhood brain tumors was associated with a maternal family history of birth defects. Kuijten and coworkers[75] found a modestly increased risk of childhood cancers only in relatives of patients with primitive neuroectodermal tumors; for relatives of astrocytoma patients, the risk was not significantly increased.

## GLIAL TUMORS

Gliomas are a heterogeneous group of mostly sporadic neoplasms derived from glial cells. They account for about 40% to 45% of all intracranial tumors and thus are the most common tumors among the primary CNS neoplasms.[1] Depending on morphological appearence and presumed histogenesis, gliomas are subdivided into several subgroups, the most important being astrocytic tumors (including the glioblastoma), oligodendroglial tumors, mixed gliomas (oligoastrocytomas), and ependymal tumors. With the exception of certain benign types such as the pilocytic astrocytoma, very few gliomas can be cured by the presently available therapeutic options (operation, radiotherapy, chemotherapy). Thus, the prognosis for most glioma patients, particularly for those with a glioblastoma, is still poor.[76,77]

A genetic predisposition for the development of gliomas is seen in NF1 and NF2, Li-Fraumeni syndrome, tuberous seleosis, and Turcot's syndrome. The specific type of glioma and its location may vary depending on the disorder. For example, pilocytic astrocytoma of the optic nerve is typical for NF1, whereas ependymoma of the spinal cord is characteristic for NF2. Of 282 children with astrocytoma examined by Kibirige and associates,[78] 21 had a diagnosis of NF1, and 4 had TS. Familial glioma not associated with a specific genetic syndrome does occur but is infrequent, and it is exceedingly rare to see more than two first-degree relatives with glioma. Vieregge and colleagues[79] reviewed 39 reports of familial glioma and concluded that 60% involved affected siblings.

### Astrocytic Gliomas

The astrocytic gliomas may be subdivided into two major groups (*1*) the more common group of diffusely infiltrating tumors, comprising astrocytoma, anaplastic astrocytoma, and glioblastoma; and (*2*) the less common group of tumors with more circumscribed growth consisting of pilocytic astrocytoma, pleomorphic xanthoastrocytoma (PXA), and subependymal giant cell astrocytoma of TS. Tumors of the second group typically occur in children and young adults, grow slowly, and have a limited potential for malignant progression. Thus, they are usually associated with a more favorable prognosis. In contrast, diffusely infiltrating astrocytomas preferentially manifest in adult patients, have an inherent tendency to undergo malignant progression, and are associated with a more ominous prognosis. Diffuse astrocytomas account for almost 50% of all primary intracranial tumors in adults. Thus far, most studies investigating the molecular genetics of astrocytic gliomas have concentrated on the common diffuse astrocytomas.

#### PILOCYTIC ASTROCYTOMA AND PLEOMORPHIC XANTHOASTROCYTOMA

The most frequent genetic abnormality in pilocytic astrocytomas identified thus far is loss of alleles on the long arm of chromosome 17 encompassing the *NF1* gene locus. About 20% of sporadic pilocytic astrocytomas were found to carry this alteration.[80] In view of the known predisposition of NF1 patients for the development of pilocytic astrocytomas, it is possible that somatic *NF1* alterations are also involved in the pathogenesis of sporadic pilocytic astrocytomas.

Molecular genetic analysis of eight cases of benign and malignant PXAs revealed mutation of the *p53* tumor suppressor gene in two tumors and epidermal growth factor receptor gene (*EGFR*) amplification in one glioblastoma, which was the second recurrence of a PXA.[81] No losses on chromosomes 10 and 19 were found. The authors concluded that the genetic alterations in PXAs may differ from those in diffuse astrocytomas.

## ASTROCYTOMA

Astrocytomas of WHO grade II preferentially occur in the cerebral hemispheres of patients around 35 to 45 years of age. With computer tomography (CT), they appear as ill-defined areas of low density that generally lack significant contrast enhancement. Histologically, astrocytomas are well-differentiated tumors of low to moderate cellularity that diffusely infiltrate the brain parenchyma. Microcystic degeneration is a common feature. Signs of anaplasia such as increased mitotic activity, necroses, or microvascular proliferations are absent. On the basis of the predominant cell type, three common histological variants can be distinguished: fibrillary, protoplasmic, and gemistocytic.[6]

Despite the relatively high differentiation and slow growth of WHO grade II astrocytomas, the median survival of these patients is only about 8 years, and most patients are dead within 10 years after diagnosis.[82,83] This rather poor prognosis of astrocytomas is related to their diffusely infiltrating growth, which does not allow complete resection, as well as to their inherent tendency for malignant progression. It has been shown that most WHO grade II astrocytomas undergo progression to anaplastic astrocytoma or glioblastoma and that this phenomenon represents the major cause of tumor-related deaths in astrocytoma patients.[82] The standard treatment for astrocytomas consists of surgical excision. Adjuvant radiotherapy is either given after the first operation or, more commonly, postponed until malignant progression has become evident upon recurrence.

## MOLECULAR GENETICS OF ASTROCYTOMAS

The genetic alterations in astrocytomas, anaplastic astrocytomas, and glioblastomas are summarized in Figure 8–1. The two most common molecular abnormalities in astrocytomas of WHO grade II are gain of chromosome 7 or 7q and allelic loss on chromosome 17p, the latter often combined with mutation of the *p53* gene at 17p13.1. For many years, trisomy 7 has been recognized as a frequent cytogenetic abnormality in astrocytic gliomas.[84,85] A more recent study with comparative genomic hybridization (CGH) has corroborated gain of 7 or 7q in 50% of low-grade astrocytomas.[86] This alteration thus represents a frequent and early event in astrocytoma formation. It remains to be determined, however, which gene(s) on chromosome 7 may provide a selective growth advantage, presumably by virtue of the gain in gene copy number resulting in increased expression.

Loss of alleles on 17p is found in about 30% to 50% of astrocytomas and is frequently but not invariably associated with mutation of the remaining *p53* allele.[45,87,88] According to Hermanson and coworkers,[89] astrocytomas (as well as anaplastic astrocytomas and glioblastomas) with loss of alleles on 17p frequently show elevated expression of the α-type receptor for platelet-derived growth factor. The precise mechanism for this association is unclear at present. The occasional finding of astrocytomas with LOH on 17p in the absence of *p53* mutation or LOH on distal 17p not involving the *p53* locus has been interpreted as evidence of a second tumor suppressor gene on 17p acting in a subset of astrocytomas.[90,91] One candidate gene is *HIC1*, a zinc-finger transcription factor gene located telomeric to *p53* at 17p13.3.[92] This gene is ubiquitously expressed in normal tissues whereas certain tumors, including a fraction of astrocytomas, lack detectable expression.

Other genetic alterations detected at more than random frequencies in low-grade

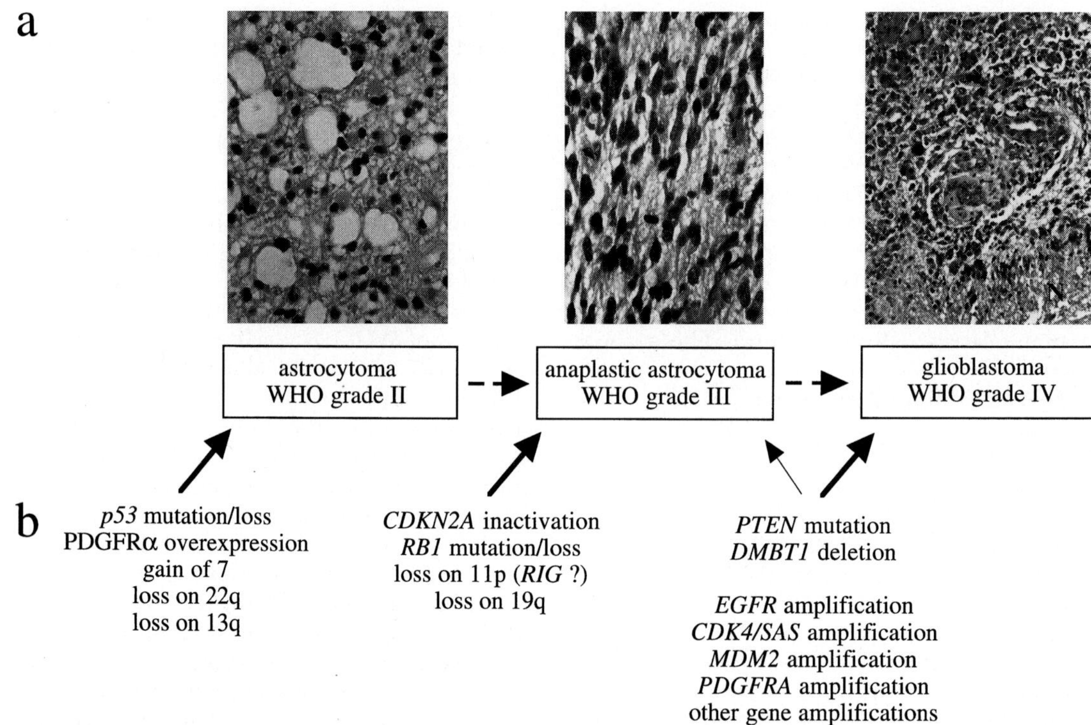


**Figure 8–1.** Histopathology and genetic alterations of diffuse astrocytomas. *(A)* Typical histopathological appearence of an astrocytoma with low cellurity and microcyst formation (left); an anaplastic astrocytoma with increased cellularity, nuclear atypia, and mitoses (middle); and a glioblastoma with microvascular proliferation and necrosis (N) (right). All sections are stained with H&E (×260, ×260, ×100). *(B)* Summary of the most common genetic abnormalities associated with the initiation and progression of diffuse astrocytic gliomas. The genetic and chromosomal aberrations are given before the malignancy grade in which they are first found at significant frequency (thick arrows). Some changes, including amplification of *EGFR, CDK4,* or *MDM2,* are not only associated with glioblastomas but may already be detected in a fraction of anaplastic astrocytomas. This fact is illustrated by a thin arrow.

diffuse astrocytomas are losses of 22q, 13q, and the sex chromosomes.[93] Mutational analysis of the *NF2* gene in low-grade and high-grade astrocytomas with LOH on 22q did not reveal mutations of this tumor suppressor gene, indicating that another gene on 22q is likely to be involved in astrocytic tumors.[94,95] The LOH on 13q observed in a subset of low-grade astrocytomas usually involved the *RB1* locus, but mutations of the *RB1* gene have not yet been found in these tumors.[96,97]

## ANAPLASTIC ASTROCYTOMA

Anaplastic astrocytomas (WHO grade III) preferentially occur in the cerebral hemispheres of patients on average a decade older than those with WHO grade II astrocytomas.[9] Radiographically, these tumors frequently show at least focal enhancement on CT scans after intravenous administration of contrast agents. Microscopically, anaplastic astrocytomas are characterized by signs of focal or diffuse anaplasia such as increased cellularity, pleomorphism, nuclear atypia, and mitotic activity.[6] The typical histological hallmarks of glioblastoma (i.e., vascular proliferations and necroses) are not yet present, but anaplastic astrocytomas tend to rapidly progress to glioblastoma. The median survival after surgery and radiotherapy is in the range of only 2 to 3 years.[77,98]

## MOLECULAR GENETICS OF ANAPLASTIC ASTROCYTOMAS

The molecular alterations described above for astrocytomas of WHO grade II (i.e., gain of 7q and loss of 17p associated with *p53* mutation) are present at similar frequencies in anaplastic astrocytomas. In addition, these tumors frequently show loss of alleles on 9p, 11p, and 19q.[99–102] The suspected tumor suppressor gene on 19q is still unknown. A candidate tumor suppressor gene on 11p is *RIG* ("regulated in glioma"), which has been found to be altered in about 25% of glioma cell lines.[103] The critical gene on 9p has been identified as the *CDKN2A (MTS1)* tumor suppressor gene at 9p21.[104,105] *CDKN2A* codes for a negative regulator of cell cycle progression from G1 to S phase (p16) which acts by the inhibition of complexes between D-type cyclins and cyclin-dependent kinases cdk4 or cdk6 (Fig. 8–2).[106,107] Schmidt and associates[108] found homozygous deletion of both *CDKN2A* alleles in 3 of 16 anaplastic astrocytomas (19%) and loss of one *CDKN2A* allele in 2 of 16 tumors (12.5%). Interestingly, about 15% of anaplastic astrocytomas were found to have amplification and overexpression of the *CDK4* (cyclin-dependent kinase 4) gene at 12q13–q14, and this alteration occurs preferentially in tumors without *CDKN2A* deletion or mutation.[96,108,190] In addition, a subset of anaplastic astrocytomas with no abnormality of *CDK4* or *CDKN2A* carries mutations in the retinoblastoma gene (*RB1*). Thus, more than 60% of anaplastic astrocytomas have aberrations of at least one of these three genes.[96]

Anaplastic astrocytomas may show amplification of proto-oncogenes, including *CDK4* and *SAS* (sarcoma amplified sequence) in about 15%, *MDM2* (murine double minute gene 2) in about 8% to 10%, and *EGFR* in less than 10% of the tumors.[25] A CGH study by Weber and coworkers[110] identified additional amplification sites on 12p13, 12q22-qter, and 18p.

## GLIOBLASTOMA

The most malignant type of glioma, the glioblastoma (WHO grade IV), is also the most common, accounting for close to 50% of all gliomas.[111] The incidence of glioblastomas peaks between 45 and 60 years of age. In adults, glioblastomas share a preferential supratentorial location with the other diffuse

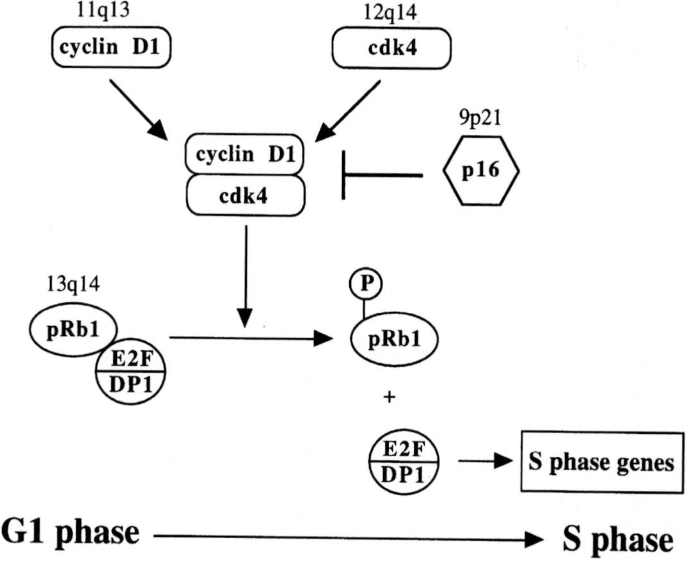


**Figure 8–2.** Simplified schematic representation of the interactions of cell cycle regulatory proteins at the G1/S phase transition in human cells. Under physiological conditions, complex formation of cyclin D1 and cdk4 results in activation of the cdk4 kinase. One important substrate of cdk4 is the retinoblastoma gene product pRb1. Underphosphorylated pRb1 can complex transcription factors of the E2F and DP1 families and thereby block their function. Upon phosphorylation, E2F and DP1 are released from pRb1 and can induce the transcription of a set of S-phase genes necessary for cell cycle progression into S phase. The *CDKN2A* gene product p16 is a potent inhibitor of cyclin D1–cdk4 complexes and can thereby block phosphorylation of pRb1 by cdk4 and induce a cell cycle arrest. Disturbances of this regulatory system are found in anaplastic astrocytomas and most glioblastomas.

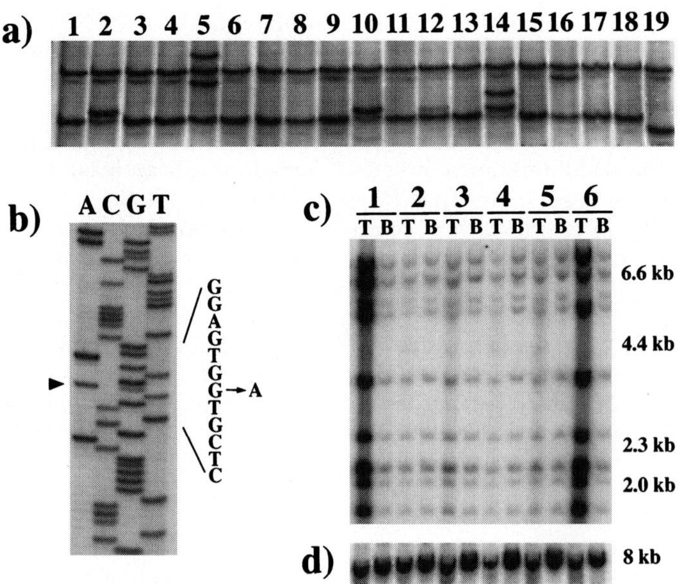


**Figure 8–3.** Examples of molecular abnormalities in glioblastomas. *(A)* Screening for mutations in the *p53* tumor suppressor gene by single-strand conformation polymorphism analysis (SSCP). Parts of the *p53* gene (exon 8) were amplified by polymerase chain reaction (PCR) from glioblastomas (lanes 1–17), leukocyte DNA (lane 18), and the A437 cell line (lane 19). The PCR products were separated on 10% nondenaturing polyacrylamide gels. Aberrant SSCP bands indicating mutations are seen in five glioblastomas (lanes 2, 5, 10, 12, and 14) as well as in the control line A431 (lane 19). *(B)* Conformation of *p53* mutation in a glioblastoma by DNA sequencing. Shown is part of a sequencing autoradiogram with a point mutation resulting in a G to A change as indicated. Because the sequence shown is that of the noncoding strand, this mutation results in a change of codon 297 (CAC to TAC). This mutation results in a histidine to tyrosine amino acid substitution. *(C, D)* Demonstration of *EGFR* amplification in glioblastomas by Southern blotting. A Southern blot with tumor (T) and leukocyte DNA (B) from six glioblastoma patients was hybridized with a radioactively labeled probe for EGFR (C). As a control for DNA loading, the same blot was rehybridized with a probe for ERBB3 (D). Note the strong increase in signal intensity for *EGFR* in the tumor DNAs of patients 1 and 6 indicating *EGFR* gene amplification.

astrocytomas. With CT, these tumors usually appear as a ring structure with a hypodense center (necrosis) surrounded by a ring of contrast-enhancing vital tumor tissue and edema. Macroscopically, typical glioblastomas are largely necrotic masses with a peripheral zone of fleshy gray tumor tissue. Intratumoral hemorrhage is a frequent finding. Histologically, glioblastomas are cellular tumors that may show a variety of tissue and cell differentiation patterns. Essential for the diagnosis is the presence of prominent vascular proliferation and/or necroses.[69]

The prognosis of glioblastoma patients is extremely poor, with a median postoperative survival time of only 12 months.[76] The standard therapy consists of neurosurgical tumor resection and postoperative radiation therapy. The benefit of adjuvant chemotherapy is disputed. Various experimental therapies, including immunotherapy and somatic gene therapy, are currently being investigated, but thus far none of these novel approaches has resulted in a significant improvement of the poor prognosis.

## ALLELIC LOSS AND TUMOR SUPPRESSOR GENES

Loss of alleles on 17p and/or *p53* mutation (Fig. 8–3) is found in about 25% to 30% of glioblastomas and is thus less frequent as in astrocytomas and anaplastic astrocytomas.[45,87] Gain of chromosome 7 also represents a common finding in glioblastomas.[84] In contrast to astrocytomas and anaplastic astrocytomas, glioblastomas typically lose genetic material from chromosome 10, commonly due to deletion of one entire chromosome (monosomy 10) and more rarely due to partial deletions. The incidence of chromosome 10 loss in glioblastomas varies in different studies, ranging from 60% to over 90% of the cases.[87] Three different regions on both arms of chromosome 10 have been implicated as potential sites of glioblastoma-associated tumor suppressor genes.[112] The region most frequently deleted is located at distal 10q and spans approximately 5 cM between the loci *D10S587* and *D10S216*.[113]

A candidate tumor suppressor gene designated *DMBT1* ("deleted in malignant brain tumors 1") has recently been cloned and mapped to this region.[114] Intragenic homozygous deletions in *DMBT1* were found in about 23% of glioblastomas.[114] Another candidate gene from distal 10q is the *MXI1* gene, which codes for a negative regulator of the Myc oncoprotein. Mutations of *MXI1* have been detected in prostate cancer.[115] Glioblastomas have not been studied in detail for *MXI1* mutations. In contrast, somatic mutations in the *PTEN* tumor suppressor gene at 10q23 have been detected in about one-third of glioblastomas.[116–118] The *PTEN* gene, also known as *MMAC1* ("mutated in multiple advanced cancers 1"),[118] is altered not only in glioblastomas but also in many other types of human malignant tumors, including breast carcinomas, prostate carcinomas, and malignant melanomas.[117,118]

In addition to loss of chromosome 10, glioblastomas frequently show deletions of one or both copies of the *CDKN2A* tumor suppressor gene on 9p21. Schmidt and associates[108] found homozygous deletion of *CDKN2A* in 41% and hemizygous loss of *CDKN2A* in 28% of primary glioblastomas. In glioblastoma cell lines, the incidence of homozygous *CDKN2A* loss seems to be even higher, reaching 70%.[119] In addition, inactivation of *CDKN2A* either by point mutation or by 5' CpG island methylation has been found in some glioblastomas.[96,120]

Other genetic alterations observed at more than random frequencies in glioblastomas are allelic losses on chromosomes 6, 11p, and 22q.[93,99,101,121] Comparative genomic hybridization studies have revealed various other deletion sites in individual glioblastomas that may involve virtually each chromosome.[110,122–125] These studies indicate that the number of genomic alterations detectable by CGH in a glioblastoma is about 10 on average. Because CGH has a limited spatial resolution and cannot detect more subtle changes such as point mutations or small deletions, the actual number of genetic abnormalities per tumor is certainly even higher.

Recent studies have provided evidence for the production and secretion of a number of angiogenic growth factors by the tumor cells and their involvement in the typical vascular proliferations in glioblastomas.[126] Among these, the most important one appears to be the vascular endothelial growth factor (VEGF). Tumor cell–derived VEGF has been shown to act in a paracrine growth–stimulating manner on vascular endothelial cells by binding to and activating VEGF receptors expressed on these cells.[126] Blocking of the VEGF system can suppress glioma growth in different experimental systems *in vivo*,[127,128] suggesting a potential value of antiangiogenic therapy for human glioblastomas.

## AMPLIFICATION OF PROTO-ONCOGENES

In addition to having lost genetic information from various chromosomes, glioblastomas are characterized by a high frequency of gene amplification.[25] The most commonly amplified gene in glioblastomas is the epidermal growth factor receptor *EGFR* gene on chromosome 7p12 (Fig. 8–3 *C* and *D*). This gene codes for a transmembrane receptor protein with tyrosine kinase activity. Its extracellular domain can bind EGF, transforming growth factor (TGF)-α, and some other polypeptide growth factors. Activation of EGFR by ligand binding has been associated with cell growth and proliferation in several *in vitro* systems, and expression of EGFR at high levels can transform cells in culture in a ligand-dependent manner.[129,130] The *EGFR* gene is amplified in about 40% of glioblastomas, and about half of these tumors additionally show genomic rearrangements of the amplified gene. Most frequently, rearrangements are deletions affecting the 5' end (coding for the extracellular domain) and, more rarely, the 3'-end (coding for the intracellular domain).[25] The most common of these rearrangements, an in-frame deletion of 801 bp resulting in the aberrant splicing of exons 1 to 8, causes the expression of a truncated receptor molecule lacking parts of the extracellular domain necessary for ligand binding. Functional characterization of this EGFR variant has revealed that it shows constitutive tyrosine kinase activity and may thereby confer enhanced tumorigenicity on human glioma cells.[25] One study suggested an altered subcellular localization of the truncated receptor protein in the endoplasmatic reticulum.[131]

Amplification of the *EGFR* gene in glioblastomas consistently results in overexpression of EGFR mRNA and protein. EGFR, however, is also overexpressed in a number of glioblastomas and even lower grade gliomas without gene amplification.[132] In addition to EGFR, gliomas generally express the mRNAs for pre-pro-EGF and/or pre-pro-TGF-α, suggesting the possibility of autocrine and paracrine growth stimulation.[132]

The second most frequent amplification site in glioblastomas is located at 12q13–q15 and may involve multiple genes such as *CDK4, SAS, MDM2, GADD153, GLI,* and *A2MR*.[109] Among these, *MDM2* (amplified in about 8% to 10% of glioblastomas) and *CDK4* (amplified in about 15% of glioblastomas) most likely represent the genes driving the amplification.

A number of other genes has been identified as being amplified in generally low fractions (<10%) of glioblastomas and glioblastoma cell lines. These include *MYCN, MYC, MET, PDGFRA, GLI, MYB,* and *KRAS*.[25] Several recent reports of CGH used for the analysis of gliomas and glioma cell lines have further stressed the importance of gene amplification in glioblastomas.[110,122–125,133] Together, these studies have identified more than 30 amplified chromosomal regions in malignant gliomas, for most of which the actual target genes remain to be identified.

## AMPLIFICATION OF PROTO-ONCOGENES AS AN ALTERNATIVE MOLECULAR MECHANISM TO INACTIVATION OF TUMOR SUPPRESSOR GENES IN GLIOBLASTOMAS

Recent studies have shown that the gene products of certain proto-oncogenes and tumor suppressor genes are interacting with each other and functioning as positive or negative regulators in cell cycle regulatory pathways. One example is the MDM2 protein, which was found to be a cellular regulator of wild-type *p53* function. Binding of MDM2 to p53 may conceal the activation domain of p53 and can thereby inhibit at least one of its important functions (i.e., transactivation of other genes).[134,135] Furthermore, transfection studies have shown that overexpression of MDM2 protein can overcome wild-type p53 suppression of transformed cell growth.[136] Thus, it is likely that *MDM2* amplification with consequent overexpression can function as an alternative mechanism to p53 mutation in tumors. This would explain why malignant gliomas with *MDM2* amplification generally do not show p53 mutations and vice versa.[137]

Another example of alternative molecular abnormalities in malignant glioma is the finding that *CDK4* amplification and deletion of *CDKN2A* are virtually exclusive alterations in anaplastic astrocytomas and glioblastomas.[108,119] More recent studies substantiated these reports and provided evidence that genetic alterations of the *RB1* gene represent a further alternative mechanism because *RB1* mutation and loss of pRb1 expression was preferentially found in glioblastomas without deletion of *CDKN2A* or amplification of *CDK4*.[96,97,138] Thus, the vast majority of glioblastomas have altered at least one of the genes *CDK4, CDKN2,* and *RB1*. The respective gene products are all functionally interacting components of the G1–S cell cycle regulatory checkpoint (see Fig. 8–2). Disturbance of the normal function of the G1–S cell cycle checkpoint thus represents a major molecular mechanism contributing to the malignant phenotype of high-grade astrocytic gliomas.

## GENETIC ALTERATIONS IN PRIMARY VERSUS SECONDARY GLIOBLASTOMA

Glioblastomas can either develop by progression from less malignant gliomas (secondary glioblastomas) or, more frequently, develop rapidly in a *de novo* manner without a history of a previous lesion of lower malignancy (primary glioblastomas). Morphologically, primary and secondary glioblastomas cannot be distinguished.[76] Clinically, secondary glioblastomas tend to occur in younger patients and are associated with a somewhat better prognosis.[139] Based on molecular genetic analyses of common alterations in glioblastomas (i.e., loss of alleles on 17p and 10, *p53* mutation, and *EGFR* gene amplification), several authors have suggested the existence of genetically distinct subsets of glioblastoma.[140–142] From these studies it appeared that loss on 17p and *p53* mutation occur significantly more often in glioblastomas without *EGFR* amplification and vice versa. Glioblastomas with loss on 17p and *p53* mutation were found in patients significantly younger on average than those having a glioblastoma with *EGFR* amplification.[140–142] It has therefore been suggested that the glioblastomas with 17p loss and *p53* mutation might represent secondary glioblastomas that had developed by progression from less malignant astrocytomas while amplification of the *EGFR* gene characterizes primary (*de novo*) glioblastomas.[141,142]

In line with this assumption, *p53* mutations were detected in 70% to 80% of glioblastomas that had developed by progression from lower grade astrocytomas, whereas *EGFR* amplification was not found in these tumors.[143,144] In addition, secondary glioblastomas more frequently than primary glioblastomas demonstrated loss of expression of the putative tumor suppressor gene *DCC* ("deleted in colorectal cancer").[145] Despite these remarkable differences, primary and secondary glioblastomas also have a number of genomic alterations in common. These include abnormalities in the p16/cdk4/pRb1 cell cycle regulatory system as well as deletions on 10q and 11p, which were found with similar frequencies in both primary and secondary glioblastomas.[110,125,146] It also needs to be emphasized that demonstration of a *p53* mutation in a particular glioblastoma does not necessarily mean that this tumor represents a secondary glioblastoma because about 25% to 30% of all primary glioblastomas also carry mutations in this tumor suppressor gene. Furthermore, giant cell glioblastomas, a rare variant of primary glioblastoma, are characterized by frequent *p53* mutations and rare *EGFR* gene amplification.[147]

## Oligodendroglial Tumors

The frequency of oligodendroglial tumors is estimated to be between 5% and 18% of all gliomas.[1, 10] The peak incidence occurs in the fifth and sixth decades of life. The vast majority of oligodendrogliomas grow in the cerebral hemispheres, with preference for the frontal and temporal lobes. Less commonly, oligodendrogliomas may originate in the brain stem, cerebellum, or spinal cord. The WHO classification lists two subtypes in the group of oligodendroglial tumors, namely, the oligodendrogliomas of WHO grade II and the anaplastic (malignant) oligodendrogliomas of WHO grade III.

Histologically, WHO grade II oligodendrogliomas are moderately cellular neoplasms characterized by uniformity of cellular and nuclear size and shape. The tumor cells typically have round hyperchromatic nuclei, an artifactually swollen clear cytoplasm, and a well-defined plasma membrane. This characteristic "fried-egg" or "honeycomb" appearence is a very distinctive diagnostic feature of oligodendrogliomas. Other histological hallmarks include focal calcifications and a typical capillary vascularization pattern often referred to as "chicken-wired." Anaplastic oligodendrogliomas are characterized by signs of increased anaplasia such as high cellularity, nuclear polymorphism, increased mitotic activity, vascular proliferations, and foci of necrosis.[6] In some anaplastic oligodendrogliomas, polymorphic multinucleated giant cells may be numerous.[10]

The primary treatment of oligodendroglial tumors consists of surgical resection, frequently followed by radiation therapy either as part of the initial therapy or at relapse. These therapeutic approaches are usually not curative, as indicated by the reported 10-year survival rates that vary between 10% and 38%.[148–151] Postoperative chemotherapy with procarbazine, lomustine, and vincristine (PCV) has been found to significantly prolong survival of patients with anaplastic oligodendroglial tumors.[152, 153]

Most oligodendendroglial tumors are sporadic neoplasms. Occasional cases of familial clustering have been reported by Parkinson and Hall (oligodendroglioma in two brothers),[154] Roosen and coworkers[155] (oligodendroglioma in a mother and her daughter), Roelvink and associates[156] (oligodendroglioma in twin sisters), and Ferraresi and associates[157] (oligodendroglioma in a father and his son). In addition, a family with polymorphous oligodendrogliomas in a brother and sister has been reported.[158]

## MOLECULAR GENETICS

The molecular genetic alterations in oligodendroglial tumors are summarized in Figure 8–4. The most frequent aberration in these tumors is LOH on the long arm of chromosome 19. The incidence of LOH on 19q varies among different studies, ranging from 50% to more than 80% of the cases.[159–162] In most oligodendrogliomas, the losses involve all informative loci on 19q, suggesting that most of the arm or the entire arm had been deleted. Individual cases demonstrating partial or interstitial losses, however, have been reported. This phenomenon allowed Reifenberger and coworkers[161] to assign a commonly deleted region to the area distal to the *CYP2a* gene and proximal to the *D19S22* locus corresponding to bands 19q13.2–13.4. Meanwhile, this region has been narrowed to an approximately 900 kb long segment at 19q13.3–q13.4 between the markers *D19S412* and *STD.*[163] Studies aimed at the positional cloning of the suspected tumor suppressor gene from this region are ongoing and may soon lead to the identification of this gene.

The second most frequent genetic alteration in oligodendroglial neoplasms is the loss of alleles on the short arm of chromosome 1. In the series of Reifenberger and colleagues,[161] LOH on 1p was detected in 67% (14/21) of the tumors. Bello and colleagues[164] found LOH on 1p in six of six oligodendrogliomas and in five of six anaplastic oligodendrogliomas. Kraus and coworkers[160] detected it in three of nine oligodendrogliomas and three of six anaplastic oligodendrogliomas. Allelic loss on 1p showed a striking association with

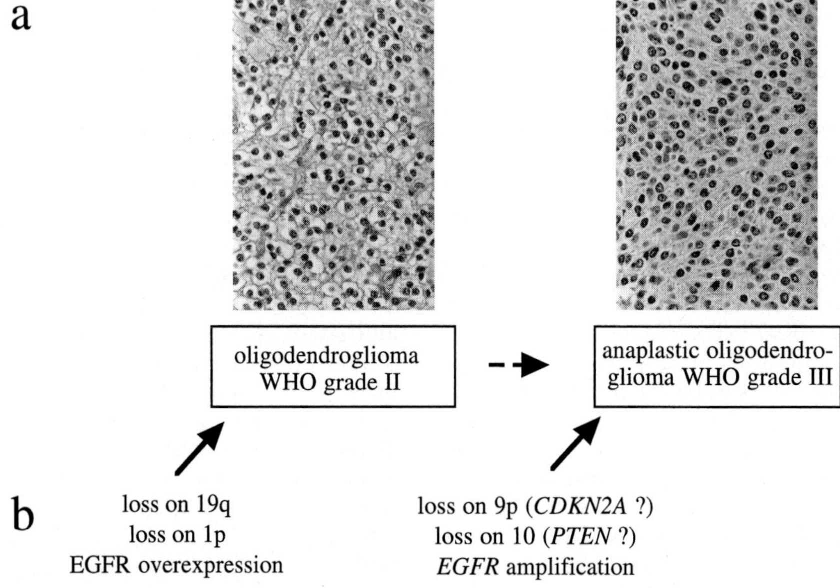


**Figure 8–4.** Histopathology and genetic alterations alterations of oligodendroglial tumors. *(A)* Typical microscopic appearance of an oligodendroglioma with moderate density of isomorphous tumor cells showing round nuclei and clear cytoplasm (left). Anaplastic oligodendrogliomas show increased cellularity, nuclear atypia, and mitoses (right). Both sections are stained with H&E (×260). *(B)* Summary of common genetic abnormalities associated with the initiation and progression of oligodendroglial tumors.

LOH on 19q, which suggests a synergistic effect of both alterations in providing a selective growth advantage.[159–161]

The localization of the suspected tumor suppressor gene on 1p is still poorly defined. Reifenberger and colleagues[161] found a common region of deletion distal to the *NGFB* locus (i.e., 1p13-pter). Bello and coworkers[164] reported one oligodendroglioma with a terminal retention of heterozygosity at the *D1Z2* locus (1p36.3) and a glioblastoma with an interstitial deletion between *D1S57* and *D1Z2* (1p32–36.3). More recently, the same group found evidence for two distinct regions, one located distal at 1p36 and the other more centromeric at 1p35–p36.[165]

Another frequent alteration in both low-grade and anaplastic oligodendrogliomas is overexpression of EGFR mRNA and protein in the absence of *EGFR* gene amplification. Reifenberger and coworkers[166] found increased levels of EGFR mRNA compared with non-neoplastic brain tissue in 6 of 13 oligodendrogliomas and in 10 of 19 anaplastic oligodendrogliomas. All tumors with increased EGFR mRNA expression showed strong immunoreactivity for EGFR protein. The precise mechanism responsible for the increased transcription of the *EGFR* gene in these tumors is unknown.

In contrast to the astrocytic tumors, LOH on 17p is rare in oligodendroglial tumors.[161] Mutations of *p53* are also less frequent. Ohgaki and asosciates[167] found *p53* mutations in 2 of 17 oligodendrogliomas (12%). Rasheed and coworkers[168] detected LOH on 17p and mutation of *p53* in 1 of 11 oligodendrogliomas (9%). Thus, alterations of the *p53* gene are of minor significance in oligodendroglial tumors.

### GENETIC ALTERATIONS ASSOCIATED WITH THE PROGRESSION OF OLIGODENDROGLIAL TUMORS

The data discussed thus far indicates that the primary genetic alterations in oligodendroglial tumors differ significantly from those associated with the development of astrocytomas. When it comes to alterations related to the progression from low-grade (WHO grade II) to high-grade (WHO-grade III and IV) lesions, however, gliomas appear to utilize common pathways. This assumption is based on the finding that anaplastic oligodendrogliomas may show additional LOH on 9p or 10.[161] Both are genetic alterations that are also typical for malignant astrocytic tumors. It is likely that the *CDKN2A* gene on 9p21 represents the critical target on 9p also in anaplastic oligodendrogliomas, but this hypothesis needs corroboration.

In addition to specific chromosomal losses, anaplastic oligodendroglial tumors show an increased incidence of multiple allelic losses on several different chromosomes.[161] Furthermore, these tumors may occasionally demonstrate amplification of proto-oncogenes. In a series of 21 anaplastic oligodendrogliomas, one tumor showed coamplification of *EGFR* and the renin gene while another tumor had coamplification of the *MYC* gene with *CDK4* and *SAS*.[161–169] In addition, individual cases of anaplastic oligodendrogliomas with amplification of *EGFR*, coamplification of *EGFR* and *MYCN*, or coamplification of *GLI* and *MYCN* have been reported.[169] This data indicates that the frequency of gene amplification in anaplastic oligodendroglial tumors is much lower than in glioblastomas, but may approximately equal the incidence in anaplastic astrocytomas.

## Oligoastrocytomas

Oligoastrocytomas are the most common mixed gliomas. These tumors are composed of a conspicuous mixture of two distinct neoplastic cell types morphologically resembling the tumor cells in oligodendroglioma or astrocytoma. The oligodendroglial and astroglial components may be either diffusely intermingled or separated into geographically distinct areas. Two malignancy grades are distinguished: well-differentiated oligoastrocytomas of WHO grade II and anaplastic oligoastrocytomas of WHO grad III.[6] Like the other gliomas, most oligoastrocytomas are sporadic tumors. Only single cases of familial clustering have been reported.[170,171]

The genetic alterations in oligoastrocytomas appear to be more heterogeneous than those in "pure" oligodendrogliomas. No consistent genetic abnormalities have been detected that would allow a clear distinction of oligoastrocytomas from oligodendrogliomas on the one hand and astrocytomas on the other hand.[161] About 30% to 50% of oligoastrocytomas are characterized by loss of genetic information from 19q and 1p.[160,161,172] Kraus and coworkers[160] have microdissected oligodendroglial and astrocytic tumor parts in three oligoastrocytomas and found loss of alleles on 1p and 19q in both components in all three cases. This finding strongly suggests that oligoastrocytomas are monoclonal neoplasms originating from a single precursor cell rather than composition tumors that had developed simultaneously.

About 30% of oligoastrocytomas carry genetic aberrations frequently found in astrocytomas (i.e., mutations of the *p53* gene and LOH on 17p).[161,172] Interestingly, those oligoastrocytomas with *p53* mutations and LOH on 17p do not have LOH on 1p and 19q and *vice versa*.[161,172] This data indicates that oligoastrocytomas are genetically heterogeneous. One subset appears to be genetically related to oligodendroglial tumors while another subset is genetically related to astrocytomas. With respect to progression-associated genetic abnormalities, anaplastic oligoastrocytomas have been found to share many alterations also implicated in the progression of astrocytomas and oligodendrogliomas, including loss of genetic information on 9p, 10, and 11p, as well as amplification of the *EGFR* gene.[161]

## Ependymal Tumors

Ependymal tumors are neoplasms composed predominantly of neoplastic ependymal or subependymal cells. Several types with different histopathological appearences, predilection sites, and biological behavior may be distinguished. The most benign ependymal tumors are the subependymoma and the myxopapillary ependymoma (both WHO grade I lesions). The "classic" ependymoma (including the clear cell, papillary, and the cellular variants) is a WHO grade II tumor. Anaplastic ependymomas, characterized by high cellularity, nuclear atypia, marked mitotic activity, vascular proliferations, and necroses, correspond to WHO grade III.[6] In accordance with their presumed histogenesis, ependymal tumors preferentially occur in or close to the ventricles, the central canal, or the filum terminale.

The present knowledge about the genetic abnormalities in ependymal tumors is rather limited because systematic molecular genetic studies on large case numbers have not been performed thus far. The vast majority of ependymal tumors are sporadic, but patients with NF2 have an increased likelihood for the development of ependymomas, in particular of the spinal cord. In addition, rare instances of familial ependymoma in the absence of other stigmata of NF2 have been reported.[173–175] Because ependymomas are the most frequent type of glioma in patients with NF2, and loss of chromosome 22q has been found in a fraction of sporadic ependymomas,[176–178] the *NF2* gene seemed a likely candidate for a tumor suppressor gene involved in the pathogenesis of ependymal tumors. Rubio and colleagues,[95] however, found mutation of the *NF2* gene in only one of eight ependymomas, and Slavc and coworkers[179] observed no *NF2* mutations in seven ependymomas. In contrast, Birch and coworkers[180] detected somatic *NF2* mutations in five of seven spinal ependymomas.

Immunocytochemical investigation of ependymomas with antibodies directed against the *NF2* gene product (schwannomin/merlin) has provided evidence of two groups of ependymomas: one group with lack of staining suggesting that inactivation of both *NF2* alleles had occurred and a second group with normal staining suggesting the presence of at least one intact *NF2* allele.[181] Thus, although *NF2* alterations may be involved in some ependymomas, other gene loci must contribute to the formation and progression of these tumors. This assumption is supported by cytogenetic and molecular genetic analyses showing abnormalities of various other chromosomes, including 1, 6, 9p, 11q, 16, 17, and 19q, in variable fractions of ependymal tumors.[176,178,182,183] In addition, genetic linkage analysis of a family with autosomal dominant meningiomas and ependymomas has suggested an ependymoma locus other than *NF2*.[184]

In contrast to the diffuse astrocytomas, mutations of the *p53* gene are rare in ependymomas.[167] Metzger and associates[185] reported a germline mutation in codon 242 of the *p53* gene in a patient with a malignant ependymoma of the posterior fossa. Several of the relatives had died at a young age from a variety of cancers, indicating that this patient may in fact belong to a family affected by Li-Fraumeni syndrome.

## Molecular Predictors of Glioma Progression and Prognosis

Although quite a number of genetic abnormalities have been found in the various types of gliomas, only a few studies have addressed the significance of these changes as potential indicators of glioma progression and survival time. With respect to spontaneous malignant progression from primary low-grade to secondary high-grade glioma, evidence has accumulated that *p53* mutation may be an important predisposing factor in the group of diffuse astrocytomas.[143,186] In a long-term follow-up study of 52 patients with low-grade astrocytomas, Iuzzolino and coworkers[187] found a trend toward more aggressive growth for patients with p53 immunopositive tumors. Five years after diagnosis, the survival estimate with the Kaplan-Meier method was 21% for patients with a p53-positive tumor, but 46% for patients whose tumors lacked p53 immunoreactivity. A similar tendency was reported by Chozick and coworkers[188] whereas Kraus and colleagues[189] observed no correlation between *p53* alteration and clinical outcome. In childhood malignant gliomas, the presence of *p53* mutations has been reported to be associated with shorter survival.[190]

Contradictory results have also been published about the prognostic significance of *EGFR* gene amplification in malignant gliomas. Two studies found no difference in survival time for glioblastomas with or without *EGFR* amplification.[191,192] In contrast, Hurtt and associates[193] reported a statistically significant association of *EGFR* amplification with shortened survival. This study, however, was based on only 14 patients, which all had been treated in different ways. Schlegel and asosciates[194] observed a relationship between the presence of *EGFR* amplification and more rapid postoperative regrowth of glioblastomas (as evaluated neuroradiologically), but a significant correlation with survival time was also not found.

From a series of 94 well-documented and similarly treated glioblastoma patients, Weber and colleagues[125] selected the ten patients with the best outcome (subgroup A) and the ten patients with the worst outcome (subgroup B), and analyzed their tumors for genomic alterations by CGH. They found that gain/amplification of 12q14–q21 (*MDM2/CDK4*) and gain of chromosome 19 were more frequent in subgroup A tumors, whereas loss of 6q16-qter, loss of parts of chromosome 13, and gain of chromosome 20 were more common in subgroup B. In contrast, gain of chromosome 7, loss of chromosomes 9p, 10, and 22q, and amplification of 7p12 (*EGFR*) were found with similar frequencies in both subgroups. The major problem of all the clinicomolecular studies is the limited number of patients analyzed. To evaluate the usefulness of molecular abnormalities as prognostic factors for glioma patients in a meaningful way, well-controlled studies of large numbers of patients are needed.

# PRIMITIVE NEUROECTODERMAL TUMORS

The WHO classification defines primitive neuroectodermal tumors (PNETs) as small cell, malignant tumors of childhood with predominant location in the cerebellum and a noted capacity for divergent differentiation, including neuronal, astrocytic, ependymal, muscular, and melanotic.[6] The cerebellar PNETs are traditionally classified as medulloblastomas. Medulloblastomas account for most PNETs and make up about 20% to 25% of all intracranial tumors in children.[1] The incidence is approximately 1/100,000 per year and peaks between 3 and 5 years of age. Histologically, medulloblastomas are malignant, embryonal childhood tumors composed of densely packed cells with round to oval or carrot-shaped nuclei and scanty cytoplasm. Several variants can be distinguished, including desmoplastic medulloblastoma, medullomyoblastoma, and melanotic medulloblastoma.[6] Immunohistochemically, most medulloblastomas express neuronal marker proteins (synaptophysin, neuron-specific enolase), but a smaller percentage may contain tumor cells positive for glial differentiation antigens such as glial fibrillary acidic protein.

Most PNETs are sporadic tumors. Only occasional cases of familial clustering have been reported.[195–197] Several hereditary syndromes are known to be associated with a predisposition for the development of medulloblastoma. These include Turcot's syndrome, in particular when caused by *APC* germline mutations,[52] Rubinstein-Taybi syndrome,[198] and Gorlin's syndrome.[53,56,57] In addition, a few medulloblastoma patients have been encountered in families with a germline mutation in the *p53* gene.[199] A recent study detected a *p53* germline mutation in two siblings with cerebral PNETs.[200] A single patient with von Hippel-Lindau disease and a PNET with multipotent differentiation has been reported.[201]

The most frequent cytogenetic abnormality in medulloblastomas is isochromosome 17q, which has been detected in about 30% to 50% of the tumors.[202,203] Isochromosome 17q results in the loss of one copy of 17p, and molecular studies have indeed confirmed LOH on 17p in a similar percentage of medulloblastomas.[177,204,205] Loss of 17p in medulloblastomas however, is usually not associated with *p53* mutation.[167,204,206–209] The infrequent mutation of *p53* together with the finding of LOH at distal 17p not including the *p53* locus suggest the existence of a second, not yet identified, tumor suppressor gene located at 17p13.3.[206,210] The *HIC1* gene[92] is a good candidate for this suspected tumor suppressor gene, but further studies are needed to substantiate the role of this gene in PNETs.

Other common genetic abnormalities in medulloblastomas are gains of portions of chromosome 1 and deletions of 1q, 6q, 11p and 16q.[99,203,211,212] A CGH study identified gains of 4p, 5, 7q, 8q, and 9p as recurrent genomic imbalances in PNETs.[213] LOH of chromosome 9q involving the Gorlin's syndrome gene locus at 9q22 (*PTCH*) has been found in a subset of medulloblastomas, including desmoplastic variants.[214,215] More recently, somatic mutations in the *PTCH* gene have been found in about 10% to 15% of medulloblastomas.[61,216]

Furthermore, occasional medulloblastomas may carry a missense mutation in the *SMOH* gene.[217] The *SMOH* gene product is a transmembrane protein that forms a complex with the PTCH protein. In the absence of the Sonic hedgehog signaling protein (SHH), PTCH inhibits the activity of SMOH. Binding of SHH to PTCH can relieve this inhibition of SMOH, which in turn results in the transduction of the SHH signal and activation of members of the TGF-β, GLi, and WNT protein families.[218] Thus, alteration of the SHH signaling pathway by mutation of *PTCH* or *SMOH* represents an important mechanisms in the pathogenesis of PNETs. Further evidence for a role of developmental control genes in these tumors has been provided by the finding that *PAX5* is aberrantly expressed in most medulloblastomas.[219]

Gene amplification is present in a subset of medulloblastomas and medulloblastoma cell lines and may involve the protooncogenes *MYC*, *MYCN* or *EGFR*.[220] In contrast, neither *MDM2* nor *CDK4* amplification has been found in these tumors.[109] Finally, a role for activating *K-ras* mutations in postirradiation PNETs in children has been reported.[221]

With respect to possible prognostic implications of molecular abnormalities, expression of the oncoprotein erbb2 has been suggested as an indicator of poor prognosis for medulloblastoma patients.[222] In addition, intense nuclear immunoreactivity for p53 has been reported to correlate with shorter survival.[223] Batra and coworkers[224] observed a statistically significant association between LOH of 17p and a shortened survival period. On the contrary, expression of the neurotrophin receptor TrkC was found to be associated with a better outcome.[225] It remains to be elucidated, however, which of these various parameters can be corroborated as an independent prognostic factor in well-controlled prospective studies on a large number of cases.

## MENINGIOMAS

Meningiomas are the most common benign brain tumors and account for about 15% of intracranial and 25% of intraspinal tumors. The incidence of meningioma increases with advancing age, and meningiomas are more common in women. Although meningiomas are frequently attached to the dural membranes, they may occur in unusual sites (e.g., intraventricularly). Histologically, meningiomas are tumors composed of neoplastic meningeal cells. Several histological variants are recognized, the most common being meningothelial, fibrous (fibroblastic), and transitional meningioma.[6]

The biological behavior of most meningiomas is benign and corresponds with WHO grade I. However, a subset of meningiomas are histologically characterized by increased mitotic activity, high cellularity, small cells with high nuclear cytoplasmic ratios and/or prominent nucleoli, uninterrupted patternless or sheet-like growth, and foci of necrosis.[6] These tumors are designated as atypical meningiomas (WHO grade II) and are associated with an increased tendency to recurrence. Finally, rare cases of meningioma may show histological features of frank anaplasia far in excess of the findings in atypical meningiomas, including gross brain invasion. Such tumors are classified as anaplastic (malignant) meningioma and correspond to WHO grade III.[6] In a retrospective series of 1799 surgical specimens of meningiomas from 1582 patients, Maier and associates classified 87.6% as classic benign meningioma, 7.2% as atypical meningioma, 2.4% as anaplastic meningioma, and 2.8% as papillary meningioma or hemangiopericytoma.[226]

Meningiomas are a hallmark of NF2.[31,227] Less frequently, meningiomas develop in patients with Werner's syndrome or Gorlin's syndrome. Many reports of familial meningioma may represent patients with NF2 who were inadequately evaluated for the presence of small vestibular or spinal schwannomas or lens opacities. Dominantly inherited meningioma without other evidence of NF2, however, does occur.[184,228]

Zang and Singer[229] for the first time demonstrated loss of chromosome 22 as a clonal chromosomal abnormality in meningiomas. Since then, numerous cytogenetic and molecular genetic studies have confirmed the significance of 22q loss in these tumors. More recent studies have shown that the *NF2* gene represents the meningioma tumor suppressor gene on 22q. Inactivating mutations of *NF2* have been found in about 40% to 50% of sporadic meningiomas and are frequently associated with loss of the second allele.[230–232] Immunohistochemical analysis of schwannomin expression in meningiomas also revealed lack of expression in approximately half of sporadic meningiomas.[181] The frequency of *NF2* mutations and LOH on 22q depends on the histological subtype of meningioma; significantly higher percentages were found in fibroblastic and transitional tumors than in meningothelial variants.[232,233]

In addition to the *NF2* gene, there is evidence that additional genes on 22q are involved in the pathogenesis of some meningiomas. Cloning of the breakpoint of a translocation t(4;22) observed in a meningioma cell line led to the identification of a novel gene, dubbed *MN1*, which is located centromeric to the *NF2* gene.[234] *MN1* is also involved in the pathogenesis of certain leukemias in which it may be translocated to the *TEL* gene.[235] In meningiomas, however, *MN1* alterations appear to be restricted to individual cases.[234] Another gene identified in the vicinity of *NF2* is the *BAM22* gene, a member of the β-adaptin gene family, which was found to be homozygously deleted in one meningioma.[236] The same authors found loss of *BAM22* expression in 8 of 70 sporadic meningiomas. Further evidence for the existence of an additional meningioma locus besides *NF2* was provided by genetic linkage analysis of a pedigree with autosomal dominant meningiomas and ependymomas.[184] This study excluded the *NF2* region and also the region centromeric to *NF2* containing the *MN1* gene.

Progression of benign meningiomas to atypical and anaplastic tumors is associated with abnormalities on various chromosomes. According to Weber and associates, atypical meningiomas frequently demonstrate losses on 1p, 6q, 10, 14q, and 18q, as well as gains on 1q, 9q, 12q, 15q, 17q, and 20q.[237] In anaplastic meningiomas, most of these alterations were also found, but the frequencies of losses on 6q, 10, and 14q were even higher. In addition, anaplastic meningiomas may show homozygous deletions of the *CDKN2A* gene at 9p21, as well as gene amplification on the long arm of chromosome 17.[237] Despite the considerable genomic instability in atypical and anaplastic meningiomas, mutations in the *p53* gene are exceedingly rare in these tumors. Based on the most common aberrations identified in meningiomas of different malignancy grades, a model for the genetic alterations associated with meningioma progression has been proposed (Fig. 8–5).[237] It remains to be determined whether the genetic changes detected in advanced meningiomas may be relevant as independent prognostic factors for recurrence and survival time. Furthermore, the individual genes targeted by the various chromosomal losses and gains in atypical and anaplastic meningiomas remain to be identified.

## SCHWANNOMAS

Schwannomas (neurilemmomas, neurinomas) are encapsulated and sometimes cystic, benign (WHO grade I) tumors composed of spindle-shaped neoplastic Schwann cells.[6] Histologically, schwannomas may show different architectural patterns, such as cellular areas of spindle cells often demonstrating palisading (Antoni A pattern) and more loosely textured, less cellular areas of cells often containing lipid (Antoni B pattern). Schwannomas account for about 8% of intracranial tumors and 29% of intraspinal tumors. Vestibular schwannomas are also (somewhat erroneously) referred to as *acoustic* schwannomas or neuromas and occur commonly as single tumors of the vestibular branch of the eighth cranial nerve. They have an incidence of around 13 per 1 million per year.[238] In patients with NF2, vestibular schwannomas are often bilateral and occur at a much earlier age than in patients with sporadic unilateral tumors. About 4% of

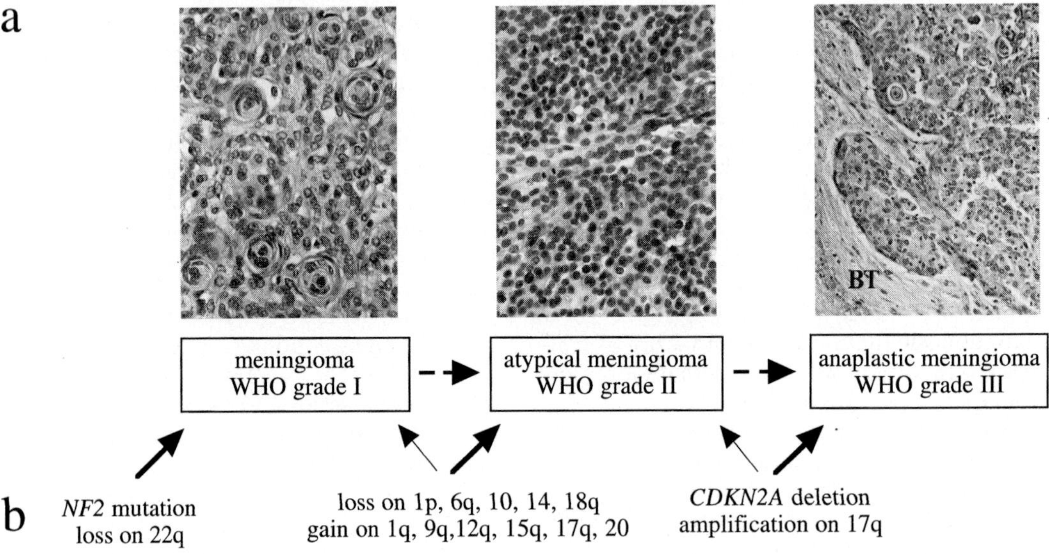


**Figure 8–5.** Histopathology and genetic alterations of meningiomas. *(A)* Typical microscopic appearance of a benign meningioma with numerous meningothelial whorls (left); an atypical meningioma with increased cellularity, nuclear atypia, and mitoses (middle); and an anaplastic meningioma with invasion of brain tissue (BT) (right). All sections are stained with H&E (×260, ×260, ×100). *(B)* Summary of common genetic abnormalities associated with the initiation and progression of meningiomas (according to Weber et al.[237]). The genetic and chromosomal aberrations are given before the malignancy grade in which they are first found at a frequency of more than 30% (thick arrows). Some changes may already be found in a smaller fraction of lower grade tumors. This fact is illustrated by thin arrows.

vestibular schwannomas are bilateral, and virtually all of these patients have NF2.

Frequent loss of alleles from 22q in sporadic vestibular schwannomas and NF2-associated tumors indicated a common pathogenetic mechanism for these tumors.[239] These findings were further supported by establishing linkage of NF2 to genetic markers on chromosome 22.[240] After the positional cloning of the *NF2* gene,[32,33] several studies investigated sporadic and NF2-associated schwannomas for *NF2* gene mutations.[230,241–248] Collectively, the available data indicates that the *NF2* gene is altered in nearly all schwannomas.

This was further corroborated by immunocytochemical studies demonstrating absence of schwannomin expression in vestibular schwannomas.[181,247] Experimental reduction of schwannomin synthesis in Schwann cells by use of antisense oligonucleotides has been shown to lead to morphological changes and loss of cell attachment.[249] In addition to mutation of the *NF2* gene, cytogenetic studies have revealed evidence for the involvement of other chromosomal abnormalities in schwannomas, including loss of one sex chromosome, losses of chromosomes 15 and 12, and gains of chromosomes 5, 7, and 20.[250] The significance of these alterations in terms of the involved genes remains to be elucidated.

## SUMMARY

Molecular genetic studies have brought important new insights into the pathogenesis of primary tumors of the nervous system. As summarized in this chapter, most of the tumor suppressor genes responsible for the hereditary tumor syndromes of the nervous system have been identified and cloned. Many of these genes, including *NF1, NF2, VHL, PTCH, PTEN,* and *p53,* also play important roles in certain types of sporadic nervous system tumors (e.g., schwannomas, meningiomas, capillary hemangioblastomas, PNETs, and gliomas). In addition, studies of sporadic brain tumors, with either molecular genetic techniques for the analysis of loss of heterozygosity and gene amplification or molecular cytogenetic methods such as comparative genomic hybridization, have identified a variety of chromosomal regions suspected to contain yet-unidentified tumor suppressor genes or proto-oncogenes involved in the initiation and/or progression of nervous system tumors. Future studies will aim at the identification and cloning of these novel genes and at the elucidation of the functional implications of their gene products for neoplastic cell growth. These studies will likely lead to the refinement of morphological tumor classification as well as the identification of novel prognostic factors. In addition, a better understanding of the molecular genetics of nervous system tumors will provide important clues for the development of new and better therapeutic approaches. Thus, molecular genetic findings will certainly have a major impact on both diagnostic and clinical neuro-oncology.

## REFERENCES

1. Russell D, Rubinstein LJ: Pathology of Tumors of the Nervous System, ed 5. Edward Arnold, London, 1989.
2. Miller RW, Young JL, Novakovic B: Childhood cancer. Cancer 75:395–405, 1995.
3. Grieg NH, Ries LG, Yancik R, Rapoport SI: Increasing annual incidence of primary malignant brain tumors in the elderly. J Natl Cancer Inst 82:1621–1624, 1990.
4. Polednak AP, Flannery JT: Brain, other central nervous system, and eye cancer. Cancer 75:330–337, 1995.
5. Desmeules M, Middelsen T, Mao Y: Increasing incidence of primary malignant brain tumors: Influence of diagnostic methods. J Natl Cancer Inst 84: 442–445, 1992.
6. Kleihues P, Burger PC, Scheithauer BW: Histological Typing of Tumours of the Central Nervous System, ed 2. Springer-Verlag, Heidelberg, 1993.
7. Bigner DD, Swenberg JA: Jänisch and Schreiber's Experimental Tumors of the Central Nervous System, 1st English ed. Upjohn Co., Kalamazoo, MI 1977.
8. Walker JS, Bigner DD: Virus induced brain tumors. In Wilkins RM, Rengachary SS (eds): Neurosurgery. McGraw-Hill, New York, 1985, pp522–525.
9. Burger PC, Scheithauer BW: Tumors of the Central Nervous System. Atlas of Tumor Pathology, 3rd Series, Fasc. 10. Armed Forces Institute of Pathology, Washington, DC, 1994.
10. Zülch KJ: Brain Tumors. Their Biology and Pathology, ed 3. Springer-Verlag, Berlin, 1986.
11. Neglia JP, Meadows AT, Robison LL, et al.: Second neoplasms after acute lymphoblastic leukemia in childhood. N Engl J Med 325:1330–1336, 1991.
12. Bondy ML, Kyritsis AP, Gu J, et al.: Mutagen sen-

sitivity and risk of gliomas: A case–control study. Cancer Res 56:1484–1486, 1996.

13. Nowell P: The clonal evolution of tumor cell populations. Science 194:23–28, 1976.
14. Nowell P: Mechanisms of tumor progression. Cancer Res 46:2203–2207, 1986.
15. Fearon ER, Vogelstein B: A genetic model for colorectal tumorigenesis. Cell 61:759–767, 1990.
16. Levine AJ: The tumor suppressor genes. Annu Rev Biochem 62:623–651, 1993.
17. Milner J, Medcalf EA: Cotranslation of activated mutant p53 with wild-type drives the wild-type p53 protein into the mutant conformation. Cell 65: 765–774, 1991.
18. Herman JG, Latif F, Weng Y, et al.: Silencing of the *VHL* tumour-suppressor gene by DNA methylation in renal carcinoma. Proc Natl Acad Sci USA 91: 9700–9704, 1994.
19. Herman JG, Merlo A, Mao L, et al.: Inactivation of the *CDKN2/p16/MTS1* gene is frequently associated with aberrant methylation in all common human cancers. Cancer Res 55:4525–4530, 1995.
20. Merlo A, Herman JG, Mao L, Lee DJ, Gabrielson E, Burger PC, Baylin SB, Sidransky D: 5' CpG island methylation is associated with transcriptional silencing of the tumour suppressor *p16/CDKN2/MTS1* in human cancers. Nature Med 1:686–692, 1995.
21. Knudson AG: Mutation and cancer: Statistical study of retinoblastoma. Proc Natl Acad Sci USA 68:820–823, 1971.
22. Lasko D, Cavenee W, Nordenskjöld M: Loss of constitutional heterozygosity in human cancer. Annu Rev Genet 25:281–314, 1991.
23. Bishop JM: Molecular themes in oncogenesis. Cell 64:235–248, 1991.
24. Cantley LC, Auger KR, Carpenter C, et al.: Oncogenes and signal transduction. Cell 64:281–302, 1991.
25. Collins VP: Gene amplification in human gliomas. Glia 15:289–296, 1995.
26. Bigner SH, Mark J, Bigner DD: Cytogenetics of human brain tumors. Cancer Genet Cytogenet 47: 141–154, 1990.
27. Bigner SH, Vogelstein B, Bigner DD: Chromosomal abnormalities and gene amplification in malignant gliomas. ISI Atlas Sci Biochem 1:333–336, 1988.
28. Brison O: Gene amplification and tumor progression. Biochim Biophys Acta 1155:25–41, 1993.
29. Viskochil D, Buchberg AM, Xu G, et al.: Deletions and a translocation interrupt a cloned gene at the neurofibromatosis type 1 locus. Cell 62:187–192, 1990.
30. Riccardi VM: Neurofibromatosis: Phenotype, Natural History and Pathogenesis, ed 2. Baltimore, Johns Hopkins University Press, 1992.
31. Evans DGR, Huson SM, Donnai D, et al.: A genetic study of type 2 neurofibromatosis in the United Kingdom. I. Prevalence, mutation rate, fitness, and confirmation of maternal transmission effect on severity. J Med Genet 29:841–846, 1992.
32. Rouleau G, Merel P, Lutchman M, et al.: Alteration in a new gene encoding a putative membrane-organizing protein causes neurofibromatosis type 2. Nature 363:515–521, 1993.
33. Trofatter JA, MacCollin MM, Rutter JL, et al.: A novel moesin-, ezrin-, radixin-like gene is a candidate for the neurofibromatosis 2 tumor suppressor. Cell 72:791–800, 1993.
34. Mautner VF, Lindenau M, Baser ME, et al.: The neuroimaging and clinical spectrum of neurofibromatosis 2. Neurosurgery 38:880–885, 1996.
35. Louis DN, Ramesh V, Gusella JF: Neuropathology and molecular genetics of neurofibromatosis 2 and related tumors. Brain Pathol 5:163–172, 1995.
36. Mautner VF, Tatagiba M, Lindenau M, et al.: Spinal tumors in patients with neurofibromatosis type 2. MR imaging study of frequency, multiplicity, and variety. Am J Roentgenol 165:951–955, 1995.
37. Filling-Katz MR, Choyke PL, Oldfield E, et al.: Central nervous system involvement in von Hippel-Lindau disease. Neurology 41:41–46, 1991.
38. Latif F, Tory K, Gnarra J, et al.: Identification of the von Hippel-Lindau disease tumor suppressor gene. Science 260:1317–1320, 1993.
39. Short MP, Richardson EP, Haines JL, Kwiatkowski DJ: Clinical, neuropathological and genetic aspects of the tuberous sclerosis complex. Brain Pathol 5: 173–179.
40. Povey S, Burley MW, Attwood J, et al.: Two loci for tuberous sclerosis: One on 9q34 and one on 16p13. Ann Hum Genet 58:107–127, 1994.
41. The European Chromosome 16 Tuberous Sclerosis Consortium: Identification and characterization of the tuberous sclerosis gene on chromosome 16. Cell 75:1305–1315, 1993.
42. van Slegtenhorst M, de Hoogt R, Hermans C, et al.: Identification of the tuberous sclerosis gene *TSC1* on chromosome 9q34. Science 277:805–808, 1997.
43. Jones AC, Daniells CE, Snell RG, et al.: Molecular genetic and phenotypic analysis reveals differences between *TSC1* and *TSC2* associated familial and sporadic tuberous sclerosis. Hum Mol Genet 6: 2155–2161, 1997.
44. Malkin D, Li FP, Strong LC, et al.: Germ line *p53* mutations in a familial syndrome of breast cancer, sarcomas, and other neoplasms. Science 250:1233–1238, 1990.
45. Bögler O, Huang HJS, Kleihues P, Cavenee WK: The *p53* gene and its role in human brain tumors. Glia 15:308–327, 1995.
46. Kyritsis AP, Bondy ML, Xiao M, et al.: Germline *p53* gene mutations in subsets of glioma patients. J Natl Cancer Inst 86:344–348, 1994.
47. Van Meyel DJ, Ramsey DA, Chambers AF, Macdonald DR, Cairncross JG: Absence of hereditary mutations in exons 5 through 9 of the *p53* gene and exon 24 of the neurofibromin gene in families with glioma. Ann Neurol 35:120–122, 1994.
48. Lasser DM, De Vivo DC, Garvin J, Wilhelmsen KC: Turcot's syndrome: Evidence for linkage to the adenomatous polyposis coli *(APC)* locus. Neurology 44:1083–1086, 1994.
49. Mori T, Nagase H, Horii A, et al.: Germ-line and somatic mutations of the *APC* gene in patients with Turcot syndrome and analysis of *APC* mutations in brain tumors. Genes Chromosomes Cancer 9:168–172, 1994.
50. Munden PM, Sobol WM, Weingeist TA: Ocular

findings in Turcot syndrome (glioma-polyposis). Ophthalmology 98:111–114, 1991.

51. Tops CM, Vasen HF, van de Klift HM, et al.: Genetic evidence that Turcot syndrome is not allelic to familial adenomatous polyposis. Am J Med Genet 43:888–893, 1992.
52. Hamilton SR, Liu BO, Parsons RE, et al.: The molecular basis of Turcot's syndrome. N Engl J Med 332:839–847, 1995.
53. Gorlin RJ: Nevoid basal-cell carcinoma syndrome. Medicine 66:98–113, 1987.
54. Hogan RE, Tress B, Gonzales MF, King JO, Cook MJ.: Epilepsy in the nevoid basal-cell carcinoma syndrome (Gorlin syndrome): Report of a case due to a focal neuronal heterotopia. Neurology 46:574–576, 1996.
55. Albrecht S, Goodman JC, Rajagopolan S, Levy M, Cech DA, Colley LD: Malignant meningioma in Gorlin's syndrome: Cytogenetic and *p53* gene analysis. Case report. J Neurosurg 81:466–471, 1994.
56. Evans DG, Birch JM, Orton CI: Brain tumours and the occurrence of severe invasive basal cell carcinoma in first degree relatives with Gorlin syndrome. Br J Neurosurg 5:643–646, 1991.
57. Evans DG, Farndon PA, Burnell LD, Gattamaneni HR, Birch JM: The incidence of Gorlin syndrome in 173 consecutive cases of medulloblastoma. Br J Cancer 64:959–961, 1991.
58. Hahn H, Wicking C, Yaphiropoulos PG, et al.: Mutations in the human homolog of Drosophila *patched* in the nevoid basal cell carcinoma szndrome. Cell 85:841–851, 1996.
59. Johnson RL, Rothman AL, Xie J, et al.: Human homolog of *patched*, a candidate gene for the basal cell nevus syndrome. Science 272:1668–1671, 1996.
60. Stone DM, Hynes M, Armanini M, et al.: The tumour-suppressor gene *patched* encodes a candidate receptor for Sonic hedgehog. Nature 384: 129–134, 1996.
61. Wolter M, Reifenberger J, Sommer C, Ruzicka T, Reifenberger G: Mutations in the human homologue of the *Drosophila* segment polarity gene *patched (PTCH)* in sporadic basal cell carcinomas of the skin and primitive neuroectodermal tumors of the central nervous system. Cancer Res 57:2581–2585, 1997.
62. Xie J, Johnson RL, Zhang X, et al.: Mutations of the *PATCHED* gene in several types of sporadic extracutaneous tumors. Cancer Res 57:2369–2372, 1997.
63. Vinchon M, Blond S, Lejeune JP, et al.: Association of Lhermitte-Duclos and Cowden disease: Report of a new case and review of the literature. J Neurol Neurosurg Psychiatry 57:699–704, 1994.
64. Lyons CJ, Wilson CB, Horton JC: Association between meningioma and Cowden's disease. Neurology 43:1436–1437, 1993.
65. Hanssen AM, Fryns JP: Cowden syndrome. J Med Genet 32:117–119, 1995.
66. Weary PE, Gorlin RJ, Gentry WC, Comer JE, Greer KE: Multiple hamartoma syndrome (Cowden's disease). Arch Dermatol 106:682–690, 1972.
67. Liaw D, Marsh DJ, Li J, et al.: Germline mutations of the *PTEN* gene in Cowden disease, an inherited breast and thyroid cancer syndrome. Nat Genet 16: 64–67, 1997.
68. Yu CE, Oshima J, Fu YH, et al.: Positional cloning of the Werner's syndrome gene. Science 272:258–262, 1996.
69. Epstein CJ, Martin GM, Schultz AL, et al.: Werner's syndrome: A review of its symptomatology, natural history, pathologic features, genetics and relationship to the natural aging process. Medicine 45: 177–221, 1966.
70. Laso FJ, Vasquez G, Pastor I, Procel C, Santos-Briz A: Werner's syndrome and astrocytoma. Dermatologica 178:118–120, 1989.
71. Tsuchiya H, Tomita K, Ohno M, Inaoki MR, Kawashima A: Werner's syndrome combined with quintuplicate malignant tumors: A case report and review of literature data. Jpn J Clin Oncol 21:135–142, 1991.
72. Choi NW, Schuman IM, Gullen WH: Epidemiology of primary central nervous system neoplasms. II. case–control study. Am J Epidemiol 91:467–485, 1970.
73. Burch JD, Craib KJP, Choi BCK, Miller AB, Risch HA, Howe GR: An exploratory case–control study of brain tumors in adults. J Natl Cancer Inst 78: 601–609, 1987.
74. Gold EB, Leviton A, Lopez R, et al.: The role of family history in risk of childhood brain tumors. Cancer 73:1302–1311, 1994.
75. Kuijten RR, Strom SS, Rorke LB, et al.: Family history of cancer and seizures in young children with brain tumors: A report from the Childrens Cancer Group (United States and Canada). Cancer Causes Control 4:455–464, 1993.
76. Burger PC, Green SB: Patient age, histologic features and length of survival in patients with glioblastoma multiforme. Cancer 59:1617–1625, 1987.
77. Nelson DF, Nelson JS, Davis DR, Chang CH, Griffin TW, Pajak TF: Survival and prognosis of patients with astrocytoma with atypical or anaplastic features. J Neurooncol 3:99–103, 1985.
78. Kibirige MS, Birch JM, Campbell RH, Gattamaneni HR, Blair V: A review of astrocytoma in childhood. Pediatr Hematol Oncol 6:319–329, 1989.
79. Vieregge P, Gerhard L, Nahser HC: Familial glioma: Occurrence within the familial cancer syndrome and systemic malformations. J Neurol 234: 220–232, 1987.
80. von Deimling A, Louis DN, Menon AG, et al.: Deletions on the long arm of chromosome 17 in pilocytic astrocytoma. Acta Neuropathol 86:81–85, 1993.
81. Paulus W, Lisle DK, Tonn JC, et al.: Molecular genetic alterations in pleomorphic xanthoastrocytomas. Acta Neuropathol 91:293–297, 1996.
82. McCormack BM, Miller DC, Budzilovic GN, Voorhees GJ, Ransohoff J: Treatment and survival of low-grade astrocytoma in adults—1977–1988. Neurosurgery 31:636–642, 1992.
83. Piepmeier JM: Observations on the current treatment of low-grade astrocytic tumors of the cerebral hemispheres. J Neurosurg 67:177–181, 1987.
84. Bigner SH, Mark J, Burger PC, et al.: Specific chromosomal abnormalities in malignant human gliomas. Cancer Res 88:405–411, 1988.
85. Jenkins RB, Kimmel DW, Moertel CA, et al.: A cytogenetic study of 53 human gliomas. Cancer Genet Cytogenet 39:253–279, 1989.

86. Schröck E, Blume C, Meffert MC, et al.: Recurrent gain of chromosome arm 7q in low-grade astrocytic tumors studied by comparative genomic hybridization. Genes Chromosomes Cancer 15: 199–205, 1996.
87. Collins VP, James CD: Gene and chromosomal alterations associated with the development of human gliomas. FASEB J 7:926–930, 1993.
88. Louis DN: The *p53* gene and protein in human brain tumors. J Neuropathol Exp Neurol 53:11–21, 1994.
89. Hermanson M, Funa K, Koopmann J, et al.: Association of loss of heterozygosity on chromosome 17p with high platelet-derived growth factor alpha receptor expression in human malignant gliomas. Cancer Res 56:164–171, 1996.
90. Frankel R, Bayonu W, Koslow M, Newcomb EW: *p53* mutations in human malignant gliomas: Comparison of loss of heterozygosity with mutation frequency. Cancer Res 52:1427–1433, 1992.
91. Saxena A, Clark WC, Robertson JT, Ikejiri B, Oldfield EH, Ali IU: Evidence for the involvement of a potential second tumor suppressor gene on chromosome 17 distinct from *p53* in malignant astrocytomas. Cancer Res 52:6716–6721, 1992.
92. Wales MM, Biel MA, el Deiry W, et al.: *p53* activates expression of HIC-1, a new candidate tumour suppressor gene on 17p13.3. Nature Med 1: 570–577, 1995.
93. James CD, Carlbom E, Dumanski JP, et al.: Clonal genomic alterations in glioma malignancy stages. Cancer Res 48:5546–5551, 1988.
94. Hoang-Xuan K, Merel P, Vega F, et al.: Analysis of the *NF2* tumor-suppressor gene and chromosome 22 deletions in gliomas. Int J Cancer 60: 478–481, 1995.
95. Rubio MA, Correa KM, Ramesh V, et al.: Analysis of the neurofibromatosis 2 gene gene in human ependymomas and astrocytomas. Cancer Res 54: 45–47, 1994.
96. Ichimura K, Schmidt EE, Goike HM, Collins VP: Human glioblastomas with no alterations of the *CDKN2A (p16INK4A, MTS1)* and *CDK4* genes have frequent mutations of the retinoblastoma gene. Oncogene 13:1065–1072, 1996.
97. Ueki K, Ono Y, Henson JW, Efird JT, von Deimling A, Louis DN: *CDKN2/p16* or *RB* alterations occur in the majority of glioblastomas and are inversely correlated. Cancer Res 56:150–153, 1996.
98. Burger PC, Vogel FS, Green SB, Strike TA: Glioblastoma multiforme and anaplastic astrocytoma: Pathologic criteria and prognostic implications. Cancer 56:1106–1111, 1985.
99. Fults D, Petronio J, Noblett BD, Pedone CA: Chromosome 11p15 deletions in human malignant astrocytomas. Genomics 14:799–801, 1992.
100. James CD, He J, Carlbom E, Nordenskjold M, Cavenee WK, Collins VP: Chromosome 9 deletion mapping reveals interferon alpha and interferon beta-1 gene deletions in human glial tumors. Cancer Res 51:1684–1688, 1991.
101. Sonoda Y, Iizuka M, Yasuda J, et al.: Loss of heterozygosity at 11p15 in malignant glioma. Cancer Res 55:2166–2168, 1995.
102. von Deimling A, Bender B, Jahnke R, et al.: Loci associated with malignant progression in astrocytomas: A candidate on chromosome 19q. Cancer Res 54:1397–1401, 1994.
103. Ligon AH, Pershouse MA, Jasser SA, Yung WKA, Steck PA: Identification of a novel gene product, *RIG*, that is down-regulated in human glioblastoma. Oncogene 14:1075–1081, 1997.
104. Kamb A, Gruis NA, Weaver-Feldhaus J, et al.: A cell cycle regulator potentially involved in genesis of many tumor types. Science 264:436–440, 1994.
105. Nobori T, Miura K, Wu DJ, Lois A, Takabayashi K, Carson DA: Deletions of the cyclin-dependent kinase-4 inhibitor gene in multiple human cancers. Nature 368:753–756, 1994.
106. Serrano M, Hannon GJ, Beach D: A new regulatory motif in cell-cycle control causing specific inhibition of cyclin D/CDK4. Nature 366:704–707, 1993.
107. Sherr CJ: G1 phase progression: Cycling on cue. Cell 79:551–555, 1994.
108. Schmidt EE, Ichimura K, Reifenberger G, Collins VP: *CDKN2 (p16/MTS1)* gene deletion or CDK4 amplification occurs in the majority of glioblastomas. Cancer Res 54:6321–6324, 1994.
109. Reifenberger G, Reifenberger J, Ichimura K, Meltzer PM, Collins VP: Amplification of multiple genes from chromosomal region 12q13–14 in human malignant gliomas: Preliminary mapping of the amplicons shows preferential involvement of *CDK4, SAS* and *MDM2.* Cancer Res 54:4299–4303, 1994.
110. Weber RG, Sabel M, Reifenberger J, et al.: Characterization of genomic alterations associated with glioma progression by comparative genomic hybridization. Oncogene 13:983–994, 1996.
111. Walker AE, Robins M, Weinfeld FD: Epidemiology of brain tumors: The national survey of intracranial neoplasms. Neurology 35:219–226, 1985.
112. Karlbom AE, James CD, Boethius J, et al.: Loss of heterozygosity in malignant gliomas involves at least three distinct regions on chromosome 10. Hum Genet 92:169–174, 1993.
113. Rasheed BK, McLendon RE, Friedman HS, et al.: Chromosome 10 deletion mapping in human gliomas: A common deletion region in 10q25. Oncogene 10:2243–2246, 1995.
114. Mollenhauer J, Wiemann S, Scheurlen W, et al.: *DMBT1*, a new member of the SRCR superfamily, on chromosome 10q25.3–26.1 is deleted in malignant brain tumours. Nat Genet 17:32–39, 1997.
115. Eagle LR, Yin X, Brothman AR, Williams BJ, Atkin NB, Prochownik EV: Mutation of the *MX11* gene in prostate cancer. Nat Genet 9:249–255, 1995.
116. Boström J, Cobbers JMJL, Wolter M, et al.: Mutation of the *PTEN (MMAC1)* tumor suppressor gene in a subset of glioblastomas but not in meningiomas with loss of chromosome arm 10q. Cancer Res 58:29–33, 1998.
117. Li J, Yen C, Liaw D, et al. *PTEN*, a putative protein tyrosine phosphatase gene mutated in human brain, breast, and prostate cancer. Science 275: 1943–1947, 1997.
118. Steck PA, Pershouse MA, Jasser SA, et al.: Identification of a candidate tumour suppressor gene, *MMAC*, at chromosome 10q23 that is mutated in multiple advanced cancers. Nat Genet 15:356–362, 1997.

119. He J, Allen JR, Collins VP, et al.: *CDK4* amplification is an alternative mechanism to *p16* gene homozygous deletion in glioma cell lines. Cancer Res 54:5804–5807, 1994.
120. Costello JF, Berger MS, Huang HJS, Cavenee WK: Silencing of p16/CDKN2 expression in human gliomas by methylation and chromatin condensation. Cancer Res 56:2405–2410, 1996.
121. Liang BC, Ross DA, Greenberg HS, Meltzer PS, Trent JM: Evidence of allelic imbalance of chromosome 6 in human astrocytomas. Neurology 44: 533–536, 1994.
122. Kim DH, Mohapatra G, Bollen A, Waldman FM, Feuerstein BG: Chromosomal abnormalities in glioblastoma multiforme tumors and glioma cell lines detected by comparative genomic hybridization. Int J Cancer 60:812–819, 1995.
123. Mohapatra G, Kim DH, Feuerstein BG: Detection of multiple gains and losses of genetic material in ten glioma cell lines by comparative genomic hybridization. Genes Chromosomes Cancer 13:86–93, 1995.
124. Schröck E, Thiel G, Lozanova T, du Manoir S, et al.: Comparative genomic hybridization of human malignant gliomas reveals multiple amplification sites and nonrandom chromosomal gains and losses. Am J Pathol 144:1203–1218, 1994.
125. Weber RG, Sommer C, Albert FK, Kiessling M, Cremer T: Clinically distinct subgroups of glioblastoma multiforme studied by comparative genomic hybridization. Lab Invest 74:108–119, 1996.
126. Plate KH, Breier G, Risau W: Molecular mechanisms of developmental and tumor angiogenesis. Brain Pathol 4:207–218, 1994.
127. Cheng SY, Huang HJ, Nagane M, et al.: Suppression of glioblastoma angiogenicity and tumorigenicity by inhibition of endogenous expression of vascular endothelial growth factor. Proc Natl Acad Sci USA 93:8502–8507, 1996.
128. Millauer B, Shawver LK, Plate KH, Risau W, Ullrich A: Glioblastoma growth inhibited *in vivo* by a dominant-negative *Flk-1* mutant. Nature 367: 576–579, 1994.
129. DiFiore PP, Pierce JH, Fleming TP, et al.: Overexpression of the human EGF receptor confers an EGF-dependent transformed phenotype to NIH 3T3 cells. Cell 51:1063–1070, 1987.
130. Velu TJ, Beguinot L, Vass WC, et al.: Epidermal growth factor receptor-dependent transformation by a human EGF receptor proto-oncogene. Science 238:1408–1410, 1987.
131. Ekstrand AJ, Liu L, He J, et al.: Altered subcellular location of an activated and tumor-associated epidermal growth factor receptor. Oncogene 10: 1455–1460, 1995.
132. Ekstrand AJ, James CD, Cavenee WK, Seliger B, Pettersson RF, Collins VP: Genes for epidermal growth factor receptor, transforming growth factor alpha, and epidermal growth factor and their expression in human gliomas *in vivo.* Cancer Res 51:2164–2172, 1991.
133. Muleris M, Almeida A, Dutrillaux AM, et al.: Oncogene amplification in human gliomas: A molecular cytogenetic analysis. Oncogene 9:2717–2722, 1994.
134. Momand J, Zambetti GP, Olson DC, George D, Levine AJ: The mdm-2 oncogene product forms a complex with the p53 protein and inhibits p53-mediated transactivation. Cell 69:1237–1245, 1992.
135. Oliner JD, Pietenpol JA, Thiagalingam S, Gyuris J, Kinzler KW, Vogelstein B: Oncoprotein MDM2 conceals the activation domain of tumour suppressor p53. Nature 362:857–860, 1993.
136. Finlay CA: The *mdm-2* oncogene can overcome wild-type p53 suppression of transformed cell growth. Mol Cell Biol 13:301–306, 1993.
137. Reifenberger G, Liu L, Ichimura K, Schmidt EE, Collins VP: Amplification and overexpression of the *MDM2* gene in a subset of human malignant gliomas without *p53* mutations. Cancer Res 53: 2736–2739, 1993.
138. He J, Olson J, James CD: Lack of $p16^{INK4}$ or retinoblastoma protein (pRb), or amplification-associated overexpression of cdk4 is observed in distinct subsets of malignant glial tumors and cell lines. Cancer Res 55:4833–4836, 1995.
139. Winger MJ, Macdonald DR, Cairncross JG: Supratentorial anaplastic gliomas in adults. The prognostic importance of extent of resection and prior low-grade glioma. J Neurosurg 71:487–493, 1989.
140. Lang FF, Miller DC, Pisharody S, Koslow M, Newcomb EW: Pathways leading to glioblastoma multiforme: A molecular analysis of genetic alterations in 65 astrocytic tumors. J Neurosurg 81:427–436, 1994.
141. Leenstra S, Bijlsma EK, Troost D, et al.: Allele loss on chromosomes 10 and 17p and epidermal growth factor receptor gene amplification in human malignant astrocytoma related to prognosis. Br J Cancer 70:684–689, 1994.
142. von Deimling A, von Ammon K, Schoenfeld D, Wiestler OD, Seizinger BR, Louis DN: Subsets of glioblastoma multiforme defined by molecular genetic analysis. Brain Pathol 3:19–26, 1993.
143. Reifenberger J, Ring GU, Gies U, et al.: Analysis of *p53* mutation and epidermal growth factor receptor amplification in recurrent gliomas with malignant progression. J Neuropathol Exp Neurol 55:824–833, 1996.
144. Watanabe K, Tachibana O, Sato K, Yonekawa Y, Kleihues P, Ohgaki H: Overexpression of EGF receptor and *p53* mutations are mutually exclusive in the evolution of primary and secondary glioblastomas. Brain Pathol 6:217–223, 1996.
145. Reyes-Mugica M, Rieger-Christ K, Ohgaki H, et al.: Loss of *DCC* expression and glioma progression. Cancer Res 57:382–386, 1997.
146. Biernat W, Tohma Y, Yonekawa Y, Kleihues P, Ohgaki H: Alterations of cell cycle regulatory genes in primary *(de novo)* and secondary glioblastomas. Acta Neuropathol (Berl) 94:303–309, 1997.
147. Meyer-Puttlitz B, Hayashi Y, Waha A, et al.: Molecular genetic analysis of giant cell glioblastomas. Am J Pathol 151:853–857, 1997.
148. Celli P, Nofrone I, Palma L, Cantore G, Fortuna A: Cerebral oligodendroglioma: Prognostic factors and life history. Neurosurgery 35:1018–1035, 1994.
149. Ludwig CL, Smith MT, Godfrey AD, Armbrust-

macher VW: A clinicopathological study of 323 patients with oligodendrogliomas. Ann Neurol 19: 15–21, 1986.

150. Mørk SJ, Lindegaard KF, Halvorson TB, Lehmann EH, Solgaard T, Hatlevoll R, Harvei S, Ganz J: Oligodendroglioma: Incidence and biological behavior in a defined population. J Neurosurg 63: 881–889, 1985.

151. Sun ZM, Genka S, Shitara N, Akanuma A, Takakura K: Factors possibly influencing the prognosis of oligodendroglioma. Neurosurgery 22: 886–891, 1988.

152. Cairncross JG, Macdonald DR, Ramsay DA: Aggressive oligodendroglioma: A chemosensitive tumor. Neurosurgery 31:78–82, 1992.

153. Glass J, Hochberg FH, Gruber ML, Louis DN, Smith D, Rattner B: The treatment of oligodendrogliomas and mixed oligodendroglioma-astrocytomas with PCV chemotherapy. J Neurosurg 76:741–745, 1992.

154. Parkinson D, Hall CW: Oligodendrogliomas. Simultaneous appearance in frontal lobes of siblings. *J Neurosurg* 19:424–426, 1962.

155. Roosen N, De La Porte C, Van Vyve M, Solheid C, Sclosse P: Familial oligodendroglioma. Case report. J Neurosurg 60:848–849, 1984.

156. Roelvink NCA, Kamphorst W, Lindhout D, Ponssen H: Concordant cerebral oliodendroglioma in identical twins. J Neurol Neurosurg Psychiatry 49: 706–708, 1986.

157. Ferraresi S, ServeHo D, De Lorenzi L, Allegranza A: Familial frontal lobe oligodendroglioma. J Neurosurg Sci 33:317–318, 1989.

158. Kros JM, Lie ST, Stefanko SZ: Familial occurrence of polymorphous oligodendroglioma. Neurosurgery 34:732–736, 1994.

159. Bello MJ, Leone PE, Vaquero J, et al.: Allelic loss at 1p and 19q frequently occurs in association and may represent early oncogenic events in oligodendroglial tumors. Int J Cancer 57:172–175, 1995.

160. Kraus JA, Koopmann J, Kaskel P, et al.: Shared allelic losses on chromosomes 1p and 19q suggest a common origin of oligodendroglioma and oligoastrocytoma. J Neuropathol Exp Neurol 54:91–95, 1995.

161. Reifenberger J, Reifenberger G, Liu L, James CD, Wechsler W, Collins VP: Molecular genetic analysis of oligodendroglial tumors shows preferential allelic losses on chromosome arms 19q and 1p. Am J Pathol 145:1175–1190, 1994.

162. von Deimling A, Louis DN, von Ammon K, Petersen I, Wiestler OD, Seizinger BR: Evidence for a tumor suppressor gene on chromosome 19q associated with human astrocytomas, oligodendrogliomas, and mixed gliomas. Cancer Res 52:4277–4279, 1992.

163. Rosenberg JE, Lisle DK, Burwick JA, et al.: Refined deletion mapping of the chromosome 19q glioma tumor suppressor gene to the *D19S412-STD* interval. Oncogene 13:2483–2485, 1996.

164. Bello MJ, Vaquero J, de Campos JM, et al.: Molecular analysis of chromosome 1 abnormalities in human gliomas reveals frequent loss of 1p in oligodendroglial tumors. Int J Cancer 57:172–175, 1994.

165. Bello MJ, Leone PE, Nebreda P, et al.: Allelic status of chromosome 1 in neoplasms of the nervous system. Cancer Genet Cytogenet 83:160–164, 1995.

166. Reifenberger J, Reifenberger G, Wechsler W, Collins VP: Epidermal growth factor receptor expression in oligodendroglial tumors. Am J Pathol 149: 29–35, 1996.

167. Ohgaki H, Eibl RH, Wiestler OD, Yasargil MG, Newcomb EW, Kleihues P: *p53* mutations in nonastrocytic human brain tumors. Cancer Res 51: 6202–6205, 1991.

168. Rasheed BKA, McLendon RE, Herndon JE, et al.: Alterations of the *TP53* gene in human gliomas. Cancer Res 54:1324–1330, 1994.

169. Reifenberger G, Reifenberger J, Liu L, James CD, Wechsler W, Collins VP: Molecular genetics of oligodendroglial tumors. In Nagai M (ed): Brain Tumor Research and Therapy. Springer-Verlag, Tokyo, 1996, pp187–201.

170. Challa VR, Goodman HO, Davis CH Jr: Familial brain tumors: Studies of two families and review of the recent literature. Neurosurgery 12:18–23, 1983.

171. Fairburn B, Urich H: Malignant gliomas occurring in identical twins. J Neurol Neurosurg Psychiatry 34:718–722, 1971.

172. Maintz D, Fiedler K, Koopmann J, et al.: Molecular genetic evidence for subtypes of oligoastrocytomas. J Neuropathol Exp Neurol 56:1098–1104, 1997.

173. Gilchrist DM, Savard ML: Ependymomas in two sisters and a maternal male cousin. Am J Med Genet 45(suppl): A22, 1989.

174. Honan WP, Anderson M, Carey MP, Williams B: Familial subependymomas. Br J Neurosurg 1:317–321, 1987.

175. Nijssen PC, Deprez RH, Tijssen CC, et al.: Familial anaplastic ependymoma: Evidence of loss of chromosome 22 in tumour cells. J Neurol Neurosurg Psychiatry 57:1245–1248, 1994.

176. Bijlsma EK, Voesten AM, Bijleveld EH, et al.: Molecular analysis of genetic changes in ependymomas. Genes Chromosomes Cancer 13:272–277, 1995.

177. James CD, He J, Carlbom E, et al.: Loss of genetic information in central nervous system tumors common to children and young adults. Genes Chromosomes Cancer 2:94–102, 1990.

178. Rogatto SR, Casartelli C, Rainho CA, Barbieri-Neto J. Chromosomes in the genesis and progression of ependymomas. Cancer Genet Cytogenet 69:146–152, 1993.

179. Slavc I, MacCollin MM, Dunn M, et al.: Exon scanning for mutations of the *NF2* gene in pediatric ependymomas, rhabdoid tumors and meningiomas. Int J Cancer 64:243–247, 1995.

180. Birch BD, Johnson JP, Parsa A, et al.: Frequent type 2 neurofibromatosis gene transcript mutations in sporadic intramedullary spinal cord ependymomas. Neurosurgery 39:135–140, 1996.

181. Huynh DP, Mautner V, Baser ME, Stavrou D, Pulst SM: Immunohistochemical detection of schwannomin and neurofibromin in vestibular schwannomas, ependymomas and meningiomas. J Neuropathol Exp Neurol 56:382–390, 1997.

182. Sainati L, Montaldi A, Putti MC, et al.: Cytoge-

netic (11;17) (q13; q21) in a pediatric ependymoma. Is 11q13 a recurring breakpoint in reported in ependymoma? Cancer Genet Cytogenet 59:213–216, 1992.
183. Sawyer JR, Sammartino G, Husain M, Boop FA, Chadduck WM: Chromosome aberrations in four ependymomas. Cancer Genet Cytogenet 74:132–138, 1994.
184. Pulst SM, Rouleau G, Marineau MS, Fain P, Sieb JP: Familial meningioma is not allelic to neurofibromatosis 2. Neurology 43:2096–2098, 1993.
185. Metzger AK, Sheffield VC, Duyk G, Daneshvar L, Edwards MS, Cogen PH: Identification of a germline mutation in the *p53* gene in a patient with an intracranial ependymoma. Proc Natl Acad Sci USA 88:7825–7829, 1991.
186. Van Meyel DJ, Ramsay DA, Casson AG, Keeney M, Chambers AF, Cairncross JG: *p53* mutation, expression, and DNA ploidy in evolving gliomas: Evidence for two pathways of progression. J Natl Cancer Inst 86:1011–1017, 1994.
187. Iuzzolino P, Ghimenton C, Nicolato A, et al.: p53 protein in low-grade astrocytomas: Study with long term follow up. Br J Cancer 69:586–591, 1994.
188. Chozick BS, Pezzullo JC, Epstein MH, Finch PW: Prognostic implications of p53 overexpression in supratentorial astrocytic tumors. Neurosurgery 35:831–838, 1994.
189. Kraus JA, Bolin C, Wolf HK, et al.: *TP53* alterations and clinical outcome in low grade astrocytomas. Genes Chromosomes Cancer 10:143–149, 1994.
190. Pollack IF, Hamilton RL, Finkelstein SD, et al.: The relationship between *TP53* mutations and overexpression of p53 and prognosis in malignant gliomas of childhood. Cancer Res 57:304–309, 1997.
191. Bigner SH, Burger PC, Wong AJ, et al.: Gene amplification in malignant human gliomas: Clinical and histopathological aspects. J Neuropathol Exp Neurol 47:191–205, 1988.
192. Hawkins RA, Killen ER, Jack WJ, Chetty U. Epidermal growth factor receptors in intracranial and breast tumors: Their clinical significance. Br J Cancer 63:553–560, 1991.
193. Hurtt MR, Moossy J, Donovan-Peluso M, Locker J. Amplification of epidermal growth factor receptor gene in gliomas: Histopathology and prognosis. J Neuropathol Exp Neurol 51:84–90, 1992.
194. Schlegel J, Merdes A, Stumm G, Albert FK, Forsting M, Hynes N, Kiessling M. Amplification of the epidermal growth factor receptor gene correlates with different growth behaviour in human glioblastoma. Int J Cancer 56:72–77, 1994.
195. Hung KL, Wu CM, Huang JS, How SW: Familial medulloblastoma in siblings: Report in one family and review of the literature. Surg Neurol 33:341–346, 1990.
196. Scheurlen W, Sorensen N, Roggendorf W, Kuhl J. Molecular analysis of medulloblastomas occurring simultaneously in monozygotic twins. Eur J Pediatr 155:880–884, 1996.
197. Tijssen CC, Halprin MR, Endtz LJ: Familial Brain Tumors. A Commented Register. Matinus Nijhoff Publishers, The Hague, pp10–73, 1982.
198. Miller RW, Rubinstein JH: Tumors in Rubinstein-Taybi syndrome. Am J Med Genet 56:112–115, 1995.
199. Kleihues P, Schäuble B, zur Hausen A, Esteve J, Ohgaki H: Tumors associated with *p53* germline mutations: A synopsis of 91 families. Am J Pathol 150:1–13, 1997.
200. Reifenberger J, Janssen G, Weber RG, et al.: Primitive neuroectodermal tumors of the cerebral hemispheres in two siblings with *TP53* germline mutation. J Neuropathol Exp Neurol 57 179–187, 1998.
201. Becker R, Bauer BL, Mennel HD, Plate KH: Cerebellar primitive neuroectodermal tumor with multipotent differentiation in a family with von Hippel-Lindau disease. Case report. Clin Neuropathol 12:107–111, 1993.
202. Biegel JA, Rorke LB, Packer RJ, et al.: Isochromosome 17q in primitive neuroectodermal tumors of the central nervous system. Genes Chromosomes Cancer 1:139–147, 1989.
203. Bigner SH, Mark J, Friedman HS, Biegel JA, Bigner DD: Structural chromosomal abnormalities in human medulloblastoma. Cancer Genet Cytogenet 30:91–101, 1988.
204. Cogen PH, Daneshvar L, Metzger AK, Edwards MS: Deletion mapping of the medulloblastoma locus on chromosome 17p. Genomics 8:279–285, 1990.
205. Raffel C, Gilles FE, Weinberg KI: Reduction to homozygosity and gene amplification in central nervous system primitive neuroectodermal tumors of childhood. Cancer Res 50:587–591, 1990.
206. Biegel JA, Burk CD, Barr FG, Emanuel BS: Evidence for a 17p tumor related locus distinct from *p53* in pediatric primitive neuroectodermal tumors. Cancer Res 52:3391–3395, 1992.
207. Cogen PH, Daneshvar L, Metzger AK, Duyk G, Edwards MS, Sheffield VC: Involvement of multiple chromosome 17 p loci in medulloblastoma tumorigenesis. Genetics 50:584–589, 1992.
208. Phelan CM, Liu L, Ruttledge MH, Müntzing K, Ridderheim PA, Collins VP: Chromosome 17 abnormalities and lack of *TP53* mutations in paediatric central nervous system tumours. Hum Genet 96:684–690, 1995.
209. Saylors III RL, Sidranski D, Friedman HS, et al.: Infrequent *p53* mutations in medulloblastomas. Cancer Res 51:4721–4723, 1991.
210. McDonald JD, Daneshvar L, Willert JR, Matsumura K, Waldman F, Cogen PH: Physical mapping of chromosome 17p13.3 in the region of a putative tumor suppressor gene important in medulloblastoma. Genomics 23:229–232, 1994.
211. Kraus JA, Koch A, Albrecht S, von Deimling A, Wiestler OD, Pietsch T: Loss of heterozygosity at locus F13B on chromosome 1q in human medulloblastoma. Int J Cancer 67:11–15, 1996.
212. Thomas GA, Raffel C: Loss of heterozygosity on 6q, 16q, and 17p in human central nervous system primitive neuroectodermal tumors. Cancer Res 51:639–643, 1991.
213. Schütz BR, Scheurlen W, Kraus J, du Manoir S, Joos S, Bentz M, Lichter P: Mapping of chromosomal gains and losses in primitive neuroectodermal tumors by comparative genomic hybridiza-

tion. Genes Chromosomes Cancer 16:196–203, 1996.
214. Albrecht S, von Deimling A, Pietsch T, et al.: Microsatellite analysis of loss of heterozygosity on chromosome 9q, 11p and 17p in medulloblastomas. Neuropathol Appl Neurobiol 20:74–81, 1994.
215. Schofield D, West DC, Anthony DC, Sklar J: Correlation of loss of heterozygosity at chromosome 9q with histological subtype in medulloblastomas. Am J Pathol 146:472–480, 1995.
216. Raffel C Jenkins RB, Frederick L, et al.: Sporadic medulloblastomas contain *PTCH* mutations. Cancer Res 57:842–845, 1997.
217. Reifenberger J, Wolter M, Weber RG, et al.: Missense mutations in *SMOH* in sporadic basal cell carinomas of the skin and primitive neuroectodermal tumors of the central nervous system. Cancer Res 58:1798–1803, 1998.
218. Alcedo J, Noll M: Hedgehog and its patched-smoothened receptor complex: A novel signalling mechanism at the cell surface. Biol Chem 378: 583–590, 1997.
219. Kozmik Z, Sure U, Ruedi D, Busslinger M, Aguzzi A: Deregulated expression of PAX5 in medulloblastoma. Proc Natl Acad Sci USA 92:5709–5713, 1995.
220. Wasson JC, Saylors RL, Zelter P, et al.: Oncogene amplification in pediatric brain tumors. Cancer Res 50:2987–2990, 1990.
221. Brüstle O, Oghaki H, Schmidt HP, Walter GF, Ostertag H, Kleihues P: Primitive neuroectodermal tumors after prophylactic central nervous system irradiation in children. Association with an activated K-ras gene. Cancer 69:2385–2392, 1992.
222. Gilbertson RJ, Pearson ADJ, Perry RH, Jaros E, Kelly PJ: Prognostic significance of the *c-erbB-2* oncogene product in childhood medulloblastoma. Br J Cancer 71:473–477, 1995.
223. Jaros E, Lunec J, Perry RH, Kelly PJ, Pearson AD: p53 protein overexpression identifies a group of central primitive neuroectodermal tumours with poor prognosis. Br J Cancer 68: 801–807, 1993.
224. Batra, SK, McLendon RE, Koo JS, et al.: Prognostic implications of chromosome 17p deletions in human medulloblastomas. J Neurooncol 24:39–45, 1995.
225. Segal RA, Goumnerova LC, Kwon YK, Stiles CD, Pomeroy SL: Expression of the neurotrophin receptor TrkC is linked to a favorable outcome in medulloblastoma. Proc Natl Acad Sci USA 91: 12867–12871, 1994.
226. Maier H, Öfner D, Hittmair A, Kitz K, Budka H: Classic, atypical, and anaplastic meningioma: Three histopathological subtypes of clinical relevance. J Neurosurg 77:616–623, 1992.
227. Parry DM, Eldridge R, Kaiser-Kupfer MI, Bouzas EA, Pikus A, Patronas N: Neurofibromatosis 2 (NF2): Clinical characteristics of 63 affected individuals and clinical evidence for heterogeneity. Am J Med Genet 52:450–461, 1994.
228. Bolger GB, Stamberg J, Kirsch IL: Chromosome translocation t(14;22) and oncogene (c-sis) variant in a pedigree with familial meningioma. N Engl J Med 312:564–567, 1980.
229. Zang KD, Singer H: Chromosomal constitution of meningiomas. Nature 216:84–85, 1967.
230. Lekanne-Deprez RH, Bianchi AB, Groen NA, et al.: Frequent *NF2* gene transcript mutations in sporadic meningiomas and vestibular schwannomas. Am J Hum Genet 54:1022–1029, 1994.
231. Ruttledge MH, Sarrazin J, Rangaratnam S, et al.: Evidence for the complete inactivation of the *NF2* gene in the majority of sporadic meningiomas. Nat Genet 6:180–184, 1994.
232. Wellenreuther R, Kraus JA, Lenartz D, et al.: Analysis of the neurofibromatosis gene reveals molecular variants of meningioma. Am J Pathol 146: 827–832, 1995.
233. Ruttledge MH, Xie YG, Han FY, et al.: Deletions on chromosome 22 in sporadic meningioma. Genes Chromosomes Cancer 10:122–130, 1994.
234. Lekanne-Deprez RH, Riegman PHJ, Groen NA, et al.: Cloning and characterization of MN1, a gene from 22q11, which is disrupted by a balanced translocation in a meningioma. Oncogene 10: 1521–1528, 1995.
235. Buijs A, Sherr S, van Baal S, et al.: Translocation (12;22)(p13; q11) in myeloproliferative disorders results in fusion of the *ETS*-like *TEL* gene on 12p13 to the *MN1* gene on 22q. Oncogene 10: 1511–1519, 1995.
236. Peyrard M, Fransson I, Xie YG, et al.: Characterization of a new member of the human beta-adaptin gene family from chromosome 22q12, a candidate meningioma gene. Hum Mol Genet 3: 1393–1399, 1994.
237. Weber RG, Boström J, Wolter M, et al.: Analysis of genomic alterations in benign, atypical, and anaplastic meningiomas: Towards a genetic model of meningioma progression. Proc Natl Acad Sci USA 94:14719–14724, 1997.
238. Tos M, Thomsen J: Epidemiology of acoustic neuromas. J Laryngol Otol 98:685–692, 1984.
239. Seizinger BR, Rouleau GA, Ozelius LJ, et al.: Common pathogenic mechanism for three tumor types in bilateral acoustic neurofibromatosis. Science 236:317–319, 1987.
240. Rouleau, GA, Wertelecki W, Haines JA, et al.: Genetic linkage of bilateral acoustic neurofibromatosis to a DNA marker on chromosome 22. Nature 329:246–248, 1987.
241. Bianchi AB, Hara T, Ramesh V, et al.: Mutations in transcript isoforms of the neurofibromatosis 2 gene in multiple human tumor types. Nat Genet 6:185–192, 1994.
242. Bijlsma EK, Merel P, Bosch DA, et al.: Analysis of mutations in the *SCH* gene in schwannomas. Genes Chromosomes Cancer 11:7–14, 1994.
243. Irving RM, Moffat DA, Hardy DG, Barton DE, Xuereb JH, Maher R: Somatic *NF2* gene mutations is familial and non-familial vestibular schwannoma. Hum Mol Genet 3:347–350, 1994.
244. Jacoby LB, MacCollin M, Louis DN, et al.: Exon scanning for mutation of the *NF2* gene in schwannomas. Hum Mol Genet 3:413–419, 1994.
245. Sainz J, Figueroa K, Baser M, Mautner VF, Pulst SM: High frequency of nonsense mutations in the *NF2* gene caused by transitions in five CGA codons. Hum Mol Genet 4:137–139, 1995.
246. Sainz J, Figueroa K, Pulst SM: Identification of

three *NF2* gene mutations in vestibular schwannomas. Hum Genet 97:121–123, 1996.
247. Sainz J, Huynh P, Figueroa K, Ragge N, Baser M, Pulst SM: Mutations of the neurofibromatosis type 2 gene and lack of the gene product in vestibular schwannomas. Hum Mol Genet 3:885–891, 1994.
248. Twist EC, Ruttledge M, Rousseau M, et al.: The neurofibromatosis type 2 gene is inactivated in schwannomas. Hum Mol Genet 3:147–151, 1994.
249. Huynh DP, Pulst SM: NF antisense oligodeoxynucleotides induce reversible inhibition of schwannomin synthesis and cell adhesion in STS26T and T98G cells. Oncogene 13:73–84, 1996.
250. Stenman G, Kindblom LG, Johansson M, Angervall L: Clonal chromosome abnormalities and *in vitro* growth characteristics of classical and cellular schwannomas. Cancer Genet Cytogenet 57:121–131, 1991.

Chapter 9

# PHAKOMATOSES

Stefan-M. Pulst, MD, Dr Med
David Gutmann, MD, PhD



The name *phakomatoses* is derived from the Greek *phakos,* meaning spot; all phakomatoses are associated with cutaneous or retinal abnormalities. Of the five major disorders in this group, neurofibromatosis types 1 and 2, tuberous sclerosis, von Hippel-Lindau disease (VHL), and Sturge-Weber syndrome, only the first four are discussed because Sturge-Weber syndrome occurs only sporadically and is not known to be passed on to offspring. The other four diseases share several features, including autosomal dominant inheritance, high penetrance, and variable expression of the phenotype. In addition to lesions on the skin or in the fundus of the eye, these four diseases predispose to the formation of tumors ranging from benign hamartomas to the development of malignant renal cancer in VHL. Although screening and follow-up of known gene carriers are important for all four diseases, the specific protocols vary greatly.

## NEUROFIBROMATOSIS 1

### Clinical Features

Neurofibromatosis 1 (NF1) is a common autosomal dominant disorder that affects 1 in 3000 individuals of all races and ethnic backgrounds and both genders.[1,2] People with NF1 manifest a wide variety of clinical symptoms both related and unrelated to tumor formation. The clinical features of NF1 include abnormalities of pigmentation, bone growth, and blood vessel integrity as well as learning disabilities and an increased frequency of tumor formation (Table 9–1). Pigmentary abnormalities include café-au-lait (CAL) spots (hyperpigmented macules

Table 9–1. **Clinical Features of Neurofibromatosis 1**

| Feature | Frequency (%) in Adults* |
|---|---|
| Café-au-lait spots† | |
| Six or more 0.5 cm in diameter before puberty | |
| Six or more 1.5 cm in diameter after puberty | |
| Axillary or inguinal freckling† | |
| Lisch's nodules (iris hamartomas)† | |
| Optic pathway glioma† | |
| Neurofibroma† | |
| Peripheral neurofibroma | |
| Plexiform neurofibroma | 27 |
| Neurofibrosarcoma | |
| Bony abnormalities† | |
| Dysplasia of the long bones/pseudarthrosis | 3 |
| Sphenoid wing dysplasia | |
| Short stature | |
| First-degree family relative† | |
| Learning disabilities | |
| Other tumors | |
| Pheochromocytoma | 1 |
| Rhabdomyosarcoma | |
| Juvenile chronic myeloid leukemia | |
| Juvenile xanthogranulomas | 1 |
| Epilepsy | 4 |
| Renal artery stenosis | 2 |

*Frequencies of recognized complications of NF1 (taken from Huson and coworkers).[2] CAL spots, freckling, and Lisch nodules were used to establish diagnosis.
†NIH diagnostic criterion for NF1. Two or more such diagnostic features are sufficient for a diagnosis of NF1.

on the skin), freckling in non-sun–exposed areas (axilla and groin), and pigmented hamartomas (benign collection of pigmented cells) of the iris (Lisch's nodules). Although individuals without NF1 may have CAL spots, rarely will an unaffected individual manifest more than four of these macules. In contrast, individuals with NF1 have six of more CAL spots of a particular size (see Table 9–1). There are other inherited disorders in which affected individuals manifest CAL spots. These include Noonan's syndrome,[3] Russell-Silver syndrome,[4] and McCune-Albright syndrome,[5] which are all distinguished from NF1 by the presence of other specific clinical features.

Lisch's nodules represent hamartomas of the iris that do not interfere with vision or evolve into benign or malignant tumors.[6] They may be apparent on visual inspection in individuals with light-colored irides, but often require slit-lamp examination by an experienced ophthalmologist. Many abnormalities of bone growth are seen in NF1. Most commonly, individuals with NF1 present with scoliosis or kyphosis.[7] Radiographic examination of the spine may demonstrate scalloping of the vertebral bodies characteristic of NF1. Other more worrisome skeletal abnormalities of NF1 include sphenoid wing dysplasia and abnormalities of the long bones in the arms and legs. Dysplasia of the long bones can manifest by cortical thinning or bony cysts that can lead to fracture with resulting nonunion. This nonunion may presage the development of a false joint (or pseudarthrosis), which is often very difficult to correct satisfactorily.[8]

Learning disabilities are commonly observed in children with NF1.[9,10,10a] Although visuospatial learning may be impaired, other forms of learning disability are also common, including lower fine motor coordination scores.[11] For this reason, any child suspected of learning disabilities with NF1 should be evaluated early and begin treatment promptly. In addition to learning disabilities, many children with NF1 manifest attention deficit disorder and may benefit from treatment with stimulant medication. Nearly half of individuals affected with NF1 demonstrate high-signal-intensity lesions on $T_2$-weighted magnetic resonance images (MRI) of the brain.[12,13] These lesions appear as well circumscribed, nonenhancing bright lesions, sometimes referred to as "unidentified bright objects" (UBOs) in the basal ganglia, cerebellum, and brain stem regions. The clinical significance of these UBOs is still debated, and their pathological basis is unclear (Fig. 9–1). Recent studies have demonstrated an association between the presence of UBOs on brain MRI and learning disabilities or low IQ scores in children with NF1, but other studies have failed to confirm this association.[14,15] Pathological analyses of a limited number of these lesions have demonstrated increased water content but no evidence of dysplasia or hamartomata.[16] Mice with only one functional *Nf1* allele show an increased numbers of astrocytes expressing high levels of glial fibrillary acidic protein in medial regions of the periaqueductal gray, in the nucleus accumbens, and in the hippocampus.[17]

Vascular abnormalities have been reported to occur in NF1 and include renal artery dysplasia, coarctation of the aorta, and cerebral artery dysplasias.[18] Hyperplasia of the vascular smooth muscle layer in the renal arteries can lead to narrowing of the arterial lumen and diminution of the blood supply to the kidneys. This can result in the development of renal artery hypertension.[19] Similar abnormalities of the cerebral blood vessels can lead to arterial occlusion and cerebral ischemia.[20] In addition, narrowing of the luminal diameter of large intracranial vessels can stimulate the sprouting of collateral vessels, leading to the characteristic "moya-moya" radiographic appearance of these vessels on cerebral angiography.

The hallmark of NF1 is the development of benign and malignant tumors, most typically neurofibromas and optic pathway gliomas.[21] The multidisciplinary management of NF1 has recently been reviewed.[22] Neurofibromas represent benign growths composed of Schwann cells, fibroblasts, and mast cells. They can occur in any location and may present as cutaneous, subcutane-

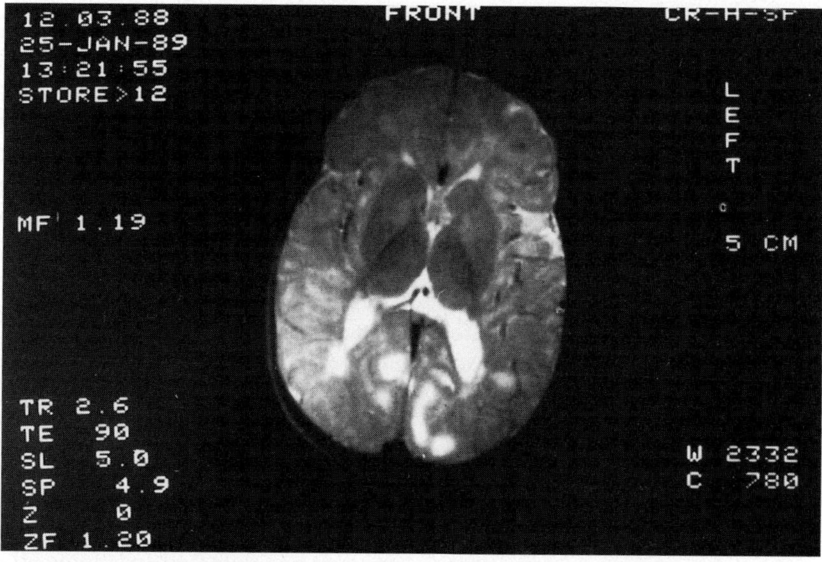


**Figure 9–1.** Typical high signal intensity lesion in an infant with NF1.

ous, or visceral tumors. Typically they begin to increase in both size and number during puberty and pregnancy, perhaps being related to hormonal influences. Less commonly, neurofibromas can grow as poorly defined tumors that interdigitate among normal structures. These neurofibromas are termed *plexiform neurofibromas* and, because of their growth pattern, are difficult to resect surgically. In addition, they may be highly vascular. Rarely, malignant transformation can occur within these plexiform neurofibromas, leading to the development of a neurofibrosarcoma, a malignant Schwann cell tumor. The development of persistent pain in a plexiform neurofibroma should be aggressively investigated for the presence of a malignant tumor.

Other tumors associated with NF1 include optic pathway glioma, pheochromocytoma and rhabdomyosarcoma. Optic pathway gliomas are seen in 15% of individuals with NF1.[23,24] Most commonly, they are detected as incidental findings on brain MRI. Only half of children who had a radiographically identifiable tumor ultimately developed any signs or symptoms from their tumors. The period of greatest risk for the development of symptomatic optic pathway gliomas is during the first 6 years of life. Demonstrable progression after the tumor is detected is uncommon. Management options include radiotherapy and chemotherapy.[25] Surgery plays a limited role in the management of these tumors. Pheochromocytomas and rhabdomyosarcomas are rare tumors in NF1.

Several families have been reported in the literature with multiple CAL spots but lacking other features of NF1 required to make the diagnosis.[26] One study failed to demonstrate linkage to chromosome 17q where the *NF1* gene resides.[27] Another family was shown to be linked to the *NF1* locus.[28] NF1 can also present in a nongeneralized form, called *segmental (or mosaic) NF1*, in which affected individuals develop pigmentary lesions (CAL spots, Lisch's nodules, and freckling) and neurofibromas in a segmental distribution.[29]

NF1 is readily distinguishable from other disorders that present with CAL spots (see earlier) or related syndromes such as Proteus syndrome, neurofibromatosis 2 (NF2), and tuberous sclerosis (TS). Joseph Merrick, who was referred to as "the elephant man," had Proteus syndrome with its characteristic overgrowth of limbs, digits, and trunk; bulky hamartomas and lipomas; and epidermal nevi.[30] The clinical features of NF2 and TS are discussed later.

## Identification of the *NF1* Gene Product

With positional cloning strategies, the *NF1* gene was identified in 1990 on the long arm of chromosome 17.[31–33] Proof that this gene represented the disease gene responsible for NF1 required the identification of mutations in this gene from individuals affected with NF1. Many such mutations have been identified thus far (see later under Genetic Testing). The *NF1* gene is a large gene spanning over 300,000 nucleotides of genomic DNA and directing the transcription of a an 11,000 to 13,000 nucleotide messenger RNA and a 2818 amino acid protein termed *neurofibromin*.[34] (Figure 9–2) Sequence analysis of neurofibromin demonstrated sequence similarities between a small region of the protein (~ 10%) and a family of proteins involved in the regulation of the *p21-ras* proto-oncogene (see later under The Function of Neurofibromin).[35] No functions have been ascribed to the remainder of the neurofibromin protein.

With the identification of the *NF1* gene, several groups developed antibodies against neurofibromin to facilitate analysis of its function.[36–41] Neurofibromin is a 220 to 250 kDa protein expressed at greatest levels in neurons (peripheral and central neurons), Schwann cells, oligodendrocytes, adrenal medullary cells, and leukocytes. Lower levels of neurofibromin expression have been detected in other tissues. Within the cells, neurofibromin is associated with cytoplasmic microtubules in several cell types, suggesting novel cytoskeletal-related functions for neurofibromin.[42,42a,42b] In other cell types, neurofibromin is found in the cytoplasm.[39,41]

During embryonic development in the mouse, chick, and rat, neurofibromin expression is detected in almost all tissues examined, including developing muscle, lung, kidney, and heart.[43–47] This high level of embryonic neurofibromin expression is dramatically reduced after the first week or two of postnatal life. This pattern of neurofibromin expression suggests that neurofibromin as a negative growth regulator might function during specific intervals of differentiation when cells are actively committing to differentiation (growth arrest). Experiments in several paradigms have demonstrated that neurofibromin expression increases during *in vitro* cell growth arrest and the onset of differentiation. To this end, *NF1* gene expression increases in astrocytes,[48,49] Schwann cells,[50] and myoblasts[51] stimulated to differentiate *in vitro* concomitant with the expression of other proteins characteristic of differentiation. In addition, *NF1* gene expression is upregulated when cells undergo growth arrest, one of the prerequisites for cellular differentiation.[52]

To better understand how neurofibromin dysfunction might result in the development of the clinical features associated with NF1, two groups successfully generated genetically engineered mice lacking *NF1* gene expression.[53,54] Mice with both copies of the *NF1* gene disrupted by mutation die during embryonic development of a cardiac vessel defect. This cardiac vessel defect, termed *double outlet right ventricle* (both the aorta and pulmonary artery arise as a single fused vessel), has been observed in chick embryos in which a population of neural crest cells have been ablated.[55] This phenotype in the NF1-deficient mice argues that neurofibromin plays a critical (perhaps indispensable) role in neural crest development. It should be noted that several of the cell types affected in NF1 derive from the neural crest (e.g., Schwann cells, adrenal medullary cells). Mice with one functional and one disrupted copy of the *NF1* gene develop tumors not commonly associated with NF1.[54] These heterozygous mice are analogous to humans with NF1 in that they possess one normal and one mutated *NF1* gene.

## The Function of Neurofibromin

As mentioned earlier, analysis of the *NF1* predicted protein sequence demonstrated similarity between a small portion of neurofibromin and the active subregion of proteins involved in the regulation of the *p21-ras* proto-oncogene (GTPase activating proteins [GAPs]). Proof for this structural similarity was provided by biochemical studies demonstrating that full-length neurofibromin, as well as the GAP-related domain of neurofibromin alone, could regulate *p21-ras* both *in vitro* and *in vivo*.[56–62] Ras proteins are active when complexed to GTP and inactive in a GDP-bound form (Fig. 9–2). Activated ras in many cells provides a growth-stimulatory signal.[63] Fibroblasts in which activated p21-ras has been introduced have growth properties characteristic of transformed tumor cells. Inactivation of ras by converting ras from its active GTP-bound form to an inactive GDP-bound conformation is accomplished by GAP molecules like neurofibromin. Loss of neurofibromin in cells would be predicted to result in increased levels of activated (GTP-bound) ras and increased cell proliferation.

*NF1* as a tumor suppressor gene functions to regulate cell growth negatively such that loss of neurofibromin expression would be associated with increased cell growth and the development of tumors. Each cell in an individual without NF1 harbors two functioning copies of the *NF1* gene that, in relevant tissues, results in normal levels of neurofibromin. In individuals with NF1, one copy of the *NF1* gene is functional while the other has been rendered nonfunctional by a DNA mutation. In cases where NF1 is inherited, the nonfunctional (mutant) *NF1* gene is inherited from the affected parent. Loss of the one remaining *NF1* gene by an additional (somatic) mutation would result in absent neurofibromin expression and the development of a neurofibroma or optic pathway glioma. This two-hit (mutation) hypothesis, first proposed by Alfred Knudson,[64] has been proven for all previously reported tumor suppressor genes.

Loss of *NF1* expression has been reported for a wide variety of human tumors (Table 9–2). Examination of tumors from individuals with NF1 has demonstrated loss of neurofibromin expression in neurofibrosarcoma,[46,56,65] leukemia,[66–68] and pheochromocytoma cells.[69,70] In the case of the neurofibrosarcoma and leukemic cells, loss of neurofibromin expression was associated

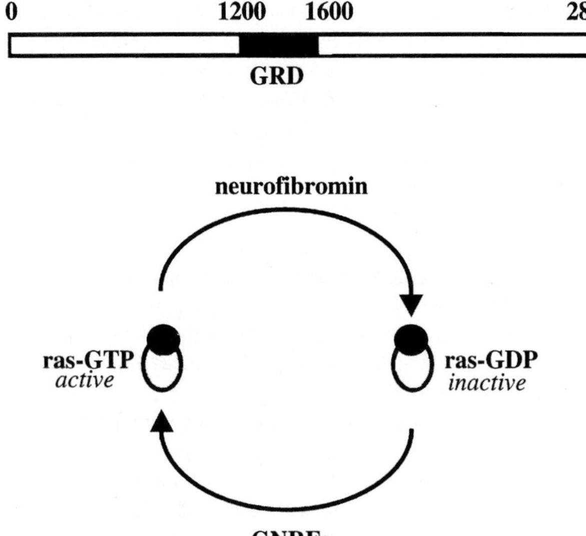


**Figure 9–2.** Schematic representation of the *NF1* gene product, neurofibromin. Neurofibromin is a 2818 amino acid protein with a small central portion with sequence and functional similarity to a family of proteins that regulate p21-ras, termed GTPase-activating proteins (GAPs). This GAP-related domain is located between residues 1200 and 1600. GAP molecules interact with GTP-bound p21-ras (activated p21-ras) and accelerate its conversion to its inactive GDP-bound form. GDP-bound p21-ras is then reactivated by guanosine nucleotide replacing factors (GNRFs). The cycling p21-ras between active and inactive conformations has been termed the "ras cycle."

with increased levels of activated p21-ras.[56,57,62] Reduction of p21-ras activity with pharmacological treatments (farnesyltransferase inhibitors) results in decreased neurofibrosarcoma tumor cell growth in experimental animals.[71] Schwann cells grown in culture from mice genetically engineered to lack *NF1* expression also demonstrate increased levels of activated p21-ras.[72] Accumulating evidence also suggests that neurofibromin expression is reduced in human neurofibromas, specifically in the Schwann cells and not the fibroblasts (J. Lynn Rutkowski and D. H. Gutmann, unpublished observations). In these tumors, there are mildly elevated levels of activated p21-ras.[73] A neurofibroma from a patient with a constitutional deletion of the entire *NF1* gene showed a 4 bp deletion in the second allele providing evidence for inactivation of both *NF1* alleles in this benign tumor.[74]

Neurofibromin expression is also reduced in tumors from individuals without NF1, suggesting that loss of neurofibromin is associated with the progression to malignancy in many different cell types. These tumors include malignant melanoma, neuroblastoma, and pheochromocytomas.[75–78] In these tumors, the association between neurofibromin loss and p21-ras activation is less clear. The lack of a correlation between *NF1* expression and p21-ras regulation suggests that neurofibromin might regulate cell growth through mechanisms unrelated to its ability to function as a GAP.[75,79] An additional observation relevant to this ras-independent function of neurofibromin comes from studies that examined the expression of neurofibromin in astrocytomas.[80] (77). Individuals with NF1 develop astrocytomas most commonly affecting the optic nerve and chiasm. Resting astrocytes, however, express little or no neurofibromin. In contrast, astrocytes activated *in vitro* or *in vivo* dramatically upregulate their expression of neurofibromin.[48,49] Similarly, there is a 3- to 10- fold increase in neurofibromin expression in astrocytomas of all WHO grades.[80,81] This increased expression of neurofibromin results from an activation of p21-ras, such that p21-ras in turn regulates *NF1* gene expression. This regulation of *NF1* gene expression may reflect a negative feedback loop between p21-ras and neurofibromin. Recent studies have dem-

Table 9–2. **Loss of *NF1* Gene Expression in Tumors**

| Patients with NF1 | Patients Without NF1 |
|---|---|
| Neurofibrosarcomas | Pheochromocytomas |
| Neurofibromas | Malignant melanomas |
| Pheochromocytomas | Neuroblastomas |
| Leukemias | |

onstrated that reduced *NF1* expression in *NF1* +/− heterozygous mice is associated with increased astrocyte proliferation *in vitro* and *in vivo.* In *NF1*+/− astrocytes, this increased cell proliferation is inhibited by blockade of the ras signaling pathway.[81a]

## The Relationship Between Neurofibromin and Clinical Features of NF1

In the case of NF1-related malignancies, it is clear that loss of neurofibromin expression is associated with the progression to tumor formation. Individuals with NF1, however, also develop learning disabilities, skeletal abnormalities, and vascular abnormalities—clinical features not obviously related to abnormal cell growth regulation. Recent work has demonstrated that neurofibromin is expressed in vascular smooth muscle cells (VSMCs) and endothelial cells.[82,83] Future work demonstrating that reduced *NF1* gene expression in VSMCs leads to vascular smooth muscle proliferation and luminal narrowing would advance our understanding of the pathophysiology underlying these NF1-associated abnormalities.

The role of neurofibromin in the maturation of central nervous system neurons has also attracted much attention. Neurons from mice genetically engineered to lack *NF1* gene expression are able to survive *in vitro* in the absence of neurotrophins (e.g., nerve growth factor), suggesting that neurofibromin might be important in the maturation of neurons.[84] (84a). Recently, a neuron-specific form of *NF1* mRNA that is developmentally regulated has been identified in the brain.[82] Further work on the role of neurofibromin in the brain and its contribution to learning in experimental mouse model systems will be required. Recently, *Nf1*$^{+/-}$ mice were shown to have deficits in specific learning tasks.[86] Little is known about the expression or function of neurofibromin in the developing skeleton.

## Genetic Testing

The *NF1* gene is a large gene spanning 60 exons and 300,000 nucleotides of genomic DNA. Mutational analysis of individuals with NF1 have failed to demonstrate common mutations. The mutations in NF1 are scattered throughout the entire gene without any "hot spots" (Fig. 9–3). In this fashion, altered *NF1* gene expression can result from large deletions or insertions, small deletions or insertions, chromosomal translocations, as well as missense and nonsense mutations. In several individuals with dysmorphic facial features, low intelligence, and NF1, large megabase deletions of the *NF1* gene have been reported.[87] Additionally, there is evidence for other genes that may modify the expression of the disease.[88]

Genetic testing for NF1 requires a combination of techniques ranging from linkage analysis in multigenerational families to fluorescent *in situ* hybridization (FISH) chromosomal analysis and and conventional mutation analysis. Recently, a protein truncation test (PTT) for NF1 has been developed.[89] In the PTT technique, *NF1* mRNA is amplified by the polymerase chain reaction in several different reactions to generate *NF1* fragments that represent the entire *NF1* coding sequence. This resulting mRNA is converted into protein *in vitro* and the protein fragments separated on polyacrylamide gels according to size. Any difference between the expected fragment size and the observed fragment size suggests that a mutation exists within that interval of the gene. It is essential that the mutation is confirmed by direct sequencing of that region. Despite the availability of these techniques, the diagnosis of NF1 is still made on clinical grounds. In such situations as prenatal diagnosis, the availability of such a test (e.g. PTT) may enable a couple to decide whether to terminate a pregnancy. Because the test cannot detect large deletions or some subtle missense mutations, however, it should be used cautiously.

Finally, the identification of a mutation in the *NF1* gene does not provide any prognostic information, because both severely and mildly affected individuals may have the identical DNA mutation. Moreover, because half of all cases of NF1 arise spontaneously without a prior family history, genetic testing is unlikely to detect all potential cases of NF1. Evaluation of individuals suspected of having NF1, based on

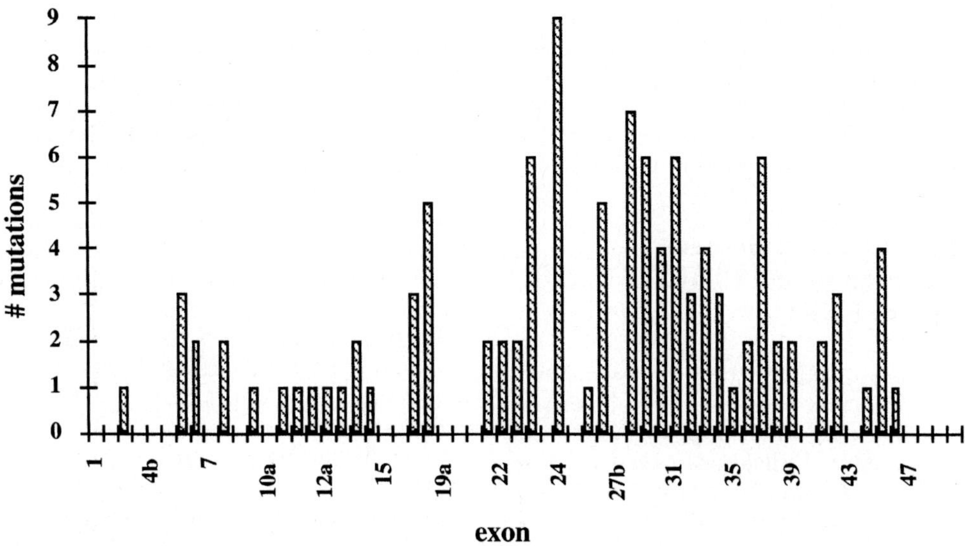


**Figure 9–3.** Graphic representation of NF1 gene mutations. This histogram plots the number of identified mutations in the *NF1* gene for each of the 60 NF1 exons. The larger number of mutations present in the C terminus of the gene reflects collection bias because genetic analysis of this region of the gene predated the availability of good DNA probes for the N-terminal end. Exons 24 to 34 have been studied more frequently than most other exons. These numbers also do not take into account large deletions or chromosomal translocations described for the *NF1* gene.

a positive family history, should include a careful physical examination with attention to the presence of CAL spots, freckling, and neurofibromas, as well as a detailed ophthalmological evaluation. Experience with DNA testing has demonstrated that it is a useful adjuvant to the clinical evaluation.[90]

## NEUROFIBROMATOSIS 2

Neurofibromatosis type 2 (NF2) is a rare autosomal dominant genetic disorder with an incidence of approximately 1:35,000 individuals and a prevalence of 0.9 per 100,000.[91] It is thus much rarer than NF1. NF2 is characterized by an increased predisposition to specific tumors of the nervous system. New mutations occur at a relatively high frequency and account for the 40% to 50% of cases with a negative family history. Although the disease has variable clinical expressivity, it is genetically homogeneous, caused by mutation of a single gene on human chromosome 22. The *NF2* gene has been identified and encodes a recessive tumor suppressor protein. Somatic mutations in the *NF2* gene are important in the pathogenesis of *sporadic* schwannomas, meningiomas, and ependymomas.

### Diagnostic Criteria and Clinical Features

The hallmark of NF2 is the occurrence of bilateral vestibular schwannomas (Fig. 9–4 *A*). When thin-section MRI is used, these tumors occur in more than 90% of patients with NF2, including patients in the pediatric age group.[92–94] Spinal tumors, usually schwannomas of the nerve roots, also occur in more than 90% of patients, although the majority of these tumors are asymptomatic (Fig. 9–4 *B*). Schwannomas of other cranial nerves, often in a bilateral distribution, occur as well. For example, Mautner and coworkers[93] found bilateral trigeminal schwannomas in 6 of 48 patients and unilateral trigeminal tumors in 8 of 48 patients. In the same study, multiple meningiomas were seen in 18 patients, and an additional 10 patients had a solitary meningioma. Most of the meningiomas were supratentorial. Ad-

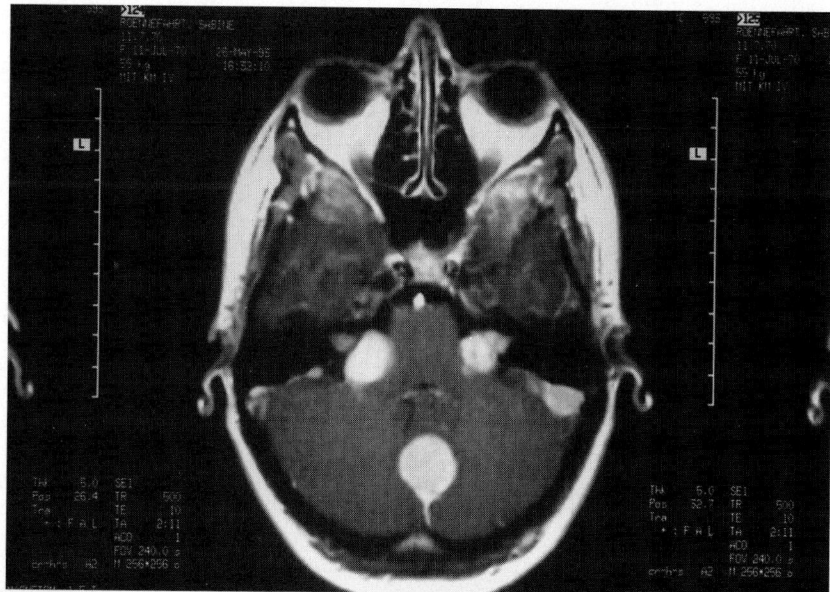


A

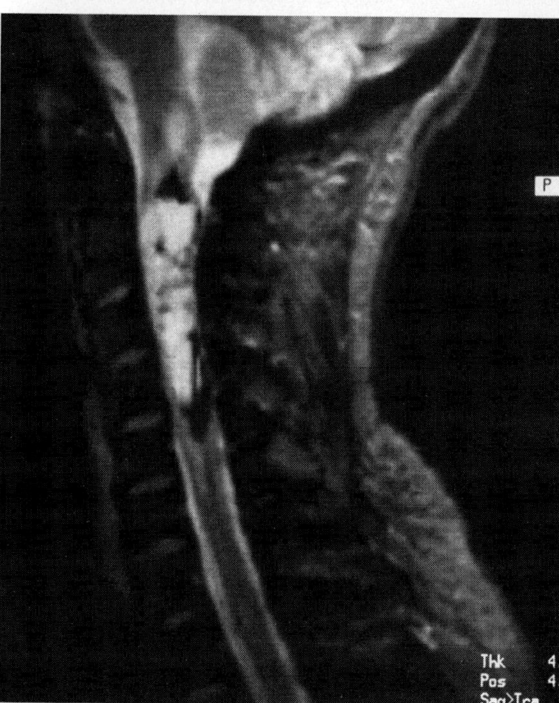


B

**Figure 9–4.** *(A)* Contrast-enhanced $T_1$-weighted (TR, 500 msec; TE, 10 msec) MRI of the posterior fossa in a 25-year-old woman with NF2. Bilateral vestibular schwannomas and a midline enhancing mass, presumably a meningioma, are shown. *(B)* Contrast-enhanced $T_1$-weighted MRI (TR, 500 msec; TE, 15 msec) of the cervical spine showing a histologically confirmed ependymoma extending from C1 to C4. The multinodular tumor has a syrinx at its cranial border.

ditionally, tumors such as brain stem and spinal cord gliomas and ependymomas and nerve root neurofibromas may also develop. Vestibular schwannomas and meningiomas occur at an earlier age than their sporadic counterparts. Skin tumors occur commonly and may be the presenting sign. Although CAL spots are found in about half of the patients, only 2% to 4% of patients have more than six CAL spot.[93–95]

A significant number of patients with NF2 have nontumor features. Cataracts occur in

60% to 80% of patients and retinal hamartomas in 8% to 22%.[93–99] In the study by Mautner and associates,[93] only 6% of patients were without ocular abnormalities. Detailed studies of the clinical and MRI features of NF2 in England, Germany, and the United States have been published.[93–95]

Based on the prevalence of these manifestation, a consensus panel convened by the U.S. NIH established diagnostic criteria for the diagnosis of NF2 (Table 9–3). Although these criteria may be highly specific and sensitive for familial cases, it is now clear that the requirement of bilateral vestibular schwannomas may lead to underdiagnosis of NF2 in patients with *de novo NF2* gene mutations. Therefore, several authors have suggested criteria for probable NF2 (Table 9–4). As in the other phakomatoses, penetrance is age dependent but virtually 100% by age 60 years, with the appropriate imaging techniques, asymptomatic gene carriers can be detected at a young age.[99]

## The NF2 Gene and Protein

Molecular genetic studies in sporadic and NF2-associated meningiomas and schwannomas originally suggested a common pathogenic mechanism for these tumors by the loss of heterozygosity for distinct chromosome 22 loci.[100] Using genetic linkage analysis in NF2 pedigrees, Rouleau and colleagues[101] in 1987 confirmed that the *NF2* locus resides also on chromosome 22 near the locus *D22S1*. The *NF2* gene was subsequently identified with classic positional cloning strategies. After refinement of the genetic location in several NF2 families and narrowing of the physical location with tumor samples, a cosmid contig spanning the region between the flanking markers was constructed. This region was screened for chromosome rearrangements by hybridization of single-copy probes to DNA of NF2 patients separated by pulse-field gel electrophoresis. Two probes detected abnormal fragment sizes in two unrelated NF2 patients. One of these was phylogenetically conserved, suggesting that a gene may be encoded within this DNA fragment. This clone was used to screen a human fetal DNA library, and a cDNA clone with sequence homology to other known genes was isolated. DNAs from NF2 patients contained several independent mutations in this gene.[102] The same gene was independently identified by another group.[103]

The *NF2* gene consists of at least 17 exons and spans approximately 100 kb of genomic sequence (Fig. 9–5). The cDNA sequence predicts a protein of 595 amino acids with an estimated molecular weight of 65 kDa. The NF2 protein, called *schwannomin* or *merlin*, belongs to a superfamily of proteins that includes band 4.1 protein in erythrocytes, talin, and the moesin-ezrin-radixin (MER) family and also shows homologies to the family of protein tyrosine phosphatases. This superfamily is thought to be involved in linking membrane proteins to the cytoskeleton. These proteins, except the protein tyrosine phosphatase family, have a common structural organization: a globular N-

Table 9–3. **Diagnostic Criteria for Neurofibromatosis 2**

NF2 may be diagnosed when one of the following is present:

1. Bilateral vestibular schwannomas seen by MRI with gadolinium
2. Family history of NF2 plus

   Unilateral vestibular schwannoma or any one of the following:

   - Meningioma
   - Neurofibroma
   - Glioma
   - Schwannoma
   - Posterior subcapsular lenticular opacities

Table 9–4. **Criteria for Probable NF2**

1. Unilateral vestibular schwannoma plus one or more of the following:
    - Neurofibroma
    - Meningioma
    - Glioma
    - Schwannoma of any cranial or peripheral nerve
    - Posterior subcapsular cataract or opacity at a young age
2. Multiple meningiomas (two or more) plus at least one of the following:
    - Neurofibroma
    - Glioma
    - Schwannoma
    - Posterior subcapsular cataract or opacity at a young age

terminal domain followed by a long α-helical structure and a charged C-terminal domain. Schwannomin interacts with several cellular proteins by coimmunoprecipitation[104] and forms a homodimer.[105] Using the yeast-2-hybrid system, Scoles and associates[106] recently confirmed self-interaction of schwannomin and showed, in addition, that schwannomin interacts with βII-spectrin at its C-terminus. Schwannomin also interacts with the regulatory cofactor of the $Na^+$-$H^+$ exchanger (NHE-RF).[107]

By *in situ* hybridization and immunocytochemical analysis, the *NF2* gene is widely expressed. Schwannomin is localized in the cytoplasm of neuronal cells and tissues of neuroectodermal origin, including motor and sensory neurons and Schwann cells.[108,109,109a] Expression is found in embryonic and adult tissues.[109,110]

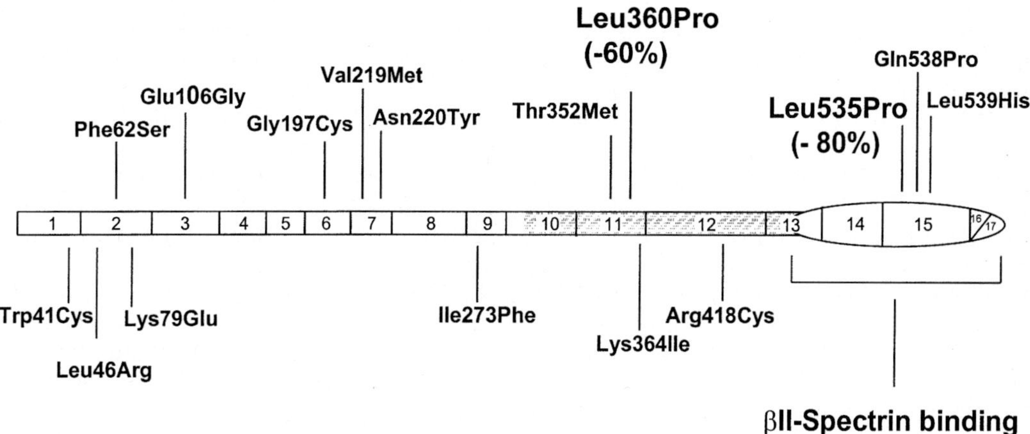


**Figure 9–5.** Structure of schwannomin, the *NF2* gene product, and location of missense mutations. The numbered boxes indicate the locations of exons. Although most NF2 mutations result in truncated schwannomins, occasional missense mutations are observed and may be related to milder phenotypes. Missense mutations occurring in the germline are indicated above the protein, somatic mutations below. The values in parentheses under two missense mutations indicate the reduction of βII-spectrin binding. (From Scoles et al.[106])

## Germline Mutational Analysis and Phenotypes

At least in some pedigrees the course of NF2 may be relatively uniform, leading to the distinction of a mild Gardner and a severe Wishart phenotype.[111] On the other hand, pedigrees with significant intrafamilial heterogeneity have been reported as well.[99] As described later, the NF2 phenotype is only in small part determined by the specific *NF2* mutation, but modifying alleles and stochastic factors may play a role.

Analysis of germline mutations in the NF2 coding region detects only 30% to 50% of mutations.[112,113] Most mutations consist of small deletions or insertions and are predicted to result in truncated schwannomins. Splice site mutations and missense mutations also occur (see Fig 9–5). Except for an increased mutation rate in CpG dinucleotides and mutations resulting in skipping of exons 2 or 4, recurrent mutations are rare.[112,114] Because genetic linkage studies of NF2 pedigrees have indicated that *NF2* is genetically homogeneous (no evidence of linkage to other loci), the unaccounted mutations likely occur within the promoter or other regulatory sequences or represent large deletions that are not detected by polymerase chain reaction screening methods.

Germline mutation analyses performed to correlate genotype to phenotype have not been conclusive, and it is not clear if mutant schwannomins are stable and partially functional.[112,115] Although the degree of truncation of mutated schwannomins may not correlate with the severity of the phenotype, some studies have suggested that mild manifestations of NF2 may be associated with missense or splice-site mutations. In one pedigree segregating an NF2 missense mutation, however, gene carriers had both mild and severe phenotypes.[114,114a,116,116a,116b]

In general, phenotypes vary widely within families. For example, in one pedigree in which the proband had severe early onset NF2, two middle-aged adults who carried the same mutation had normal cranial and spinal MRIs and normal eye examinations.[99] In the same study a pedigree with a severely affected adolescent is described whose mother, aged 48 years, had only bilateral cataracts since adolescence. Variable phenotypes associated with the same mutation may also be due to somatic mosaicism.[116] In some families, however, mild phenotypes may cluster, pointing to the influence of other alleles on the phenotype.[111]

Studies of monozygotic twins provide the opportunity to dissect the relative contribution of *NF2* mutations and modifying genes on the one hand and stochastic and environmental factors on the other hand. Baser and coworkers[117] performed a detailed clinical study of three pairs of monozygotic twins with NF2. Although concordant for age of onset and general severity of symptoms, the pairs were discordant for most specific clinical manifestations such as number and type of tumors or ocular findings. This study emphasized the importance of environmental and stochastic mechanisms in determining the NF2 phenotype.

## Schwannomin as a Recessive Tumor Suppressor Protein

The mechanisms of recessively acting tumor suppressor genes are discussed in Chapters 1 and 8. Loss of heterozygosity of chromosome 22 alleles in schwannomas and meningiomas had strongly suggested that schwannomin was a tumor suppressor protein.[100,118] Indeed, inactivation of both *NF2* alleles was demonstrated in most schwannomas and about 50% of meningiomas.[108,119–122,122a] Frequently, a mutation was detected in one *NF2* allele, and the second allele was lost. In some tumors that had retained heterozygosity, mutations were detected in both *NF2* alleles. Immunoreactivity for schwannomin was absent in most schwannomas, indicating that tumor cells contained little or no functional schwannomin.[108,117,122a] Somatic *NF2* mutations are further discussed in the chapter on brain tumors.

A tumor suppressor role for schwannomin is consistent with cellular phenotypes observed when schwannomin is overexpressed or underexpressed in cell lines.[123,124,124a,124b] Transfection of the full-length cDNA in NIH3T3 fibroblasts results in phenotypic changes such as extension of varying numbers of thin processes, and the growth rate decreases to one-third of normal. Similarly, transfection of the full-length NF2 cDNA into *v-Ha-ras*–transformed NIH3T3 cells has been shown to reverse the Ras-induced anchorage-independent growth of these cells in soft agar.[123] In an alternative strategy, Huynh and Pulst[124] reduced schwannomin expression by treating Schwann-like STS26T cells with antisense oligonucleotides. Treated cells showed morphological changes, loss of attachment to the substratum, and increased proliferation.

## Genetic Testing and Presymptomatic Diagnosis

Because no mutational hot spots (except for CpG dinucleotides)[114] have been identified in the *NF2* gene, direct testing for *NF2* mutations in a symptomatic individual to confirm the diagnosis or in an individual at risk is currently advisable only for selected cases. Even then, as discussed earlier, at least 50% of mutations are not detected when the coding region is examined by amplification of individual exons (see later). When a strategy is used that can detect large deletions involving several exons, however, the detection rate increases to around 80%.[125]

When DNAs from at least two clinically affected individuals are available, the abundance of microsatellite markers closely flanking the *NF2* gene will allow diagnosis by segregation analysis with a high degree of accuracy in most cases.[99,111,122] Bijlsma and colleagues,[127] however, pointed to the problems with linkage-based predictive testing in a family in which the proband's mother had NF2 but was a mosaic for an *NF2* mutation.

Most adult asymptomatic gene carriers are found to show signs of NF2 when the proper imaging studies and ocular examinations are initiated. Baser and associates,[99] however, identified two individuals, aged 26 and 38 years, from a pedigree with severe early onset NF2 who were asymptomatic and had normal MRIs of the entire neuraxis and normal ocular examinations. In a pedigree with a mild NF2 phenotype, Sainio and colleagues[111] identified three asymptomatic adult *NF2* gene carriers, aged 29 to 41 years, who had normal cranial and spinal MRIs.

## Variant Phenotypes

### SCHWANNOMATOSIS

A disease presenting with Schwann cell tumors that include multiple cutaneous and spinal neurilemmomas has been described in the Japanese literature as neurilemmomatosis,[128] and also in Caucasians.[129] It was thought to be distinct from NF2 because of the absence of other NF2 features. Germline *NF2* mutations, however, have been identified in some of these patients. Kluwe and coworkers[130] described a 47-year-old patient with schwannomatosis. Several first-degree relatives were asymptomatic. Mutational analysis of the proband revealed a 163 bp deletion in the *NF2* gene. The same mutation was present in three other offspring, two of whom had bilateral vestibular schwannomas. It is rare for patients with spinal schwannomatosis to have offspring with the same phenotype. One pedigree with multiple spinal tumors in two generations without the development of vestibular schwannomas or cataracts, however, has been described. The mutation in this pedigree was excluded from the *NF1* locus and likely linked to the *NF2* locus (S. M. Pulst et al., unpublished data).[131]

The finding of multiple spinal tumors in a patient poses several problems with regard to classification and genetic counseling because these patients may harbor germline mutations in the *NF1* or *NF2* genes or germline mutations in other as yet unidentified genes.[132,133] Alternatively, these patients may be mosaics or harbor somatic mutations.[129] When patients with schwannomatosis are counseled for recurrence risk, consideration needs to be given to the presence of an *NF2* germline mutation due to the potentially grave implications of such a diagnosis. Whenever possible, the proband *and* first-degree relatives should be evaluated with a complete physical examination, including skin and ocular examinations and complete neuraxis MRIs.

### MULTIPLE MENINGIOMATOSIS

Many patients presenting with familial meningioma or multiple meningiomas will have NF2 when properly examined (see Table 9–4). For example, Delleman and associates[134] reported a family with four members in two generations who had meningiomas. Other signs of NF2 were missing. A fifth member of the pedigree, however, had multiple meningiomas and vestibular schwannomas. On the other hand, dominantly inherited meningioma without other evidence of NF2 does occur.[135,136] In one pedigree with meningiomas and ependymomas located above and below the foramen magnum, linkage to the *NF2* region was excluded. This established that germline mutations in a gene other than the *NF2* gene may give rise to familial meningioma.[136] These patients did not have the ocular findings typical for NF2.

## Work-Up of Symptomatic and Asymptomatic Patients

### THE SYMPTOMATIC PATIENT

The work-up and treatment of symptomatic NF2 patients is dictated by symptoms and tumor location, but should always include gadolinium-enhanced MRI of the brain with thin sections through the posterior fossa and slit-lamp and fundus examinations for the presence of cataracts and hamartomas. A detailed MRI protocol is described by Mautner and coworkers.[93] An MRI of the spine may also be performed even in the absence of symptoms, but should definitely be undertaken before posterior fossa surgery.

In contrast to sporadic unilateral vestibular schwannoma, there is currently no clear consensus about timing of operations and surgical approach to the tumors in the presence of bilateral schwannomas.[136a,137,138] One extreme position is to delay the operation until the tumor has destroyed hearing or caused other neurologic signs and then approach the tumor, sacrificing the eighth nerve, thus giving the patient the longest possible time of hearing. At the other extreme, one can operate as early as possible with the attendant risk of deterioration or loss of hearing. Factors that may influence the decision are age of the patient, level of hearing in the ear to be operated on, size of the tumor, and growth rate of the tumor. Other important factors are the level of hearing in the contralateral ear and the size of the contralateral tumor.

### THE ASYMPTOMATIC PATIENT

It is not known how frequently asymptomatic NF2 patients should be screened. Tumors of the eighth nerve in NF2 may have rapid and unexpected growth patterns, but may also enter long periods of seeming dormancy (F. V. Mautner and S. M. Pulst, unpublished data). We currently recommend MRI of the brain every 1 to 2 years, accompanied by a careful physical examination. There is not sufficient information to determine whether asymptomatic small vestibular schwannomas should be removed or carefully observed. In three tumors that were asymptomatic preoperatively, hearing was lost after the operation.[138] Our personal experience and that of others[136a] support the NIH consensus[137] of watchful waiting if there is hearing remaining in the affected ear.

### THE ASYMPTOMATIC AT-RISK INDIVIDUAL

As described earlier, molecular testing may be a highly accurate and cost-efficient approach when the *NF2* mutation segregating in the family is known or when analysis by linked genetic markers is possible. Very often, however, this approach is not possible and the individual will need clinical examination. A typical problem may be that of an asymptomatic adolescent with a parent with NF2 whose mutation is unknown. Initially, a careful physical examination is warranted because more than half of NF2 patients have skin tumors. This should be followed by contrast-enhanced cranial MRI and ocular examinations. When these do not show changes, contrast-enhanced spinal MRI should be undertaken. If all these examinations are negative, the risk that the individual is a carrier of an *NF2* mutation is considerably decreased, but certainly not reduced to 0 because middle-aged gene carriers with negative ocular and imaging studies have been described.[99,111]

## Animal Models

In mice, the NF2 homologue encodes a 596 amino acid protein of 65 kDa that is 98% identical to human schwannomin.[110,139] Due to the high conservation of the gene, insights on schwannomin function may be derived from studies in mice. The *NF2* gene is widely expressed in adult and embryonic rodents. Several strains of mice heterozygous and homozygous for inactivating mutations in the *NF2* gene have been created. *Nf2*$^{-/-}$ mice are embryonic lethals due to the absence of extraembryonic ectoderm.[140] Mice heterozygous for a mutation at the *Nf2* locus are viable, however, but develop a range of highly metastatic tumors.[141] Two tumor types, osteosarcoma and hepatocellular carcinoma, were observed more commonly than in wild-type animals. In these tumors, loss of the second *NF2* allele indicated that loss of *NF2* function was causal in tumor development.

# TUBEROUS SCLEROSIS

## Clinical Features

Tuberous sclerosis (TS) is an autosomal dominant disorder with an estimated frequency of 1 in 30,000.[142] This figure, however, likely underestimates the true frequency of TS, which may be age dependent (e.g., 1 in 7500 for children under 5 years of age). Affected individuals manifest mental retardation, seizures, hamartomous growths and tumors (Table 9–5).[143,143a] The diagnostic criteria for TS are undergoing a redefinition based on new information derived from molecular genetic studies.[144] No single sign is present in all affected patients. Some clinical signs once regarded as pathognomonic for TS complex are now known to be less specific. Family history was removed as a diagnostic criterion, a decision that certainly merits further study.

Several skin manifestations are characteristic of TS. These include adenoma sebaceum, more than three hypopigmented macules (Shagreen patches and ash leaf macules), and fibromas under the tongue and fingernails. Adenoma sebaceum presents as dome-shaped papules symmetrically distributed on the nasolabial folds, cheeks, and chin. It typically develops after 4 years of age, ultimately affecting most individuals with TS. Shagreen patches appear as flesh-colored wrinkled lesions that resemble pigskin. Hypopigmented lesions are one of the earliest signs of TS. They may vary in shape (''mountain ash leaf'' lesion) and are best appreciated with a Wood's lamp. Histologically, these lesions contain normal numbers of melanocytes, but the melanosomes are small and partially or totally deficient in melanin. Subungual fibromas are most commonly seen after puberty.

Central nervous system manifestations of TS include seizures, mental retardation, and cerebral calcifications. Seizures occur in 70% of affected individuals, and mental retardation affects 60%. Multiple tumor-like nodules are seen in subependymal regions, often projecting into the ventricles. Radiographically, these lesions appear as ''candle guttering.'' In the same regions, individuals with TS can develop an uncommon glioma, the subependymal giant cell astrocytoma. Cerebral calcifications are also common, affecting 50% to 60% of all individuals with TS. Other tumors seen in association with TS include renal angiomyolipomas, cardiac rhabdomyosarcomas, and hamartomas of any organ. Angiomyolipomas are often multiple or bilateral, whereas rhabdomyosarcomas can present as single or multiple lesions.

## Identification of the *TSC* Genes

Analyses of families with TS have demonstrated the existence of two distinct genetic loci, one on chromosome 9 and the other on chromosome 16.[145] There are no major differences in the clinical features of individuals from families with chromosome 9– versus chromosome 16–linked TS. The gene for TS on chromosome 9 is termed *TSC1* (tuberous sclerosis complex 1) and the chromosome 16–linked TS gene, *TSC2*. The *TSC2* gene was identified in 1993[146] and the *TSC1* gene in 1997.[147]

Table 9–5. **Revised Diagnostic Criteria for Tuberous Sclerosis Complex**

*Major Features*
Facial angiofibromas or forehead plaque
Nontraumatic ungual or periungual fibromas
Cortical tuber
Subependymal nodule
Subependymal giant cell astrocytoma
Multiple retinal nodular hamartomas
Shagreen patch
Hypomelanotic macules (three or more)
Cardiac rhabdomyoma, single or multiple
Lymphangiomyomatosis
Renal angiomyolipoma

*Minor Features*
Multiple, randomly distributed enamel pits in dental enamel
Harmartomatous rectal polyps
Bone cysts
Cerebral white matter radial migration lines
Gingival fibromas
Nonrenal hamartoma
Retinal achromic patch
'Confetti' skin lesions
Multiple renal cysts

*Definite TS*
Either two major features or one major plus two minor features

*Probable TSC*
One major plus one minor feature

*Possible TSC*
Either one major or two or more minor features

**Source:** Roach et al.[143a]

The *TSC1* gene is located on chromosome 9q34 and encodes a 8.6 kb transcript. It is widely expressed and encodes a 130 kDa protein designated *hamartin.*[147] The majority of mutations were truncating. In one renal cell carcinoma from a TS patient, mutations in both alleles were identified, confirming a recessive tumor suppressor role for *TSC1*. *TSC1* has homologies with a yeast gene of unknown function, and hamartin appears to be located in cytoplasmic vesicles.[148] Mental retardation appears to be less common in patients with *TSC1* mutations.[149]

Hamartin has been recently identified and found to physically associate with tuberin.[149a,149b] Although no function has been ascribed to hamartin, it may form a functional complex with tuberin to modulate intracellular signaling pathways related to cell proliferation.

The *TSC2* gene is composed of 41 exons transcribed as a 5500 nucleotide mRNA present at some level in most mammalian tissues.[146,150,151] Proof that the *TSC2* gene was the gene responsible for TS in chromosome 16–linked families required the identification of mutations in the *TSC2* gene.[146,152,153] Many such mutations have been identified to date without evidence for common mutations or clustering of mutations within particular regions of the gene. Furthermore, loss of heterozygosity has been reported in the benign hamartomas associated with TS, supporting the idea that the *TSC2* gene is a tumor suppressor gene.[154]

The *TSC2* gene encodes a 1784 amino acid protein, termed *tuberin.* In addition to several membrane-spanning regions of the protein, a small 58 amino acid region in the C terminus of tuberin shares striking sequence with a family of proteins that regulate p21-rap1 (Fig. 9–6).[155,156] Rap1 is another small GTPase protein, like p21-ras, that is active in its GTP-bound conformation and inactive when bound to GDP. Tuberin is therefore predicted to function as a GAP protein for rap1. Subsequent biochemical studies have demonstrated that tuberin indeed catalyzes the conversion of rap1 from an active GTP-bound form to an inactive GDP-bound form *in vitro.*[157] In this regard, tuberin is specific for rap1 without any significant GAP activity toward other related ras-like proteins. Recently, Gutmann and associates[158,158a] found increased rap1 expression or reduced tuberin expression in approximately 60% of sporadic gliomas.

As with neurofibromin, it is unclear what the rest of the tuberin protein does. Recent evidence suggests that the carboxyl terminus of tuberin (not containing the rap 1GAP region) may activate DNA transcription by localizing to the nucleus.[159] Further studies are required to demonstrate whether tuberin functions to regulate DNA transcription *in vivo.* In addition, recent studies have demonstrated that expression of tuberin or of its catalytically active C-terminal fragment can inhibit cell growth, anchorage-independent growth, and tumor formation in nude mice.[160] In addition to rap1 regulation, there are data to support a role for tuberin in regulating endocytosis by modulating rab5 activity, transcription, and cell cycle progression.[160a–c]

The *TSC2* gene is highly expressed in brain tissues in adult rats and mice, whereas it is expressed in many tissues during development.[161–163] *TSC2* gene expression is observed in the adult cerebellum, hippocampus, and olfactory bulb. During embryonic development, there is abundant expression in the spinal cord that becomes restricted to anterior motor neurons in the adult. Its high level of expression in the brain may reflect the frequency of mental retardation and seizures in this patient population. Similar studies on the protein level have demonstrated high levels of tuberin expression in the developing and adult rodent brain.[164]

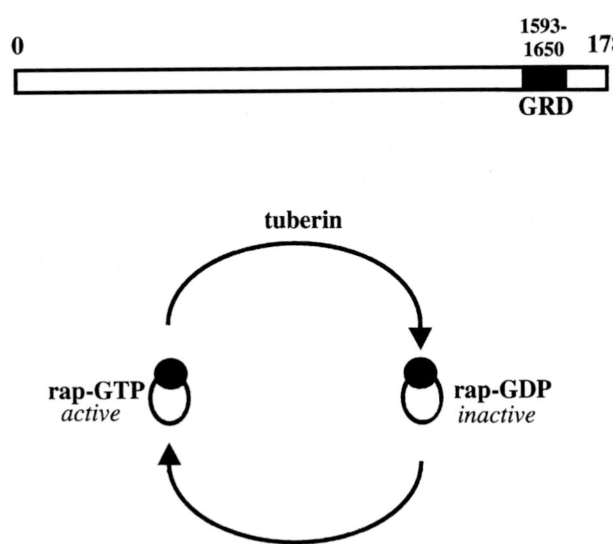


**Figure 9–6.** Schematic representation of the *TSC2* gene product, tuberin. Tuberin is a 1784 amino acid protein with a small C-terminal portion with sequence and functional similarity to a family of proteins that regulate rap proteins, termed GTPase-activating proteins (GAPs). This rap1GAP-related domain is located between residues 1593 and 1650. GAP molecules interact with GTP-bound p21-rap1 (activated p21-rap1) and accelerate its conversion to its inactive GDP-bound form. GDP-bound p21-rap1 is then reactivated by guanosine nucleotide replacing factors (GNRFs).

## Animal Models

A spontaneously occurring rat model of TS, the Eker rat strain, has been identified.[165] These rats develop bilateral renal carcinomas and, less frequently, tumors of the uterus and spleen. Genetic studies on the Eker rat strain have demonstrated that the rat *Tsc2* gene homologue harbors an insertional mutation in intron 30 that would be predicted to render tuberin nonfunctional. No tuberin has been found in the tumors from these rats. Eker rats with both copies of the rat *Tsc2* containing this inactivating mutation die *in utero*, as previously reported for the genetically engineered *Nf1* mutant mice. Future work aimed at characterizing the functional properties of tuberin and its role in cell differentiation and tumor formation will likely expand our understanding of this important tumor suppressor gene.

## Genetic Testing

Diagnostic DNA testing will be difficult due to the genetic (nonallelic) heterogeneity with at least two known genes and the large size of the genes.[166] For the near future, diagnostic testing will likely remain restricted to research laboratories. The possibility of somatic and germline mosaicism needs to be considered in genetic counseling.[167]

# VON HIPPEL-LINDAU DISEASE

von Hippel-Lindau disease is an autosomal dominant genetic disorder with variable expression and age-dependent penetrance. Its prevalence is estimated at approximately 1 in 40,000. Estimates for the frequency of new mutations vary greatly from 6% to 50% of all cases.[168,169] The combination of retinal angiomata (angiomatosis retinae) and cerebellar hemangioblastoma represents the classic manifestation of VHL syndrome. The *VHL* gene has been identified and encodes a recessively acting transcription factor. Somatic mutations in the *VHL* gene are important in the pathogenesis of *sporadic* hemangioblastomas.

## Diagnostic Criteria and Clinical Features

The hallmark of VHL are retinal angiomas and hemangioblastomas of the posterior fossa and spinal cord. Renal lesions, however, are as frequent as hemangiomas of the eye.[170] Other organ systems such as the pancreas, the adrenal gland and paraganglia, and the epididymis are frequently involved as well. Typical manifestations of the disease in these organs range from cysts (kidney, pancreas, epididymis) to histologically benign tumors (pheochromocytoma, pancreatic cystadenoma) to malignant clear cell renal carcinoma.[171] Retinal lesions are usually the first signs, with a mean age of diagnosis of 25 years.[172]

In contrast to NF2, in which schwannomas of cranial or spinal nerves are present in more than 90% of patients, the incidence of capillary hemangioblastomas of the central nervous system in VHL shows strong interfamilial variability and ranges from 21% to 72% (see later).[168] The cerebellum is the most common site for these tumors, followed by the brain stem and the spinal cord. Capillary hemangioblastomas in VHL patients tend to manifest in younger patients than do sporadic capillary hemangioblastomas and are more often multifocal.[173] Most investigators use the criteria developed by Melmon and Rosen[174] for diagnosis (Table 9–6). About 50% of VHL patients have only one manifestation of the disease. Renal and epididymal cysts are too common in the general population to be reliable markers of the disease by themselves.

Nonexpression of the VHL phenotype in obligate gene carriers older than 60 years of age is rare. Davies and colleagues[175] describe a 65-year-old woman who did not show any sings of VHL even after extensive screening. Unfortunately, an MRI of the spine was not performed.

## The VHL Gene and Protein

Linkage studies in VHL families have revealed that the von Hippel-Lindau gene (*VHL*) is located at 3p25–p26.[176] *VHL* was

Table 9–6. **Diagnostic Criteria for VHL Disease**

VHL may be diagnosed if two of the findings in column A are present or one from column A and one from column B are present. With a family history of VHL, one finding from either column is sufficient.

| Column A | Column B |
|---|---|
| Retinal angioma | Pheochromocytoma |
| Cerebellar hemangioma | Pancreatic cyst |
| Spinal hemangioma | Epididymal cyst |
| | Renal cyst |
| | Renal cancer |

**Source:** Melmon and Rosen.[174]

positionally cloned in 1993.[177] There are two transcription start sites encoding proteins of 18 and 24 kDa.[178] The *VHL* gene shows expression in many tissues, including the brain and kidney. Southern blot analysis for deletions detected abnormalities in 28 of 221 unrelated VHL patients. Although initial sequence comparison of the VHL protein (pVHL) with other known proteins provided no clues regarding its function, subsequent studies showed that pVHL is a nuclear protein, binds to elongins B and C, and inhibits transcriptional activity.[179,180] Recently, it was shown that pVHL may regulate the accumulation of hypoxia-inducible mRNAs.[181]

## Germline Mutational Analysis and Phenotypes

Many different mutations cause VHL, and mutations are scattered throughout the gene. About half of the mutations are predicted to result in a truncated gene product. Using genomic polymerase chain reaction (PCR) and single-stranded-conformation polymorphism (SSCP) analyses, Whaley and associates[182] detected variant conformers in 22 of 61 samples. Mutations were detected in all three exons and included deletions, insertions, and splice site mutations, as well as missense and nonsense mutations. Point mutations constituted a significant percentage of the mutations; 45% were missense mutations. Recurring mutations were seen in codons 136, 147, 169, 229, and 238 (amino acid numbers according to Latif and colleagues[177]). Chen and coworkers[183] identified germline mutations in 85 of 114 (75%) families with VHL. Mutations were found in all three exons. Codon 238 was identified as a mutational hotspot, resulting in Arg to Trp or Arg to Gln substitutions in 8% of families.

The types of mutations responsible for VHL without pheochromocytoma (VHL type 1) differed from those responsible for VHL with pheochromocytoma (VHL type 2); 56% of the mutations responsible for VHL type 1 were microdeletions/insertions, nonsense mutations, or deletions; 96% of the mutations responsible for VHL type 2 were missense mutations. Specific mutations in codon 238 accounted for 43% of the mutations responsible for VHL type 2. Members of a large family with a T505C substitution had pheochromocytomas, angiomas, and hemangioblastomas, but lacked renal cell carcinomas or pancreatic cysts.[184] A 709 G to T transversion was seen in a three-generation family with pheochromocytomas. In one individual, who also had a chemodectoma, a cerebellar hemangioblastoma was discovered 25 years after the pheochromocytoma.[185] In a series of 68 patients with apparently sporadic pheochromocytomas, six carried germline mutations in the *VHL* gene.[186]

Estimates of *de novo* mutations have varied from a low of $0.18 \times 10^{-6}$ gametes per generation to a high of $4.4 \times 10^{-6}$.[169] The higher rate of new mutations is supported by the fact that few identical mutations are found on chromosomes with identical haplotypes. Software and a database for the analysis of VHL mutations have been created.[187]

## Mutations in the *VHL* Gene in Sporadic Hemangioblastomas

Although a frequent manifestation of VHL syndrome, most capillary hemangioblastomas are solitary sporadic lesions that grow in patients without further stigmata of VHL disease or a family history.[168] However, hemangioblastomas occurring at a young age should initiate a work-up for VHL. Both sporadic and hereditary capillary hemangioblastomas are slowly growing, benign neoplasms that are histologically graded as WHO grade I. Despite their benign nature, capillary hemangioblastomas of the cerebellum and brain stem are associated with a considerable mortality rate, and many patients require emergency treatment.[168] In addition, capillary hemangioblastomas not infrequently recur after operation with a reported mean rate of recurrence around 16%.[188] Recent studies have shown that sporadic hemangioblastomas commonly demonstrate somatic mutations of the VHL gene.[189,190] Lee and coworkers[191] identified mutations in selectively procured stromal (as opposed to vascular) cells, providing evidence that this cell type is a neoplastic component of hemangioblastoma.

## Presymptomatic Molecular Diagnosis

Similar to the other phakomatoses, direct molecular analysis is difficult due to the fact that different mutation types cause VHL disease. The relatively small size of the cDNA, however, makes direct testing feasible in selected cases.

Indirect genetic testing using linked molecular markers is possible in pedigrees with at least two affected individuals. Glenn and associates[192] examined 48 asymptomatic individuals at risk of developing VHL. DNA polymorphism analysis predicted nine carriers of a mutant VHL allele and 33 individuals with the wild-type (normal) allele. All nine individuals predicted to carry the disease allele had evidence of occult disease on clinical examination. There was no clinical evidence of disease in individuals predicted to carry the wild-type allele. This was also recently confirmed in a family segregating a codon 238 missense mutation with the identification of a premalignant renal cyst in an asymptomatic gene carrier.[193] Due to the expense and time of screening studies, molecular diagnosis is cost-effective.

## Work-Up of Symptomatic and Asymptomatic Patients

Screening of at-risk individuals and known *VHL* gene carriers is even more involved than the screening undertaken in NF2. The screening recommendations of three groups treating a large number of VHL patients was recently reviewed.[172] The screening methods include imaging studies, blood chemistries, and ophthalmological examinations. Although there are differences in the use of specific tests, all protocols share screening throughout life, beginning in infancy.

Urinary catecholamine levels should be checked every 1 to 2 years, beginning in infancy. Ophthalmoscopy is recommended yearly beginning at age 5 to 6 years, with fluorescein angiography recommended by some. Enhanced MRI scans of brain and spine should be undertaken every 2 to 3 years, beginning in adolescence. Screening for renal lesions should begin in adolescence. The use of ultrasonography versus the more sensitive abdominal CT is still debated, but, at the minimum, abdominal ultrasonography should be performed every year and abdominal CT scanning every other year. It is likely that MRIs of the kidneys will play an increasing role in the future.

## SUMMARY

The genes for the four major phakomatoses have been identified by positional cloning, and major advances have been made in understanding the function of the gene products. For some of the diseases, genotype–

phenotype correlations have been established, whereas for others the type of mutation seems only to exert a minor influence on the phenotype, which appears to be more dependent on stochastic events and other genetic modifying alleles. Mouse models generated by homologous recombination may recapitulate some, but not all, of the features of the human disease. Follow-up studies of known gene carriers as well as screening methods for asymptomatic first-degree relatives differ for the four diseases. Molecular genetic testing can aid in identifying presymptomatic gene carriers.

## REFERENCES


1. Riccardi VM: Neurofibromatosis: Past, present and future. N Engl J Med 324:1283–1285, 1991.
2. Huson SM, Harper PS, Compston DA: von Recklinghausen neurofibromatosis: A clinical and population study in South East Wales. Brain 111:1355–1381, 1988.
3. Noonan JA: Hypertelorism with Turner phenotype: A new syndrome with associated congenital heart disease. Am J Dis Child. 116:373–380, 1968.
4. Tanner JM, Lejarraga H, Cameron N: The natural history of the Silver-Russell syndrome: A longitudinal study of thirty-nine cases. Pediatr Res 9:611–623, 1975.
5. Albright F, Butler AM, Hampton AO, Smith P: Syndrome characterized by osteitis fibrosa disseminata, areas of pigmentation and endocrine dysfunction, with precocious puberty in 'females. N Engl J Med 17:727–746, 1937.
6. Lubs M-LE, Bauer MS, Formas ME, Djokic B: Lisch nodules in neurofibromatosis type 1. N Engl J of Med 324:1264–1266, 1991.
7. Disimone RE, Berman AT, Schwentker EP: The orthopedic manifestation of neurofibromatosis. Clin Orthop Rel Res 230:277–283, 1988.
8. Brown GA, Osebold WR, Ponseti IV: Congenital pseudarthrosis of long bones. Clin Orthop and Rel Res 128:228–242, 1977.
9. Stine SB, Adams WV: Learning problems in neurofibromatosis patients. Clin Orthop Rel Res 245: 43–50, 1989.
10. Hofman KJ, Harris EL, Bryan N, Denckla MB: Neurofibromatosis type 1: the cognitive phenotype. J Pediatr 124:S1–S8, 1994.

10a. North KK, Riccardi V, Samango-Sprouse C, Ferner R, Moore B, Legius E, Ratner N, Denckla MB: Cognitive function and academic performance in neurofibromatosis 1: Consensus statement from the NF1 Cognitive Disorders Task Force. Neurology 48:1121–1127, 1997.

11. Chapman CA, Waber DP, Bassett N, Urion DK, Korf BR: Neurobehavioral profiles of children with neurofibromatosis 1 referred for learning disabilities are sex-specific. Am J Med Genet 67:127–132, 1996.
12. Duffner PK, Cohen ME, Seidel FG, Shucard DW: The significance of MRI abnormalities in children with neurofibromatosis. Neurology 39:373–378, 1989.
13. Menor F, Marti-Bonmati L, Arana E, Poyatos C, Cortina H: Neurofibromatosis type 1 in children: MR imaging and follow-up studies of central nervous system findings. Eur J Radiol 26:121–131, 1998.
14. Moore BD, Slopis JM, Schomer D, Jackson EF, Levy BM: Neuropsychological significance of areas of high signal intensity on brain MRIs of children with neurofibromatosis. Neurology 46:1660–1668, 1996.
15. North K, Joy P, Yuille D, et al.: Specific learning disability in children with neurofibromatosis type 1: Significance of MRI abnormalities. Neurology 44:878–883, 1994.
16. DiPaolo DP, Zimmerman RA, Rorke LB, Zackai EH, Bilaniuk LT, Yachnis AT: Neurofibromatosis type 1: Pathologic substrate of high signal intensity foci in the brain. Radiology 195:721–724, 1995.
17. Rizvi TA, Akunuru S, de Courten-Myers G, et al.: Region-specific astrogliosis in brains of mice heterozygous for mutations in the neurofibromatosis type 1 (Nfl) tumor suppressor. Brain Res 16:111–123, 1999.
18. Greene JF, Fitzwater JE, Burgess J: Arterial lesions associated with neurofibromatosis. Am J Clin Pathol 62:481–487, 1974.
19. Halpern M, Currarino G: Vascular lesions causing hypertension in neurofibromatosis. N Engl J Med 273:248–252, 1965.
20. Rizzo JF, Lessell S: Cerebrovascular abnormalities in neurofibromatosis type 1. Neurology 44:1000–1002, 1994.
21. Bader JL: Neurofibromatosis and cancer. Ann NY Acad Sci 486:57–65, 1986.
22. Gutmann DH, Alsworth A, Carey JC, et al.: The diagnostic evaluation and multidisciplinary management of neurofibromatosis 1 and neurofibromatosis 2. JAMA 278:51–57, 1997.
23. Duffner PK, Cohen ME: Isolated optic nerve gliomas in children with and without neurofibromatosis. Neurofibromatosis 1:201–211, 1988.
24. Listernick R, Darling C, Greenwald M, Strauss L, Charrow J: Optic pathway tumors in children: The effect of neurofibromatosis type 1 on clinical manifestations and natural history. J Pediatr 127:718–722, 1995.
25. Listernick R, Louis DN, Packer RJ, Gutmann DH: Optic pathway gliomas in children with neurofibromatosis 1: Consensus statement from the optic pathway glioma task force. Ann Neurol 41:143–149, 1997.
26. Arnsmeier SL, Riccardi VM, Paller AS: Familial multiple cafe-au-lait spots. Arch Dermatol 130: 1425–1426, 1994.
27. Charrow J, Listernick R, Ward K: Autosomal dominant multiple cafe-au-lait spots and neurofibromatosis-1: Evidence of non-linkage. Am J Med Genet 45:606–608, 1993.
28. Abelovich D, Gelman-Kohan Z, Silverstein S, et al: Familial cafe au lait spots: A variant of neurofibromatosis type 1. J Med Genet 32:985–986, 1995.

29. Moss C, Green SH: What is segmental neurofibromatosis? Bri J Dermatol 130:106–110, 1994.
30. Cohen MM: Further diagnostic thought about the elephant man. Am J Hum Genet 29:777–782, 1988.
31. Viskochil D, Buchberg AM, Xu G, et al.: Deletions and a translocation interrupt a cloned gene at the neurofibromatosis type 1 locus. Cell 62:187–192, 1990.
32. Cawthon RM, Weiss M, Xu G, et al.: A major segment of the neurofibromatosis type 1 gene: cDNA sequence, genomic structure, and point mutations. Cell 62:193–201, 1990.
33. Wallace MR, Marchuk DA, Andersen LB, et al.: Type 1 neurofibromatosis gene: Identification of a large transcript disrupted in three NF1 patients. Science 249:181–186, 1990.
34. Marchuk DA, Saulino AM, Tavakkol R, et al: cDNA cloning of the type 1 neurofibromatosis gene: Complete sequence of the *NF1* gene product. Genomics 11:931–940, 1991.
35. Xu G, O'Connell P, Viskochil D, et al: The neurofibromatosis type 1 gene encodes a protein related to GAP. Cell 62:599–608, 1990.
36. DeClue JE, Cohen BD, Lowy DR: Identification and characterization of the neurofibromatosis type 1 gene product. Proc Natl Acad Sci USA 88:9914–9918, 1991.
37. Daston MM, Scrable H, Norlund M, Sturbaum AK, Nissen LM, Ratner N: The protein product of the neurofibromatosis type 1 gene is expressed at highest abundance in neurons, Schwann cells and oligodendrocytes. Neuron 8:415–428, 1992.
38. Gutmann DH, Wood DL, Collins FS: Identification of the neurofibromatosis type 1 gene product. Proc Natl Acad Sci USA 88:9658–9662, 1991.
39. Golubic M, Roudebush M, Dobrowolski S, Wolfman A, Stacey DW: Catalytic properties, tissue, and intracellular distribution of the native neurofibromatosis type 1 protein. Oncogene 7:2151–2159, 1992.
40. Huynh DP, Lin CT, Pulst SM: Expression of neurofibromin, the neurofibromatosis type 1 gene product: studies in human neuroblastoma cells and rat brain. Neuroscience Letters 143:233–236, 1992.
41. Nordlund M, Gu X, Shipley MT, Ratner N: Neurofibromin is enriched in the endoplasmic reticulum of CNS neurons. J Neuroscience 13:1588–1600, 1993.
42. Gregory PE, Gutmann DH, Boguski M, et al: The neurofibromatosis type 1 gene product, neurofibromin, associates with microtubules. Somatic Cell and Molecular Genetics 19:265–274, 1993.
42a. Bollag G, McCormick F, Clark R: Characterization of full-length neurofibromin: Tubulin inhibits Ras GAP activity. EMBO J 12:1923–1927, 1993.
42b. Xu H-M, Gutmann DH: Mutations in the GAP-related domain impair the ability of neurofibromin to associate with microtubules. Brain Research 759: 149–152, 1998.
43. Stocker KM, Baizer L, Coston T, Sherman L, Ciment G: Regulated expression of neurofibromin in migrating neural crest cells of avian embryos. J Neurobiol 27:535–552, 1995.
44. Huynh DP, Nechiporuk T, Pulst SM: Differential expression and tissue distribution of type I and type II neurofibromins during mouse fetal development. Develop Biol 161:538–551, 1994.
45. Gutmann DH, Cole JL, Collins FS: Expression of the neurofibromatosis type 1 (NF1) gene during mouse embryonic development. Progress in Brain Research 105:327–335, 1995.
46. Gutmann DH, Geist RT, Wright DE, Snider WD: Expression of the neurofibromatosis 1 (NF1) isoforms in developing and adult rat tissues. Cell Growth and Development 6:315–322, 1995.
47. Daston MM, Ratner N: Neurofibromin, a predominantly neuronal GTPase activating protein in the adult, is ubiquitously expressed during development. Developmental Dynamics 195:216–226, 1993.
48. Hewett SJ, Choi DW, Gutmann DH: Increased expression of the neurofibromatosis 1 (NF1) tumor suppressor gene protein, neurofibromin, in reactive astrocytes *in vitro*. Neuroreport 6:1505–1508, 1995.
49. Giordano MJ, Mahadeo DK, He YY, Geist RT, Hsu C, Gutmann DH: Increased expression of the neurofibromatosis 1 (NF1) gene product, neurofibromin, in astrocytes in response to cerebral ischemia. J Neurosci Res 43:246–253, 1996.
50. Gutmann DH, Tennekoon GI, Cole JL, et al.: Modulation of the neurofibromatosis type 1 gene product, neurofibromin, during Schwann cell differentiation. J. Neurosci Res 36:216–223, 1993.
51. Gutmann DH, Cole JL, Collins FS: Modulation of neurofibromatosis type 1 *(NF1)* gene expression during *in vitro* myoblast differentiation. J Neurosci Res 37:398–405.
52. Norton KK, Geist RT, Mahadeo DK, Gutmann DH: Expression of the neurofibromatosis 1 (NF1) tumor suppressor gene product, neurofibromin, during growth arrest in fibroblasts. Neuroreport 7: 601–604, 1996.
53. Brannan CI, Perkins AS, Vogel KS, et al.: Targeted disruption of the neurofibromatosis type-1 gene leads to developmental abnormalities in heart and various neural crest–derived tissues. Genes Dev 8: 1019–1029, 1994.
54. Jacks T, Shih TS, Schmitt EM, Bronson RT, Bernards A, Weinberg RA: Tumor predisposition in mice heterozygous for a targeted mutation in NF1. Nat Genet 7:353–361, 1994.
55. Kirby ML, Gale TF, Stewart DE: Neural crest cells contribute to normal aorticopulmonary septation. Science 220:1059–1061, 1983.
56. Basu TN, Gutmann DH, Fletcher JA, Glover TW, Collins FS, Downward J: Aberrant regulation of ras proteins in tumor cells from type 1 neurofibromatosis patients. Nature 356:713–715, 1992.
57. DeClue JE, Papageorge AG, Fletcher JA, et al.: Abnormal regulation of mammalian p21$^{ras}$ contributes to malignant tumor growth in von Recklinghausen (type 1) neurofibromatosis. Cell 69:265–273, 1992.
58. Golubic M, Tanaka K, Dobrowski S, et al.: The GTPase stimulatory activity of the neurofibromatosis type 1 and yeast IRA2 proteins are inhibited by arachidonic acid. EMBO J 10:2897–2903, 1991.
59. Gutmann DH, Boguski M, Marchuk D, Wigler M, Collins FS, Ballester R: Analysis of the neurofibro-

matosis type 1 (NF1) GAP-related domain by site-directed mutagenesis. Oncogene 8:761–769, 1993.
60. Ballester R, Marchuk DA, Boguski M, Saulino AM, Letcher R, Wigler M, Collins FS: The *NF1* locus encodes a protein functionally related to mammalian GAP and yeast IRA proteins. Cell 63:851–859, 1990.
61. Xu G, Lin B, Tanaka K, et al.: The catalytic domain of the neurofibromatosis type 1 gene product stimulates *ras* GTPase and complements ira mutants of *S. cerevisiae.* Cell 63:835–841, 1990.
62. Martin GA, Viskochil D, Bollag G, et al.: The GAP-related domain of the neurofibromatosis type 1 gene product interacts with *ras* p21. Cell 63:843–849, 1990.
63. Bollag G, McCormick F: Regulators and effectors of *ras* proteins. Annu Rev Cell Biol 7:601–632, 1991.
64. Knudson AG: Mutation and cancer: Statistical study of retinoblastoma. Proc Natl Acad Sci USA 68:820–823, 1971.
65. Legius E, Marchuk DA, Collins FS, Glover TW: Somatic deletion of neurofibromatosis type 1 gene in a neurofibrosarcoma supports a tumor suppressor gene hypothesis. Nature Genetics 3:122–126, 1993.
66. Shannon KM, O'Connell P, Martin GA, et al.: Loss of the normal NF1 allele from the bone marrow of children with type 1 neurofibromatosis and malignant myeloid disorders. N Engl J Med 330:597–601, 1994.
67. Bollag G, Clapp DW, Shih S, et al.: Loss of NF1 results in activation of the Ras signaling pathway and leads to aberrant growth in haematopoietic cells. Nat Genet 12:144–148, 1996.
68. Largaespada DA, Brannan CI, Jenkins NA, Copeland NG: Nf1 deficiency causes Ras-mediated granulocyte/macrophage colony stimulating factor hypersensitivity and chronic myeloid leukaemia. Nat Genet 12:137–143, 1996.
69. Xu W, Mulligan LM, Ponder MA, et al.: Loss of *NF1* alleles in phaeochromocytomas from patients with type 1 neurofibromatosis. Genes Chromosomes Cancer 4:337–342, 1992.
70. Gutmann DH, Cole JL, Stone WJ, Ponder BAJ, Collins FS: Loss of neurofibromin in adrenal gland tumors from patients with neurofibromatosis type 1. Genes Chromosomes Cancer 10:55–58, 1993.
71. Yan N, Ricca C, Fletcher JA, Glover T, Seizinger BR, Manne V: Farnesyltransferase inhibitors block the neurofibromatosis type 1 (NF1) malignant phenotype. Cancer Res 55:3569–3575, 1995.
72. Kim HA, Rosenbaum T, Marchionni MA, Ratner N, DeClue JE: Schwann cells from neurofibromin-deficient mice exhibit activation of p21-ras, inhibition of cell proliferation and morphological changes. Oncogene 11:325–335, 1995.
73. Guha A, Lau N, Huvar I, Gutmann DH, Provias J, Pawson T, Boss G: Ras-GTP levels are elevated in human NF1 peripheral nerve tumors. Oncogene 12:507–513, 1996.
74. Sawada S, Florell S, Purandare SM, Ota M, Stephens K, Viskochil D: Identification of NF1 mutations in both alleles of a dermal neurofibroma. Nat Genet 14:110–112, 1996.
75. Johnson MR, Look AT, DeClue JE, Valentine MB, Lowy DR: Inactivation of the *NF1* gene in human melanoma and neuroblastoma cell lines without impaired regulation of GTP-Ras. Proc Natl Acad Sci USA 90:5539–5543, 1993.
76. Andersen LB, Fountain JW, Gutmann DH, et al.: Mutations in the neurofibromatosis 1 gene in sporadic malignant melanomas. Nat Genet 3:118–121, 1993.
77. Gutmann DH, Geist RT, Rose K, Wallin G, Moley JF: Loss of neurofibromatosis type 1 (NF1) gene expression in pheochromocytomas from patients without NF1. Genes Chromosomes Cancer 13:104–109, 1995.
78. The I, Murthy AE, Hannigan GE, et al.: Neurofibromatosis type 1 gene mutations in neuroblastoma. Nat Genet 3:62–66, 1993.
79. Johnson MR, DeClue JE, Felzmann S, et al.: Neurofibromin can inhibit Ras-dependent growth by a mechanism independent of its GTPase-accelerating function. Mol Cell Biol 14:641–645, 1994.
80. Gutmann DH, Giordano MJ, Mahadeo DK, Lau N, Silbergeld D, Guha A: Increased neurofibromatosis 1 gene expression in astrocytic tumors: Positive regulation by p21-ras. Oncogene 12: 2121–2127, 1996.
81. Platten M, Giordano MJ, Dirven CM, Gutmann DH, Louis DN: Upregulation of specific NF1 gene transcripts in sporadic pilocytic astrocytomas. Am J Pathol 149(2):621–627, 1996.
81a. Gutmann DH, Loehr A, Zhang Y, Kim J, Henkemeyer M, Cashen A: Haploinsufficiency for the neurofibromatosis 1 (NF1) tumor suppressor results in increased astrocyte proliferation. Oncogene (in press).
82. Norton KK, XU J, Gutmann DH: Expression of the neurofibromatosis 1 gene product, neurofibromin, in blood vessel endothelial cells and smooth muscle: Neurobiol Dis 2:13–21, 1995.
83. Ahlgren-Beckendorf JA, Maggio WW, Chen F, Kent TA: Neurofibromatosis 1 mRNA expression in blood vessels. Biochem Biophys Res Commun 197: 1019–1024, 1993.
84. Vogel KS, Brannan CI, Jenkins NA, Copeland NG, Parada LF: Loss of neurofibromin results is neurotrophin-independent survival of embryonic sensory and sympathetic neurons. Cell 82:733–742, 1995.
84a. Vogel KS, Parada LF: Sympathetic neuron survival and proliferation are prolonged by loss of p53 and neurofibromin. Molecular and Cellular Neuroscience 11, 19–28, 1998.
85. Danglot G, Regnier V, Fauvet D, Vassal G, Kujas M, Bernheim A: Neurofibromatosis 1 (NF1) mRNAs expressed in the central nervous system are differentially spliced in the 5' part of the gene. Hum Mol Genet 4:915–920, 1995.
86. Silva AJ, Frankland PW, Marowitz Z, et al.: A mouse model for the learning and memory deficits associated with neurofibromatosis type 1. Nat Genet 15:281–284, 1997.
87. Kayes LM, Burke W, Riccardi V, Stephens K: Deletions spanning the neurofibromatosis 1 gene: Identification and phenotype of five patients. Am J Med Genet 54:424–436, 1994.
88. Easton DF, Ponder MA, Huson SM, Ponder BAJ: An analysis of variation in expression of neurofi-

bromatosis (NF) type 1 (NF1): Evidence for modifying genes. Am J Hum Genet 53:305–311, 1993.

89. Heim RA, Silverman LM, Farber RA, Kam-Morgan LNW, Luce MC: Screening for truncated NF1 proteins. Nat Genet 8:218–219, 1994.

90. Hofman KJ, Boehm CD: Familial neurofibromatosis 1: Clinical experience with DNA testing. J Pediatr 120:394–398, 1992.

91. Evans DGR, Huson SM, Donnai D, et al.: A genetic study of type 2 neurofibromatosis in the United Kingdom I. Prevalance, mutation rate, fitness and confirmation of material transmission effect on severity. J Med Genet 29:841–846, 1992.

92. Mautner FV, Tatagiba M, Guthoff RK, Samii M, Pulst SM: Neurofibromatosis 2 in the pediatric age group. Neurosurgery 33:92–96, 1993.

93. Mautner FV, Lindenau M, Hazim W, et al.: The neuroimaging and ocular spectrum of neurofibromatosis 2. Neurosurgery 38:880–886, 1996

94. Parry DM, Eldridge R, Kaiser-Kupfer MI, Bouzas EA, Pikus A, Patronas B: Neurofibromatosis 2 (NF2): Clinical characteristics of 63 affected individuals and clinical evidence for heterogeneity. Am J Med Genet 52:450–461, 1994.

95. Evans DGR, Huson SM, Donnai D, et al.: A clinical study of type 2 neurofibromatosis QJM 304: 603–618, 1992.

96. Mautner VF, Tatagiba M, Lindenau M, et al.: Spinal tumors in patients with neurofibromatosis type 2: MR imaging study of frequency, multiplicity and variety. Am J Roentgen 165:951–955, 1995.

97. Kaiser-Kupfer MI, Freidlin V, Datiles MB, et al.: The association of posterior capsular lens opacities with bilateral acoustic neuromas in patients with neurofibromatosis type 2. Arch Ophthalmol 107:541–544, 1989.

98. Ragge NK, Baser ME, Klein J, et al.: Ocular abnormalities in neurofibromatosis 2. Am J Ophthalmol 120:634–641, 1995.

99. Baser M, Mautner VF Ragge N, et al.: Presymptomatic diagnosis in neurofibromatosis 2 using linked genetic markers, neuroimaging, and ocular examinations. Neurology 47:1269–1277, 1996.

100. Seizinger BR, Rouleau G, Ozelius LJ, et al.: Common pathogenetic mechanism for three tumor types in bilateral acoustic neurofibromatosis. Science 236:317–319 1987.

101. Rouleau GA, Wertelecki W, Haines JL, et al.: Genetic linkage of bilateral acoustic neurofibromatosis to DNA marker on chromosome 22. Nature 329:246–248, 1987.

102. Rouleau GA, Merel P, Lutchman M, et al.: Alteration in a new gene encoding a putative membrane-organizing protein causes neurofibromatosis type 2. Nature 363:515–521, 1993.

103. Trofatter JA, MacCollin MM, Rutter JL, et al.: A novel moesin-, radixin-like gene is a candidate for the neurofibromatosis 2 tumor suppressor. Cell 72:791–800, 1993.

104. Takeshima H. Izawa I, Lee PSY, Safdar N, Levin VA, Saya H et al.: Detection of cellular proteins that interact with the NF2 tumor suppressor gene product. Oncogene 9:2135–2144, 1994.

105. Sherman L, Xu HM, Geist RT, et al: Interdomain binding mediates tumor growth suppression by the NF2 gene product. Oncogene 15:2505–2509, 1997.

106. Scoles DR, Huynh D, Marcos PA, Coulsell E, Robinson NGG, Tamanoi F, Pulst SM: Neurofibromatosis 2 tumour suppressor schwannomin interacts with βII-spectrin. Nature Genet 18:354–359, 1998.

107. Murthy A, Gonzalez-Agosti C, Cordero E, et al.: NHE-RF, a regulatory cofactor for Na(+)-H+ exchange, is a common interactor for merlin and ERM (MERM) proteins. J Biol Chem 273:1273–1276, 1998.

108. Sainz J, Huynh D, Figueroa K, Ragge NK, Baser M, Pulst SM: Mutations of the neurofibromatosis type 2 gene and lack of the gene product in vestibular schwannomas. Hum Mol Genet 3:885–891, 1994.

109. Gutmann DH, Wright DE, Geist RT, Snider WD: Expression of the neurofibromatosis 2 (NF2) gene isoforms during rat embryonic development. Hum Mol Genet 4:471–478, 1995.

109a. Scherer SS, Gutmann DH: Expression of the neurofibromatosis 2 tumor suppressor gene product, merlin, in Schwann cells. J Neurosci Res 46: 595–605, 1996.

110. Huynh D, Tran M, Nechiporuk T, Pulst SM: Expression of neurofibromatosis 2 transcript and gene product during mouse fetal development. Cell Growth Differ 7:11, 1551–1561, 1996.

111. Sainio M, Strachan T, Blomstedt G, et al.: Presymptomatic DNA and MRI diagnosis of neurofibromatosis 2 with mild clinical course in an extended pedigree. Neurology 45:1314–1322, 1995.

112. MacCollin M, Ramesh V, Jacoby LB, et al.: Mutational analysis of patients with neurofibromatosis 2. Am J Hum Genet 55:314–320, 1994.

113. Merel P, Hoang-Xuan K, Sanson M, et al.: Screening for germ-line mutations in the NF2 gene. Genes Chromosomes Cancer. 12:117–127, 1995.

114. Sainz, Figueroa K, Mautner V, Baser M, Pulst SM: High frequency of nonsense mutations in the NF2 gene caused by C to T transitions in five CGA codons. Hum Mol Genet 4:137–139, 1995.

114a. Scoles DR, Baser ME, Pulst SM: A missense mutation in the neurofibromatosis 2 gene occurs in patients with mild and severe phenotypes. Neurology 47:544–546, 1996.

115. Huynh DP, Mautner V, Baser ME, Stavrou D, Pulst SM: Immunohistochemical detection of schwannomin and neurofibromin in vestibular schwannomas, ependymomas and meningiomas. J Neuropathol Exp Neurol 56:382–390, 1997.

116. Bourn D, Carter SA, Evans DG, Goodship J, Coakham H, Strachan T: A mutation in the neurofibromatosis type 2 tumor-suppressor gene, giving rise to widely different clinical phenotypes in two unrelated individuals. Am J Hum Genet 55:69–73, 1994.

116a. Ruttledge M, Andermann A, Phelan C, et al.: Type of mutation in the neurofibromatosis type 2 gene (NF2) frequently determines severity of disease. Am J Hum Genet 59:331–342, 1996.

116b. Parry D, MacCollin M, Kaiser-Kupfer M, et al.: Germ-line mutations in the neurofibromatosis 2 gene: Correlations with disease severity and retinal abnormalities. Am J Hum Genet 59:529–539, 1996.

117. Baser M, Ragge N, Riccardi V, Janus T, Gantz B, Pulst SM: Phenotypic variability in monozygotic twins with neurofibromatosis 2. Am J Med Genet 64:563–567, 1994.

118. Seizinger R, Monte SDI, Atkins L, Gusella JF, Martuza RL: Molecular genetic approach to human meningioma: Loss of genes on chromosome 22. Proc Natl Acad Sci 84:5419–5423, 1987.

119. Ruttledge MH, Sarrazin J, Rangaratnam S, et al.: Evidence for the complete inactivation of the *NF2* gene in the majority of sporadic menigiomas. Nat Genet 6:180–184, 1994.

120. Lekanne-Deprez RH, Bianchi AB, Groen NA, et al.: Frequent *NF2* gene transcript mutations in sporadic meningiomas and vestibular schwannomas. Am J Hum Genet 54:1022–1029, 1994.

121. Bijlsma EK, Merel P, Bosch DA, et al.: Analysis of mutations in the SCH gene in schwannomas. Genes Chromosomes Cancer 11:7–14, 1994.

122. Papi L, De Vitis LR, Vitelli F, et al.: Somatic mutations in the neurofibromatosis type 2 gene in sporadic meningiomas. Hum Genet 95:347–351, 1995.

122a. Gutmann DH, Giordano MJ, Fishback AS, Guha A: Loss of merlin expression in sporadic meningiomas, ependymomas and schwannomas. Neurology 48:267–270, 1997.

123. Lutchman M, Rouleau GA: The neurofibromatosis type 2 gene product schwannomin, suppresses growth of NIH 3T3 cells. Cancer Res 55:2270–2274, 1995.

124. Huynh D, Pulst SM: NF2 antisense oligodeoxynucleotides induce reversible inhibition of schwannomin synthesis and cell adhesion in STS26T and T98G cells. Oncogene 13:73–84, 1996.

124a. Gutmann DH, Sherman L, Seftor L, Haipek C, Lu KH, Hendrix M: Increased expression of the NF2 tumor suppressor gene product, merlin, impairs cell motility, adhesion and spreading. Human Molecular Genetics 8:267–275, 1999.

124b. Gutmann DH, Geist RT, Xu H-M, Kim JS, Saporito-Irwin S: Defects in neurofibromatosis 2 protein function can arise at multiple levels. Human Molecular Genetics 7:335–345, 1998.

125. Zucman-Rossi J, Legoix P, Der Sakissian, et al.: *NF2* gene in neurofibromatosis type 2 patients. Hum Mol Genet 7:2095–2101, 1998.

126. Evans DG, Bourn D, Wallace A, Ramsden RT, Mitachell JD, Strachan T: Diagnostic issues in a family with late onset type 2 neurofibromatosis. J Med Genet 32:470–474, 1995.

127. Bijlsma EK, Wallace AJ, Evans DG: Misleading linkage results in an NF2 presymptomatic test owing to mosaicism. J Med Genet 34:934–936, 1997.

128. Honda M, Arai E, Sawada S, Ohta A, Niimura M: Neurofibromatosis 2 and neurilemmomatosis gene are identical. J Invest Dermatol 104:74–77, 1995.

129. Jacoby LB, Jones D, Davis K, et al.: Molecular analysis of the NF2 tumor-suppressor gene in schwannomatosis. Am J Hum Genet 61:1293–1302, 1997.

130. Kluwe L, Pulst SM, Koppen J, Mautner VF: A 163-bp deletion in the neurofibromatosis 2 (NF2) gene associated with variant phenotypes. Hum Genet 95:443–446, 1995.

131. Pulst SM, Riccardi VM, Fain P, Barker D, Korenberg JR: Familial spinal neurofibromatosis: Clinical and DNA linkage studies. Neurology 41:1923–1927, 1991.

132. MacCollin M, Woodfin W, Kronn D, Short MP: Schwannomatosis: A clinical and pathologic study. Neurology 46:1072–1079, 1996.

133. Pulst S, Riccardi V, Mautner V: Spinal schwannomatosis. Neurology 48:787–788, 1997.

134. Delleman J, Dejong JGY, Bleekr GM: Meningiomas in five members of a family over two generations in one member simultaneously with acoustic neurinomas. Neurology 28:567–570, 1978.

135. Bolger GB, Stamberg J, Kirsch IL: Chromosome translocation t (14;22) and oncogene (c-sis) variant in a pedigree with familial meningioma. N Engl J Med 312:564–567, 1980.

136. Pulst SM, Fain P, Rouleau GA, Sieb JP: Familial meningioma is not allelic to NF2. Neurology 43: 2096–2098, 1993.

136a. Briggs RJ, Brackmann DE, Baser ME, Hitselberger WE: Comprehensive management of bilateral acoustic neuromas. Current perspectives. Arch Otolaryngol Head Neck Surg 120:1307–1314, 1994.

137. Consensus Development Panel (CDP) 1994 National Institutes of Health Consensus Development Conference Statement on Acoustic Neuroma, December 11–13, 1991. Arch Neurol 51: 201, 1994.

138. Evans DGR, Ramsden R, Huson SM, Harris R, Lye R, King TT: Type 2 neurofibromatosis. The need for supraregional care? J Laryngol Otol 107:401–406, 1993.

139. Claudio JO, Lutchman M, Rouleau GA: Widespread but cell type specific expression of the mouse neurofibromatosis type 2 gene. Neuroreport 6:1942–1946, 1995.

140. McClatchey AI, Saotome I, Ramesh V, Gusella JF, Jacks T: The NF2 tumor suppressor gene product is essential for extraembryonic development immediately prior to gastrulation. Genes Dev 11: 1253–1265, 1997.

141. McClatchey AI, Saotome I, Mercer K, et al.: Mice heterozygous for a mutation at the *Nf2* tumor suppressor locus develop a range of highly metastatic tumors. Genes Dev 12:1121–33, 1998.

142. Gomez MR: Tuberous Sclerosis, ed 5. New York: Raven Press 1988.

143. Roach ES, Smith M, Huttenlocher P, Bhat M, Alcorn D, Hawley L: Diagnostic criteria: Tuberous sclerosis complex. J Child Neurol 7:221–224, 1992.

143a. Roach ES, Gomez MR, Northrup H: Tuberous sclerosis complex consensus conference: Revised diagnostic criteria. J. Child Neurology 13:624–628, 1998.

144. Roach ES, Gomez MR, Northrup H: Tuberous sclerosis complex consensus conference: Revised clinical diagnostic criteria. J Child Neurol 13:624–628, 1998.

145. Haines JL, Short MP, Kwiatkowski DJ, et al.: Localization of one gene for tuberous sclerosis

within 9q32–34 and further evidence for heterogeneity. Am J Hum Genet 49:764–772, 1991.
146. European Chromosome 16 Tuberous Sclerosis Consortium: Identification and characterization of the tuberous sclerosis gene on chromosome 16. Cell 75:1305–1315, 1993.
147. van Slegtenhorst M, de Hoogt R, Hermans C, et al.: Identification of the tuberous sclerosis gene *TSC1* on chromosome 9q34. Science 277:805–808, 1997.
148. Plank TL, Yeung RS, Henske EP: Hamartin, the product of the tuberous sclerosis 1 *(TSC1)* gene, interacts with tuberin and appears to be localized to cytoplasmic vesicles. Cancer Res 58:4766–4770, 1998.
149. Jones AC, Daniells CE, Snell RG, et al.: Molecular genetic and phenotypic analysis reveals differences between TSC1 and TSC2 associated familial and sporadic tuberous sclerosis. Hum Mol Genet 12:2155–2161, 1997.
149a. Plank TL, Yeung RS, Henske EP: Hamartin, the product of the tuberous sclerosis 1 (TSC1) gene, interacts with tuberin and appears to be localized to cytoplasmic vesicles. Cancer Research 58:4766–4770, 1998.
149b. van Slegtenhorst M, Nellist M, Nagelkerken B, Cheadle J, Snell R, van den Ouweland A, Reuser A, Sampson J, Halley D, van der Sluijs P: Interaction between hamartin and tuberin, the TSC1 and TSC2 gene products. Human Molecular Genetics 7:1053–1057, 1998.
150. Maheshwar MM, Sandford R, Nellist M, et al.: Comparative analysis and genomic structure of the tuberous sclerosis 2 *(TSC2)* gene in human and pufferfish. Hum Mol Genet 5:131–137, 1996.
151. Kobayashi T, Nishizawa M, Hirayama Y, Kobayashi E, Hino O: cDNA structure, alternative splicing and exon–intron organization of the predisposing tuberous sclerosis *(Tsc2)* gene of the Eker rat model. Nucleic Acids Res 23:2608–2613, 1995.
152. Wilson PJ, Ramesh V, Kristiansen A, Bove C, Jozwiak S, Kwiatkowski DJ, Short MP, Haines JL: Novel mutations detected in the *TSC2* gene from both sporadic and familial TSC patients. Hum Mol Genet 5:249–256, 1996.
153. Kumar A, Wolpert C, Kandt RS, Segal J, Pufky J, Roses AD, Pericak-Vance MA, Gilbert JR: A *de novo* frame-shift mutation in the tuberin gene. Hum Mol Genet 4:1471–1472, 1995.
154. Green AJ, Yates JRW: Loss of heterozygosity on chromosome 16p in hamartomata from patients with tuberous sclerosis. Am J Hum Genet 53S:244, 1993.
155. Rubinfeld B, Crozier WJ, Albert I, Conroy L, et al.: Localization of the rap1 GAP catalytic domain and sites of phosphorylation by mutational analysis. Mol Cell Biol 12:4634–4642, 1992.
156. Rubinfeld B, Munemitsu S, Clark R, et al.: Molecular cloning of a GTPase activating protein specific for the Krev-1 protein, p21-rap1. Cell 65: 1033–1042, 1991.
157. Wienecke R, Konig A, DeClue JE: Identification of tuberin, the tuberous sclerosis-2 product: Tuberin possesses specific Rap1GAP activity. J Biol Chem 270:16409–16414, 1995.
158. Gutmann DH, Saporito-Irwin S, DeClue JE, Wienecke R, Guha A: Alterations in the rap 1 signaling pathway are common in human gliomas. Oncogene 15:1611–1616, 1997.
158a. Wienecke R, Guha A, Maize JC, Heideman RL, DeClue JE, Gutmann DH: Reduced TSC2 RNA and protein in sporadic astrocytomas and ependymomas. Annals of Neurology 42:230–235, 1997.
159. Tsuchiya H, Orimoto K, Kobayashi T, Hino O: Presence of potent transcriptional activation domains in the predisposing tuberous sclerosis *(Tsc2)* gene product of the Eker rat model. Cancer Res 56:429–433, 1996.
160. Jin F, Wienecke R, Xiao G-H, Maize JC, DeClue JE, Yeung RS: Suppression of tumorigenicity by the wild-type tuberous sclerosis 2 *(Tsc2)* gene and its C-terminal region. Proc Natl Acad Sci USA 93: 9154–9159, 1996.
160a. Xiao G-H, Shoarinejad F, Jin F, Golemis EA, Yeung RS: The tuberous sclerosis 2 gene product, tuberin, functions as a Rab5 GTPase activating protein (GAP) in modulating endocytosis. J Biol Chem 272:6097–6100, 1997.
160b. Soucek T, Pusch O, Weinecke R, DeClue JE, Hengstschlager M: Role of the tuberous sclerosis gene 2 product in cell cycle control. J Biol Chem 272:29301–23308, 1997.
160c. Henry KW, Yuan X, Koszewski NJ, Onda H, Kwiatkowski DJ, Noonan DJ: Tuberous sclerosis gene 2 product modulates transcription mediated by steroid hormone receptor family members. J Biol Chem 273:20535–20539, 1998.
161. Xiao G-H, Jin F, Yeung RS: Identification of tuberous sclerosis 2 messenger RNA splice variants that are conserved and differentially expressed in rat and human tissues. Cell Growth Diff 6:1185–1911, 1995.
162. Xu L, Sterner C, Maheshwar MM, Wilson PJ, Nellist M, Short PM, Haines JL, Sampson JR, Ramesh V: Alternative splicing of the tuberous sclerosis 2 *(TSC2)* gene in human and mouse tissues. Genomics 27:475–480, 1995.
163. Geist RT, Gutmann DH: The tuberous sclerosis 2 gene is expressed at high levels in the adult cerebellum and developing spinal cord. Cell Growth Differ 6:1477–1483, 1995.
164. Geist RT, Reddy AJ, Zhang J, Gutmann DH: Expression of the tuberous sclerosis 2 gene product, tuberin, in adult and developing nervous system tissues. Neurobiol Dis 3:111–120, 1996.
165. Yeung RS, Xiao GH, Jin F, Lee WC, Testa JR, Knudson AG: Predisposition to renal cell carcinoma in the Eker rat is determined by germline mutation of the tuberous sclerosis 2 *(TCS2)* gene. Proc Natl Acad Sci USA 91:11413–11416, 1994.
166. Au KS, Rodriguez JA, Finch JL, et al.: Germ-line mutational analysis of the *TSC2* gene in 90 tuberous-sclerosis patients. Am J Hum Genet 62: 286–294, 1998.
167. Yates JRW, van Bakei I, Sepp T, et al.: Female germline mosaicism in tuberous sclerosis confirmed by molecular genetic analysis. Hum Mol Genet 6:2265–2269, 1997.
168. Neumann HP, Lips CJ, Hsia YE, Zbar B: von Hippel Lindau syndrome. Brain Pathol 5:181–193, 1995.
169. Richards FR, Payne SJ, Zbar B, Affara NA,

Ferguson-Smith MA, Maher ER: Molecular analysis of *de novo* germline mutations in the von Hippel-Lindau disease gene. Hum Mol Genet 4: 2139–2143, 1995.

170. Karsdop N, Elderson A, Wittebol-Post D, et al.: von Hippel-Lindau disease: New strategies in early detection and treatment. Am J Med 97:158–168, 1994.
171. Maher ER, Yates JR: Familial renal cell carcinoma: clinical and molecular genetic aspects. Br J Cancer 63:176–179, 1991.
172. Choyke P L, Glenn GM, Walther MM, Patronas NJ, Linehan WM, Zbar B: von Hippel-Lindau disease: Genetic, clinical and imaging features. Radiology 194:629–642, 1995.
173. Filling-Katz MR, Choyke PL, Oldfield E, at al.: Central nervous involvement in von Hippel-Lindau disease. Neurology 41–46, 1991.
174. Melmon KL, Rosen SW: Lindau's disease: Review of the literature and study of a large kindred. Am J Med 36:595–617, 1964.
175. Davis DR, Norman AM, Whitehouse RW, Evans DGR: Non-expression of von Hippel-Lindau phenotype in an obligate gene carrier. Clin Genet 45: 104–106, 1994.
176. Seizinger BR, Rouleau GA, Ozelius LJ, et al.: von Hippel-Lindau disease maps to the region of chromosome 3 associated with renal cell carcinoma. Nature 332:268–269, 1988.
177. Latif F, Tory K, Gnarra J, et al.: Identification of the von Hippel-Lindau disease tumor suppressor gene. Science 260:1317–1320, 1993.
178. Schoenfeld A, Davidowitz EJ, Burk RD: A second major native von Hippel-Lindau gene product, initiated from an internal translation start site, functions as a tumor suppressor. Proc Natl Acad Sci USA 95:8817–8822, 1998.
179. Duan DR, Pause A, Burgess WH, et al.: Inhibition of transcription elongation by the VHL tumor suppressor protein. Science 269:1402–1406, 1995.
180. Kibel A, Iliopoulos O, DeCaprio JA, Kaelin WG: Binding of the von Hippel-Lindau tumor suppressor protein to elongin B and C. Science 269: 1444–1446, 1995.
181. Lonergan KM, Iliopoulos O, Ohh M, et al.: Regulation of hypoxia-inducible mRNAs by the von Hippel-Lindau tumor suppressor protein requires binding to complexes containing elongins B/C and Cul2. Mol Cell Biol 18:732–741, 1998.
182. Whaley JM, Naglich J, Gelbert L, et al.: Germ-line mutations in the von Hippel-Lindau tumor-suppressor gene are similar to somatic von Hippel-Lindau aberrations in sporadic renal cell carcinoma. Am J Hum Genet 55:1092–1103, 1994.
183. Chen F, Kishida T, Tao M, et al.: Germ line mutations in the von Hippel-Lindau disease tumor suppressor gene: correlations with phenotype. Hum Mutat 5:66–75, 1995.
184. Brauch H, Kishida T, Glavac D, et al.: von Hippel-Lindau (VHL) disease with pheochromocytoma in the Black Forest region of Germany: Evidence for a founder effect. Hum Genet 95:551–556, 1995.
185. Gross DJ, Avishai N, Meiner V, Filon D, Zbar B, Abeliovich D: Familial pheochromocytoma associated with a novel mutation in the von Hippel-Lindau gene. J Clin Endocrinol Metab 81:147–149, 1996.
186. van der Harst E, de Krijger RR, Dinjens WN, Weeks LE, Bonjer HJ, Bruining HA, Lamberts SW, Koper JW: Germline mutations in the vhl gene in patients presenting with phaeochromocytomas. Int J Cancer 77:337–340, 1998.
187. Beroud C, Joly D, Gallou C, Staroz F, Orfanelli MI, Junien C: Software and database for the analysis of mutations in the VHL gene. Nucleic Acids Res 26:256–258, 1998.
188. Constans JP, Meder F, Maiuri F, et al.: Posterior fossa hemangioblastomas. Surg Neurol 25:269–275, 1986.
189. Kanno H, Kondo K, Ito S: Somatic mutations of the von Hippel-Lindau tumor suppressor gene in sporadic central nervous system hemangioblastomas. J Cancer Res 54:4845–4847, 1994.
190. Oberstraß J, Reifenberger G, Reifenberger J, Wechssler W, Collins VP: 6 Mutation of the von Hippel-Lindau tumor suppressor gene in capillary hemangioblastomas of the central nervous system. J Pathol 179:151–156, 1996.
191. Lee JY, Dong SM, Park WS, et al.: Loss of heterozygosity and somatic mutations of the VHL tumor suppressor gene in sporadic cerebellar hemangioblastomas. Cancer Res 58:504–508, 1998.
192. Glenn GM, Linehan WM, Hosoe S, et al.: Screening for von Hippel-Lindau disease by DNA polymorphism analysis. JAMA 267:1226–1231, 1992.
193. Curley SA, Lott ST, Luca JW, Frazier ML, Killary AM: Surgical decision-making affected by clinical and genetic screening of a novel kindred with von Hippel-Lindau disease and pancreatic islet cell tumors. Ann Surg 227:229–235, 1998.

Chapter 10

# PRION DISEASES

Otto Windl, PhD
H. A. Kretzschmar, MD



## PRION DISEASES

Prion diseases have been known for a long time. Scrapie in sheep was first described 200 years ago in Germany and in Great Britain and in 1936 was shown to be experimentally transmissible.[1] Human prion diseases were recognized as rare neurodegenerative entities in the 1920s by Hans Gerhard Creutzfeldt[2] and Alfons Jakob.[3] One of the early cases published by Jakob[4] and Meggendorfer[5] was a familial Creutzfeldt-Jakob disease case that later was shown to carry the D178N mutation.[6] Thus spongiform encephalopathies for a long time were considered as neurodegenerative and hereditary disorders. It was not until the 1960s, after William Hadlow[7] first noticed similarities between scrapie in sheep and kuru, a deadly neurological disease of humans in New Guinea, and after kuru had been transmitted to apes that Creutzfeldt-Jakob disease was also shown to be a transmissible disease by D. C. Gajdusek, J. Gibbs, and M. Alpers.[8] Hereditary spongiform encephalopathies were first transmitted to monkeys in 1981.[9]

## THE PRION HYPOTHESIS

The nature of the infectious agent of spongiform encephalopathies has been the subject of heated debate for many years. The assumption that seemed natural in the early 1970s, that the agent must be some "unconventional" or "slow virus", was challenged by the failure to detect viral nucleic acids or an immunological response to a hypothetical virus. The term *prion* was proposed to distinguish the infectious pathogen from viruses or viroids. Albeit not formally proven, the prion hypothesis is supported by many lines of evidence.

Prions are defined as small proteinaceous particles that resist inactivation by procedures that modify nucleic acids.[10] The change of a normal protein encoded by the host genome, the cellular isoform of the prion protein ($PrP^C$), into an altered isoform, the scrapie isoform of the prion protein ($PrP^{Sc}$), is at the heart of this hypothesis, which more than 15 years after its introduction is still not proven beyond doubt. Whether the conversion of $PrP^C$ to $PrP^{Sc}$ involves an as yet unidentified chemical modification or whether it only involves a conformational change remains to be established. The existence of various scrapie strains with distinct combinations of pathological changes has not been satisfactorily explained by the prion hypothesis. On the other hand, the fact that mutations in the prion protein gene result in the generation of a transmissible disease is most plausibly explained by this hypothesis. A host of other findings also favor the prion hypothesis.[11]

The pathogenesis of prion diseases is poorly understood. Because mice lacking the prion protein gene develop and live without major abnormalities, a "gain of function" of $PrP^{Sc}$ during the course of the disease has been thought to cause pathological changes. Others have argued that the fundamental pathogenic process may be the loss of function of $PrP^C$.[12]

Six human prion diseases have been described to date:

1. Kuru, a disease formerly transmitted through ritual cannibalism in New Guinea
2. Creutzfeldt-Jakob disease (CJD), which in a small percentage is inherited as an autosomal dominant trait (it may also be accidentally [iatrogenically] transmitted, but most cases are sporadic, with no known infectious source)
3. Gerstmann-Sträussler-Scheinker syndrome (GSS), which in all cases is a hereditary disorder
4. Fatal familial insomnia (FFI), which is also inherited as an autosomal dominant trait
5. Atypical prion disease, which has been reported as a heritable trait in a small number of families with insertion mutations
6. New variant CJD (nvCJD), a new variant of CJD that has been described in the United Kingdom[13] (it may be caused by bovine spongiform encephalopathy (BSE) and shows an unusual combination of clinical and neuropathological features)

Historical names may in the future be replaced by more specific terms, for example, "familial prion disease with a P102L mutation and predominant ataxia" or "GSS-P102L" (Table 10–1).

## CREUTZFELDT-JAKOB DISEASE

Sporadic CJD most often affects patients in their 60s. It usually presents with dementia and various neurologic signs, most often ataxia. The clinical criteria established by Masters and colleagues.[14] have been modified and adopted by a large CJD surveillance group in Europe.[15] The definite diagnosis can only be made on neuropathological or biochemical examination of the brain. The clinical diagnostic criteria are listed in Table 10–2.

## GERSTMANN-STRÄUSSLER-SCHEINKER SYNDROME

Gerstmann-Sträussler-Scheinker syndrome was first described in 1928[16,17] and is caused by various mutations of the human prion protein gene *(PRNP)* (see Table 10–3, later). Patients may show signs of ataxia, dysphagia, dysarthria, hyporeflexia, and mental deterioration, which sometimes may be mild. GSS is thought to be distinguisha-

Table 10–1. **Human Prion Diseases**

| New Nomenclature | Traditional Nomenclature |
|---|---|
| Sporadic prion disease | CJD |
| Inherited prion diseases | |
| GSS-P102L | GSS |
| GSS-P105L | GSS |
| GSS-A117V | GSS |
| GSS-Y145* | GSS |
| With N171S | Schizophrenic or schizoaffective disorder |
| CJD-D178N | Familial CJD |
| FFI-D178N | FFI |
| CJD-V180I | Familial CJD |
| With T183A | Familial progressive dementia |
| GSS-F198S | GSS |
| CJD-E200K | Familial CJD |
| GSS-D202N | GSS |
| CJD-R208H | Familial CJD |
| CJD-V210I | Familial CJD |
| GSS-Q212P | GSS |
| GSS-Q217R | GSS |
| CJD-M232R | Familial CJD |
| With extra repeats (+1, +2, . . . , +9) | Familial CJD, GSS, atypical |
| Acquired prion diseases | Kuru<br>Iatrogenic CJD<br>nvCJD |

Table 10–2. **Diagnostic Criteria for CJD**

Sporadic CJD
- Probable CJD
  - Progressive dementia of less than 2 years duration and
  - Typical EEG and
  - At least two out of four clinical features
    - Myoclonus
    - Visual or cerebellar disturbance
    - Pyramidal or extrapyramidal dysfunction
    - Akinetic mutism
- Possible CJD
  - Clinical features identical to 'probable CJD' but no typical EEG

Accidentally transmitted CJD
- Progressive cerebellar syndrome in a pituitary hormone recipient
- Sporadic CJD with a recognized exposure risk (e.g., dura mater transplant)

Familial CJD
- Definite or probable CJD plus definite or probable CJD in a first-degree relative
- Neuropsychiatric disorders plus disease-specific *PRNP* mutations

ble from CJD by its predominance of ataxia, whereas dementia and myoclonus are more prominent in CJD. The clinical manifestations of CJD and GSS, however, may occur in carriers of the same mutation in one family. Neuropathologically, GSS is quite distinct and is characterized by large multicentric PrP-containing amyloid plaques; spongiform change is variable (for details, see Ghetti and colleagues[18]).

## FATAL FAMILIAL INSOMNIA

Patients with FFI often present with insomnia and dysautonomia and later show signs of ataxia, dysarthria, myoclonus, and pyramidal tract dysfunction. In the later stages, patients exhibit total insomnia and dementia, rigidity, dystonia, and mutism. The patients die after approximately 13 months of disease in a state of stupor or coma. Neuropathologically, FFI is characterized by neuronal loss and astrocytic gliosis preferentially affecting the ventral anterior and medial dorsal nuclei of the thalamus. The disease is caused by a D178N mutation of *PRNP* associated with a methionine codon at position 129 of the same allele[19,20] (for details, see Montagna and coworkers[21] and Parchi and colleagues[22]). The detection of 14–3-3 protein in the cerebrospinal fluid, which is highly sensitive and specific for the diagnosis of sporadic CJD, largely failed for FFI cases.[23,24] It is tempting to speculate that this difference is due to the different localization of the lesions or to the rate of neuronal loss.

## NEUROPATHOLOGY OF HUMAN PRION DISEASES

The classic constellation of neuropathological changes in CJD consists of spongiform degeneration (spongiform change and status spongiosus), neuronal loss, and astrocytic gliosis (Figs. 10–1 through 10–6 show typical changes). Of these changes, only spongiform degeneration has some claim to specificity. Notably even the first descriptions of CJD lack a reference to spongiform degeneration,[3] and the absolute requirement of spongiform degeneration for diagnosis is debatable. Kuru plaques and other forms of PrP-containing amyloid plaques, although pathognomonic of prion disease, are found only in a minority of sporadic cases where they are almost exclusively associated with a valine codon at position 129 of *PRNP*. Multicentric plaques are a regular finding in GSS (Fig. 10–5).

Spongiform degeneration comprises a spectrum of changes with variable diagnostic significance. First, spongiform change consists of a delicate vacuolation of the neuropil. The vacuoles, which often have an opaque appearance, range in size from 2 to 20 μm. Spongiform change may be focal and must be distinguished from vacuolar change often observed in the second corti-

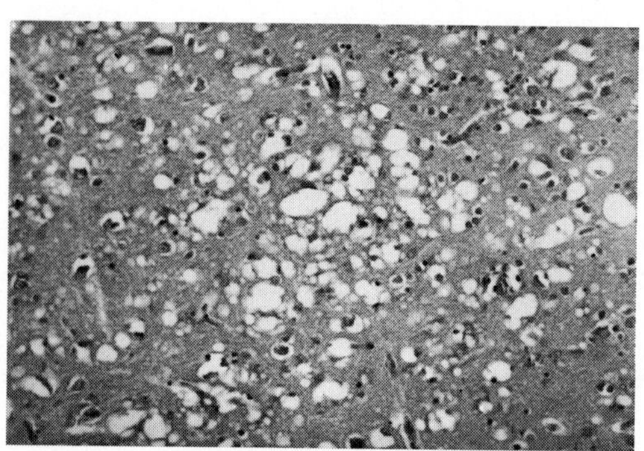

**Figure 10–1.** Spongiform change in the neocortex of a CJD patient. Small round vacuoles coalescing in places are seen. H&E; original magnification, ×30.

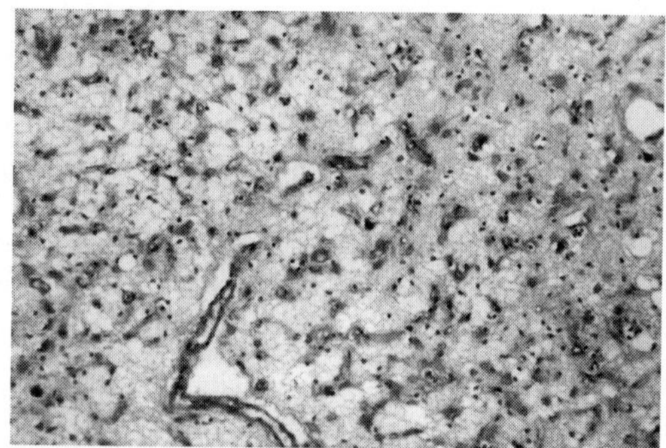

**Figure 10–2.** Status spongiosus in the cerebral cortex of a CJD patient. In this case most neurons are lost. There is marked rarefaction of the tissue and astrocytic gliosis. H&E; original magnification, ×30.

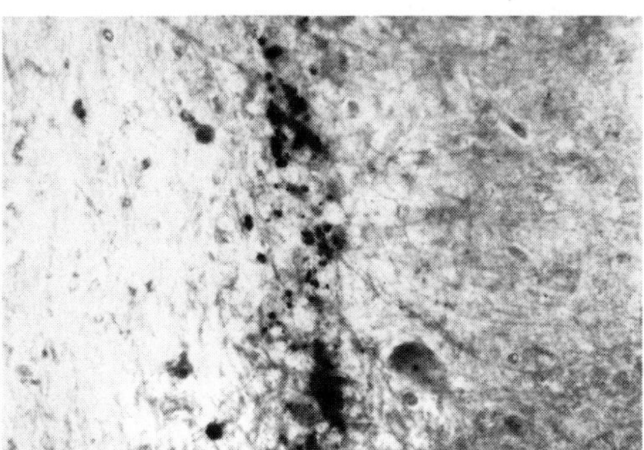

**Figure 10–3.** Granular deposition of prion protein in the granular cell layer of the cerebellum of a CJD patient. Immunohistochemistry with an antibody against PrP. Original magnification, ×10.

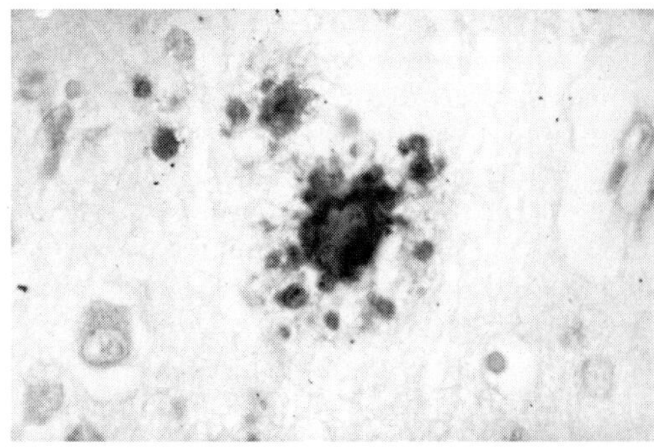

**Figure 10–5.** Multicentric plaque in the cerebral cortex in a GSS patient with a P102L mutation. Immunohistochemistry with an antibody against PrP. Original magnification, ×100.

cal layer in various disorders associated with cortical atrophy. Second, status spongiosus describes a condition in which the small vacuoles of spongiform change appear to coalesce, forming large multilobulated vacuoles. This condition typically is accompanied by severe astrocytic gliosis and pronounced nerve cell loss. It is, however, also observed in late stages of other neurodegenerative diseases and other disorders. Third, spongy degeneration with vacuoles in the perikaryon of neurons is rarely observed in human prion disease and is of low diagnostic value. It was, however, noted in early descriptions of the disease and is more often seen in prion disease of animals. Fourth, spongiform degeneration of the white matter has been reported in the "panencephalopathic variant" of CJD.[25] Although delicate spongiform change may be pathognomonic of CJD, other forms of spongiform degeneration are not.

Modern neuropathological diagnosis of human prion diseases is based on the use of antibodies against PrP combined with various tissue pretreatment regimens and immunohistochemical techniques to specifically detect $PrP^{Sc}$ in histological sections of the brain (for details, see Kretzschmar and associates[26]).

## NEW VARIANT CREUTZFELDT-JAKOB DISEASE

In 1996, a new variant of CJD (nvCJD) was described in 10 patients in the United King-

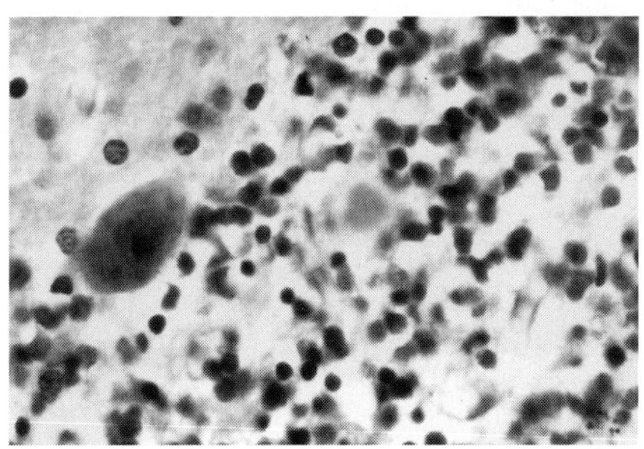

**Figure 10–4.** Kuru plaque in the granular layer of a CJD patient. H&E; original magnification, ×100.

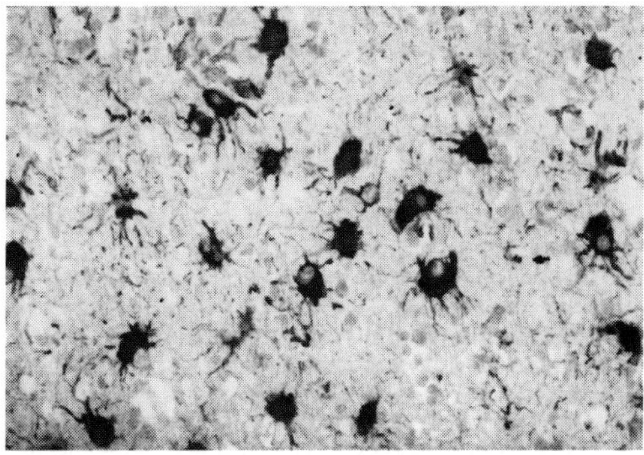

**Figure 10–6.** Marked astrocytic gliosis in the white matter of a sporadic CJD case. Immunohistochemistry with an antibody against GFAP. Original magnification, ×40.

dom.[13] These patients had a mean age of 29 years and presented with psychiatric disturbances such as depression and withdrawal. Signs more typical of CJD developed only later in the course. The electroencephalograms (EEGs) in these patients did not show typical changes. Pathological changes at autopsy were exceptional, showing extensive depositions of the prion protein in various areas of the brain in a fashion that hitherto had only been described in hereditary disease. In addition, there were "florid" plaques with central PrP plaques and surrounding vacuoles that had not been seen in human prion disease before.

None of the nvCJD cases carried a pathogenic mutation in the coding region of *PRNP*, and all patients were homozygous for methionine at codon 129, whereas in sporadic "classic" cases of CJD, PrP plaques are almost exclusively associated with valine at codon 129 of *PRNP* on at least one allele.[27–29] This finding, on the one hand, adds further evidence for the existence of a new disease phenotype and, on the other hand, underscores the importance of genetic studies in apparently sporadic cases of CJD. In addition to PrP plaques in the central nervous system, some lymphoid organs of the nvCJD cases showed PrP deposits, a finding thus far unseen in other human prion diseases.[30,31]

The hypothesis that these new cases might have been caused by the consumption of BSE-infected foodstuff was strengthened, albeit not proven, by several experimental findings. *(1)* Macaques intracerebrally infected with BSE showed pathological changes very similar to those of the new variant of CJD.[32] *(2)* The protease-resistant PrP derived from brain material of nvCJD patients was analyzed by immunoblot and showed a glycopattern that was not found in any other CJD case, but showed similarities to $PrP^{Sc}$ from BSE-infected cattle.[33] *(3)* Transmission of nvCJD to wild-type and transgenic mice showed incubation times and pathology indistinguishable from transmission studies with BSE, but dissimilar to transmission of various other CJD cases.[34,35] To date, 35 cases of nvCJD have been reported, but the magnitude of the number of people eventually succumbing to nvCJD can at present not be estimated.[36]

## THE HUMAN PRION PROTEIN GENE AND THE CELLULAR PRION PROTEIN

The human PrP gene *(PRNP)* is located on the short arm of chromosome 20 (20pter-12). It has a simple genomic structure and consists of two exons and a single intron of 13 kb in length. The entire protein-coding region or open reading frame (ORF) is located at exon 2.[37] All other known *PrP* genes in mammals and birds have a similar genomic structure, and the ORF is never interrupted by intronic sequences.[38–40] The degree of homology in the protein-coding region of the human gene with its mammalian counterparts is high on the amino acid level (nonhuman primates, 92.9% to 99.6%[41]; rodents, 91% to 92%[39,42]; ruminants, 92% to 93%[43,44]). This evolutionary conservation argues for an important function of the protein. Yet the cellular function of $PrP^{C}$ is still elusive.

The cellular human $PrP^{C}$ is a membrane protein mainly expressed in neurons but also in astrocytes and in a number of other cell types.[45–47] $PrP^{C}$ consists of 253 amino acid residues with two N-linked glycosylation sites at amino acids 181 and 197 and a disulfide bond between two cysteines at positions 179 and 214.[48] As formally shown in the maturation of hamster PrP, a signal peptide of 22 amino acids is cleaved off at the N terminus and a peptide of 23 residues is removed from the C terminus when a glycosyl phospholipid inositol (GPI) anchor is added to serine residue 230.[49]

Nuclear magnetic resonance (NMR) studies on a recombinant PrP ranging from amino acids 121 to 231 have shown that in this region there is a two-stranded antiparallel β-sheet (residues 128 to 131 and 161 to 164) and three α-helices (residues 144 to 154, 179 to 193, and 200 to 217).[50] Recent NMR examinations on full-length recombinant murine and hamster PrP have confirmed this structure C-terminally to amino acid 121, but have shown that the N terminus is flexibly disordered.[51,52] Yet other experimental approaches have defined the N terminus with its five octapeptide repeats as the copper-binding domain of $PrP^{C}$ *in vitro* and *in vivo*.[53,54]

## PATHOGENIC MUTATIONS

In families with inherited prion diseases, 16 different point mutations and 15 types of insertions have been described in the ORF of *PRNP* (Fig. 10–7; Table 10–3).). The insertional mutations are all situated in the N-terminal half of the protein in an octapeptide repeat region, whereas the point mutations cluster in the central and the C-terminal regions of the protein.

The frequencies of various pathogenic mutations in cases of inherited prion disease are not equally distributed. Some mutations share the major load of known patients and are generally associated with certain phenotypes. The P102L substitution is responsible for most of the GSS cases, the E200K mutation accounts for around 50% of familial CJD cases, and the D178N mutation is causative in most FFI cases and a considerable percentage of cases of familial CJD. Finally, the phenotypically highly heterogenous group of various insertion mutations accounts for a substantial proportion of cases of inherited prion diseases as well. The following sections discuss the known point mutations, following the PrP amino acid sequence from the N to the C terminus. The chapter closes with a discussion of the different insertion mutations.

## P102L

The proline (CCG) → leucine (CTG) substitution at codon 102 is the mutation most frequently associated with GSS. More than 30 families in countries of the Northern hemisphere have been described to date.[55] This was the first mutation to be formally linked to a human prion disease[56] and was

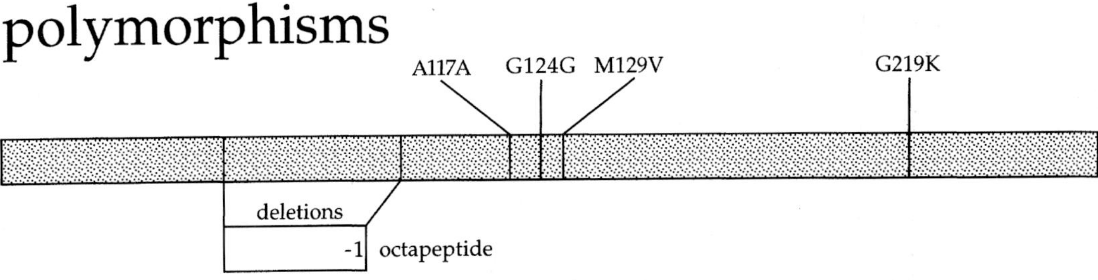


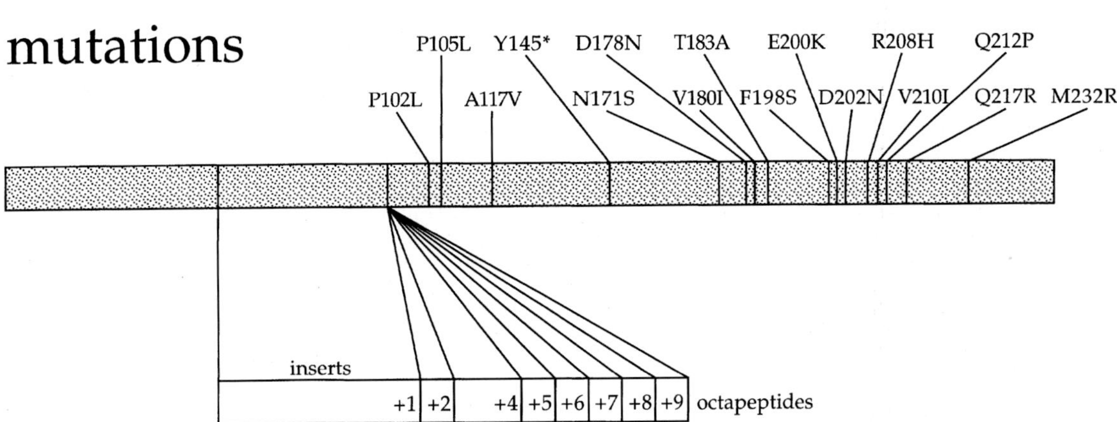


**Figure 10–7.** Polymorphisms and mutations of *PRNP*. The coding region of *PRNP* is denoted by shaded bars. The position of polymorphisms and mutations of *PRNP* are indicated. The single letter code is used for amino acids. The letter preceding the codon number represents the normal protein; the letter following the codon number represents the mutated allele. The asterisk at position 145 indicates a stop codon.

Table 10–3. ***PRNP* Mutations Associated with Inherited Prion Diseases**

| Location | Amino Acid Change | Reference | Genetic Linkage Shown | No. of Families | Traditional Name | Trans-mission Shown |
|---|---|---|---|---|---|---|
| 102 | P→L | Hsiao[56] | + | >30 | GSS | + |
| 105 | P→L | Kitamoto[63] | | 4 | GSS | |
| 117 | A→V | Doh-ura[67] | | 3 | GSS | |
| 145 | Y→* | Kitamoto[72] | | 1 Patient | GSS | |
| 171 | N→S | Samaia[75] | | 1 | Psychiatric disorder | |
| 178 | D→N | Goldfarb[78] | + | ≥7 | CJD | + |
| 178 | D→N | Medori[19] | + | ≥21 | FFI | + |
| 180 | V→I | Kitamoto[63] | | 4 Patients | CJD | |
| 183 | T→A | Nitrini[93] | | 1 | Dementia | |
| 198 | F→S | Hsiao[96] | + | 1 | GSS | |
| 200 | E→K | Goldgaber[100] | + | ≥50 | CJD | + |
| 202 | D→N | Piccardo[119] | | 1 Patient | GSS | |
| 208 | R→H | Mastrianni[120] | | 1 Patient | CJD | |
| 210 | V→I | Ripoll[121] | | 6 | CJD | nd |
| 212 | Q→P | Young[126] | | 1 Patient | GSS | |
| 217 | Q→R | Hsiao[96] | | 1 | GSS | |
| 232 | M→R | Kitamoto[63] | | 11 Patients | CJD | + |
| 51–91: inserts | | | | | | |
| +1×24 bp | +8 | Laplanche[138] | | 1 Patient | CJD | nd |
| +2×24 bp | +16 | Goldfarb[139] | | 1 | CJD | nd |
| +4×24 bp | +32 | Laplanche[138] | | 1 Patient | CJD | nd |
| +4×24 bp | +32 | Campbell[140] | | 1 Patient | CJD | nd |
| +5×24 bp | +40 | Goldfarb[133] | | 1 | CJD | + |
| +5×24 bp | +40 | Cochran[145] | | 1 | CJD | nd |
| +6×24 bp | +48 | Owen[129] | + | 1 | Dementia | |
| +6×24 bp | +48 | Nicholl[134] | | 1 | Dementia | nd |
| +6×24 bp | +48 | Oda[135] | | 1 | Dementia | nd |
| +6×24 bp | +48 | Capellari[136] | | 1 | Dementia | nd |
| +7×24 bp | +56 | Goldfarb[133] | | 1 | CJD | + |
| +8×24 bp | +64 | Goldfarb[133] | | 1 | GSS | + |
| +8×24 bp | +64 | Van Gool[141] | | 1 | Dementia | nd |
| +9×24 bp | +72 | Duchen[143] | | 1 | Dementia | nd |
| +9×24 bp | +72 | Krasemann[144] | | 1 | CJD | nd |

also found in the family originally described by Gerstmann, Sträussler, and Scheinker in 1936.[17,57]

The pathology of patients with this mutation is characterized by multicentric PrP plaques. Clinical signs are mainly of cerebellar origin, with ataxia as the most prominent feature. In all but one case the P102L mutation was found in coupling with methionine at codon 129. The one case with valine at this polymorphic position showed a very different clinicopathological presentation (very long duration of the disease, seizures, no spongiform changes), exemplifying the influence of the amino acid at codon 129 on the phenotype of an inherited prion disease.[58]

Aside from codon 129, the type of

protease-resistant PrP in the diseased brain correlates with distinct pathology as demonstrated in several cases with the P102L-129M haplotype.[59] Brain tissue from P102L cases was used for transmission of spongiform encephalopathy to small rodents[60] and primates,[9] thus clearly demonstrating the infectious nature of the genetic disease. Transgenic mice expressing the mouse gene with the genetically engineered P102L mutation developed a spontaneous neurodegenerative disease that was transmissible to other rodents (see also "Transgenic Animals" in "Experimental Studies").[61,62]

## P105L

The proline (CCA) → leucine (CTA) mutation at codon 105 was described in six patients in four families with GSS in Japan[63,64] and to date has not been identified elsewhere. Clinically, patients present with spastic paraparesis. Histopathology reveals PrP plaques in the cerebral cortex. Compared with GSS patients with the P102L mutation, plaques were infrequent in the cerebellum.[65] Transmission experiments by inoculating brain tissue from two cases with this mutation in small rodents were not successful or are still inconclusive.[66]

## A117V

An alanine (GCA) → valine (GTG) substitution at codon 117 was originally found in a French GSS patient.[67] This mutation has now been found in three families, but the lod scores are still too low for formal genetic linkage.[68] Clinically, the patients of two families present with dementia, and the term *telencephalic GSS* has been introduced to distinguish these cases from the ataxic form of GSS associated with the P102L mutation.[69] One patient of the third family with the A117V substitution clearly showed the ataxic phenotype, however, and also had numerous plaques in the cerebellum.[70] Another patient of one of the first two families had neurofibrillary tangles in various brain regions.[71] The cause for the different clinical and pathological presentations of GSS-A117V patients is not known.

## Y145*

In the Y145* mutation, the tyrosine codon 145 is replaced by an amber codon (TAG), resulting in a translational stop. Only one GSS patient, a Japanese woman, showed this mutation on one *PRNP* allele.[72] The patient presented clinically with an unusually long disease duration of over 20 years and progressive dementia.

Detailed histological and biochemical studies were performed on brain material from this patient and revealed a unique deposition of PrP in cerebral blood vessel walls in conjunction with tau protein–positive neurofibrillary tangles (NFTs) in neurons.[73] Therefore, the term *PrP cerebral amyloid angiopathy* (PrP-CAA) was proposed for this phenotype. Biochemical studies showed that the deposits are mainly composed of a 7.5 kDa fragment and that they bind antibodies directed against PrP epitopes between amino acids 90 and 147. In contrast to findings in F198S and Q217R,[74] in the Y145* mutation the wild-type as well as the mutant PrP seems to contribute to the deposits. Transmission studies with brain material from this patient have been unsuccessful.[66]

## N171S

The asparagine (AAC) to serine (AGC) substitution at codon 171 was reported in a Brazilian family with a high incidence of schizophrenic or schizoaffective disorders.[75] Yet this mutation was found in an unaffected family member and in a normal control of another CJD study as well.[76] At the moment, therefore, there is no formal proof of an association between the psychiatric disorder and this particular mutation in *PRNP*.[77] It remains to be seen whether this mutation is truly pathogenic and might lead to a considerable widening of the clinical phenotypes caused by mutations in *PRNP* or whether it is a rare polymorphism.

## CJD-D178N

The aspartic acid (GAC) → asparagine (AAC) substitution at codon 178 was first reported in a large Finnish pedigree of familial CJD.[78] Meanwhile, at least seven families of European origin with familial CJD and this particular mutation have been reported, and genetic linkage studies have been performed with two families.[79] One family of Flemish descent is of particular historical interest, as this family was the first in which the familial form of CJD was described.[5,6]

Clinically, the disease is characterized by early cognitive impairment, early disease onset, and duration longer than in sporadic CJD.[80] In addition, the periodic sharp wave complexes seen in sporadic CJD are typically absent in D178N patients. The neuropathological features are dominated by severe spongiform degeneration of the cerebral cortex, whereas no PrP plaques are identified. The infectivity of the brain material of several patients has been shown by transmission to primates.[80]

## FFI-D178N

A clinically and pathologically distinct entity, FFI has also been found to be associated with the D178N mutation.[19] Fatal familial insomnia is inherited in an autosomal dominant fashion, and genetic linkage with the D178N mutation has been shown for one family. At least 21 kindreds with this mutation and phenotype have been reported to date.[81] It is manifested clinically by progressive insomnia and pathologically by selective thalamic atrophy. FFI has also been successfully transmitted to wild-type and transgenic mice.[82,83]

The disease phenotype of the D178N mutation seems to be determined by a polymorphism at codon 129, which encodes either methionine or valine (see Fig. 10–7).[20,84] Valine at codon 129 of the mutant allele (D178N) is associated with familial CJD. Methionine at codon 129 in conjunction with the D178N mutation causes the FFI phenotype (Fig. 10–8). Patients with FFI homozygous for methionine at codon 129 show a more rapid progression of disease than heterozygous patients.[21] In CJD-D178N with homozygosity for valine at codon 129, the disease course is more rapid, and the age of onset is earlier.[85] Codon 129 on the mutant allele therefore specifies the phenotype of the disease, and on the normal allele it modulates the severity of each of the two phenotypes.

Biochemical analyses of the protease-resistant PrP in brain material from FFI and CJD-D178N patients revealed differences both in the relative abundance of glycosylated forms and in the size of the protease-resistant fragments,[86,22] yet the allelic origin of the protease-resistant PrP is exclusively the mutant allele for both diseases.[87] It was hypothesized that the combination of the mutation at codon 178 and the polymorphism at codon 129 determines the disease phenotype by producing two altered conformations of the prion protein. The NMR structure of recombinant murine $PrP^C$ showed a close vicinity of the residues at codon 178 and codon 129, suggesting a structural basis for the influence of the amino

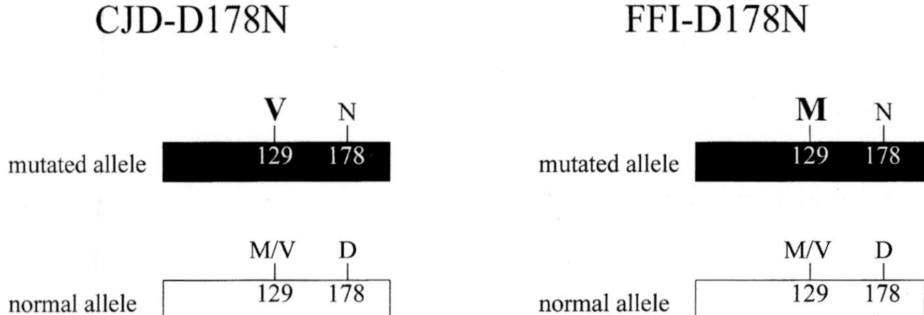


**Figure 10–8.** Genotype of CJD-D178N and FFI-D178N. The coding region of *PRNP* is denoted by bars. Both the normal and the mutated alleles of *PRNP* are shown. Amino acids at codon 129 and 178 are indicated with the single letter code. Codon 129 in the mutated allele, which codetermines the phenotype, is enlarged.

acid at codon 129 on the disease phenotype.[88]

Although it is indisputable that the FFI phenotype is found in most carriers with the genotype D178N-129M, there are recent publications about cases with the same genotype but a phenotype more reminiscent of CJD.[89–91] The reason for this phenotypical divergence is not clear, and it remains to be seen whether these cases are rare exceptions or again define a specific disease subtype.

## V180I

V180I is a very rare valine (GTC) → isoleucine (ATC) mutation; it has been described in only four Japanese patients with nonfamilial CJD.[63] One of the patients additionally presented with the M232R substitution.[92] Clinically and pathologically, these patients are very similar to those with sporadic CJD but do not show periodic synchronous discharges on EEG examination. The mutation was not found in 100 normal Japanese individuals, but the possibility that V180I is a rare polymorphism cannot be ruled out at present.

## T183A

A threonine (ACA) to alanine (GCA) substitution at codon 183 was found in a Brazilian family.[93] The predominant clinical sign was a progressive dementia that occurred early in life (mean age at onset of 44.8 years) and a long disease duration. Neuropathologically, severe spongiform changes but minimal gliosis were detectable in the cortical layers and the putamen. Yet the PrP immunoreactivity was restricted to the putamen and the cerebellum. If formally proven as an inherited prion disease by genetic linkage and transmission studies, the disease caused by the T183A mutation might well be termed a novel subtype of prion disease. The T183A mutation is the only point mutation in *PRNP* whose biochemical consequences for the cellular PrP are known, as one of the two consensus sequences for N-glycosylation is destroyed and therefore the glycosylation of $PrP^C$ is incomplete. This was in fact demonstrated in tissue culture as well as in transgenic mice.[94,95]

## F198S

In one large family with autosomally inherited GSS, the "Indiana kindred," a phenylalanine (TTC) → serine (TCC) substitution was described at codon 198.[96] This missense mutation was clearly genetically linked to the disease[97] and was in coupling with valine at codon 129. In affected members of this family, the wild-type allele of *PRNP* can carry either methionine or valine at 129, but for homozygous patients (F198S; $129^{Val/Val}$) the onset of disease is about 10 years earlier than for heterozygous patients (F198S; $129^{Met/Val}$).

The hallmark of the pathological phenotype associated with this mutation is PrP plaques in the grey matter of the cerebrum, cerebellum, and midbrain in close association with Alzheimer-type NFTs.[98] Clinically, these patients present with progressive ataxia and dementia. Biochemical analyses of the PrP plaques revealed a major component of 11 kDa stretching from residue 58 to around 150.[99] This protein does not contain the mutated amino acid residue. Nevertheless, with the help of the valine residue at codon 129 it was possible to show that only mutated PrP accumulates in the plaque-type deposits.[74] Inoculation of brain material from several patients into rodents and primates has hitherto not shown transmission of disease.[18]

## E200K

The most frequent mutation in inherited human prion diseases is the glutamic acid (GAG) → lysine (AAG) change at codon 200.[100] This mutation is the major cause of familial CJD and has been found in more than 50 families worldwide.[101] The largest known cluster is among Libyan Jews living in Israel, who have an incidence of CJD 100 times higher than the population worldwide.[102] Further clusters are known from Slovakia,[101] Chile,[101] Italy,[103] and France,[104] but CJD-E200K has also been found in Japan.[105] Originally, the higher incidence of

CJD in the Libyan Jewish population was thought to be due to the consumption of lightly cooked sheep brains or eyeballs,[106] but in recent years it has become clear that each CJD case in the Libyan Jews had at least one *PRNP* allele carrying the E200K mutation and that the E200K allele is genetically linked to CJD.[102,107] Five patients homozygous for E200K[102,108,109] are the only known patients homozygous for any of the pathogenic *PRNP* mutations. In their clinical courses, the homozygous patients did not differ from the heterozygous patients, suggesting that inherited CJD (at least CJD-E200K) is a true dominant disorder.

The penetrance of the E200K mutation was estimated as 0.56,[101] whereas all other *PRNP* mutations are thought to be fully penetrant (V210I might turn out to be yet another exception; see later). Closer inspection of the cluster within Libyan Jews using life table analysis revealed a penetrance of almost 100%.[110,111] It seems that this inherited disease may largely affect gene carriers of old age and that this may in fact be the difference from the other *PRNP* mutations. Most recently, the analysis of the Italian cluster showed a penetrance again of 0.6, and it was suggested that for CJD-E200K the penetrance is variable in clusters of different ethnic origin.[103]

In age distribution as well as in clinical manifestations and pathology, many cases of inherited CJD-E200K very closely resemble sporadic CJD.[105] These patients present with rapidly progressing dementia and have typical periodic synchronous discharges on EEG examination. Histologically, there are no PrP plaques in brain sections. Immunohistochemistry shows the synaptic type of PrP deposition.[112] PrP deposits have also been analyzed biochemically, and it has been shown that they consist of both the wild-type and the mutant protein, but only the mutant PrP contributes to the protease resistance.[113] Brain material from several CJD-E200K patients was injected into primates and the disease was successfully transmitted in most trials,[114] a finding that again is very similar to sporadic CJD.[115]

Recently, several reports were published that widened the clinical and pathological spectrum usually observed in CJD-E200K.[116] One patient from the Libyan Jewish cluster showed FFI clinically and pathologically but carried the E200K mutation and no D178N mutation.[117] Another patient, who was of French origin, presented, in addition to CJD, with a demyelinating peripheral neuropathy.[118]

## D202N

In a case of GSS that was clinically diagnosed as Alzheimer's disease, an aspartate to asparagine change at codon 202 was demonstrated.[119] Abundant PrP deposits were detectable in the cerebrum and the cerebellum, but spongiform changes were absent. Additionally, NFTs were present in the cerebral cortex. Due to the limited information on this case, it is currently not possible to state whether D202N is a truly pathogenic mutation.

## R208H

The arginine (CGC) → histidine (CAC) substitution at codon 208 was found in a patient with pathologically confirmed CJD but a negative familial history for a dementing disease.[120] Clinically and pathologically, the patient presented with characteristics of typical CJD. At present, it cannot be said whether R208H is causative, but this mutation has not been found in healthy control subjects.

## V210I

A more common point mutation in *PRNP* associated with familial CJD is the valine (GTT) → isoleucine (ATT) substitution at codon 210. This mutation was reported in one French and several Italian patients, two of them members of a family with a known history of CJD.[121,122] More recently, this mutation was also found in a Japanese patient and a Chinese family with CJD,[123,124] arguing for its worldwide occurrence. In one Italian family, two carriers of the mutation aged over 80 years are unaffected by CJD. This may indicate incomplete penetrance of this particular mutation. As with the E200K mutation, seemingly incomplete penetrance may be the sole recognizable effect of the late onset of this inherited disease,[110] but a detailed analysis requires a much higher patient number carrying this mutation.

Clinically and pathologically, the CJD-V210I mutation is indistinguishable from that of sporadic CJD. The biochemical characterization of brain material of CJD-V210l patients showed that both mutated and normal PrP contribute to its protease-resistant isoform.[125] With the notable exception of insertion mutations,[87] this is unlike most other *PRNP* mutations analyzed for this feature, where only the mutated protein was converted.[74,87,113] The reasons for this mutation-specific difference in the allelic origin of the protease-resistant PrP are currently not understood.

## Q212P

In one case of GSS, a glutamine (CAG) → proline (CCG) substitution at codon 212 was described.[126] There was no familial history of a dementing disease, but one related assymptomatic mutation carrier of old age was found. Clinically, an olivopontocerebellar degeneration was diagnosed, but neuropathologically PrP immunopositive deposits were seen and the immunoblot revealed protease-resistant PrP.[119]

## Q217R

Two GSS patients in one Swedish family show a glutamine (CAG) → arginine (CGG) mutation at codon 217.[96] The disease is very similar to the P198S phenotype ("Indiana kindred"). Neuropathology revealed massive PrP plaques in the cerebrum and the cerebellum and the presence of NFTs mainly in the cerebral cortex and several subcortical nuclei.[74] Yet another parallel with the F198S mutation is that only mutant PrP is converted to the protease-resistant isoform.

## M232R

A methionine (ATG) → arginine (AGG) change at codon 232 was reported in at least 11 Japanese CJD patients, most of them with no family history.[63] Therefore, it is still unclear whether this variant is a mutation with low penetrance or a rare polymorphism.[66] One patient carried the V180I variant, in addition to the M232R mutation, making it impossible to judge which mutation may have caused the disease.[92] The clinicopathological features of the CJD-M232R patients are very similar to those of sporadic CJD, and the disease was transmitted to mice.[127]

## Inserts

A completely different type of mutation in *PRNP* is the various insertion mutations on one allele of the gene. The normal protein carries five repeats (one nonarepeat, four octarepeats; amino acids 51 to 91) in this region, whereas the mutated proteins have between one and nine additional octarepeats (see Fig. 10–7, Table 10–3). In fact, the first mutation found in familial cases of CJD was an insertion[128] that subsequently turned out to have *six additional octarepeats.*[129] The same mutation was found in four families in southeast England, and it was demonstrated that all four families were part of one sibship dating back to the early nineteenth century.[130] Genetic linkage studies delivered a LOD score of around 11, demonstrating highly significant, tight linkage between the disease and this particular mutation.

The clinical and pathological features assigned to this mutation vary widely, ranging from patients presenting with classic CJD or GSS to patients with no morphological phenotype who only show progressive dementia.[131,132] A long-standing personality disorder followed by slowly progressive dementia seems to be the common denominator. The variable clinicopathological picture within this family was one of the major arguments for revising the traditional nomenclature of inherited prion diseases. The mutated allele in this sibship is in coupling with methionine at codon 129. The wild-type allele can have either valine or methionine in affected patients, but patients with methionine on both alleles have a significantly lower age at death.[130]

The order of repeats in the normal *PRNP* allele is R1, R2, R2, R3, R4, where R1 stands for the nonapeptide and R2 to R4 for the octapeptides (Table 10–4).[129] The octapeptides are identical on the amino acid level but have silent changes at the nucleic acid level. The mutated alleles in families with insertion mutations carry either additional R2 or R3 repeats or repeats that are not found in the normal allele and are named R2a, R2c, and R3g.[133] Again R2a, R2c, and R3g are identical to R2 to R4 on the amino acid level but show changes on the nucleic acid level. According to this nomenclature, the sibship from southeast England has the order R1, R2, R2, R2, R3, R2, R3g, R2, R2, R3, R4 (see Table 10–4).[129] Three further families with *six additional octapeptides* have been found, one of them in Britain,[134] one in Japan,[135] and the third in the Basque provinces.[136] Yet, the arrangement of repeats in all three families is different from that in the southeast England family, reflecting that they have evolved independently. Nevertheless, the clinicopathological pictures in those families are comparable to the southeast England family.

After the report on this family, a large survey of the CJD case collection of the National Institutes of Health (Bethesda, MD) showed three additional families with insertions of different size, that is, *five, seven,* and *eight additional octapeptides.*[133] Affected persons of all three families presented clinically with progressive dementia and were pathologically classified as either CJD (*five* and *seven additional octapeptides*) or GSS (*eight additional peptides*). Another case was reported with *four additional octapeptides,* but no indication of an inherited prion disease. This finding gave rise to speculation that a certain threshold of repeats has to be overrun to be pathogenic, as in trinucleotide repeat expansion diseases.[137] This hypothesis must be dismissed after reports on various patients with prion diseases carrying *one, two,* or *four additional octapeptides* on one allele of *PRNP.*[138–140] An insertion with *two additional octapeptides* was found in connection with a history of dementing illnesses in one family, indicating a true pathogenic mutation.[139] In contrast, the insertion with one and the two different insertions with four additional octapeptides were found in allegedly sporadic cases of CJD, but have not been found in the normal population to date.[138,140]

The disease phenotype in all of these cases with a low number of extra repeats is characterized by late onset and short duration of a progressive dementia, as in sporadic CJD. This is in contrast to the diseases

Table 10–4. **Inherited Prion Disease with Extra Repeats**

| ***PRNP* Allele** | **Reference** | **Order of Repeats** | | | | | | | | | | | | | |
|---|---|---|---|---|---|---|---|---|---|---|---|---|---|---|---|
| Normal | Kretzschmar[48] | R1 | R2 | R2 | R3 | — | — | — | — | — | — | — | — | — | R4 |
| Insertions | | | | | | | | | | | | | | | |
| +1×24 bp | Laplanche[138] | R1 | R2 | R2 | R2 | R3 | — | — | — | — | — | — | — | — | R4 |
| +2×24 bp | Goldfarb[139] | R1 | R2 | R2 | R3 | R2a | R2a | — | — | — | — | — | — | — | R4 |
| +4×24 bp | Laplanche[138] | R1 | R2 | R2 | R3 | R2 | R2 | R2 | R3 | — | — | — | — | — | R4 |
| +4×24 bp | Campbell[140] | R1 | R2 | R2 | R2 | R2 | R2 | R2 | R2 | — | — | — | — | — | R4 |
| +5×24 bp | Goldfarb[133] | R1 | R2 | R2 | R3 | R2 | R3g | R2 | R2 | R3 | — | — | — | — | R4 |
| +5×24 bp | Cochran[145] | R1 | R2 | R2 | R3 | R2 | R2 | R2 | R2 | R3 | — | — | — | — | R4 |
| +6×24 bp | Owen[129] | R1 | R2 | R2 | R2 | R3 | R2 | R3g | R2 | R2 | R3 | — | — | — | R4 |
| +6×24 bp | Nicholl[134] | R1 | R2 | R2 | R3 | R2 | R3g | R2 | R3g | R2 | R3 | — | — | — | R4 |
| +6×24 bp | Oda[135] | R1 | R2 | R2 | R3g | R2 | R2 | R3g | R2 | R2 | R3 | — | — | — | R4 |
| +6×24 bp | Capellari[136] | R1 | R2 | R2 | R2 | R2 | R2 | R2 | R2 | R2 | R3 | — | — | — | R4 |
| +7×24 bp | Goldfarb[133] | R1 | R2 | R2c | R3 | R2 | R3 | R2 | R3 | R2 | R3g | R3 | — | — | R4 |
| +8×24 bp | Goldfarb[133] | R1 | R2 | R2 | R3 | R2 | R2 | R2 | R2 | R2 | R2 | R2 | R2a | — | R4 |
| +8×24 bp | Van Gool[141] | R1 | R2 | R2 | R3g | R3 | R2 | R2 | R2 | R2 | R2 | R2 | R3 | — | R4 |
| +9×24 bp | Duchen[143] | R1 | R2 | R2 | R3 | R2 | R3g | R2a | R2 | R2 | R2 | R3g | R2 | R3 | R4 |
| +9×24 bp | Krasemann[144] | R1 | R2 | R2 | R3 | R2 | R3 | R3g | R2 | R2a | R2 | R3 | R2 | R3 | R4 |

caused by five or more extra repeats, which have an early onset and long duration.

Recently, more families with longer repeats have been described, one American family with *five additional octapeptides*, one Dutch family with *eight additional octapeptides* and one English and one German family with nine *extra repeats*.[141–145] The Dutch family again shows no clear genotype–phenotype relationship. The onset of disease varies between ages 21 and 54 years and the duration between 5 months and 6 years. Clinically, one patient presented with classic CJD, whereas most affected family members resembled the GSS phenotype. The two patients examined at autopsy showed GSS-type PrP deposits. In the Dutch family, valine at codon 129 was found, in coupling with the mutated allele. All other insertion mutations are coupled with methionine at codon 129, as far as this particular feature was analyzed.

Identical arrangements of octapeptides have never been observed in independent families, which indicates diverse origins of these extra repeats. The mechanism of the formation of extra repeats is thought to be unequal crossover and recombination.[133] To generate more than four extra repeats, more than one round of crossover would have been necessary. Both the diverse origin of the extra repeats and the probability of several rounds of recombination within one family suggest that the octapeptide region is genetically unstable. Yet the rarity of extra repeats in the population and the existence of one large family whose mutated allele has not changed over six generations[130] argue against this.

## POLYMORPHISMS

Aside from the pathogenic mutations in the *PRNP* ORF, several polymorphisms have been described that are found in CJD patients as well as in the normal population. Of high significance is the common polymorphism at amino acid position 129 (either methionine or valine), which has consequences for the occurrence of sporadic CJD and the clinical and neuropathological phenotypes of the sporadic and inherited types of the disease.

### Deletions

The postulated generation of insertions by unequal crossover implicates the simultaneous generation of repeat regions that lack one (or more) repeats. In fact, *PRNP* alleles with one missing repeat have been found in suspected and confirmed CJD cases as well as in the normal population.[146–148] Even in the publication of the genomic structure of the human *PRNP* gene, a *PRNP* allele with only four repeats was described.[37] Four variants with different locations of the deletion within the repeat region have been identified.[149,150] The deletion of one repeat is now generally considered to be a nonpathogenic polymorphism on around 0.5% of the *PRNP* alleles in the normal population, but it is not excluded that it might predispose to prion disease or affect the phenotype of other neurologic conditions.[150]

### A117A

The silent GCA → GCG change at codon 117 was detected as a *Pvu*II restriction fragment length polymorphism before pathogenic mutations in *PRNP* were identified.[151] The prevalence of this polymorphism in the normal population is about 5%. It is conceivable that the pathogenic A117V (GCA → GTG) substitution occurred on an allele carrying the GCG change.[68] Methodical problems arose through the fact that an additional polymorphism within the sequence of the standard primer 5' to the coding region (e.g., primer K, as reported by Hsiao and coworkers[56]) cosegregates with the silent polymorphism at codon 117.[152] Therefore, in the polymerase chain reaction with this or similar primers, the allele carrying the polymorphic codon (GCG instead of GCA) is amplified preferentially, and the other allele may be missed by the analysis.

### G124G

The silent GGC → GGG change has only been reported twice in conjunction with the Q217R mutation.[96] In the one patient analyzed in detail, it was shown that the silent mutation is not in coupling with the Q217R allele. It has not been found in the normal population. On the other hand, we have recently found three CJD patients with this silent mutation.[153]

## M129V

Frequently, a change from methionine (ATG) → valine (GTG) is found at position 129 of *PRNP*.[84] This common polymorphism clearly influences susceptibility to the sporadic and iatrogenic type of prion diseases and furthermore determines in part the phenotype of the sporadic as well as of some inherited prion diseases. The distribution of the different genotypes in the normal Caucasian population was determined in several countries and occurs in 37.5% to 45% homozygotes for methionine, 10% to 15% homozygotes for valine, and 40% to 51% heterozygotes.[28,154–158] Consequently, the allele frequencies are between 0.6 and 0.65 for methionine and 0.35 and 0.4 for valine in the different European and North American populations. The allele frequency in Japan is vastly different, with 0.96 for methionine and 0.04 for valine. Therefore, more than 90% of the Japanese population is homozygous for methionine.[159]

The difference in allele frequencies may be the cause of a dispute over the influence of homozygosity at codon 129 on the susceptibility to sporadic CJD. Several European studies have revealed a marked overrepresentation of homozygotes (mainly for methionine) at this position in cases of sporadic CJD compared with the normal population.[156,158,160,161] This was not the case in Japan, but a similar shift in distribution might be masked by the high incidence of homozygotes for methionine in the normal Japanese population.[162]

Patients, homozygous at codon 129 also show a higher susceptibility to iatrogenic CJD.[155,157,163,164] A French study showed that the heterozygous patients had a delay of 5 years in disease onset.[164]

Not only the susceptibilty to sporadic CJD but also the phenotype of the disease are influenced by codon 129. As originally found in Japan and now confirmed by two European studies, the appearance of PrP plaques in sporadic cases of CJD is almost exclusively associated with at least one *PRNP* allele carrying valine at position 129.[27–29] This finding turned out to be particularly important in the analysis of nvCJD, which is probably caused by ingestion of BSE-contaminated meat.[13] These patients showed PrP plaques as well, but all of them were homozygous for methionine at codon 129, which adds further evidence for a new disease phenotype. One important question concerns the pathological and clinical phenotypes in patients heterozygous or homozygous for valine at codon 129 and whether such persons are susceptible at all.[164–166]

Codon 129 is not the sole facor that influences the disease phenotype of sporadic CJD. As shown by Parchi and colleagues,[167] another important factor is the type of protease-resistant PrP.[167] $PrP^{Sc}$ types 1 and 2 differ in size by 2 kDa and, taken together with the 129 polymorphism, define six subtypes of CJD.[168]

Codon 129 influences the phenotype of some inherited prion diseases, as outlined earlier (see "P102L," "D178N," "F198S," and "Inserts"). In contrast, in CJD-E200K there is no detectable influence on the phenotype and course of the disease.[102]

## E219K

Recently, a glutamic acid (GAG) → lysine (AAG) change at codon 219 was found in the Japanese population with an allele frequency of 6%.[169] In sporadic CJD, heterozygosity at this position seems to serve as a protecting factor similar to codon 129 in the Caucasian population.[170] In inherited prion disorders, lysine at codon 219 has thus far only been found in coupling with P102L.[169] Four patients in one such family were analyzed in detail. Two patients did not present cerebellar signs, and the one patient autopsied showed only a small number of PrP plaques. Both findings are in contrast to the usual GSS-P102L phenotype. Therefore, a new variant of GSS with the constellation P102L and E219K was postulated. In the Caucasian population, the search for this polymorphism has been unsuccessful.[171]

## OTHER GENES AND LOCI

At present, there is no strong indication for the involvement of genes other than *PRNP* as a cause of or predisposing factor for human prion diseases. In humans, the apolipoprotein E (ApoE) gene allele ε4 was first identified as a risk factor for late-onset Alzheimer's disease (AD), where it acts as a dose-dependent modifier of the age of onset of disease.[172] The latter finding prompted several groups to examine the ApoE allele distribution in sporadic and inherited prion diseases. A study with French patients found a higher risk for CJD in humans with the ε4 allele and delayed death in carriers of the ε2 allele, which would be similar to the findings in late-onset AD.[173] These findings, however, were not reproduced in several studies in Japan, Germany, and the United States.[174–177] It was claimed that in the latter studies the choice of patients, with exclusion of familial cases and controls who were age matched, was more appropriate to address the problem. Recently, a small study in British CJD patients again did not detect a higher risk in carriers of the ε4 allele but found delayed onset in patients with the ε2 allele.[178] This was not confirmed by the study in the United States.[176] Conclusive evidence is yet to be given as to whether any ApoE allele has an influence on prion diseases, but it is likely that the potential effects will be subtle. Studies with large and very carefully selected patient samples are necessary to clarify this problem.

## EXPERIMENTAL STUDIES

The prion diseases are an area of intense experimental efforts ranging from the more traditional infection studies to highly sophisticated biophysical methodology. The experimental approach to the nature of the inherited types of disease has been mainly by transgenic studies and, more recently, by tissue culture studies. Transgenic technology has furthermore allowed insight into the phenomenon of the species barrier and the normal function of the cellular PrP ($PrP^C$) as well as the role of $PrP^C$ in disease pathology.

### Transgenic Animals

The nature of the species barrier was in the first instance examined by introducing the hamster *PrP* gene into the germline of mice.[179,180] These transgenic mice became readily susceptible to the hamster agent and produced the homologous type of agent when infected with material from either hamster or mouse.[181] The situation was more complicated when human *PRNP* was introduced into mice. Only after a chimeric gene with murine N and C termini and the central part of *PRNP* (codons 96 to 167) was expressed in transgenic animals did these mice become susceptible to human prion.[182] This data conflicts with findings of another group who succeeded in breaking the species barrier by introducing unmodified *PRNP* into mice.[183] More recently, a bovine *PrP* gene was introduced into transgenic mice, and these mice were shown to be much more susceptible to the BSE agent than were wild-type mice.[184] Unexpectedly, mice carrying a chimeric mouse/bovine *PrP* gene similar to the chimeric mouse/human mice[182] were resistant to the BSE agent.[184]

The exact requirements in the *PrP* sequence for the species barrier are currently not fully understood and may vary from one species-to-species transmission to another. Nevertheless, the transgenic animals carrying PrP of nonmurine species are precious resources for the understanding and diagnosis of human and animal prion diseases. This was highlighted by the study of Hill and colleagues[34] on the similarity of the nvCJD to the BSE agent.[34] Another study with transgenic animals (the mouse/human chimeras[182]) showed that characteristics in the immunoblot pattern and pathology of various human agents (FFI-D178N, CJD-E200K, or sporadic CJD) are mimicked after inoculation in those mice.[185] This finding supported the idea that different strains of prions are reflected by different conformations of the protease-resistant PrP.

The role of cellular PrP in the course of infection and its normal function was in part unraveled by destroying the murine *PrP* gene via homologous recombination (*PrP$^{0/0}$* mice). The three *PrP$^{0/0}$* mouse lines that were generated by different targeting strategies proved to be resistant to infection with mouse-adapted scrapie.[186–190] Therefore, the presence of the normally expressed PrP, PrP$^C$, is necessary for agent replication. Also, neuronal loss in prion disease seems to depend on the expression of PrP$^C$ as shown by two very different experimental approaches with either transplants of PrP-synthesizing mouse brain in *PrP$^{0/0}$* mice[191] or primary neuronal cultures derived from *PrP$^{0/0}$* mice.[192] In contrast, the normal function of PrP$^C$ has not been clarified. *PrP$^{0/0}$* mice are grossly normal, a finding that is quite surprising for a gene of high evolutionary conservation.[40] Several subtle phenotypes, however, have been detected. Electrophysiological examination of two of these *PrP$^{0/0}$* mouse lines revealed slight changes in hippocampal long-term potentiation and GABA$_A$ receptor-mediated responses.[12,193] These findings were not confirmed by other groups in one of the two *PrP$^{0/0}$* lines.[194,195] The role of PrP$^C$ in synaptic plasticity, therefore, appears to be debatable. More recently, two further phenotypes were reported. In two of the three *PrP$^{0/0}$* mice lines, there were subtle changes in the circadian rhythm,[196] and in the third line there was loss of Purkinje cells in aged animals.[190] The reason for this variation in the phenotypes of the different *PrP$^{0/0}$* lines is at present unknown.

On the cellular level, cerebellar neurons derived from *PrP$^{0/0}$* mice showed less resistance to oxidative stress, and a reduced activity of superoxide dismutase (SOD-1) was found in the brain tissue of *PrP$^{0/0}$* mice compared with wild-type mice.[197] As PrP is a copper-binding protein,[53,54] the concept of its involvement in the cellular copper metabolism and its influence on the activity of copper-binding enzymes such as SOD-1 is intriguing.

The most exciting data concerning inherited prion diseases was provided by experiments with mice overexpressing a murine *PrP* gene with a homologue of the GSS-P102L mutation (Tg[MoPrP-P101L]H). These mice spontaneously developed a neurodegenerative disease reminiscent of GSS.[61] Accumulation of protease-resistant PrP, however, was not found. The infectious nature of the generated disease was shown by serial transmission to hamsters (10% of animals) and transgenic mice expressing low levels of the mutated protein (40% of animals),[62] while the disease could not be transmitted to normal mice. Again, protease-resistant PrP was not detectable in the brains of any of the infected animals.

Although the successful transmission of the disease of Tg(MoPrP-P101L)H mice to some hamsters but not to normal mice remains puzzling, the transmission to mice carrying low copies of the mutated protein supports the idea that homologous protein–protein interaction favors transmissibility. This concept was strengthened by studies with mice overexpressing a mouse/human chimeric gene with the P102L mutation on *PrP$^{0/0}$* background. These mice became ill after a much shorter incubation time when infected with GSS-P102L material than when infected with material from a sporadic CJD case.[182] In addition, most of these mice became spontaneously ill late in life. A further reduction in incubation time and a highly synchronous onset of disease was achieved by crossing the Tg(MoPrP-P101L)H transgene on *PrP$^{0/0}$* background.[198]

It was reported in the same study that mice overexpressing the murine PrP gene with the E200K mutation did not develop any central nervous system disorder. Furthermore, transgenic animals with the T183A mutation in the *PrP* gene of the Syrian hamster did not develop a spontaneous disease, but showed a general mislocation of the mutated protein.[95] Some mice carrying *PrP* genes with other mutations (D178N and F198S) have been generated,[113] but data on long-term survival and potential spontaneous diseases is not availbable. Therefore, the recent findings on a transgenic mouse carrying a *PrP* gene with nine octapeptide insertions is of importance, as these mice developed a neurodegenerative disorder and showed some biochemical properties reminiscent of PrP$^{Sc}$.[199] It remains to be seen whether this disease is transmissible and therefore fully reproduces the disease phenotype of the Tg(MoPrP-P101L)H animals.

Astonishingly, the pathogenic potential of mutated *PrP* genes in transgenic animals is not restricted to the known human mutations. Two different sets of point mutations in the central part of the *PrP* gene (around A117V) gave rise to a neurodegenerative disease when transgenic animals expressed such genes.[200] A divergent topology of the mutated PrP molecules was proposed as a cause that might also be applicable to the generation of GSS-A117V. Large deletions in the C-terminal part of the *PrP* gene also led to fatal central nervous system illnesses,[201] as do large deletions in the N-terminal part spanning from amino acids 32 to 121 or 134.[202] The latter phenotype was only detectable on *PrP*$^{0/0}$ background and was rescuable by one allele of the normal full-length *PrP* gene.

To complicate the matter further, some transgenic lines overexpressing various normal *PrP* genes developed a lethal spontaneous disease late in life as well.[203] This disease was characterized by degeneration of the skeletal muscle and peripheral nerves, but also by spongiform changes in the brain. It was claimed that this disease may be transmissible, yet no protease-resistant PrP was found. To avoid potential confusion in discriminating between the disease caused by overexpression of normal PrP genes and the disease caused by a specific mutation in the same gene, some experiments are underway that employ gene replacement strategies.[204,205] In these experiments the endogenous murine *PrP* gene (*Prn-p*) was replaced in embryonic stem cells by *Prn-p* carrying the P101L mutation[204] or the human *PRNP* carrying the Y145* mutation.[205] It will be interesting to see what the consequences of these subtle changes are in regard to the normal function of PrP and particularly whether the generated transgenic animals will develop spontaneous prion disease.

## Tissue Culture Studies

Analyses of the expression of mutant *PrP* genes in cell cultures have shown promising results. The insertion of six additional octapeptides in the octapeptide repeat region of the murine gene and the subsequent expression in Chinese hamster ovary cells resulted in a protein that could not be released from the cell surface with phosphatidylinositol-specific phospholipase C (PIPLC) and that post-translationally acquired protease resistance.[206,207] Similar findings were also observed after the expression of the mouse *Prn-p* gene carrying point mutations corresponding to the P102L, D178N, and E200K mutations in *PRNP*.[208]

It was shown that the conversion of the mutant PrP to a protease-resistant isoform proceeds through a series of identifiable biochemical intermediates.[209] PrP molecules with the T183A mutation again acquired protease resistance, but additionally exhibited perturbated N-glycosylation and did not reach the cell surface.[94] Protease resistance and detergent insolubility are properties of PrP$^{Sc}$, which is part of the infectious agent; however, the degree of protease resistance of the mutant PrP molecules in tissue culture is at least 1000-fold lower than that of authentic PrP$^{Sc}$.[210] It has not been shown whether the expression of pathogenic *PRNP* genes in tissue culture results in the production of infectious prions. Other groups have published results that by and large confirm these findings, but show distinct differences that might be due to the different cell lines used.[211,212]

Expression of *PRNP* carrying the D178N mutation together with either valine or methionine at codon 129 (the CJD-D178N or the FFI-D178N constellation) in a human neuroblastoma cell line resulted in neither spontaneous generation of protease-resistant PrP nor abnormal association with the cell membrane. Instead, underrepresentation of the unglycosylated form of PrP was detected in these cells, which is reminiscent of the finding in brain material from patients with either CJD-D178N or FFI-D178N.[86,211] Mutant PrP molecules carrying the Q217R mutation showed increased aggregation and protease resistance compared with wild-type PrP[212]. The increased aggregation behavior of the mutant protein was reverted when the cells were incubated at low temperature, indicating an altered folding of the mutant PrP. Although studies in genetically manipulated tissue cultures cannot address all aspects of the disease process, they will most likely provide valuable insights into the cellular consequences of the expression of mutant *PrP* genes in a much shorter time than the transgenic approach.

## OUTLOOK

Human prion diseases constitute a group of rare, deadly neurologic disorders, with an incidence of approximately 1 case per 1 million people per year, of which 10% to 15% percent are hereditary and have a mutation of the prion protein gene. With the recognition that prion diseases can be familial and the description of a great number of mutations in the prion protein gene, it has now become possible to offer genetic counseling to affected families. In the wake of BSE and the worldwide scare of a possible transmission of this disease to humans, it is now mandatory to perform rigorous epidemiological studies in the human population. These studies must include genetic examinations to distinguish hereditary from sporadic cases and specifically to recognize possible new variants of the disease.

In quite a different way, prion diseases and in particular hereditary prion diseases offer the opportunity to study neurodegeneration and nerve cell death in animal models and cell culture systems with the ultimate aims of understanding the pathogenesis and divising therapeutic strategies. In addition, it seems to be clear that there are great similarities in the pathogeneses of many neurodegenerative diseases such as Alzheimer's disease, Parkinson's disease, and amyotrophic lateral sclerosis. Prion diseases are one of the best understood type of neurodegenerative disease today. They may therefore serve as a model to address many questions of pathogenesis and therapy in neurodegenerative diseases.

## SUMMARY

Prion diseases, or spongiform encephalopathies, are transmissible neurodegenerative disorders that have been observed in a great number of mammalian species. The outbreak of a prion disease in cattle (BSE) in the United Kingdom about 10 years ago and the appearance of a new variant of CJD in humans in 1995 have raised major public fears of a possible spread of BSE to humans.

The infectious agent of spongiform encephalopathies, termed *prion*, is thought to consist of an altered isoform ($PrP^{Sc}$) of a host-encoded protein ($PrP^{C}$). According to the prion hypothesis,[10,11] $PrP^{C}$ undergoes conformational changes in the infectious process that eventually enable it to confer the same changes to other $PrP^{C}$ molecules, a process that results in the perpetual generation of $PrP^{Sc}$ and thus the propagation of infection.

Human prion diseases can be sporadic or hereditary. They have also been transmitted iatrogenically and by ritual cannibalism. Prion diseases, including hereditary variants, are experimentally transmissible to mammals. Although the total number of inheritable prion diseases is small, they are of great interest scientifically, medically, and epidemiologically. More than ten point mutations and a great number of various insertion mutations of the human prion protein gene have been associated with hereditary human prion diseases (i.e., familial CJD, GSS, and FFI). These classic names may in the future be replaced by more specific terms that indicate the clinical picture and the specific mutation, such as GSS-P102L for a proline-to-leucine mutation at codon 102 of the *PRNP* gene.

Transgenic animals with a mutation of the prion protein gene have been shown to spontaneously develop a transmissible disease. Other transgenic animals are used for transmission experiments and as models of various aspects of the disease. Prion diseases nowadays may be the best understood neurodegenerative diseases and may therefore lead the way to understanding the mechanisms of cell death in neurodegenerative diseases.

## REFERENCES

1. Cuillé J, Chelle P-L: La maladie dite tremblante du mouton est-elle inoculable? C R Acad Sci III 203: 1552–1554, 1936.

2. Creutzfeldt HG: Über eine eigenartige herdförmige Erkrankung des Zentralnervensystems. Z Ges Neurol Psychiatrie 57:1–18, 1920.
3. Jakob A: Über eigenartige Erkrankungen des Zentralnervensystems mit bemerkenswertem anatomischem Befunde (spastische Pseudosklerose-Encephalomyelopathie mit disseminierten Degenerationsherden). Dtsch Z Nervenheilkd 70: 132–146, 1921.
4. Jakob A: Spastische Pseudosklerose, In Jakob A (ed): Die extrapyramidalen Erkrankungen. Springer, Berlin, 1923, pp215–245.
5. Meggendorfer F: Klinische und genealogische Beobachtungen bei einem Fall von spastischer Pseudosklerose. Z Ges Neurol Psychiatrie 128:337–341, 1930.
6. Kretzschmar HA, Neumann M, Stavrou D: Codon 178 mutation of the human prion protein gene in a German family (Backer family): Sequencing data from 72 year-old celloidin-embedded brain tissue. Acta Neuropathol (Berl) 89:96–98, 1995.
7. Hadlow WJ: Scrapie and kuru. Lancet 2:289–290, 1959.
8. Gajdusek DC, Gibbs CJ, Alpers M: Experimental transmission of a kuru-like syndrome to chimpanzees. Nature 209:794–796, 1966.
9. Masters CL, Gajdusek DC, Gibbs CJ Jr: Creutzfeldt-Jakob disease virus isolations from the Gerstmann-Sträussler syndrome: With an analysis of the various forms of amyloid plaque deposition in the virus-induced spongiform encephalopathies. Brain 104:559–588, 1981.
10. Prusiner SB: Novel proteinaceous infectious particles cause scrapie. Science 216:136–144, 1982.
11. Prusiner SB, Scott MR, DeArmond SJ, Cohen FE: Prion protein biology. Cell 93:337–348, 1998.
12. Collinge J, Whittington MA, Sidle KCL, Smith CJ, Palmer MS, Clarke AR, Jefferys JGR: Prion protein is necessary for normal synaptic function. Nature 370:295–297, 1994.
13. Will RG, Ironside JW, Zeidler M, Cousens SN, Estibeiro K, Alperovitch A, Poser S, Pocchiari M, Hofman A, Smith PG: A new variant of Creutzfeldt-Jakob disease in the UK. Lancet 347:921–925, 1996.
14. Masters CL, Harris JO, Gajdusek DC, Gibbs CJ Jr, Bernoulli C, Asher DM: Creutzfeldt-Jakob disease: Patterns of worldwide occurrence and the significance of familial and sporadic clustering. Ann Neurol 5:177–188, 1979.
15. Concerted Action of the EU: Surveillance of Creutzfeldt-Jakob disease in the European community. Minutes of the second meeting in Rome, July 3, 1993, and the third meeting in Paris, April 29–30, 1994.
16. Gerstmann J: Über ein noch nicht beschriebenes Reflexphänomen bei einer Erkrankung des zerebellaren Systems. Wien Med Wochenschr 78:906–908, 1928.
17. Gerstmann J, Sträussler E, Scheinker I: Über eine eigenartige hereditär-familiäre Erkrankung des Zentralnervensystems. Zugleich ein Beitrag zur Frage des vorzeitigen lokalen Alterns. Z Neurol 154:736–762, 1936.
18. Ghetti B, Dlouhy SR, Giaccone G, Bugiani O, Frangione B, Farlow MR, Tagliavini F: Gerstmann-Sträussler-Scheinker disease and the Indiana kindred. Brain Pathol 5:61–75, 1995.
19. Medori R, Tritschler H-J, LeBlanc A, Villare F, Manetto V, Chen HY, Xue R, Leal S, Montagna P, Cortelli B, Tinuper P, Avoni P, Moghi M, Baruzzi A, Hauw JJ, Ott J, Lugaresi E, Gambetti P: Fatal familial insomnia, a prion disease with a mutation at codon 178 of the prion protein gene. N Engl J Med 326:444–449, 1992.
20. Goldfarb LG, Petersen RB, Tabaton M, Brown P, Leblanc AC, Montagna P, Cortelli P, Julien J, Vital C, Pendelbury WW, Haltia M, Wills PR, Hauw JJ, McKeever PE, Monari L, Schrank B, Swergold GD, Gajdusek DC, Lugaresi E, Gambetti P: Fatal familial insomnia and familial Creutzfeldt-Jakob disease: Disease phenotype determined by a DNA polymorphism. Science 258:806–808, 1992.
21. Montagna P, Cortelli P, Avoni P, Tinuper P, Piazzi G, Gallassi R, Portaluppi F, Julien J, Vital C, Delisle MB, Gambetti P, Lugaresi E: Clinical features of fatal familial insomnia: Phenotypic variability in relation to a polymorphism at codon 129 of the prion protein gene. Brain Pathol 8:520, 1998.
22. Parchi P, Petersen RB, Chen SG, Autillo-Gambetti L, Capellari S, Monari L, Cortelli P, Montagna P, Lugaresi E, Gambetti P: Molecular pathology of fatal familial insomnia. Brain Pathol 8:539–548, 1998.
23. Zerr I, Bodemer M, Otto M, Poser S, Windl O, Kretzschmar HA, Gefeller O, Weber T: Diagnosis of Creutzfeldt-Jakob disease by two-dimensional gel electrophoresis of cerebrospinal fluid. Lancet 348: 846–849, 1996.
24. Zerr I, Bodemer M, Gefeller O, Otto M, Poser S, Wiltfang J, Windl O, Kretzschmar HA, Weber T: Detection of 14-3-3 protein in the cerebrospinal fluid supports the diagnosis of Creutzfeldt-Jakob disease. Ann Neurol 43:32–38, 1998.
25. Mizutani T, Okumura A, Oda M, Shiraki H: Panencephalopathic type of Creutzfeldt-Jakob disease: Primary involvement of the cerebral white matter. J Neurol 44:103–115, 1981.
26. Kretzschmar HA, Ironside JW, DeArmond SJ, Tateishi J: Diagnostic criteria for sporadic Creutzfeldt-Jakob disease. Arch Neurol 53:913–920, 1996.
27. De Silva R, Ironside JW, McCardle L, Esmonde T, Bell J, Will R, Windl O, Dempster M, Estibeiro P, Lathe R: Neuropathological phenotype and "prion protein" genotype correlation in sporadic Creutzfeldt-Jakob disease. Neurosci Lett 179:50–52, 1994.
28. Schulz-Schaeffer WJ, Giese A, Windl O, Kretzschmar HA: Polymorphism at codon 129 of the prion protein gene determines cerebellar pathology in Creutzfeldt-Jakob disease. Clin Neuropathol 15: 353–357, 1996.
29. Miyazono M, Kitamoto T, Dohura K, Iwaki T, Tateishi J: Creutzfeldt-Jakob disease with codon-129 polymorphism (valine): A comparative study of patients with codon-102 point mutation or without mutations. Acta Neuropathol (Berl) 84:349–354, 1992.
30. Hill AF, Zeidler M, Ironside J, Collinge J: Diagnosis of new variant Creutzfeldt-Jakob disease by tonsil biopsy. Lancet 349:99–100, 1997.
31. Hilton DA, Fathers E, Edwards P, Ironside JW, Za-

jicek J: Prion immunoreactivity in appendix before clinical onset of variant Creutzfeldt-Jakob disease. Lancet 352:703–704, 1998.
32. Lasmézas CI, Deslys J-P, Demalmay R, Adjou KT, Lamoury F, Dormont D, Robain O, Ironside J, Hauw J-J: BSE transmission to macaques. Nature 381:743–744, 1996.
33. Collinge J, Sidle KCL, Meads J, Ironside J, Hill AF: Molecular analysis of prion strain variation and the aetiology of "new variant" CJD. Nature 383:685–690, 1996.
34. Hill A, Desbruslais M, Joiner S, Sidle KC, Gowland I, Collinge J: The same prion strain causes vCJD and BSE. Nature 389:448–450, 1997.
35. Bruce ME, Will RG, Ironside JW, McConnell I, Drummond D, Suttie A, McCardie L, Chree A, Hope J, Birkett C, Cousens S, Fraser H, Bostock CJ: Transmissions to mice indicate that "new variant" CJD is caused by the BSE agent. Nature 389:489–501, 1997.
36. Ghani AC, Ferguson NM, Donnelly CA, Hagenaars TJ, Anderson RM: Estimation of the number of people incubating variant CJD. Lancet 352:1353–1354, 1998.
37. Puckett C, Concannon P, Casey C, Hood L: Genomic structure of the human prion protein gene. Am J Hum Genet 49:320–329, 1991.
38. Gabriel JM, Oesch B, Kretzschmar HA, Scott M, Prusiner SB: Molecular cloning of a candidate chicken prion protein. Proc Natl Acad Sci USA 89: 9097–9101, 1992.
39. Westaway D, Cooper C, Turner S, Da Costa M, Carlson GA, Prusiner SB: Structure and polymorphism of the mouse prion protein gene. Proc Natl Acad Sci USA 91:6418–6495, 1994.
40. Windl O, Dempster M, Estibeiro P, Lathe R: A candidate marsupial PrP gene reveals two domains conserved in mammalian PrP proteins. Gene 159: 181–186, 1995.
41. Schätzl HM, Da Costa M, Taylor L, Cohen FE, Prusiner SB: Prion protein gene variation among primates. J Mol Biol 245:362–374, 1995.
42. Oesch B, Westaway D, Wälchli M, McKinley MP, Kent SBH, Aebersold R, Barry RA, Tempst P, Teplow DB, Hood LE, Prusiner SB, Weissmann C: A cellular gene encodes scrapie PrP 27–30 protein. Cell 40:735–746, 1985.
43. Goldmann W, Hunter N, Foster JD, Salbaum JM, Beyreuther K, Hope J: Two alleles of a neural protein linked to scrapie in sheep. Proc Natl Acad Sci USA 87:2476–2480, 1990.
44. Goldmann W, Hunter N, Martin T, Dawson M, Hope J: Different forms of the bovine PrP gene have five or six copies of a short, G-C-rich element within the protein-coding exon. J Gen Virol 72: 201–204, 1991.
45. Kretzschmar HA, Prusiner SB, Stowring LE, DeArmond SJ: Scrapie prion proteins are synthesized in neurons. Am J Pathol 122:1–5, 1986.
46. Moser M, Colello RJ, Pott U, Oesch B: Developmental expression of the prion protein gene in glial cells. Neuron 14:509–517, 1995.
47. Manson J, West JD, Thomson V, McBride P, Kaufman MH, Hope J: The prion protein gene: A role in mouse embryogenesis? Development 115:117–122, 1992.
48. Kretzschmar HA, Stowring LE, Westaway D, Stubblebine WH, Prusiner SB, DeArmond SJ: Molecular cloning of a human prion protein cDNA. DNA 5:315–324, 1986.
49. Stahl N, Baldwin MA, Burlingame AL, Prusiner SB: Identification of glycoinositol phospholipid linked and truncated forms of the scrapie prion protein. Biochemistry 29:8879–8885, 1990.
50. Riek R, Hornemann S, Wider G, Billeter M, Glockshuber R, Wüthrich K: NMR structure of the mouse prion protein domain PrP (121–231). Nature 382:180–182, 1996.
51. Riek R, Hornemann S, Wider G, Glockshuber R, Wüthrich K: NMR characterization of the full-length recombinant murine prion protein, mPrP(23–231). FEBS Lett 413:282–386, 1997.
52. Donne DG, Viles JH, Groth D, Mehlhorn I, James TL, Cohen FE, Prusiner SB, Wright PE, Dyson HJ: Structure of the recombinant full-length hamster prion protein PrP(29–231): The N terminius is highly flexible. Proc Natl Acad Sci USA 94:13452–13457, 1997.
53. Hornshaw MP, McDermott JR, Candy JM: Copper binding to the N-terminal tandem repeat regions of mammalian and avian prion protein. Biochem Biophys Res Commun 207:621–629, 1995.
54. Brown DR, Qin K, Herms JW, Madlung A, Manson J, Strome R, Fraser P, Kruck T, von Bohlen A, Schulz-Schaeffer W, Giese A, Westaway D, Kretzschmar H: The cellular prion protein binds copper *in vivo*. Nature 390:684–687, 1997.
55. Young K, Jones CK, Piccardo P, Lazzarini A, Golbe LI, Zimmerman TR, Dickson DW, McLachlan DC, George-Hyslop PSt, Lennox A, Perlman S, Vinters HV, Hodes ME, Dlouhy S, Ghetti B: Gerstmann-Sträussler-Scheinker disease with mutation at codon 102 and methionine at codon 129 of PRNP in previously unreported patients. Neurology 45: 1127–1134, 1995.
56. Hsiao K, Baker HF, Crow TJ, Poulter M, Owen F, Terwilliger JD, Westaway D, Ott J, Prusiner SB: Linkage of a prion protein missense variant to Gerstmann-Sträussler syndrome. Nature 338:342–345, 1989.
57. Kretzschmar HA, Honold G, Seitelberger F, Feucht M, Wessely P, Mehraein P, Budka H: Prion protein mutation in family first reported by Gerstmann, Sträussler, and Scheinker. Lancet 337:1160–1160, 1991.
58. Young K, Clark HB, Piccardo P, Dlouhy SR, Ghetti B: Gerstmann-Sträussler-Scheinker disease with the PRNP P102L mutation and valine at codon 129. Mol Brain Res 44:147–150, 1997.
59. Parchi P, Chen SG, Brown P, Zou W, Capellari S, Budka H, Hainfellner J, Reyes PF, Golden GT, Hauw JJ, Gajdusek DC, Gambetti P: Different patterns of truncated prion protein fragments correlate with distinct phenotypes in P102L Gerstmann-Sträussler-Scheinker disease. Proc Natl Acad Sci USA 95:8322–8327, 1998.
60. Tateishi J, Ohta M, Koga M, Sato Y, Kuroiwa Y: Transmission of chronic spongiform encephalopathy with kuru plaques from humans to small rodents. Ann Neurol 5:581–584, 1979.
61. Hsiao K, Scott M, Foster D, Groth DF, DeArmond SJ, Prusiner SB: Spontaneous neurodegeneration

in transgenic mice with mutant prion protein. Science 250:1587–1590, 1990.

62. Hsiao K, Groth D, Scott M, Yang S-L, Serban H, Raff D, Foster D, Torchia M, DeArmond SJ, Prusiner SB: Serial transmission in rodents of neurodegeneration from transgenic mice expressing mutant prion protein. Proc Natl Acad Sci USA 91: 9126–9130, 1994.

63. Kitamoto T, Ohta M, Dohura K, Hitoshi S, Terao Y, Tateishi J: Novel missense variants of prion protein in Creutzfeldt-Jakob disease or Gerstmann-Straussler syndrome. Biochem Biophys Res Commun 191:709–714, 1993.

64. Kitamoto T, Amano N, Terao Y, Nakazato Y, Isshiki T, Mizutani T, Tateishi J: A new inherited prion disease (PrP-P105L mutation) showing spastic paraparesis. Ann Neurol 34:808–813, 1993.

65. Itoh Y, Yamada M, Hayakawa M, Shozawa T, Tanaka J, Matsushita M, Kitamoto T, Tateishi J, Otomo E: A variant of Gerstmann-Sträussler-Scheinker disease carrying codon 105 mutation with codon 129 plymorphism of the prion protein gene: A clinicopathological study. J Neurol Sci 127: 77–86, 1994.

66. Tateishi J, Kitamoto T: Inherited prion diseases and transmission to rodents. Brain Pathol 5:53–59, 1995.

67. Doh-ura K, Tateishi J, Sasaki H, Kitamoto T, Sakaki Y: Pro→ Leu change at position 102 of prion protein is the most common but not the sole mutation related to Gerstmann-Sträussler syndrome. Biochem Biophys Res Commun 163:974–979, 1989.

68. Tranchant C, Doh-ura K, Warter JM, Steinmetz G, Chevalier Y, Hanauer A, Kitamoto T, Tateishi J: Gerstmann-Sträussler-Scheinker disease in an Alsatian family—Clinical and genetic studies. J Neurol Neurosurg Psychiatry 55:185–187, 1992.

69. Hsiao K, Cass C, Schellenberg GD, Bird T, Devine-Gage E, Wisniewski H, Prusiner SB: A prion protein variant in a family with the telencephalic form of Gerstmann-Sträussler-Scheinker syndrome. Neurology 41:681–684, 1991.

70. Mastrianni JA, Curtis MT, Oberholtzer JC, Da Costa MM, DeArmond S, Prusiner SB, Garbern JY: Prion disease (PrP-A117V) presenting with ataxia instead of dementia. Neurology 45:2042–2050, 1995.

71. Tranchant C, Sergeant N, Wattez A, Mohr M, Warter JM, Delacourte A: Neurofibrillary tangles in Gerstmann-Sträussler-Scheinker syndrome with the A117V prion gene mutation. J Neurol Neurosurg Psychiatry 63:240–246, 1997.

72. Kitamoto T, Iizuka R, Tateishi J: An amber mutation of prion protein in Gerstmann-Straussler syndrome with mutant PrP plaques. Biochem Biophys Res Commun 192:525–531, 1993.

73. Ghetti B, Piccardo P, Spillantini MG, Ichimiya Y, Porro M, Perini F, Kitamoto T, Tateishi J, Seiler C, Frangione B, Bugiani O, Ciaccone G, Prelli F, Goedert M, Dlouhy SR, Tagliavini F: Vascular variant of prion protein cerebral amyloidosis with τ-positive neurofibrillary tangles: The phenotype of the stop codon 145 mutation in PRNP. Proc Natl Acad Sci USA 93:744–748, 1996.

74. Tagliavini F, Prelli F, Porro M, Rossi G, Giaccone G, Farlow MR, Dlouhy SR, Ghetti B, Bugiani O, Frangione B: Amyloid fibrils in Gerstmann-Straussler-Scheinker disease (Indiana and Swedish kindreds) express only PrP peptides encoded by the mutant allele. Cell 79:695–704, 1994.

75. Samaia HB, Mari JD, Vallada HP, Moura RP, Simpson AJG, Brentani RR: A prion-linked psychiatric disorder. Nature 390:241–241, 1997.

76. Fink JK, Peacock ML, Warren JT, Roses AD, Prusiner SB: Detecting prion protein gene mutations by denaturing gradient gel electrophoresis. Hum Mutat 4:42–50, 1994.

77. Samaia HB, Brentani RR: Can loss-of-function prion-related diseases exist? Mol Psychiatry 3:196–197, 1998.

78. Goldfarb LG, Haltia M, Brown P, Nieto A, Kovanen J, McCombie WR, Trapp S, Gajdusek DC: New mutation in scrapie amyloid precursor gene (at codon 178) in Finnish Creutzfeldt-Jakob kindred. Lancet 337:425–425, 1991.

79. Goldfarb LG, Brown P, Haltia M, Cathala F, McCombie WR, Kovanen J, Cervenáková L, Goldin L, Nieto A, Godec MS, Asher DM, Gajdusek DC: Creutzfeldt-Jakob disease cosegregates with the codon $178^{Asn}$ PRNP mutation in families of European origin. Ann Neurol 31:274–281, 1992.

80. Brown P, Goldfarb LG, Kovanen J, Haltia M, Cathala F, Sulima M, Gibbs CJ, Jr, Gajdusek DC: Phenotypic characteristics of familial Creutzfeldt-Jakob disease associated with the codon $178^{Asn}$ *PRNP* mutation. Ann Neurol 31:282–285, 1992.

81. Gambetti P, Lugaresi E: Conclusions of the symposium (FFI). Brain Pathol 8:571–575, 1998.

82. Tateishi J, Brown P, Kitamoto T, Hoque ZM, Roos R, Wollman R, Cervenáková L, Gajdusek DC: First experimental transmission of fatal familial insomnia. Nature 376:434–435, 1995.

83. Collinge J, Palmer MS, Sidle KCL, Gowland I, Medori R, Ironside J, Lantos P: Transmission of fatal familial insomnia to laboratory animals. Lancet 346:569–570, 1995.

84. Goldfarb LG, Brown P, Goldgaber D, Asher DM, Strass N, Graupera G, Piccardo P, Brown WT, Rubinstein R, Boellaard JW, Gajdusek DC: Patients with Creutzfeldt-Jakob disease and kuru lack the mutation in the PRIP gene found in Gerstmann-Sträussler syndrome, but they show a different double allele mutation in the same gene. Am J Hum Genet 45(suppl):A189–A189,1989.

85. Gambetti P, Parchi P, Petersen RB, Chen SG, Lugaresi E: Fatal familial insomnia and familial Creutzfeldt-Jakob disease: Clinical, pathological and molecular features. Brain Pathol 5:43–51, 1995.

86. Monari L, Chen SG, Brown P, Parchi P, Petersen RB, Mikol J, Gray F, Cortelli P, Montagna P, Ghetti B, et al.: Fatal familial insomnia and familial Creutzfeldt-Jakob disease—different prion proteins determined by a DNA polymorphism. Proc Natl Acad Sci USA 91:2839–2842, 1994.

87. Chen SG, Parchi P, Brown P, Capellari S, Zou W, Cochran EJ, Vnencak-Jones CL, Julien J, Vital C, Mikol J, Lugaresi E, Gambetti P: Allelic origin of the abnormal prion protein isoform in familial prion diseases. Nat Med 3:1009–1015, 1997.

88. Riek R, Wider G, Billeter M, Hornemann S, Glock-

shuber R, Wüthrich K: Prion protein NMR structure and familial human spongiform encephalopathies. Proc Natl Acad Sci USA 95:11667–11672, 1998.
89. McLean CA, Storey E, Gardner RJM, Tannenberg AEG, Cervenáková L, Brown P: The D178N (cis-129M) "fatal familial insomnia" mutation associated with diverse clinicopathologic phenotypes in an Australian kindred. Neurology 49:552–558, 1997.
90. Kretzschmar H, Giese A, Zerr I, Windl O, Schulz-Schaeffer W, Skworc K, Poser S: The German FFI cases. Brain Pathol 8:559–561, 1998.
91. Zerr I, Giese A, Windl O, Kropp S, Schulz-Schaeffer W, Riedemann C, Skworc K, Bodemer M, Kretzschmar HA, Poser S: Phenotypic variability in fatal familial insomnia (D178N-129M) genotype. Neurology 51:1398–1405, 1998.
92. Hitoshi S, Nagura H, Yamanouchi H, Kitamoto T: Double mutations at codon 180 and codon 232 of the PRNP gene in an apparently sporadic case of Creutzfeldt-Jakob disease. J Neurol Sci 120: 208–212, 1993.
93. Nitrini R, Rosemberg S, Passos-Bueno MR, Teixeira da Silva LS, Iughetti P, Papadopoulos M, Carrilho PM, Caramelli P, Albrecht S, Zatz M, et al.: Familial spongiform encephalopathy associated with a novel prion protein gene mutation. Ann Neurol 42:138–146, 1997.
94. Lehmann S, Harris DA: Blockade of glycosylation promotes acquisition of scrapie-like properties by the prion protein in cultured cells. J Biol Chem 272:21479–21487, 1997.
95. DeArmond S, Sanchez H, Yehiely F, Qiu Y, Ninchak-Casey A, Daggett V, Camerino AP, Cayetano J, Rogers M, Groth D, Torchia M, Tremblay P, Scott MR, Cohen FE, Prusiner SB: Selective neuronal targeting in prion disease. Neuron 19: 1337–1348, 1997.
96. Hsiao K, Dlouhy SR, Farlow MR, Cass C, Da Costa M, Conneally PM, Hodes ME, Ghetti B, Prusiner SB: Mutant prion proteins in Gerstmann-Sträussler-Scheinker disease with neurofibrillary tangles. Nat Genet 1:68–71, 1992.
97. Dlouhy SR, Hsiao K, Farlow MR, Foroud T, Conneally PM, Johnson P, Prusiner SB, Hodes ME, Ghetti B: Linkage of Indiana kindred of Gerstmann-Straussler-Scheinker disease to prion protein gene. Nat Genet 1:64–67, 1992.
98. Ghetti B, Tagliavini F, Masters CL, Beyreuther K, Giaccone G, Verga L, Farlow MR, Conneally PM, Dlouhy SR, Azzarelli B, Bugiani O: Gerstmann-Sträussler-Scheinker disease. II. Neurofibrillary tangles and plaques with PrP-amyloid coexist in an affected family. Neurology 39:1453–1461, 1989.
99. Tagliavini F, Prelli F, Ghiso J, Bugiani O, Serban D, Prusiner SB, Farlow MR, Ghetti B, Frangione B: Amyloid protein of Gerstmann-Sträussler-Scheinker disease (Indiana kindred) is an 11 kd fragment of prion protein with an N-terminal glycine at codon 58. EMBO J 10:513–519, 1991.
100. Goldgaber D, Goldfarb LG, Brown P, Asher DM, Brown WT, Lin S, Teener JW, Feinstone SM, Rubenstein R, Kascsak RJ, Boellaard JW, Gajdusek DC: Mutations in familial Creutzfeldt-Jakob-disease and Gerstmann-Sträussler-Scheinker's syndrome. Exp Neurol 106:204–206, 1989.
101. Goldfarb LG, Brown P, Mitrowa E, Cervenáková L, Goldin L, Korczyn AD, Chapman J, Galvez S, Cartier L, Rubenstein R, et al.: Creutzfeldt-Jakob disease associated with the PRNP codon 200 Lys mutation. An analysis of 45 families. Eur J Epidemiol 7:477–486, 1991.
102. Gabizon R, Rosenmann H, Meiner Z, Kahana I, Kahana E, Shugart Y, Ott J, Prusiner SB: Mutation and polymorphism of the prion protein gene in Libyan Jews with Creutzfeldt-Jakob disease (CJD). Am J Hum Genet 53:828–835, 1993.
103. D'Alessandro M, Petraroli R, Ladogana A, Pocchiari M: High incidence of Creutzfeldt-Jakob disease in rural Calabria, Italy. Lancet 352:1989–1990, 1998.
104. Chatelain J, Delasnerie-Laupretre N, Lemaire M-H, Cathala F, Launay J-M, Laplanche J-L: Cluster of Creutzfeldt-Jakob disease in France associated with the codon 200 mutation (E200K) in the prion protein gene. Eur J Neurol 5:375–379, 1998.
105. Inoue I, Kitamoto T, Doh-ura K, Shii H, Goto I, Tateishi J: Japanese family with Creutzfeldt-Jakob disease with codon 200 point mutation of the prion protein gene. Neurology 44:299–301, 1994.
106. Kahana E, Alter M, Braham J, Sofer D: Creutzfeldt-Jakob disease: Focus among Libyan Jews in Israel. Science 183:90–91, 1974.
107. Goldfarb LG, Korczyn AD, Brown P, Chapman J, Gajdusek DC: Mutation in codon 200 of scrapie amyloid precursor gene linked to Creutzfeldt-Jakob disease in Sephardic Jews of Libyan and non-Libyan origin. Lancet 336:637–638, 1990.
108. Hsiao K, Meiner Z, Kahana E, Cass C, Kahana I, Avrahami D, Scarlato G, Abramsky O, Prusiner SB, Gabizon R: Mutation of the prion protein in Libyan Jews with Creutzfeldt-Jakob disease. N Engl J Med 324:1091–1097, 1991.
109. Rosenmann H, Halimi M, Kahana E, Biran I, Gabizon R: Differential allelic expression of PrP mRNA in carriers of the E200K mutation. Neuron 49:851–856, 1997.
110. Chapman J, Ben-Israel J, Goldhammer Y, Korczyn AD: The risk of developing Creutzfeldt-Jakob disease in subjects with the PRNP gene codon 200 point mutation. Neurology 44:1683–1686, 1994.
111. Spudich S, Mastrianni JA, Wrensch M, Gabizon R, Meiner Z, Kahana I, Rosenmann H, Kahana E, Prusiner SB: Complete penetrance of Creutzfeldt-Jakob disease in Libyan Jews carrying the E200K mutation in the prion protein gene. Mol Med 1: 607–613, 1995.
112. Kitamoto T, Shin R-W, Doh-ura K, Tomokane N, Miyazono M, Muramoto T, Tateishi J: Abnormal isoform of prion proteins accumulates in the synaptic structures of the central nervous system in patients with Creutzfeldt-Jakob disease. Am J Pathol 140:1285–1294, 1992.
113. Gabizon R, Telling G, Meiner Z, Halimi M, Kahana I, Prusiner SB: Insoluble wild-type and protease-resistant mutant prion protein in brains of patients with inherited prion disease. Nat Med 2:59–64, 1996.
114. Brown P, Goldfarb LG, Gibbs CJ, Gajdusek DC:

The phenotypic expression of different mutations in transmissible familial Creutzfeldt-Jakob disease. Eur J Epidemiol 7:469–476, 1991.
115. Brown P, Gibbs CJ, Rodgers-Johnson P, Asher DM, Sulima MP, Bacote A, Goldfarb LG, Gajdusek DC: Human spongiform encephalopathy: The National Institutes of Health series of 300 cases of experimentally transmitted disease. Ann Neurol 35:513–529, 1994.
116. Korczyn AD, Chapman J: The varied manifestations of E200K Creutzfeldt-Jakob disease. In Court L, Dodet B (eds): Transmissible Subacute Spongiform Encephalopathies. Paris, Elsevier, 1996, pp417–419.
117. Chapman J, Arlazoroff A, Goldfarb LG, Cervenáková L, Neufeld MY, Werber E, Herbert M, Brown P, Gajdusek DC, Korczyn AD: Fatal insomnia in a case of familial Creutzfeldt-Jakob disease with the codon $200^{Lys}$ mutation. Neurology 46:758–761, 1996.
118. Antoine JC, Laplanche JL, Mosnier JF, Beaudry P, Chatelain J, Michel D: Demyelinating peripheral neuropathy with Creutzfeldt-Jakob disease and mutation at codon 200 of the prion protein gene. Neurology 46:1123–1127, 1996.
119. Piccardo P, Dlouhy SR, Lievens PMJ, Young K, Bird TD, Nochlin D, Dickson DW, Vinters HV, Zimmerman TR, Mackenzie IRA, Kish SJ, Ang L-C, De Carli C, Pocchiari M, Brown P, Gibbs CJ, Gajdusek DC, Bugiani O, Ironside J, Tagliavini F, Ghetti B: Phenotypic variability of Gerstmann-Sträussler-Scheinker disease is associated with prion protein heterogeneity. J Neuropathol Exp Neurol 57:979–988, 1998.
120. Mastrianni JA, Iannicola C, Myers RM, DeArmond S, Prusiner SB: Mutation of the prion protein gene at codon 208 in familial Creutzfeldt-Jakob disease. Neurology 47:1305–1312, 1996.
121. Ripoll L, Laplanche JL, Salzmann M, Jouvet A, Planques B, Dussaucy M, Chatelain J, Beaudry P, Launay JM: A new point mutation in the prion protein gene at codon 210 in Creutzfeldt-Jakob disease. Neurology 43:1934–1937, 1993.
122. Pocchiari M, Salvatore M, Cutruzzolá F, Genuardi M, Allocatelli CT, Masullo C, Macchi G, Alemá G, Galgani S, Xi YG, Petraroli R, Silvestrini MC, Brunori M: A new point mutation of the prion protein gene in Creutzfeldt-Jakob disease. Ann Neurol 34:802–807, 1993.
123. Furukawa H, Kitamoto T, Hashiguchi H, Tateishi J: A Japanese case of Creutzfeldt-Jakob disease with a point mutation in the prion protein gene at codon 210. J Neurol Sci 141:120–122, 1996.
124. Shyu WC, Hsu YD, Kao MC, Tsao WL: Panencephalitic Creutzfeldt-Jakob disease in a Chinese familiy—Unusual presentation with PrP codon 210 mutation and identification by PCR-SSCP. J Neurol Sci 143:176–180, 1996.
125. Silvestrini MC, Cardone F, Maras B, Pucci P, Barra D, Brunori M, Pocchiari M: Identification of the prion protein allotypes which accumulate in the brain of sporadic and familial Creutzfeld-Jakob disease patients. Nat Med 3:521–525, 1997.
126. Young K, Piccardo P, Kish SJ, Ang L-C, Dlouhy S, Ghetti B: Gerstmann-Sträussler-Scheinker disease (GSS) with a mutation at prion protein (PrP) residue 212. J Neuropathol Exp Neurol 57:518, 1998.
127. Hoque MZ, Kitamoto T, Furukawa H, Muramoto T, Tateishi J: Mutation in the prion protein gene at codon 232 in Japanese patients with Creutzfeldt-Jakob disease: A clinicopathological, immunohistochemical and transmission study. Acta Neuropathol 92:441–446, 1996.
128. Owen F, Poulter M, Lofthouse R, Collinge J, Crow TJ, Risby D, Baker HF, Ridley RM, Hsiao K, Prusiner SB: Insertion in prion protein gene in familial Creutzfeldt-Jakob disease. Lancet 1:51–52, 1989.
129. Owen F, Poulter M, Shah T, Collinge J, Lofthouse R, Baker H, Ridley R, McVey J, Crow TJ: An in-frame insertion in the prion protein gene in familial Creutzfeldt-Jakob disease. Mol Brain Res 7: 273–276, 1990.
130. Poulter M, Baker HF, Frith CD, Leach M, Lofthouse R, Ridley RM, Shah T, Owen F, Collinge J, Brown J, et al.: Inherited prion disease with 144 base pair gene insertion. 1. Genealogical and molecular studies. Brain 115:675–686, 1992.
131. Collinge J, Owen F, Poulter M, Leach M, Crow TJ, Rossor MN, Hardy J, Mullan MJ, Janota I, Lantos PL: Prion dementia without characteristic pathology. Lancet 336:7–9, 1990.
132. Collinge J, Brown J, Hardy J, Mullan M, Rossor MN, Baker H, Crow TJ, Lofthouse R, Poulter M, Ridley R, et al.: Inherited prion disease with 144 base pair gene insertion. 2. Clinical and pathological features. Brain 115:687–710, 1992.
133. Goldfarb LG, Brown P, McCombie WR, Goldgaber D, Swergold GD, Wills PR, Cervenáková L, Baron H, Gibbs CJ Jr, Gajdusek DC: Transmissible familial Creutzfeldt-Jakob disease associated with five, seven, and eight extra octapeptide coding repeats in the PRNP gene. Proc Natl Acad Sci USA 88:10926–10930, 1991.
134. Nicholl D, Windl O, De Silva R, Sawcer S, Dempster M, Ironside JW, Estibeiro JP, Yuill GM, Lathe R, Will RG: Inherited Creutzfeldt-Jakob disease in a British family associated with a novel 144 base pair insertion of the prion protein gene. J Neurol Neurosurg Psychiatry 58:65–69, 1995.
135. Oda T, Kitamoto T, Tateishi J, Mitsuhashi T, Iwabuchi K, Haga C, Oguni E, Kato Y, Tominaga I, Yanai K, Kashima H, Kogure T, Hori K, Ogino K: Prion disease with 144 base pair insertion in a Japanese family line. Acta Neuropathol 90:80–86, 1995.
136. Capellari S, Vital C, Parchi P, Petersen RB, Ferrer X, Jarnier D, Pegoraro E, Gambetti P, Julien J: Familial prion disease with a novel 144-bp insertion in the prion protein gene in a Basque family. Neurology 49:133–141, 1997.
137. Paulson HL, Fischbeck KH: Trinucleotide repeats in neurogenetic disorders. Annu Rev Neurosci 19: 79–107, 1996.
138. Laplanche JL, Delasnerie-Lauprêtre N, Brandel JP, Dussaucy M, Chatelain J, Launay JM: Two novel insertions in the prion protein gene in patients with late-onset dementia. Hum Mol Genet 4:1109–1111, 1995.
139. Goldfarb LG, Brown P, Little BW, Cervenáková L, Kenney K, Gibbs CJ, Gajdusek DC: A new (2-

repeat) ocatapeptide coding insert mutation in Creutzfeldt-Jakob disease. Neurology 43:2392–2394, 1993.
140. Campbell TA, Palmer MS, Will RG, Gibb WRG, Luthert PJ, Collinge J: A prion disease with novel 96-base pair insertional mutation in the prion protein gene. Neurology 46:761–765, 1996.
141. Van Gool WA, Hensels GW, Hoogerwaard EM, Wiezer JHA, Wesseling P, Bolhuis PA: Hypokinesia and presenile dementia in a Dutch family with a novel insertion in the prion protein gene. Brain 118:1565–1571, 1995.
142. Owen F, Poulter M, Collinge J, Leach M, Lofthouse R, Crow TJ, Harding AE: A dementing illness associated with a novel insertion in the prion protein gene. Mol Brain Res 13:155–157, 1992.
143. Duchen LW, Poulter M, Harding AE: Dementia associated with a 216 base pair insertion in the prion protein gene—Clinical and neuropathological features. Brain 116:555–568, 1993.
144. Krasemann S, Zerr I, Weber T, Poser S, Kretzschmar HA, Hunsmann G, Bodemer W: Prion disease associated with a novel nine octapeptide repeat insertion in the PRNP gene. Mol Brain Res 34:173–176, 1995.
145. Cochran EJ, Bennett DA, Cervenáková L, Kenney K, Bernard B, Foster NL, Benson DF, Goldfarb LG, Brown P: Familial Creutzfeldt-Jakob disease with a five-repeat octapeptide insert mutation. Neurology 47:727–733, 1996.
146. Laplanche JL, Chatelain J, Launay J-M, Gazengel C, Vidaud M: Deletion in prion protein gene in a Moroccan family. Nucleic Acids Res. 18:6745–6745, 1990.
147. Diedrich JF, Knopman DS, List JF, Olson K, Frey WH, Emory CR, Sung JH, Haase AT: Deletion in the prion protein gene in a demented patient. Hum Mol Genet 1:443–444, 1992.
148. Vnencak-Jones CL, Phillips JA: Identification of heterogeneous PrP gene deletions in controls by detection of allele-specific heteroduplexes (DASH). Am J Hum Genet 50:871–872, 1992.
149. Palmer MS, Mahal SP, Campbell TA, Hill AF, Sidle KC, Laplanche JL, Collinge J: Deletions in the prion protein gene are not associated with CJD. Hum Mol Genet 2:541–544, 1993.
150. Cervenáková L, Brown P, Piccardo P, Cummings JL, Nagle J, Vinters HV, Kaur P, Ghetti B, Chapman J, Gajdusek DC, Goldfarb LG: 24-Nucleotide deletion in the *PRNP* gene: Analysis of associated phenotypes. In Court L, Dodet B (eds): Transmissible Subacute Spongiform Encephalopathies: Prion Diseases. Paris, Elsevier, 1996, pp433–444.
151. Wu Y, Brown WT, Robakis NK, Kobkin C, Devine-Gage E, Merz P, Wisniewski HM: A *Pvu*II RFLP detected in the human prion protein (PrP) gene. Nucleic Acids Res 15:3191–3191, 1987.
152. Palmer MS, Van Leeven RH, Mahal SP, Campbell TA, Humphreys CB, Collinge J: Sequence variation in intron of prion protein gene, crucial for complete diagnostic strategies. Hum Mutat 7:280–281, 1996.
153. Weis J, Kretzschmar HA, Windl O, Podoll K, Schwarz M: Fatal spongiform encephalopathy in a patient who had handled animal feed. Lancet 348:1240, 1996.
154. Owen F, Poulter M, Collinge J, Crow TJ: Codon 129 changes in the prion protein gene in Caucasians. Am J Hum Genet 46:1215–1216, 1990.
155. Collinge J, Palmer MS, Dryden AJ: Genetic predisposition to iatrogenic Creutzfeldt-Jakob disease. Lancet 337:1441–1442, 1991.
156. Laplanche JL, Delasnerie-Lauprêtre N, Brandel JP, Chatelain J, Beaudry P, Alperovitch A, Launay J-M: Molecular genetics of prion diseases in France. Neurology 44:2347–2351, 1994.
157. Brown P, Cervenáková L, Goldfarb LG, McCombie WR, Rubenstein R, Will RG, Pocchiari M, Martinez Lage JF, Scalici C, Masullo C, Graupera G, Ligan J, Gajdusek DC: Iatrogenic Creutzfeldt-Jakob disease: An example of the interplay between ancient genes and modern medicine. Neurology 44:291–293, 1994.
158. Salvatore M, Genuardi M, Petraroli R, Masullo C, DAlessandro M, Pocchiari M: Polymorphisms of the prion protein gene in Italian patients with Creutzfeldt-Jakob disease. Hum Genet 94:375–379, 1994.
159. Doh-ura K, Kitamoto T, Sakaki Y, Tateishi L: CJD discrepancy. Nature 353:801–802, 1991.
160. Palmer MS, Dryden AJ, Hughes JT, Collinge J: Homozygous prion protein genotype predisposes to sporadic Creutzfeldt-Jakob disease. Nature 352:340–342, 1991.
161. Windl O, Dempster M, Estibeiro JP, Lathe R, De Silva R, Esmonde T, Will R, Springbett A, Campbell TA, Sidle KCL, Palmer MS, Collinge J: Genetic basis of Creutzfeldt-Jakob disease in the United Kingdom: A systematic analysis of predisposing mutations and allelic variations in the PRNP gene. Hum Genet 98:259–264, 1996.
162. Collinge J, Palmer M: CJD discrepancy. Nature 353:802, 1991.
163. Deslys J-P, Marcé D, Dormont D: Similar genetic susceptibility in iatrogenic and sporadic Creutzfeldt-Jakob disease. J Gen Virol 75:23–27, 1994.
164. Deslys J-P, Jaegly A, d'Aignaux JH, Mouthon F, De Villemeur TB, Dormont D: Genotype at codon 129 and susceptibility to Creutzfeldt-Jakob disease. Lancet 351:1251–1251, 1998.
165. Cervenakova L, Goldfarb LG, Garruto R, Lee HS, Gajdusek DC, Brown P: Phenotype–genotype studies in kuru: Implications for new variant Creutzfeldt-Jakob disease. Proc Natl Acad Sci USA 95:13239–13241, 1998.
166. McLean CA, Ironside JW, Alpers MP, Brown PW, Cervenakova L, Anderson RM, Masters CL: Comparative neuropathology of kuru with the new variant of Creutzfeldt-Jakob disease: Evidence for strain of agent predominating over genotype of host. Brain Pathol 8:429–437, 1998.
167. Parchi P, Castellani R, Capellari S, Ghetti B, Young K, Chen SG, Farlow M, Dickson DW, Sima AAF, Trojanowsky JQ, Petersen RB, Gambetti P: Molecular basis of phenotypic variability in sporadic Creutzfeldt-Jakob disease. Ann Neurol 39:767–778, 1996.
168. Parchi P, Giese A, Capellari S, Brown P, Schulz-Schaeffer W, Windl O, Budka H, Julien J, Kopp N, Poser S, Rojiani AM, Streichenberger N, Vital C, Zerr I, Ghetti B, Kretzschmar HA, Gambetti P:

The molecular and clinicopathologic spectrum of phenotypes of sporadic Creutzfeldt-Jakob disease (sCJD). Neurology 50:A336, 1998.
169. Furukawa H, Kitamoto T, Tanaka Y, Tateishi J: New variant prion protein in a Japanese family with Gerstmann-Sträussler syndrome. Mol Brain Res 30:385–388, 1995.
170. Shibuya S, Higuchi J, Shin R-W, Tateishi J, Kitamoto T: Protective prion protein polymorphisms against sporadic Creutzfeldt-Jakob disease. Lancet 351:419, 1998.
171. Petraroli R, Pocchiari M: Codon 219 polymorphism of PRNP in healthy Caucasians and Creutzfeldt-Jakob disease patients. Am J Hum Genet 58:888–889, 1996.
172. Corder EH, Saunders AM, Strittmatter WJ, Schmechel DE, Gaskell PC, Small GW, Roses AD, Haines JL, Pericak-Vance MA: Gene dose of apolipoprotein E type 4 allele and the risk of Alzheimer's disease in late onset families. Science 261: 921–923, 1993.
173. Amouyel P, Vidal O, Launay JM, Laplanche JL: The apolipoprotein E alleles as major susceptibility factors for Creutzfeldt-Jakob disease. Lancet 344:1315–1318, 1994.
174. Zerr I, Helmhold M, Weber T: Apolipoprotein E in Creutzfeldt-Jakob disease. Lancet 345:68–69, 1995.
175. Zerr I, Helmhold M, Poser S, Armstrong VW, Weber T: Apolipoprotein E phenotype frequency and cerebrospinal fluid concentration are not associated with Creutzfeldt-Jakob disease. Arch Neurol 53:1233–1238, 1996.
176. Chapman J, Cervenáková L, Peterson RB, Lee H-S, Estupinan J, Richardson S, Vnencak-Jones CL, Gajdusek DC, Korczyn AD, Brown P, Goldfarb LG: APOE in non-Alzheimer amyloidoses: Transmissible spongiform encephalopathies. Neurology 51:548–553, 1998.
177. Nakagawa Y, Kitamoto T, Furukawa H, Ogomori K, Tateishi J: Apolipoprotein E in Creutzfeldt-Jakob disease. Lancet 345:68, 1995.
178. Pickering-Brown SM, Mann DMA, Owen F, Ironside JW, De Silva R, Roberts DA, Balderson DJ, Cooper PN: Allelic variations in apolipoprotein E and prion protein genotype related to plaque formation and age of onset in sporadic Creutzfeldt-Jakob disease. Neurosci Lett 187:127–129, 1995.
179. Scott M, Foster D, Mirenda C, Serban D, Coufal F, Wälchli M, Torchia M, Groth D, Carlson G, DeArmond SJ, Westaway D, Prusiner SB: Transgenic mice expressing hamster prion protein produce species-specific scrapie infectivity and amyloid plaques. Cell 59:847–857, 1989.
180. Race RE, Priola SA, Bessen RA, Ernst D, Dockter J, Rall GF, Mucke L, Chesebro B, Oldstone MBA: Neuron-specific expression of a hamster prion protein minigene in transgenic mice induces susceptibility to hamster scrapie agent. Neuron 15: 1183–1191, 1995.
181. Prusiner SB, Scott M, Foster D, Pan K-M, Groth D, Mirenda C, Torchia M, Yang S-L, Serban D, Carlson GA, Hoppe PC, Westaway D, DeArmond SJ: Transgenetic studies implicate interactions between homologous PrP isoforms in scrapie prion replication. Cell 63:673–686, 1990.
182. Telling GC, Scott M, Mastrianni J, Gabizon R, Torchia M, Cohen FE, DeArmond SJ, Prusiner SB: Prion propagation in mice expressing human and chimeric PrP transgenes implicates the interaction of cellular PrP with another protein. Cell 83:79–90, 1995.
183. Collinge J, Palmer MS, Sidle KCL, Hill AF, Gowland I, Meads J, Asante E, Bradley R, Doey LJ, Lantos PL: Unaltered susceptibility to BSE in transgenic mice expressing human prion protein. Nature 378:779–783, 1995.
184. Scott MR, Safar J, Telling G, Nguyen O, Groth D, Torchia M, Koehler R, Tremblay P, Walther D, Cohen FE, DeArmond SJ, Prusiner SB: Identification of a prion protein epitope modulating transmission of bovine spongiform encephalopathy prions to transgenic mice. Proc Natl Acad Sci USA 94:14279–14284, 1997.
185. Telling GC, Parchi P, DeArmond SJ, Cortelli P, Montagna P, Gabizon R, Mastrianni J, Lugaresi E, Gambetti P, Prusiner SB: Evidence for the conformation of the pathologic isoform of the prion protein enciphering and propagating prion diversity. Science 274:2079–2082, 1996.
186. Büeler H, Fischer M, Lang Y, Bluethmann H, Lipp H-P, DeArmond SJ, Prusiner SB, Aguet M, Weissmann C: Normal development and behaviour of mice lacking the neuronal cell-surface PrP protein. Nature 356:577–582, 1992.
187. Büeler H, Aguzzi A, Sailer A, Greiner RA, Autenried P, Aguet M, Weissmann C: Mice devoid of PrP are resistant to scrapie. Cell 73:1339–1348, 1993.
188. Manson JC, Clarke AR, Hooper ML, Aitchison L, McConnell I, Hope J: 129/Ola mice carrying a null mutation in PrP that abolishes mRNA production are developmentally normal. Mol Neurobiol 8:121–127, 1994.
189. Manson JC, Clarke AR, McBride PA, McConnell I, Hope J: PrP gene dosage determines the timing but not the final intensity or distribution of lesions in scrapie pathology. Neurodegeneration 3: 331–340, 1994.
190. Sakaguchi S, Katamine S, Nishida N, Moriuchi R, Shigematsu K, Sugimoto T, Nakatani A, Kataoka Y, Houtani T, Shirabe S, Okada H, Hasegawa S, Miyamoto T, Noda T: Loss of cerebellar Purkinje cells in aged mice homozygous for a disrupted PrP gene. Nature 380:528–531, 1996.
191. Brandner S, Isenmann S, Raeber A, Fischer M, Sailer A, Kobayashi Y, Marino S, Weissmann C, Aguzzi A: Normal host prion protein necessary for scrapie-induced neurotoxicity. Nature 379:339–343, 1996.
192. Brown DR, Schmidt B, Kretzschmar HA: Role of microglia and host prion protein in neurotoxicity of prion protein fragment. Nature 380:345–347, 1996.
193. Manson JC, Hope J, Clarke AR, Johnston A, Black C, MacLeod N: PrP gene dosage and long term potentiation. Neurodegeneration 4:113–115, 1995.
194. Herms JW, Kretzschmar HA, Titz S, Keller BU: Patch-clamp analysis of synaptic transmission to cerebellar Purkinje cells of prion protein knockout mice. Eur J Neurosci 7:2508–2512, 1995.

195. Lledo PM, Tremblay P, DeArmond SJ, Prusiner SB, Nicoll RA: Mice deficient for prion protein exhibit normal neuronal excitability and synaptic transmission in the hippocampus. Proc Natl Acad Sci USA 93:2403–2407, 1996.
196. Tobler I, Gaus SE, Deboer T, Achermann P, Fischer M, Rülicke T, Moser M, Oesch B, McBride PA, Manson JC: Altered circadian activity rhythms and sleep in mice devoid of prion protein. Nature 380:639–642, 1996.
197. Brown DR, Schulz-Schaeffer WJ, Schmidt B, Kretzschmar HA: Prion protein–deficient cells show altered response to oxidative stress due to decreased SOD-1 activity. Exp Neurol 146:104–112, 1997.
198. Telling GC, Haga T, Torchia M, Tremblay P, DeArmond SJ, Prusiner SB: Interactions between wild-type and mutant prion proteins modulate neurodegeneration in transgenic mice. Genes Dev 10:1736–1750, 1996.
199. Chiesa R, Piccardo P, Ghetti B, Harris DA: Neurological illness in transgenic mice expressing a prion protein with an insertional mutation. Neuron 21:1339–1351, 1999.
200. Hedge RS, Mastrianni JA, Scott MR, DeFea KA, Tremblay P, Torchia M, DeArmond SJ, Prusiner SB, Lingappa VR: A transmembrane form of the prion protein in neurodegenerative disease. Science 279:827–834, 1998.
201. Muramoto T, DeArmond SJ, Scott M, Telling GC, Cohen FE, Prusiner SB: Heritable disorder resembling neuronal storage disease in mice expressing prion protein with deletion of an a-helix. Nat Med. 3:750–755, 1997.
202. Shmerling D, Hegyi I, Fischer M, Blättler T, Brandner S, Götz J, Rülicke T, Flechsig E, Cozzio A, von Mering C, Hangartner C, Aguzzi A, Weissmann C: Expression of amino-terminally truncated PrP in the mouse leading to ataxia and specific cerebellar lesions. Cell 93:203–214, 1998.
203. Westaway D, DeArmond SJ, Cayetano-Canlas J, Groth D, Foster D, Yang SL, Torchia M, Carlson GA, Prusiner SB: Degeneration of skeletal muscle, peripheral nerves, and the central nervous system in transgenic mice overexpressing wild-type prion proteins. Cell 76:117–129, 1994.
204. Moore RC, Redhead NJ, Selfridge J, Hope J, Manson JC, Melton DW: Double replacement gene targeting for the production of a series of mouse strains with different prion protein gene alterations. Bio-Technology 13:999–1004, 1995.
205. Kitamoto T, Nakamura K, Nakao K, Shibuya S, Shin R-W, Gondo Y, Katsuki M, Tateishi J: Humanized prion protein knock-in by cre-induced site-specific recombination in the mouse. Biochem Biophys Res Commun 222:742–747, 1996.
206. Lehmann S, Harris DA: A mutant prion protein displays an aberrant membrane association when expressed in cultured cells. J Biol Chem 270: 24589–24597, 1995.
207. Lehmann S, Harris DA: Two mutant prion proteins expressed in cultured cells acquire biochemical properties reminiscent of the scrapie isoform. Proc Natl Acad Sci USA 93:5610–5614, 1996.
208. Lehmann S, Harris DA: Mutant and infectious prion proteins display common biochemical properties in cultured cells. J Biol Chem 271: 1633–1637, 1996.
209. Daude N, Lehmann S, Harris DA: Identification of intermediate steps in the conversion of mutant prion protein to a scrapie-like form in cultured cells. J Biol Chem 272:11604–11612, 1997.
210. Priola SA, Chesebro B: Abnormal properties of prion protein with insertional mutations in different cell types. J Biol Chem 273:11980–11985, 1998.
211. Petersen RB, Parchi P, Richardson SL, Urig CB, Gambetti P: Effect of the D178N mutation and the codon 129 polymorphism on the metabolism of the prion protein. J Biol Chem 271:12661–12668, 1996.
212. Singh N, Zanusso G, Chen SG, Fujioka H, Richardson S, Gambetti P, Petersen RB: Prion protein aggregation reverted by low temperature in transfected cells carrying a prion protein gene mutation. J Biol Chem 272:28461–28470, 1997.

# Chapter 11

# HEREDITARY SPASTIC PARAPLEGIA

Marie-Pierre Dubé, PhD
Guy A. Rouleau, MD, PhD



Hereditary spastic paraplegia (HSP) (also known as familial spastic paraparesis and Strumpell-Lorrain syndrome) is defined by progressive weakness and spasticity of the lower limbs.[1–3] The disease comprises clinically and genetically diverse disorders, classified according to the mode of inheritance and based on whether progressive spasticity occurs in isolation, referred to as *pure* or *uncomplicated* HSP, or in combination with other neurologic abnormalities, referred to as *complicated* HSP. Features associated with complicated HSP include optic neuropathy, retinopathy, extrapyramidal disturbance, dementia, ataxia, ichthyosis, mental retardation, and deafness. Genetic studies of HSP focus on the identification of mutant genes responsible for disease expression.

It is now clear that HSP is a genetically heterogeneous set of disorders. Seven gene loci have been identified that cause pure HSP. Four have been identified in autosomal dominant HSP, two in autosomal recessive HSP, and mutations in the proteolipid protein (*PLP*) gene have been identified in X-linked HSP kindreds. The complicated forms of HSP are diverse, and, although some have been linked to loci responsible for pure HSP, it is likely that they are caused by several different gene mutations. Two complicated HSP loci have been reported; one for autosomal dominant complicated HSP was linked to markers on chromosome 10q, and a mutation in the X-linked L1CAM gene was reported. The clinical and pathological features of HSP, are reviewed in the following sections, and the advances in genetic research of uncomplicated HSP are outlined.

## CLINICAL AND NEUROPATHOLOGICAL FEATURES

HSP is clinically characterized by slow, upwardly progressive spastic weakness of the lower limbs (reviewed in 1993 by Harding[1]) Subjects develop leg stiffness and progressive gait disturbance due to difficulty with foot dorsiflexion and weakness of hip flexion. The majority of patients have onset of symptoms in the second through fourth decades of life, but the onset can occur anywhere from infancy through age 85 years. After onset, locomotion becomes gradually but progressively more impaired. Frequently, urinary urgency progresses to urinary incontinence as a late manifestation of HSP.

Neurologic examination shows the cranial nerves and fundi to be normal. The jaw jerk reflex may be brisk in older subjects, but there is no evidence of corticobulbar tract dysfunction. There are no abnormalities in upper extremity muscle tone and strength. Muscle tone, however, is increased at the hamstrings, quadriceps, and ankles in the lower extremities. Weakness is most notable at the iliopsoas, tibialis anterior, and, to a lesser extent, hamstring muscles. Muscle wasting is rare in uncomplicated HSP; however, atrophy of lower leg musculature has been observed in wheelchair-dependent elderly patients. Occasionally, there is decreased perception of pin prick pain below the knees, and vibratory sensation is often diminished in the distal lower extremities. Deep tendon reflexes may be brisk in the upper extremities, but are pathologically increased in the lower extremities. Hoffman's and Tromner's signs are often observed, and pes cavus is generally present and prominent in older subjects.

The major neuropathological feature of HSP is axonal degeneration, which is maximal in the terminal portions of the longest descending and ascending tracts. The crossed and uncrossed corticospinal tracts to the legs, fasciculus gracilis, and, to a lesser extent, spinocerebellar fibers are specifically involved. Mild loss of anterior horn cells may occur.

Electrophysiological studies of the peripheral and central nervous systems are useful in the evaluation of HSP. Subclinical sensory deficits are common in HSP and may involve peripheral nerves, spinal pathways, or both.[4] Somatosensory evoked potentials from the lower limbs may show conduction delay in dorsal column fibers. Cortical evoked potentials show reduced conduction velocity and amplitude in muscles innervated by lumbar spinal segments. Although the cortical evoked potentials show variable results, they suggest that there is loss of corticospinal tract axons reaching the lumbar spinal cord and that the remaining axons conduct more slowly.[5]

The presence or absence of associated deficits (such as ataxia, retinitis pigmentosa, peripheral neuropathy, amyotrophy, and extrapyramidal signs) is the basis for classifying HSP as uncomplicated or complicated. The diagnosis of uncomplicated HSP is generally one of exclusion. The diagnostic criteria for HSP were recently reviewed, and recommendations are presented by Fink and coworkers[6] (Table 11–1).

## GENETIC ASPECTS

Genetic penetrance is the frequency with which obligate HSP gene carriers exhibit the disorder. In HSP, penetrance is age dependent and nearly complete. Segregation ratios in large, autosomal dominant HSP kindreds approach 0.5, as predicted for completely penetrant dominant disorders. An exception, however, has been reported in an autosomal dominant uncomplicated HSP kindred in which a subject is apparently an asymptomatic carrier, past the typical age of onset for this family.[7] It is important to note that the apparently high degree of genetic penetrance of HSP may include an ascertainment bias, as autosomal dominant HSP is more readily diagnosed in large kindreds for whom the disorder is highly penetrant. This could contribute to an overrepresentation of highly penetrant HSP kindreds in published studies. Thus, there may be less penetrant forms of HSP that may be unrecognized or perhaps misdiagosed.

Age of onset is variable between and within families and ranges from early childhood to late adulthood. It was originally proposed by Harding,[1] in a study involving 19 families with "pure" autosomal dominant HSP, that two forms of the disease could be distinguished according to age of onset. As such, autosomal dominant uncomplicated HSP was referred to as type I, in which onset occurs before age 35 years, with spasticity, exceeding weakness, and slow progression; and type II, in which onset occurs after age 35 years and patients have weakness in addition to spasticity, mild distal sensory loss, urinary bladder disturbances, and faster progression. After this classification was proposed, several individual family studies showed evidence of overlapping features and age of onset within families. The classification, however, was conclusively invalidated in a study by Durr and associates[8] involving 23 families with pure autosomal dominant HSP in which a unimodal distribution of age of onset was found. The clinical manifestations of early onset and late onset disease were not significantly different. Therefore, there is no apparent genetic basis for HSP classification based entirely on age of symptoms onset.

Genetic anticipation has occasionally been reported in descriptions of HSP kindreds. Anticipation occurs when there is progressively younger age of onset or increased disease severity in succeeding generations. In a recent study by Bürger and colleagues,[9] 11 meioses out of 12 (of female germline) showed anticipation with an average of 10.8 years reduction in age of onset in a kindred linked to the chromosome 2p locus. However, not all families linked to this locus show anticipation.[9a] There has also been report of anticipation in a family linked to chromosome 14q,[10] and in an unlinked family.[10a] In a study presented by Nielsen and colleagues,[10b] the repeat expansion detection (RED) method was used to successfully associate CAG repeat expansions with HSP in six Danish families with linkage to the chromosome 2 locus. The size of the CAG repeat expansion, however, did not correlate well with age at onset of the disease. The number of CAG repeats in affected individuals was reported to be 60 repeats and above. For several neurodegenerative diseases, anticipation correlates with the expansion of CAG trinucleotide repeats, such as in Huntington's disease, spinocerebellar ataxias, and several others. The infrequent occurrence of anticipation among HSP kindreds suggests that, although possible, trinucleotide repeat mutations are probably not responsible for the majority of HSP mutations. Caution must be taken when reporting anticipation, however, because the difference in age at onset can be the result of a recruitment bias favoring families in which the disease was detected earlier in children than in parents.

## NOMENCLATURE

There are two distinct forms of X-linked HSP, designated SPG1 and SPG2. SPG1 has in fact only been found in cases of complicated HSP and is allelic to X-linked hydrocephalus (HSAS, hydrocephalus due to stenosis of the aqueduct of sylvius) and MASA syndrome (mental retardation, aphasia, shuffling gait, and adducted thumbs). These allelic conditions result from mutations in the L1 neural cell adhesion molecule (*L1CAM*) gene located at Xq28.[22] SPG2, responsible for both complicated and uncomplicated HSP, is allelic to Pelizaeus-Merzbacher disease (PMD) and results from mutations in the proteolipid protein (*PLP*) gene located at Xq22.[19] SPG3 has been used to designate autosomal dominant HSP linked to chromosome 14q, the first autosomal dominant locus found and sometimes also referred to as FSP1.[13] SPG4 refers to pure and complicated autosomal dominant HSP linked to the chromosome 2p locus, also known as FSP2.[14,15] SPG6 refers to the form of autosomal dominant HSP linked to the chromosome 15q locus, also known as FSP3.[17] SPG8 refers to the locus for autosomal dominant HSP at the 8q23–q24 locus.[10c] Finally, SPG9 refers to the recently characterized chromosomal region at 10q23.3–q24.1, linked to an autosomal dominant complicated form of HSP.[10d] Two loci for autosomal recessive HSP have been described. The first one, localized on chromosome 8p12–q13, is symbolized SPG5.[12] Recently, a novel mitochondrial metaloprotease gene *paraplegin* was associated with pure and complicated forms of autosomal recessive HSP at 16q24.3, and is referred to as SPG7.[10e,11]

## LINKAGE STUDIES

The first reported positive linkage with an HSP family was to the SPG1 locus at Xq28.[11a] The family presented complicated HSP with mental retardation and absence of extensor pollicis longus. A mutation in the L1CAM gene was later found to be responsible for the disease in this family,[22] and no other linkage of HSP has been reported to this locus. The second HSP locus identified was also X-linked, at Xq22,[19] and mutations in pure and complicated HSP families were later reported (see Proteolipid protein below).

Uncomplicated autosomal recessive HSP was mapped to chromosome 8q12–13,[12] which is also referred to as the SPG5 locus. The size of the candidate region for the location of the gene was reported to be 32 cM

Table 11–1. **Differential Diagnosis of Hereditary Spastic Paraplegia (HSP)**

| Category | Disorder | Clinical Features that Differentiate From HSP | Diagnostic Evaluation |
|---|---|---|---|
| Structural spinal cord abnormality | Arnold-Chiari malformations | Ataxia | MRI of posterior fossa |
| | Cervical or lumbar spondylosis | Involvement of upper extremities; radiculopathy | Spine radiographs and MRI |
| | Tethered cord syndrome | | MRI of conus medullaris |
| | Neoplasm involving spinal cord | Pain, loss of sensation, asymmetric involvement | MRI of spinal cord |
| | Spinal cord arteriovenous malformation | Saltatory progression; spinal sensory level | MRI, spinal arteriography |
| | Granuloma (e.g., tuberculosis) involving vertebrae with spinal cord | Back pain, subacute course | Spine radiographs and MRI |
| Degenerative diseases | Multiple sclerosis | Exacerbations, remissions, ataxia, optic neuritis, Lhermitte's sign | MRI, cerebrospiral fluid examination, visual evoked potentials |
| | Amyotrophic lateral sclerosis | Fasciculations, amyotrophy | Electromyography and nerve conduction testing |
| | Spinocerebellar ataxias, including Machado-Joseph disease | ALD and AMN are X-linked | Prominent ataxia; Machado-Joseph disease also has extrapyramidal involvement |
| Leukodystrophy | ALD, AMN | In childhood-onset ALD, progressive cognitive impairment and peripheral neuropathy accompany corticospinal tract signs. In adolescent/adult-onset AMN, cognition is normal, peripheral neuropathy is variable | Brain MRI; plasma long chain fatty acid analysis |
| | MLD | MLD (autosomal recessive) in children is typically associated with psychomotor regression and peripheral neuropathy | MRI (brain), arylsulfatase |

*(continued)*

flanked by markers PLAT and D8S279. More recently, a second recessive locus, SPG7, was identified on chromosome 16q24.3 in a pure HSP consanguineous Italian family.[10e] Subsequently, homozygous deletions were identified in this family, which led to the characterization of *paraplegin,* a novel metaloprotease gene involved in mitochondrial OXPHOS activity.[11] Frameshift mutations in the gene were also found in

Table 11–1. Continued

| Category | Disorder | Clinical Features that Differentiate From HSP | Diagnostic Evaluation |
|---|---|---|---|
| | Krabbe's (globoid cell) leukodystrophy | Krabbe's disease is an autosomal recessive disorder. Peripheral neuropathy, a feature of childhood-onset Krabbe's disease, may be absent in adolescent/adult-onset Krabbe's disease. | MRI (brain), galactocerebrosidase |
| Metabolic disorders | Subacute combined degeneration | Peripheral neuropathy, marked dorsal column involvement | Serum vitamin B12 concentration |
| | Mitochondrial encephalomyopathy | Short stature, retinitis pigmentosa, and multiple stroke-like episodes may help distinguish this diverse group of disorders from HSP | MRI (brain), serum lactate and pyruvate |
| | Abetalipoproteinemia (Bassen-Kornzweig disease) | Peripheral neuropathy | Lipoprotein electrophoresis |
| | Vitamin E deficiency | Peripheral neuropathy | Serum vitamin E concentration |
| Infectious diseases | Tertiary syphilis (hypertrophic pachymeningitis) | | VDRL, fluorescent treponemal antibody |
| | Tropical spastic paraparesis | Subacute course | Human T cell lymphotropic virus type antibodies |
| | Acquired immunodeficiency syndrome (AIDS) | Subacute course | Human immunodeficiency virus antibodies |
| Miscellaneous | Dopa-responsive dystonia | Diurnal fluctuation; response to low-dose levodopa–carbidopa | Therapeutic trial of low-dose levodopa–carbidopa |

ALD = adrenoleukodystrophy; AMN = adrenomyeloneuropathy; MLD = metachromatic leukodystrophy; VDRL = Venereal Disease Research Laboratory test.
**Source:** Fink et al.[6]

one pure HSP Italian family and one complicated HSP French family. Some families with recessive genes have been excluded from linkage to this locus, which is an indication that there may be one or several additional loci responsible for autosomal recessive HSP.

Five loci for autosomal dominant HSP have been found. The first uncomplicated autosomal dominant HSP locus was found in a large French kindred, linked to chromosome 14q11.2 (SPG3).[13] Subsequently, independent investigators identified linkage to this locus in one German family,[10] one Tibetan family,[11b] one North American family,[15] and one French family.[11c] In a recent report, the size of the candidate region was refined from 9 to 5 cM flanked by the markers D14S301 and D14S991.[11c] Two groups working independently identified a locus on chromosome 2p24-21 (SPG4)[14,15] that is linked to pure HSP in North American families,[11d,11e,15] French families,[14] a German family,[9] Danish families,[16] Belgian families,[16a] and Swiss families.[16b] The SPG4 locus was reported to be flanked by the markers D2S400 and D2S367 in a 4 cM interval.[9] Heinzlef and colleagues[16c] reported linkage of a complicated HSP French family with dementia and epilepsy, to the SPG4 locus. They reported familial recombinations that would place the SPG2 gene between markers D2S2255 and D2S2347, in an estimated 2.5Mb segment, assuming commonality of gene between the pure and complicated forms. Finally, tight linkage between a locus on chromosome 15q11.1 (SPG6) and autosomal dominant HSP was found in a large North American HSP kindred.[17] To date, this has been the only reported family whose HSP is linked to this region, which is approximately 8 cM and is flanked by markers D15S128 and D15S156. Recently, linkage to a new locus, SPG8, was demonstrated in a large autosomal dominant pure HSP family of German descent.[10c] Testing for linkage with the new loci SPG7, SPG8, and SPG9 in families for which other HSP loci were excluded or uninformative will provide helpful information on linkage frequencies to the many HSP loci. Linkage should be tested at all loci, because different mutations of a gene could result in dominant and recessive mutations.

## PARAPLEGIN

The paraplegin gene was identified in a pure autosomal recessive family segregating a 9.5 kb deletion at the linked locus on chromosome 16q14.3.[11] The novel gene encodes a metaloprotease involved in the regulation of oxidative phosphorylation of mitochondria. Analysis of muscle biopsy specimens from two patients carrying the deletion showed typical signs of mitochondrial oxidative phosphorylation defects with the presence of several ragged-red fibers and no reaction to cytochrome c oxidase. Northern analysis showed that the transcript is ubiquitously expressed in all fetal and adult tissues tested, with transcripts of alternate size in the heart and pancreas. The Paraplegin protein, which is predicted to contain 795 amino acids, is highly homologous to the yeast mitochondrial ATPases AFG3, RCA1, and YME1, which were demonstrated to have proteolytic and chaperone-like activities at the inner mitochondrial membrane. The functional domains of the yeast proteins, an ATP-binding motif and a zinc-dependent ATP-binding motif, are completely conserved in Paraplegin. The AAA (ATPases Associated with various cellular Activities) family consensus sequence is highly conserved in Paraplegin. The AAA protein superfamily is characterized by a highly conserved module including an ATP binding consensus, present in one or two copies in the AAA proteins. AAA proteins are found in all organisms and are essential for cell cycle functions, vesicular transport, mitochondrial functions, peroxisome assembly, and proteolysis.

Mitochondrial dysfunction resulting from respiratory chain or oxidative phosphorylation defects have been described in several neurodegenerative disorders. For example, Friedreich's ataxia is caused by the absence of a nuclear gene product encoding for a non-respiratory chain mitochondrial protein. In Parkinson's disease, mitochondrial DNA seems to be directly implicated in some patients.[17a] The sensitivity of the central nervous system to respiratory chain and oxidative phosphorylation system defects is noted, and may result from this tissue's dependence on aerobic metabolism.

## PROTEOLIPID PROTEIN: THE X-LINKED GENE

One of the most abundant proteins in central nervous system myelin is PLP, a 30 kDa integral membrane protein. It is post-translationally modified by the addition of long chain fatty acids via an autoacylation process. The PLP gene contains seven exons and six introns and has two gene products, PLP and DM-20. These products are generated from alternate splicing in which part of exon 3 is absent in DM-20. A family of molecules with a strong homology to PLP/DM-20 has been identified across fish and mammals, and this early evolutionary implication suggests that PLP may function as part of a dynamic molecular environment. DM-20 is the predominant isoform in oligodendrocyte progenitors and is expressed before PLP in the developing brain where it is thought to play a major role in oligodendrocyte maturation. PLP is expressed later in development and is crucial to myelin sheet compaction.

Mutations in the PLP gene have been known to cause PMD, a severe rare disorder characterized by trunk hypotonia, nystagmus, progressive pyramidal, dystonic, and cerebellar signs during the first years of life, and slow psychomotor deterioration. Histopathological examination of the central nervous systems of PMD patients revealed a severe deficit of myelin sheaths enwrapping axons and a profound loss of the oligodendrocytes associated with dysmyelination. Gow and Lazzarini[18] recently proposed that the cellular basis for the difference in disease severity between HSP and PMD is based on cellular protein trafficking of the two gene products PLP and DM-20. Several mutations are known to cause PMD by duplication of an intact PLP gene, deletion of the gene, and point mutations.[31] Interestingly, this situation is similar to that in Charcot-Marie-Tooth disease type 1A, which may be caused by duplication, deletion, or point mutation in the myelin protein gene PMP22, which is homologous to PLP, but is expressed in the peripheral nervous system.

PLP mutations can also cause HSP. X-linked pure HSP was initially linked to markers at the SPG2 locus on Xq22,[19] following which a missense mutation in the PLP gene coding sequence was found in affected males of one complicated HSP family.[20] The reported mutation in the PLP gene results in a mutant PLP product but normal DM-20. A PLP gene mutation was subsequently found in the pure HSP family from which the initial linkage was established.[21]

A mutation occurring in the major extracellular loop of the protein present in both DM-20 and PLP was found in the pure HSP family. Several other mutations were reported in the extracellular loop, one homologous to the mouse mutant *rumpshaker*,[26,26a] in Pelizaeus-Merzbacher disease and pure HSP patients. Other *PLP* mutations have been reported for complicated HSP, including one missense mutation at the PLP nucleotide 236 in exon 6 of the gene,[26b] and one missense mutation at nucleotide 506 in exon 4 of the gene.[26c] Hodes and colleagues, emphasizing that mutations in the PLP gene cause a wide range in severity of disorders, recommended a joint referral to the clinical condition of Pelizaeus-Merzbacher disease and SPG2 linked HSP, and coined the expression PMD/SPG2.[26d]

Steinmüller and colleagues[26e] report a family with HSP linked to Xq11.2–q23, harboring the SPG2 locus. They conducted extensive mutation analysis of the PLP gene without success, and report the likely presence of a third HSP gene near the PLP gene. Interestingly, a large proportion of Pelizaeus-Merzbacher disease families linked to the PLP gene region have failed to identify mutations in the gene.

In addition to PLP mutations, a complicated form of X-linked HSP has been linked to the L1 neural cell adhesion molecule (*L1CAM*) gene on chromosome Xq28 (SPG1). To date, mutations in the *L1CAM* gene have only been associated with the complicated form of the disorder.[22,23] This form is allelic to X-linked hydrocephalus (HSAS, hydrocephalus due to stenosis of the aqueduct of sylvius), MASA syndrome (mental retardation, aphasia, shuffling gait, and adducted thumbs), and complicated corpus callosum agenesis/dysgenesis (ACC/DCC). Clinical studies have indicated a large overlap in the phenotypes of these conditions and the presence of several of these phenotypes in a single family. Fransen and coworkers[24] reviewed the clinical spectrum of mutations of *L1CAM*, which they refer to as the CRASH syndrome (corpus callosum agenesis, retardation, adducted thumbs, spastic paraparesis, hydrocephalus).

## ANIMAL MODELS

*Rumpshaker* (*jp*$^{rsh}$) is an allele of the *jimpy* locus. Clinical features of *jimpy* mice are similar to those of PMD and show failure of development and differentiation of oligodendrocytes, leading to early death. Although *rumpshaker* mice are myelin deficient like other *jimpy* mutants (which can therefore serve as useful PMD models), they have normal longevity and a full complement of morphologically normal oligodendrocytes. Affected mice show a generalized tremor at about 12 days of age, which generally becomes confined to the hindlimbs.

The *rumpshaker* PLP mutation spontaneously developed in a mouse from a stock homozygous for robertsonian translocations.[25] The mutation was mapped to the PLP gene on the X chromosome, to a single base change in exon 4, resulting in an isoleucine to threonine substitution at position 186 and altering both PLP and DM-20. Interestingly, the same mutation was found to be segregating in a human HSP kindred.[26,26a] The high homology between the mouse and human PLP sequence and the similarity of the mouse *rumpshaker* and human HSP mutations will allow direct parallels to be drawn with regard to pathophysiology.

Morphological analysis of *rumpshaker* mice indicates that spinal cord axons are either unmyelinated or myelinated with disproportionately thin sheaths, whereas in the optic nerve the myelinated axons that are present have sheaths of normal thickness. Ultrastructural examination shows a majority of the myelin to be similar to wild type in appearance of its lamellar staining; however, in a small percentage of the myelin a decreased periodicity and lack of the intraperiod line is observed. Antibody staining of *rumpshaker* myelin shows decreased levels of PLP, DM-20, and myelin basic protein. Studies of *rumpshaker* heterozygous females indicate occasionally unmyelinated spinal cord axons and an overall reduction in brain and spinal cord myelin. Heterozygous optic nerves show only a slight increase in the number of oligodendrocytes.[25,27] X-ray diffraction studies indicate that the *rumpshaker* mouse has abnormalities in both myelin membrane packing and stability, correlating the biochemical abnormalities in the mutant mouse with a wider periodicity and less stable packing of the myelin.[28]

A study presented by Anderson and colleagues demonstrated that mice overexpressing at low levels the Plp mouse gene had late-onset progressive myelin loss, axonal swellings with resultant Wallerian degeneration, and marked vacuolation of the neuropil associated with ataxia, tremor, and seizures.[28a] The age of onset and severity of the phenotype was shown to correlate with Plp gene dosage.

Another animal model of PLP mutations resembling spastic paraplegia is the *shaking* pup, a defect recognized in male Springer Spaniel pups. *Shaking* pups show gross generalized tremor at about 10 to 12 days of age[29] and have severe hypomyelination throughout the central nervous system that is more marked in the brain and optic nerves than in the spinal cord; the amount of myelin increases with age. Axons are either naked or surrounded by a disproportionately thin layer of myelin. There is a marked reduction of oligodendrocytes in affected pups, with many of these cells having distended rough endoplasmic reticulum (indicating elevated rates of protein synthesis). Astrocyte numbers are normal. Many of the oligodendrocytes contain empty or granular vacuoles within the cytoplasm. It was demonstrated that PLP and DM-20 are expressed in approximately equal and greatly reduced amounts in the mutant spinal cord and are present in thin myelin sheaths. Female heterozygote dogs can develop a marked tremor that disappears with age. A mutation was identified near the first transmembrane region of PLP and DM-20, which causes the spliced transcript DM-20 to be overexpressed, disrupting the normal maturation schedule of these oligodendrocyte developmental proteins.[30]

## GENETIC COUNSELING

Genetic counseling provides information to affected individuals or family members at risk for a genetic disorders such as HSP. Several issues are discussed during genetic counseling, such as the consequences of the disorder, the probability of developing or transmitting it, and the ways in which it may be prevented or ameliorated. Recent discoveries and advances in the molecular genetics of HSP can help determine the probability of developing and transmitting HSP. For example, DNA analysis can be used for risk estimation by examining closely linked markers that are known to flank the genes for the autosomal HSP loci. It is also possible to directly detect mutations in the case of the X-linked loci. Several aspects of HSP, however, must be taken into consideration in counseling for this disorder. Of particular concern are the delayed age of onset and the rate of symptom progression.

Genetic counseling for autosomal HSP is only applicable to genetically informative families from kindreds with linkage to one of the known HSP loci. A family is informative when family members are available for the study and are heterozygous for the linked markers. Risk estimates when a gene has not been cloned can involve extensive study of several family members. This study can be complicated by the need to examine numerous polymorphic markers to collect definitive information about location, phase, and the presence of possible recombination events between markers. Each patient suspected of having HSP should undergo a thorough neurologic examination. Care must be taken in the assignment of penetrance probabilities for linkage analysis.

Counseling by direct detection of the mutation can be done if the mutation is known. Due to the heterogeneity of the disorder, however, the specific mutation type of each family must be determined. Several mutations of the PLP gene have been reported, and a single mutation each in HSP was observed for paraplegin and *L1CAM*.

Rate of symptom progression and age of onset for HSP are greatly variable between and within families. Great caution must be practiced in counseling on these aspects. It is not possible to predict with certainty whether a wheelchair will be required or if urinary incontinence will inevitably occur. In some HSP kindreds, the condition begins in childhood and is relatively nonprogressive after approximately age 10 years, and patients often remain ambulatory.

Extreme caution must be used in counseling unaffected parents of a child with suspected HSP about the risk of HSP in other progeny. Genetic markers flanking known HSP loci can only be used when there is a large kindred for whom the disorder was linked to a known locus. Assuming the diagnosis of HSP is correct, the affected child could represent a new mutation or nonpaternity (both cases resulting in a lower chance of HSP in other siblings), a rare case of incomplete penetrance in one of the parents (resulting in a higher chance of HSP in other siblings), or an autosomal recessive kindred (with a 25% chance of HSP in other siblings).

## CONCLUSIONS

Our understanding of the genetic basis of HSP has expanded greatly in the recent years. The disorder has been shown to arise from mutations at three genes: Paraplegin, *L1CAM* and *PLP*; and six loci for which gene identification is underway: 2p, 8q, 8cen, 10q, 14q, and 15q. The existence of HSP families for whom these loci are excluded indicates the existence of additional HSP loci. The high similarity in clinical characteristics observed in HSP families with linkage to different genetic loci suggests a common structure or pathway where the gene products would act together. The identification of additional genetic defects causing HSP is likely to provide important insights into factors responsible for the development and maintenance of axonal integrity.

## SUMMARY

Hereditary spastic paraplegia is a degenerative disorder of the motor system, defined by progressive weakness and spasticity of the lower limbs. Insights into the genetic basis of the disorder are expanding rapidly. The disorder can be caused by different gene mutations, and nine susceptibility loci have now been identified. Two loci for autosomal recessive HSP are known; one is on chromosome 8q, and the paraplegin gene is on chromosome 16q. Loci for autosomal dominant HSP have been identified on chromosomes 2p, 8q, 10q, 14q, and 15q. One locus, Xq22, has been identified for X-linked uncomplicated HSP and shown to be due to PLP gene mutations. Another X-linked locus at chromosome Xq28 was shown to result in complicated HSP following mutation of the *L1CAM* gene. The existence of HSP families for whom these loci are excluded indicates the existence of additional HSP loci. The high degree of similarity between HSP kindreds with linkage to different genetic loci suggests a common structure or pathway where the gene products would act together. The identification of genetic defects causing HSP is likely to provide important insights into factors responsible for the development and maintenance of axonal integrity.

## REFERENCES


1. Harding AE: Hereditary spastic paraplegia. Semin Neurol 13:333–336, 1993.
2. Sutherland JM: Familial spastic paraplegia. In Vinken PJ, Bruyn GW (eds): Handbook of Clinical Neurology, Vol 22. System Disorders and Atrophies, Part II. North Holland, Amsterdam, 1975, pp420–431.
3. Harding AE: Hereditary "pure" spastic paraplegia: A clinical and genetic study of 22 families. J Neurol Neurosurg Psychiatry 44:871–883, 1981.
4. Schady W, Scheard A: A qualitative study of sensory functions in hereditary spastic paraplegia. Brain 113:709–720, 1990.
5. Schady W, Dick JP, Sheard A, Crampton S: Central motor conduction studies in hereditary spastic paraplegia. J Neurol Neurosurg Psychiatry 54:1099–1102, 1991.
6. Fink JK, Heiman-Patterson T, Bird T, et al.: Hereditary spastic paraplegia: Advances in genetic research. Neurology 46:1507–1514, 1996.
7. Cooley WC, Rawnsley E, Melkonian G, et al.: Autosomal dominant familial spastic paraplegia: Report of a large New England family. Clin Genet 38: 57–68, 1990.
8. Durr A, Brice A, Serdaru M, et al.: The phenotype of "pure" autosomal dominant spastic paraplegia. Neurology 44:1274–1277, 1994.
9. Bürger J, Metzke H, Paternotte C, Schilling F, Hazan J, Reis A: Autosomal dominant spastic paraplegia with anticipation maps to a 4-cM interval on chromosome 2p21–p24 in a large German family. Hum Genet 98:371–375, 1996.

9a. Dürr A, Davoine CS, Paternotte C, et al.: Phenotype of autosomal dominant spastic paraplegia linked to chromosome 2. Brain 119(Pt5):1487–1496, 1996.

10. Gispert S, Santos N, Damen R, et al.: Autosomal dominant familial spastic paraplegia: Reduction of the FSP1 candidate region on chromosome 14q to 7 cM and locus heterogeneity. Am J Hum Genet 56:183–187, 1995.

10a. Fink JK, Sharp GB, Lange KM, Wu C-tB, Haley T, Otterud B, Peacock M, Leppert M: Autosomal dominant, familial spastic paraplegia, type I: Clinical and genetic analysis of a large North American family. Neurology 45:325–331, 1995.

10b. Nielsen JE, Koefoed P, Abell K, et al.: CAG repeat expansion in autosomal dominant pure spastic paraplegia linked to chromosome 2p21-p24. Hum Mol Genet 6(11):1811–1816, 1997.

10c. Hedera P, Rainier S, Alvarado D, Zhao X, Williamson J, Otterud B, Leppert M, Fink JK: Novel locus for autosomal dominant hereditary spastic paraplegia, on chromosome 8q. Am J Hum Genet 64:563–569, 1999.

10d. Seri M, Cusano R, Forabosco P, et al.: Genetic mapping to 10q23.3-q24.2, in a large Italian pedigree, of a new syndrome showing bilateral cataracts, gastroesophageal reflux, and spastic paraparesis with amyotrophy. Am J Hum Genet 64:586–593, 1999.

10e. De Michele G, De Fusco M, Cavalcanti F, et al.: A new locus for autosomal recessive hereditary spastic paraplegia maps to chromosome 16q24.3. Am J Hum Genet 63:135–139, 1998.

11. Casari G, De Fusco M, Ciarmatori S, et al.: Spastic paraplegia and OXPHOS impairment caused by mutations in paraplegin a nuclear-encoded mitochondrial metalloprotease. Cell 93:973–983, 1998.

11a. Kenwrick S, Ionasescu V, Ionasescu G, et al.: Linkage studies of X-linked recessive spastic paraplegia using DNA probes. Hum Genet 73(3):264–266, 1986.

11b. Huang S, Zhuyu, Li H, Labu, Baizhu, Lo WH, Fisher C, Vogel F: Another pedigree with pure autosomal dominant spastic paraplegia (AD-FSP) from Tibet mapping to 14q11.2-q24.3. Hum Genet 100(5–6):620–623, 1997.

11c. Paternotte C, Rudnicki D, Fizames C, et al.: Quality assessment of whole genome mapping data in the refined familial spastic paraplegia interval on chromosome 14q. Genome research 8:1216–1227, 1998.

11d. Raskind WH, Pericak-Vance MA, Lennon F, Wolff J, Lipe HP, Bird TD: Familial spastic paraparesis: Evaluation of locus heterogeneity, anticipation, and haplotype mapping of the SPG4 locus on the short arm of chromosome 2. Am J Med Genet 74: 26–36, 1997.

11e. Nance MA, Raabe WA, Midani H, et al.: Clinical heterogeneity of familial spastic paraplegia linked to chromosome 2p21. Hum Hered 48:169–178, 1998.

12. Hentati A, Pericak-Vance MA, Hung W-Y, et al.: Linkage of "pure" autosomal recessive familial spastic paraplegia to chromosome 8 markers and evidence of genetic locus heterogeneity. Hum Genet 3(8):1263–1267, 1994.
13. Hazan J, Lamy C, Melki J, Munnich A, de Recondo J, Weissenbach J: Autosomal dominant familial spastic paraplegia is genetically heterogeneous and one locus maps to chromosome 14q. Nat Genet 5: 163–167, 1993.
14. Hazan J, Fontaine B, Bruyn RPM, et al.: Linkage of a new locus for autosomal dominant familial spastic paraplegia to chromosome 2p. Hum Mol Genet 3(9):1569–1573, 1994.
15. Hentati A, Pericak-Vance MA, Lennon F, et al.: Linkage of a locus for autosomal dominant familial spastic paraplegia to chromosome 2p markers. Hum Genet 3(10):1867–1871, 1994.
16. Nielsen JE, Krabbe K, Jennum P, et al.: Autosomal dominant pure spastic paraplegia: A clinical, paraclinical, and genetic study. J Neurol Neurosurg Psychiatry 64(1):61–66, 1998.

16a. De Jonghe P, Krols L, Michalik A, et al.: Pure familial spastic paraplegia: Clinical and genetic analysis of nine Belgian pedigrees. Eur J Hum Genet 4(5):260–266, 1996.

16b. Von Fellenberg J, Paternotte C, Prud'homme JF, Weissenbach J, Hazan J, Burgunder JM: Clinical and molecular genetic analysis of 4 Swiss families with the pure form of hereditary spastic spinal paralysis. Schweiz Med Wochenschr 128(26):1043–1050, 1998.
16c. Heinzlef O, Paternotte C, Mahieux F, et al.: Mapping of a complicated familial spastic paraplegia to locus SPG4 on chromosome 2p. J Med Genet 35: 89–93, 1998.
17. Fink JK, Brocade Wu C-T, Jones SM, et al.: Autosomal dominant familial spastic paraplegia: Tight linkage to chromosome 15q. Am J Hum Genet 56: 188–192, 1995.
17a. Schapira AHV: Mitochondrial involvement in Parkinson's disease, Huntington's disease, hereditary spastic paraplegia and Friedreich's ataxia. Biochimica et Biophysica Acta 1410:159–170, 1999.
18. Gow A, Lazzarini RA: A cellular mechanism governing the severity of Pelizaeus-Merzbacher disease. Nat Genet 13:422–428, 1996.
19. Keppen LD, Leppert MF, O'Connell P, et al.: Etiological heterogeneity in X-linked spastic paraplegia. Am J Hum Genet 41:933–943, 1987.
20. Saugier-Veber P, Munnich A, Bonneau D, et al.: X-linked spastic paraplegia and Pelizaeus-Merzbacher disease are allelic disorders at the proteolipid protein locus. Nat Genet 6:257–262, 1994.
21. Cambi F, Tang X-M, Cordray P, et al.: Refined genetic mapping and proteolipid protein mutation analysis in X-linked pure hereditary spastic paraplegia. Neurology 46:1112–1117, 1996.
22. Jouet M, Rosenthal A, Armstrong G, et al.: X-linked spastic paraplegia (SPG1), MASA syndrome and X-linked hydrocephalus result from mutations in the L1 gene. Nat Genet 7:407–407, 1994.
23. Schrander-Stumpel C, Höweler C, Jones M, et al.: Spectrum of X-linked hydrocephalus (HSAS), MASA syndrome, and complicated spastic paraplegia(SPG1): Clinical review with six additional families. Am J Med Genet 57:107–116, 1995.
24. Fransen E, Vits L, Van Camp G, Willems PJ: The clinical spectrum of mutations in L1, a neuronal cell adhesion molecule. Am J Med Genet 64:73–77, 1996.
25. Griffiths IR, Scott I, McCullock MC, et al.: Rumpshaker mouse: A new X-linked mutation affecting myelination: Evidence for a defect in PLP expression. J Neurocytol 19:273–283, 1990.
26. Kobayashi H, Hoffman EP, Marks HG: The rumpshaker mutation in spastic paraplegia (Letter). Nature Genet 7:351–352, 1994.
26a. Naidu S, Dlouhy SR, Geraghty MT, Hodes ME: A male child with the rumpshaker mutation, S-linked spastic paraplegia/Pelizaeus-Merzbacher disease and lysinuria. J Inherit Dis 20(6):811–816, 1997.
26b. Donnelly A, Colley A, Crimmins D, Mulley J: A novel mutation in exon 6 (F236S) of the proteolipid protein gene is associated with spastic paraplegia. Hum Mutat 8:384–385, 1996.
26c. Hodes ME, Hadjisavvas A, Butler IJ, Aydanian A, Dlouhy SR: X-linked spastic paraplegia due to a mutation (C506T; ser169phe) in exon 4 of the proteolipid protein gene (PLP). Am J Med Genet 75: 516–517, 1998.
26d. Hodes ME, Zimmerman AW, Aydanian A, et al.: Different mutations in the same codon of the proteolipid protein gene, *PLP*, may help in correlating genotype with phenotype in Pelizaeus-Merzbacher disease/X-linked spastic paraplegia (PMD/SPG2). Am J Med Genet 82:132–139, 1999.
26e. Steinmüller R, Lantigua-Cruz A, Garcia-Garcia R, Kostrzewa M, Steinberger D, Müller U: Evidence of a third locus in X-linked recessive spastic paraplegia. Hum Genet 100:287–289, 1997.
27. Fanarranga ML, Griffiths IR, McCullock MC, et al.: Rumpshaker: An X-linked mutation causing hypomyelination: Developmental differences in myelination and glial cells between the optic nerve and spinal nerve. Glia 5:161–170, 1992.
28. Karthigasan J, Evans EL, Vouyiouklis DA, Inouye H, et al.: Effects of rumpshaker mutation on CNS myelin composition and structure. J Neurochem 66:338–345, 1996.
28a. Anderson TJ, Schneider A, Barrie JA, Klugmann M, McCulloch MC, Kirkham D, Kyriakides E, Nave KA, Griffiths IR: Late-onset neurodegeneration in mice with increased dosage of the proteolipid protein gene. J Comp Neurol 394:506–519, 1998.
29. Griffiths IR, Duncan ID, McCulloch M, Harvey MJ: Shaking pups: A disorder of central myelination in the Spaniel dog. Part 1. Clinical, genetic and light-microscopical observations. J Neurol Sci 50(3): 423–433, 1981.
30. Nadon NL, Duncan ID, Hudson LD: A point mutation in the proteolipid protein gene of the "shaking pup" interrupts oligodendrocyte development. Development 110(2):529–537, 1990.
31. Hodes ME, Pratt VM, Dlouhy SR: Genetics of Pelizaeus-Merzbacher disease. Dev Neurosci 15: 383–394, 1993.
32. Popot J-L, Pham Ding D, Dautigny A: Major myelin proteolipid: The 4-alpha-helix topology. J Membr Biol 120:233–246, 1991.

Chapter 12

# HEREDITARY ATAXIAS

Stelan-M. Pulst, MD, Dr Med
Susan Perlman, MD



Three causes of locomotor ataxia each distinguishable and unique in its spinal cord pathology, were recognized in the late nineteenth century: tabes dorsalis, multiple sclerosis, and the recessive genetic syndrome of Friedreich. Near the turn of the twentieth century, Marie's ataxia was described as a later onset, syndrome with early involvement of brain stem and cerebellum. To this day, the recessive spinocerebellar ataxias are likened to Friedreich's ataxia, and the central cerebellopontine syndromes are lumped as "Marie's ataxia" by many practitioners (Table 12–1).

Detailed clinical and pathological studies of many individuals and families over the past 100 years, however, have shown multiple variations on these two themes, resulting in a plethora of eponyms and many classifications.[1–3] "Splitting" made it easy to scatter pieces of a unique genetic illness (and divergent branches of the same family) along several eponymic byways, just as "lumping" tended to bury together genetically distinct syndromes, hiding them from further study. It became apparent that a phenotype based on multiple clinical and pathological criteria might not be specific for a unique genotype and that a specific genotype in a single pedigree may have significant clinical and pathological variations among affected individuals.

Previous classifications have relied heavily on clinicopathological correlation, generating confusing layers of terminology (Table 12–1). The current accepted classification now refers to the dominant ataxias as *spinocerebellar ataxia* (SCA) with the type defined by genetic locus (i.e., SCA1 on chromosome 6). Included in the SCAs are those ataxias accompanied by prominent retinal degeneration or dementia and the

Table 12–1. **Classifications of Progressive, Late Onset Cerebellar Ataxia**

| Greenfield (1954)[1] | Konigsmark and Weiner (1970) | Harding (1984)[3] | Current Study |
|---|---|---|---|
| Type A (Menzel): Dominant olivopontocerebellar atrophy | OPCA I (Menzel)<br>OPCA IV (Schut)<br>Type 1: FA-like<br>Type 2: cerebellar<br>Type 3: spastic | ADCA type I<br><br>(ADCAI) includes Azorean ataxia | SCA1<br>SCA1<br>SCA2<br>SCA3/MJD<br>SCA4<br>SCA5<br>SCA6 |
| With dementia | OPCA V: Dementia | | |
| With blindness | OPCA III (with retinal degeneration) | ADCA II (with retinal degeneration) | SCA7 |
| With amyotrophy | | | |
| "Special" (Becker, 1969) | | ADCA III: very late onset pure cerebellar | SCA6 and others |
| "Variant" (Eadie, 1975) | | ACDA IV: myoclonus, deafness<br>ADCA with essential tremor<br>Periodic Autosomal dominant ataxia | <br><br>Episodic Ataxia Type 1: Myokymia<br>Type 2: Nystagmus |
| Type B (Holmes): Recessive cerebelloolivary degeneration with hypogonadism | OPCA II (Fickler-Winkler) Recessive olivopontocerebellar atrophy | Autosomal Recessive cerebellar ataxia (rare) | ? |
| | OPCA VII (others; e.g., very late onset with dementia) | | ? |
| — | — | X-linked cerebellar ataxia (rarer) | ? |
| Sporadic cerebello-olivary degeneration (Marie) | OPCA VIII | Late onset idiopathic cerebellar ataxia | Inclusion body–positive SOPCA and MSA |
| Sporadic olivopontocerebellar atrophy (Dejerine-Thomas) | | Type A (Marie's)<br>Type B (with severe tremor)<br>Type C (Dejerine-Thomas) | |

OPCA = olivopontocerebellar ataxia; SCA = spinocerebellar ataxia; ADCA = autosomal dominant cerebellar ataxia; FA = Friedreich's ataxia; MJD = Machado-Joseph disease; SOPCA = sporadic olivoponto cerebellar ataxia; MSA = multiple syndrome atrophy syndrome.

Machado-Joseph disease (MJD) phenotype. Recessive ataxias with a Friedreich's-like and non-Friedreich's-like phenotype, as well as maternally transmitted ataxias (X-linked or mitochondrial), are distinguished. These categories are specific enough to allow selective use of panels of direct genetic tests especially when a positive family history is available. The molecular diagnosis of patients without a family history may require use of direct gene tests from both the SCA and the Friedreich's ataxia (FRDA) group.

## THE DOMINANT ATAXIAS

The autosomal dominant cerebellar ataxias have an incidence of about 1 to 5/100,000 in the general population.[4] These conditions share the primary clinical features of gait ataxia, dysarthria, dysphagia, and limb dysmetria and intention tremor, resulting from changes in the cerebellum and its afferent and efferent pathways (Table 12–2). There may be additional changes in other brain stem or spinal cord–associated structures (causing upper or lower motor neuron or basal ganglia signs, oculomotor palsies, bulbar palsy, peripheral and central sensory changes), as well as optic nerve or retinal disease and some subcortical dementia. The relative presence of these findings, however, depends on the particular subset of patients studied, probably reflecting ethnic differences and observer variability.

The relative frequencies shown in Table 12–2 were obtained from two independent sets of patients examined by a single observer at each site. Onset of symptoms may be from the first to seventh decade, but averages in the third decade. The course is one of slow, fairly symmetrical progression over 15 or more years. Clinically, the cerebellar features involve gait, speech, and upper extremities in fairly quick succession, with the secondary features occurring in variable proximity to the primary ones (e.g., "early" vs. "late" ophthalmoplegia). On clinical criteria alone, without the use of genetic analysis, most of the typical dominant ataxias would be indistinguishable.

In several of the SCAs the disease-causing mutation is expansion of a polymorphic CAG trinucleotide repeat (Table 12–3). The clinical hallmark of this type of mutation is anticipation, the earlier onset of disease often accompanied by more severe symptoms in succeeding generations of affected families. Anticipation of age of onset and increasing severity of disease symptoms are correlated with expansion of the CAG repeat when passed from parent to child.

## SCA1

Spinocerebellar ataxia type 1 (SCA1) was the first of the late-onset, dominantly inherited cerebellar syndromes to be linked to a known gene locus, the HLA complex on chromosome 6.[5] This finding was almost immediately used by ataxia researchers to include or exclude other ataxias in large families from this locus. The *SCA1* gene was the

Table 12–2. **Symptoms of Dominant Ataxias***

| | **SCA1 (n = 10)** | **SCA2 (Germany; n = 21)** | **SCA2 (Los Angeles; n = 12)** | **SCA3 (n = 59)** | **SCA6 (Germany; n = 22)** | **SCA6 (Los Angeles; n = 12)** |
|---|---|---|---|---|---|---|
| Cerebellar dysfunction | 100 | 100 | 100 | 100 | 100 | 100 |
| Reduced saccadic velocity | 50 | 77 | 92 | 10 | 6 | 0 |
| Myoclonus | 0 | 33 | 0 | 4 | 0 | 0 |
| Dystonia or chorea | 20 | 0 | 38 | 8 | 0 | 0 |
| Pyramidal involvement | 70 | 29 | 31 | 70 | 44 | 33 |
| Peripheral neuropathy | 100 | 94 | 44 | 80 | 44 | 16 |
| Intellectual Impairment | 20 | 25 | 37 | 5 | 0 | 0 |

Data are from Schols et al.[71,73] and Geschwind et al.[31,70] Results are given as percentages.

Table 12–3. **Spinocerebellar Ataxias and Gene Locations**

| Current Classification | Chromosomal Location | Mutational Mechanisms | Unique Features |
|---|---|---|---|
| SCA 1 | 6q22–23 | CAG-nl 16–37,* abnl 39–81 | Dysphagia, pyramidal signs, vibratory loss |
| SCA2 | 12q24.1 | CAG-nl 15–32, abnl 34–64 | Slow saccades, loss of reflexes, dementia |
| SCA3/MJD | 14q24.3–32 | CAG-nl 12–40, abnl 66–84 | Pyramidal and extrapyramidal signs, peripheral motorsensory neuropathy |
| SCA4 | 16q24-ter | Unknown | Sensory axonal neuropathy, pyramidal signs |
| SCA5 | 11cent | Unknown | Relatively benign course, pyramidal signs in early onset |
| SCA6 | 19p | CAG nl 4–19, abnl 21–29 | Predominant cerebellar symptoms |
| SCA7 | 3p | CAG nl 7–17, abnl 38–130 | Retinal degeneration |
| SCA8 | 9 | CTG nl <100, abnl 106–139 | Predominant cerebellar syndrome |
| SCA10 | 22q | Unknown | Predominant cerebellar syndrome with epilepsy |

*There are longer normal SCA1 alleles, but they carry a CAT interruption.

first ataxia gene to be identified, and the disease-causing mutation was shown to be expansion of a DNA trinucleotide repeat.[6]

## RANGE OF CLINICAL FINDINGS

Several large pedigrees with confirmed SCA1 have been studied in depth and observed over a number of generations.[7–12] Onset of mild first symptoms such as intermittent upbeat nystagmus, hand tremor, or unsteadiness may precede the progressive clinical illness by years. Onset of the complete cerebellar syndrome with ataxia, dysarthria, titubation, dysdiadochokinesis, and dysmetria was typically in the 30s and 40s. A wide range of phenotypes is associated with SCA1 in individual patients, although some similarities to SCA2 and SCA3 emerge when larger groups of patients from several pedigrees are compared (Table 12–2).

## LABORATORY AND PATHOLOGICAL FINDINGS

Computed tomography (CT), magnetic resonance imaging (MRI), single-photon emission computed tomography (SPECT), position emission tomography (PET), and proton MRI show changes in cerebellar cortex, vermis, and brain stem.[13,14] Abnormal electrophysiological studies such as changes in somatosensory evoked potentials (SSEPs) and sensory nerve conduction velocities (NCVs), brain stem auditory evoked responses (BAERs), motor NCVs, and, less commonly, visual evoked responses (VERs) and electroencephalograms (EEGs) are also seen. Occasionally, cognitive changes can be identified with neuropsychological testing. Although these studies may correlate with progression of disability, they are not diagnostic for SCA1. No definitive blood, urine, or cerebrospinal fluid biochemical markers have been found for SCA1 other than DNA-based genetic testing.

Neuropathologically, several studies[1,2,10,15] have confirmed mild to moderate neuronal loss with reactive gliosis in the Purkinje cell layer, dentate nuclei, and pontine nuclei, with reduced neuronal number in the inferior olives and marked degeneration of spinocerebellar tracts. Motor neurons of cranial nerves and anterior horn have often been involved, with neurogenic changes in muscle. Homogeneity of repeat size ranges was seen in most brain regions of patients with SCA1 in contrast to the marked somatic instability in brains from patients with dentato-rubro-pallido-luysian atrophy (DRPLA). Thus, selective neuronal vulnerability cannot be explained by repeat size variability.[16]

### THE SCA1 GENE

With a positional cloning strategy, the *SCA1* gene was identified when a 1.2 Mb cosmid contig was screened for trinucleotide repeats. Of two CAG repeats in the region, one was found to be expanded in patients with SCA1.[6] Normal alleles contain 19 to 38 repeats, whereas disease alleles have 40 to 81 CAG repeats.[11] Normal repeats contain CAT interruptions (coding for histidine instead of glutamine), whereas expanded alleles contain a perfect CAG repeat. Occasional normal alleles extend into the abnormal allele size range. These alleles contain CAT interruptions that can be detected by digestion of the polymerase chain reaction (PCR) products with *Sfi*I.

The SCA1 transcript is 10,660 bases and is transcribed from both the wild-type and SCA1 alleles. The CAG repeat, coding for a polyglutamine tract, lies within the coding region. The gene spans 450 kb of genomic DNA and is organized in nine exons. The first seven fall in the 5' untranslated region, and the last two contain the coding region and a 7,277 bp 3' untranslated region. The first four noncoding exons undergo alternative splicing in several tissues. These features suggest that the transcriptional and translational regulation of ataxin-1, the SCA1-encoded protein, may be complex. On Northern blots, an 11 kb transcript is seen that is widely expressed. The gene is organized into nine exons of which only the last two are coding. The *SCA1* gene product, designated ataxin-1, has a predominantly nuclear localization, although in Purkinje cells nuclear and cytoplasmic localization is seen.[17] Ataxin-1 interacts with nuclear matrix proteins.[18,19]

### GENOTYPE–PHENOTYPE CORRELATIONS

Large repeat abnormalities of 60 to 81 units are associated with juvenile onset (under age 18 years; more likely in paternal transmissions). Parent to child transmissions were observed with no change in the repeat number, with increases of 2 or 3 up to 12 triplets (more likely in paternal transmissions) or with decreases of 1 triplet (seen only in maternal transmissions).

In addition to age of onset, clinical course was also tied to repeat length. Shorter repeat abnormalities showed a 16 to 26 year duration, with death in the mid-50s to mid-60s. Longer repeat abnormalities ran an 8 to 23 year course, with death in the late 30s to early 50s. Juvenile patients were often moribund after 3 to 6 years of illness.

In the Siberian study of 78 patients, Goldfarb and colleagues[12] found amyotrophy of skeletal muscle and tongue, as well as dysphagia, to be absent or mild in patients with low repeat abnormalities, but to be complications of the course of illness in 15 of 22 patients with CAG repeats equal to or greater than 52. Contrary to earlier studies, this was the first evidence that repeat length could influence phenotype. This kindred also showed the first evidence of incomplete penetrance, with an asymptomatic 66-year-old female mutation carrier with 44 CAG repeats. Other kindreds had shown complete penetrance by age 52 years. In addition, in three individuals homozygous for expanded alleles, age of onset, rate of progression, and clinical manifestation corresponded to the size of the larger allele (alleles were not additive). Studies of seven large SCA1 pedigrees of diverse ethnic backgrounds suggested that additional genetic and nongenetic factors may influence CAG repeat stability and age of onset of disease.[7]

## SCA2

The dominantly inherited cerebellar ataxia in a large, homogeneous population of patients from the Holguin province of Cuba was excluded from the SCA1 locus and subsequently linked to markers on chromosome 12q24.[20] Disease in a second pedigree of Southern Italian descent was also linked to CHR 12q24.1.[21] Additional pedigrees of Italian,[22] Tunisian,[23] Austrian, and French Canadian lineage[24,25] were also shown to have disease linkage to the new SCA2 locus. SCA2 is caused by expansion of a CAG trinucleotide repeat in the coding region of a novel gene.[26–28]

## RANGE OF CLINICAL FINDINGS

In the original Cuban study, age of onset was from 2 to 65 years, with a mean in the third to fourth decades. Earliest symptoms were gait ataxia, often accompanied by leg cramps.[29] More than 50% of patients developed a kinetic or postural tremor, decreased muscle tone and tendon reflexes, and abnormal eye movements with slowed saccades progressing to nuclear ophthalmoplegia. The clinical course to inability to walk developed over 4 to 10 years (occasionally longer), with death occurring 12 to 25 years after onset. Although anticipation was not reported in the Cuban pedigree, Pulst and coworkers[21] described marked anticipation in the Southern Italian pedigree.

SCA2 shows significant interfamilial variability in both the degree of anticipation and the prominence of secondary symptoms at various stages of illness. Belal and associates[23] described a surprising 23% incidence of extrapyramidal signs in their study family, and Cancel and coworkers[30] described a 29% incidence of dementia. Geschwind and associates[31] found an even higher incidence of dystonia or chorea (38%) and dementia (37%), as well as some indication of family-specific phenotypes. Mild, primarily cerebellar symptoms appeared to segregate in some families, whereas others had an MJD-like phenotype or an early onset with dementia and chorea.

## LABORATORY AND PATHOLOGICAL FINDINGS

Computed tomography and MRI scans have shown nonspecific cerebellar or pontocerebellar atrophy. Evoked potential studies showed abnormal central auditory conduction on brain stem testing. Motor and somatosensory responses were normal except in advanced stages of disease, but abnormal peripheral nerve conduction studies were consistent with an associated axonal sensorimotor neuropathy. Nerve biopsy material has shown moderate loss of large myelinated fibers.[22]

Neuropathological studies confirmed neuronal loss in the inferior olive, pons, and cerebellum, as well as degeneration of spinal motor neurons and to a lesser extent spinocerebellar tracts and dorsal columns.[29,32] The SCA2 gene product ataxin-2 has a widespread neuronal expression and has a cytoplasmic localization in normal and SCA2 brains.[33]

## THE *SCA2* GENE

The *SCA2* gene was recently identified independently by three groups using three different approaches. Pulst and associates[26] constructed a physical map of the critical region using P1 artificial chromosomes and bacterial artificial chromosomes and then identified CAG repeat–containing sequences (Fig. 12–1). Sanpei and colleagues[27] used a novel technique to isolate DNA sequences containing expanded CAG repeats in genomic Southern blots, and Imbert and associates[28] identified polyglutamine-containing proteins in an expression library using a monoclonal antibody that recognizes extended polyglutamine repeats.

The *SCA2* gene contains a CAG trinucleotide repeat that is not highly polymorphic in the normal population. Two alleles of 22 and 23 repeats account for more than 95% of alleles. Rare normal alleles ranging from 15 to 32 repeats have also been identified.[27,28,34] Normal alleles typically show one or two CAA interruptions.

Disease alleles range from 34 to 64 repeats and carry perfect CAG repeats without interruption and can be easily identified by amplification of patient DNA with oligonucleotide primers flanking the CAG repeat (Fig. 12–1). Several individuals in SCA2 pedigrees with 34 repeats have been identified. These individuals are still asymptomatic, however, and it is not known whether they might develop symptoms within the normal human life span.

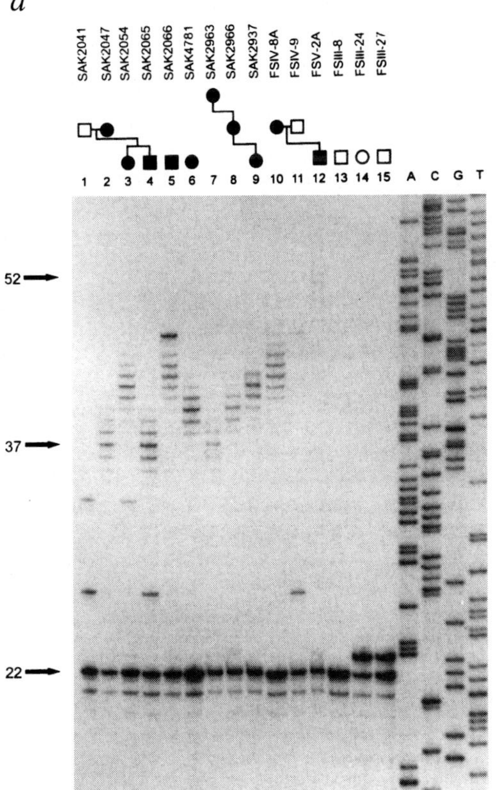


**Figure 12–1.** Analysis of the SCA2 CAG repeat. The repeat was amplified from genomic DNAs with oligonucleotide primers flanking the repeat and alleles separated according to size by polyacrylamide electrophoresis. Normal individuals (samples 1, 11, 13) are homozygous for the common 22 repeat allele; normal samples 14 and 15 are heterozygous with alleles of 22 and 23 repeats. All SCA2 patients have one normal 22 repeat allele and an expanded allele with repeats ranging from 37 to 52 repeats. Alleles were sized by comparison with a sequencing ladder using single stranded M13mp18 DNA. (Reproduced with permission from Pulst et al.[26])

## GENOTYPE–PHENOTYPE CORRELATIONS

Using direct analysis of the SCA2 repeat, Geschwind and coworkers[31] found almost universal presence of cerebellar ataxia and slow saccadic eye movements, but also a relatively high incidence of dystonia or chorea (38%) and dementia (37%). There was some indication of occurrence of specific phenotypes within families. Mild, primarily cerebellar symptoms appeared to segregate in some families, whereas others had an early onset with dementia and chorea. One patient had been clinically diagnosed as having a typical MJD-like phenotype.

Similar findings were also reported by Cancel and colleagues[30] in a series of 111 patients from 32 families of diverse origins. Slow eye movements were seen in 56%, fasciculations in 25%, and dystonia in 9%. The authors also examined which findings were correlated with disease duration and which were correlated with increasing CAG repeat length. The size of the repeat was significantly larger in patients with dystonia, myoclonus, and myokymia, whereas both CAG length and duration influenced the frequencies of decreased reflexes and vibration sense in the lower extremities, amyotrophy, fasciculations, and slow eye movements.

Schols and colleagues[36] found *SCA2* expansion in 6 of 64 families of German ancestry with autosomal dominant cerebellar ataxia. Clinical features were highly variable within and between families. Although no specific feature was sufficient to distinguish SCA2 from other SCAs, slowed saccades, postural and action tremors, myoclonus, and hyporeflexia were more common than in SCA1 and SCA3. Similar to the study reported by Geschwind and coworkers,[31] this study was remarkable in that all patients were examined by the same clinician, thus reducing interobserver variability.

Burk and associates[36] examined several SCA2 patients defined by linkage analysis and compared them with SCA1 and SCA3 patients. SCA2 patients had significantly slower saccadic speed (138°/sec) than did patients with SCA1 (244°/sec) or SCA3 (347°/sec). All eight SCA2 patients had saccadic velocities two standard deviations below the mean of a control group. Magnetic resonance imaging showed that the middle cerebellar peduncles and the pontine base were significantly smaller in SCA2 patients than in SCA1 and SCA3 patients. Similar findings were also reported by Buttner and colleagues[37] and clearly distinguished SCA2 patients from patients with expansions in the other *SCA* genes.

Storey and colleagues[38] recently analyzed cognitive impairment in seven Australian patients with SCA2. Although six patients had a Mini-Mental-Status Examination score of 25 or greater, they performed significantly below the norm on several tests sensitive to frontal-executive dysfunction. These observations point to a potential role of the cerebellum and its connections in higher cortical functions in addition to its well-established role in the motor system.

## SCA3/Machado-Joseph Disease

"Azorean disease" of the nervous system was an autosomal dominant disorder originally described as three phenotypically different diseases in three separate families from the Azores. After more careful epidemiological studies, it was confirmed to be a single illness, with diverse phenotypes occurring within each family.[39] Molecular studies have confirmed its occurrence in non-Azorean/Portuguese families of diverse ethnicity throughout the world, including a typical SCA phenotype designated SCA3. The disease-causing mutation is expansion of a CAG repeat in a gene on chromosome 14q.[40]

### RANGE OF CLINICAL FINDINGS

Since 1975, large numbers of cases of SCA3/MJD have been traced and studied through organizations and clinics in the United States, the Azores, and elsewhere. The mean age of onset is in the 20s or 30s, with a range of 6 to 70 years of age.

Classic MJD in Portuguese kindreds has four distinct presentations, sometimes occurring in successive generations of the same family.[41] Type 1 has the earliest onset (mean, 25 years) and the most rapid course, with early presentation of dystonia and a progressive akinetic-rigid syndrome with spasticity, in addition to the more typical cerebellar/supranuclear and nuclear ophthalmoplegic syndrome. Type 2 has an average age of onset of 40 years, with progression over about 20 years. Symptoms are primarily cerebellar/ophthalmoplegic, with variable pyramidal signs and minimal extrapyramidal and peripheral features. This is the most common MJD phenotype and the one similar to other SCAs. Type 3 has an onset after 50 years with initial cerebellar/ophthalmoplegic signs and a prominent peripheral component, including amyotrophy and vibratory loss or other sensory symptoms. Type 4 is a rare levodopa-responsive parkinsonian phenotype, with ataxia, distal atrophy, and sensory loss, also later in onset.[42] Not all families with dominant atypical parkinsonism and Portuguese ancestry have been found to have the SCA3/MJD mutation.[43]

Cancel and colleagues[44] found SCA3/MJD mutations in three French pedigrees with typical autosomal dominant cerebellar ataxia type I phenotypes. A pedigree with neuropathological findings suggesting the ataxochoreic form of DRPLA also carried an expanded SCA3/MJD CAG repeat.

### LABORATORY AND PATHOLOGICAL FINDINGS

Imaging studies typically show pontocerebellar and spinal atrophy, with occasional milder olivary atrophy in longer duration illness (Fig. 12–2). In type 1 MJD, mild atrophy of frontal lobes and marked atrophy of putamen and globus pallidus may be seen.[45] Abnormal electrophysiological studies (SSEPs, electromyograms [EMGs]/NCVs, BAERs, electronystagmograms [ENGs], and, less commonly VERs) are seen, but are not significantly different from the results in SCA1.[46]

Neuropathologically, severe degeneration with gliosis is described in the subthalamopallidal system, oculomotor and trochlear nuclei, pontocerebellar tract, and Clarke's column. There is mild to moderate degeneration in the substantia nigra, the hypoglossal, ambiguus, trigeminal, and vestibular nuclei, the anterior horn of the spinal cord, and anterior nerve roots. SCA3/MJD appears to have more marked changes in the subthalamopallidal system and intermediolateral column than either SCA1 or SCA2, while SCA1 and SCA 2 show Purkinje cell and inferior olivary degeneration that is rarely seen in SCA3/MJD.[46,47]. Lopes-Cendes and coworkers[48] did not find evidence of mosaicism of CAG repeat number in multiple brain regions, yielding no explanation for the selective neuronal loss in SCA3.

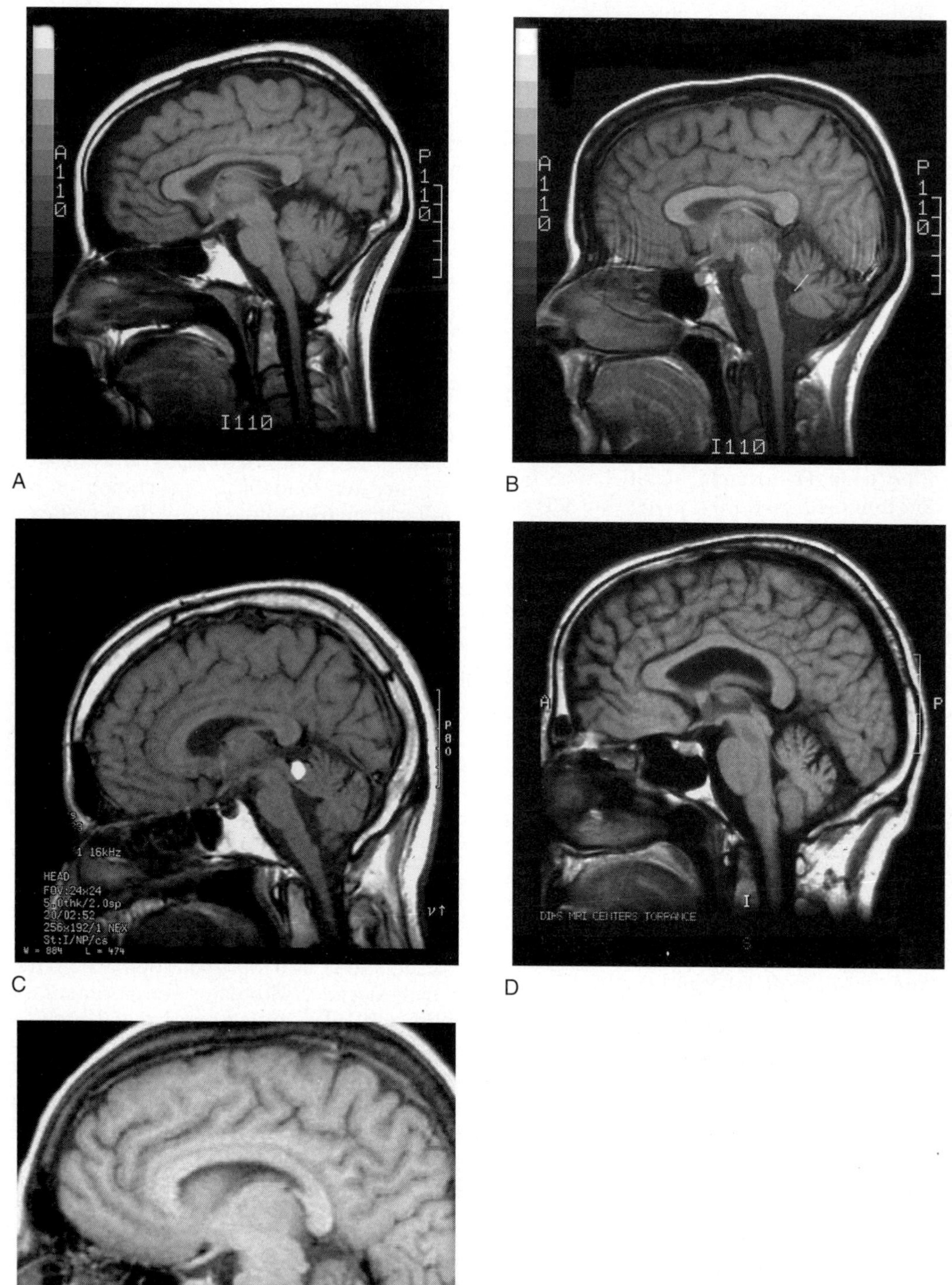


**Figure 12–2.** MRI findings in dominant ataxias and in Friedreich's ataxia. Values for TE and TR are given in parentheses. (*A*) A 29-year-old woman with SCA1 (600/15). (*B*) A 30-year-old woman with SCA2 (400/16). (*C*) A 56-year-old man with SCA3/MJD; note the incidental lipoma (383/16). (*D*) A 58-year-old patient with SCA6 (600/15). (*E*) A 37-year-old woman with Friedreich's ataxia; note sparing of the cerebellum, but marked atrophy of the spinal cord (400/16).

## THE SCA3 GENE

After mapping of the MJD gene to chromosome 14q by genetic linkage analysis,[49] a gene containing a CAG trinucleotide repeat was mapped to this region. This repeat was expanded in patients with MJD.[40] Normal alleles contain 12 to 40 CAG repeats and abnormal alleles, 61 to 84.[50–53] One patient with 56 repeats and onset at age 51 years has been reported.[54] The repeat is located in the 3'- coding region of a novel gene. The CAG repeat contains three variant triplets, CAA and AAG at three positions.

The cDNA predicts a protein of 359 amino acids. The protein, ataxin-3, does not show homology to known genes, but several related genes have been identified. When truncated MJD proteins containing 79 repeats are overexpressed in COS cells, apoptotic cell death is seen.[55] These truncated fragments may form larger complexes by covalent binding.

Ataxin-3 is widely expressed in normal and SCA3-affected brains. In normal brains it is localized to neuronal and non-neuronal cells in a predominantly cytoplasmic distribution. In diseased brain, intranuclear ubiquitinated inclusions were seen in several regions.[56] These were most frequently found in the ventral pons, a region severely affected in MJD, but also in the substantia nigra and dentate nucleus. No inclusions were seen in neurons typically spared in MJD such as the Purkinje cell layer and cortex.

## GENOTYPE–PHENOTYPE CORRELATIONS

Age of onset has been shown to be inversely correlated with the abnormal CAG repeat length,[11] accounting for about 50% of the variance in age of onset.[40,50,51,53] A contribution may also be seen from the size of the normal allele, suggesting an additive effect.[46] There was marked variation in average age of onset among different ethnic groups. Russians, Indians, Japanese, and black Americans have an onset in their 20s, whereas Chinese have a later onset in their 60s. Other genetic and environmental factors are suspected of further influence so that average mutation size alone may not account for the observed ethnic variability.[57]

Parent to child transmissions of the abnormal allele often showed no change in size, but some showed an increase of two to nine CAG repeats or, less commonly, a contraction of up to eight repeats. Unstable alleles were more likely the result of paternal transmission. These small increases in expansion size sometimes did not result in clinical evidence of anticipation.[50] Meiotic drive has also been seen in male transmissions, with the abnormal allele being preferentially transmitted to 73% of offspring.[58]

The SCA3/MJD phenotype may somewhat correlate with CAG repeat length. Expansion to 65 to 70 repeats is associated with greater than 50% occurrence of peripheral neuropathy without hyperreflexia (MJD type 3); patients with 71 to 74 repeats have peripheral neuropathy with 28% hyperreflexia (MJD type 2); patients with 75 or more repeats have an early onset at ages 21 to 33 years and greater than 50% occurrence of hyperreflexia with little peripheral neuropathy (MJD type 1). Variability is great, however, and many features such as supranuclear ophthalmoplegia, amyotrophy, sphincter disturbances, and dysphagia are seen as a result of disease progression, not CAG repeat length.[46]

Variant phenotypes have been confirmed to be due to CAG expansions at the SCA3/MJD locus. Sakai and Kawakaini[59] described a patient with spastic paraplegia with facial fasciculations and ophthalmoplegia in the fourth decade, with later development of mild cerebellar and extrapyramidal signs. A pure cerebellar syndrome with very late onset at 75 years of age was seen with an expansion of 66 repeats.[60] A multiple system atrophy (MSA) like phenotype with ataxia and orthostatic hypotension was seen in one patient with 56 repeats.[54] Homozygous individuals have very early onset (age 7 or 8 years) and an aggressive type 1 phenotype, possibly reflecting an additive effect of the two mutant alleles.[61] An asymptomatic 66-year-old female mutation carrier has recently been reported.[62]

# SCA4

Flanigan and colleagues[63] reported a unique hereditary ataxia phenotype in a

Utah kindred that has been tightly linked to a locus on chromosome 16. The family has a prominent sensory axonal neuropathy and normal eye movements, in addition to cerebellar and pyramidal tract signs. Neuropathological studies show degeneration of cerebellar Purkinje cells, dorsal root ganglion neurons, and neurons of the trigeminal ganglion. A similar pedigree with cerebellar ataxia, marked sensory loss involving the face, and reduction of sensory action potentials was described by Nachmanoff and associates,[64] although genetic linkage analysis was not carried out.

The SCA4 gene has not yet been cloned. Anticipation is not a prominent feature.

## SCA5

Ranum and coworkers[65] reported another unique hereditary ataxia phenotype in a family descended from the grandparents of President Abraham Lincoln. Age of onset ranges from 10 to 68 years, but is typically in the third or fourth decade. First symptoms are usually mild gait ataxia, arm incoordination, and slurred speech. Progression is slow over several decades. Although the adult disease is disabling, it does not shorten life, probably due to the lack of severe bulbar involvement. Two juvenile cases did have mild bulbar involvement. Magnetic resonance imaging shows pure cerebellar atrophy, consistent with the clinical presentation. Neuropathology has not been reported.

Anticipation is evident. The average decrease in age per generation is 15.7 years in maternal transmission and 9.3 years in paternal transmission. All four juvenile cases (age of onset, 10 to 18 years) were maternally inherited. This pattern is different from the paternal bias seen in other SCAs.

The gene has been mapped close to the centromere of chromosome 11 by genetic linkage analysis, but has not yet been cloned.[65]

## SCA6

The designation of SCA6 was initially reserved for a possible gene locus associated with a phenotype with prominent dementia not linked to the other SCA loci, but has recently been reassigned to a dominantly inherited ataxia mapping to chromosome 19p13. Expansion of a CAG repeat was identified in the human $\alpha_{1A}$ voltage-dependent calcium channel subunit (*CACNL1A4*) gene,[66] the same gene that contains mutations in episodic ataxia type 2 (EA-2).

### RANGE OF CLINICAL FINDINGS

Disease onset is insidious, with sensations of momentary imbalance and dizziness with quick turns or rapid movements. These sensations are reminiscent of the episodic symptoms of the milder EA-2 phenotypes. Progression of cerebellar ataxia of limbs and gait, dysarthria, nystagmus, and mild vibratory and proprioceptive sensory loss occurs over 20 to 30 years, causing the patient to become wheelchair bound. In the few older patients studied, choking suggested brain stem involvement, and in two families complications of ataxia were the cause of death.

### LABORATORY AND PATHOLOGICAL FINDINGS

Magnetic resonance imaging of the brain has shown isolated cerebellar atrophy. Detailed neuropathological studies on two deceased members of one kindred showed marked cerebellar and very mild brain stem atrophy. Microscopic examination revealed severe Purkinje cell loss, moderate loss of granule cells and dentate nucleus neurons, and mild to moderate neuronal loss in the inferior olive.[67]

### THE *SCA6* GENE

Mutations causing SCA6 are allelic with mutations causing EA-2 and familial hemiplegic migraine (FHM). In contrast to EA-2 mutations, which truncate the protein, SCA6 mutations are caused by expansion of a CAG repeat located in the coding region of three alternatively spliced transcripts of the gene encoding the human $\alpha_{1A}$ voltage-dependent calcium channel. In these isoforms, the CAG repeat is predicted to code for polyglutamine. Normal alleles have from 4 to 19 repeats, while disease alleles range in size from 21 to 27.[66,68–70]

### GENOTYPE–PHENOTYPE CORRELATIONS

SCA6 alleles with 21 to 23 repeats are associated with later disease onset and a predominantly cerebellar (autosomal dominant cerebellar ataxia type III) phenotype. Larger expansions lead to earlier onset and a phenotype seen in autosomal dominant cerebellar ataxia type I.[68–70] Patients homozygous for expanded alleles have an earlier onset and more severe disease manifestations.[68–70] Some patients experience episodic phenomena before developing a progressive ataxia.[70]

The human $\alpha_{1A}$ voltage-dependent calcium channel is important for calcium entry and homeostasis in Purkinje cells. Abnormalities in its structure may cause alterations of transmitter release or abnormal intracellular calcium concentrations leading to progressive neuronal loss rather than the episodic and minimally progressive dysfunction seen in EA-2. The overlap of EA-2, SCA6, and FHM points to a continuum of phenotypes associated with different types of mutations in *CACNL1A4.*

## Frequencies of SCA Types 1, 2, 3 and 6 Mutations in Diverse Populations

The identification of SCA genes has made it possible to investigate individuals with ataxia with no family history or pedigrees too small for genetic linkage analysis (Table 12–4). The relative percentages vary greatly with the ethnic mix of the ataxia population that is studied.

The frequency of SCA3 ranges from 11% to 23% in North American and non-Portuguese SCA pedigrees, to 27% to 50% in European families, to 84% in patients of Portuguese extraction. Combined occurrence of SCA1, SCA2, and SCA3/MJD mutations may account for roughly 50% or more of the cases of SCAs in unselected populations (Table 12–4). The frequency of SCA2 appears to lie between those of the frequent SCA3 mutation and the rare SCA1 mutation.[26,30,34,71] In one study, however, SCA2 made up 18% of mutations and was the most common autosomal dominant cerebellar ataxia.[72]

Sporadic cases (''new dominant mutations'') have been identified. For example, Schols and coworkers[71] identified expansion in the SCA2 locus in two patients with sporadic ataxia. The asymptomatic 50-year-old mother of one patient was subsequently shown to carry one allele with 34 CAG repeats, which is the smallest size for a SCA2 disease allele. Sporadic cases are quite frequent in SCA6, probably related to the relatively late onset of the disease and the meiotic stability of the repeat.[31,73,74] Although sporadic mutations appear to be rare overall, they justify genetic testing in individuals without a family history of ataxia after obvious causes for acquired ataxias have been excluded.

## SCA7

Dominantly inherited progressive SCA with early onset and atypical retinitis pigmentosa has been described in a number of families from 1951 onward and was designated autosomal dominant cerebellar ataxia type II by Harding.[3] Eight families have been studied genetically[75,76] and found to map to chromosome 3p12–p21.1. SCA7 is caused by expansion of a CAG repeat.[77]

### RANGE OF CLINICAL FINDINGS

Mean age of onset was in the third decade (range, infancy to the late 50s), with no affected child showing onset later than the affected parent. Anticipation resulted in earlier onset by as much as 38 years in the next generation. Benomar and colleagues[75] observed in French and Moroccan kindreds greater paternal than maternal transmission effects. Gouw and associates,[76] studying Caucasian and African Americans, observed an average difference in age of onset from parent to child of −24.4 years for maternal and −17.6 years for paternal transmissions. There are also occasional obligate gene car-

Table 12–4. **Distribution of Known Mutations in the Dominant Ataxias***

| Study | Ethnicity | SCA1 | SCA2 | SCA3/MJD | SCA6 | Total |
|---|---|---|---|---|---|---|
| Schols (1998) ref. 73 | German | 9 | 11 | 43 | 16 | 79 |
| Geschwind (1997) ref. 70 | North American | 6 | 13 | 23 | 12 | 54 |
| Cancel (1995, 1997) ref. 44, 30 | French, North African, West Indian | 10 | 14–15 | 28 | — | 55 |
| Lorenzetti (1997) ref. 72 | Worldwide | 8 | 18 | 8 | 5 | 39 |
| Matsumura (1997)† ref. 68 | Japanese | 3 | 6 | 39 | 31 | |
| Ranum (1995) ref. 11 | German American, African American, and others | 3 | — | 21 | 24 | |

*Only reports using direct mutation analysis were used. Results are given as percentages.
†Dentato-rubral-pallido-lysian atrophy constituted 11% of pedigrees.

riers who do not develop symptoms of the disease despite living until the age of 65 years or more, providing evidence of reduced penetrance in this disorder.[78]

The earliest symptoms were macular changes and loss of color discrimination in the tritan (blue–yellow) axis, which is rarely affected in color blindness but appears to be a sensitive and specific symptom in SCA7. This is followed by loss of vision, progressive ataxia and upper motor neuron dysfunction.[76] With disease onset before age 30 years, decreased visual acuity was often the first symptom. In later onset disease, patients noted ataxia first, but virtually all went on to suffer vision loss.

## LABORATORY AND PATHOLOGICAL FINDINGS

Computed tomography and MRIs showed cerebellar and pontine atrophy. Electroretinography confirmed associated retinal degeneration beyond the macula, but the ophthalmological examination remained the earliest determinant of macular change and associated optic atrophy.[79]

Neuropathologically, there was loss of ganglion and bipolar cells in the retina, adhesions of the retina to the choroid, and loss of pigment epithelium, with associated loss of optic nerve fibers and degeneration of lateral geniculate bodies. Neuronal loss was seen in Purkinje and granule cells of the cerebellum and in the dentate nuclei, as well as inferior olivary nuclei and basis pontis with corresponding tract atrophy including spinocerebellar fibers and middle cerebellar peduncles. There was mild atrophy in the posterior funiculus of the spinal cord.[80]

## THE *SCA7* GENE

The *SCA7* gene, identified by positional cloning, is a gene of unknown function.[77] The gene was independently identified by two other groups.[81,82] It contains a CAG repeat in the coding region that is highly variable in size in SCA7 patients, ranging from 37 to 130 repeats. In normal individuals, the repeat ranges from 4 to 35 repeats.[81,83] One child with onset of the disease at age 3 months had more than 200 repeats.[84] During meiosis the SCA7 repeat is highly unstable, especially during paternal transmissions. In addition, there is significant gonadal and somatic mosaicism.[84,85] Of the known CAG repeat–containing genes, the SCA7 repeat appears to be the most predisposed to expansion. Gouw and colleagues.[85] noticed that maternal transmission of the disease is more common, suggesting germline or embryonic effects of the repeat expansion.

## SCA8

Koob and associates[82,86] isolated an expanded CTG repeat from the DNA of a single affected individual using the RAPID cloning method. Subsequent analysis of this repeat identified five SCA families out of 178 dominant ataxia pedigrees. Affected individuals had 106 to 139 repeats, whereas normal individuals had fewer than 100 repeats. Initial symptoms include ataxia, dysarthria, and bulbar dysfunction. Severely affected individuals also develop corticospinal tract involvement and sensory neuropathy.

SCA8 was initially described as an infantile recessive ataxia.[87] However, this is now referred to as *infantile onset SCA* and is described below. SCA9 has not been mapped.

## SCA10

The association of an adult onset cerebellar ataxia associated with epilepsy in some individuals was recently described.[88] The family was of Mexican descent, and marked anticipation was observed. In five parent-child pairs, disease onset occurred earlier in the offspring by 18 to 23 years. Zu and coworkers[89] mapped the mutation to the distal long arm of chromosome 22. Subsequently, a second pedigree mapping to the same region was described.[90] Eight of 12 individuals in this pedigree had generalized motor seizures. In two, complex partial seizures were seen as well. This family was also of Mexican descent.

## Dentato-Rubral-Pallido-Luysian Atrophy

DRPLA is common in Japan, with an incidence of 0.2 to 0.7 per 100,000,[91,92] but isolated families from other ethnic backgrounds (British, Maltese, Caucasian and African American) have been described.[93] The gene on chromosome 12p contains an unstable CAG trinucleotide repeat.[91,92]

### RANGE OF CLINICAL FINDINGS

Detailed studies in Japanese pedigrees[94,95] have shown a close correlation between age of onset and clinical features. Onset before age 20 years manifests as progressive myoclonus epilepsy with dementia or mental retardation and ataxia. Onset at ages 40 to 69 years shows cerebellar ataxia, choreoathetosis, dementia, and psychiatric features, sometimes indistinguishable from the signs of Huntington's disease.[93,96] Three out of four affected individuals in a British family had a Huntington-like phenotype.[96] Danish family members had been misdiagnosed as having Huntington's disease, but the presence of seizures in some members prompted testing for DRPLA.[97] Onset between the ages of 20 and 40 years results in an intermediate phenotype of nonprogressive myoclonus epilepsy with choreoathetosis, ataxia, and dementia.

The Caucasian American family,[93] while having a phenotype similar to that in the Japanese pedigrees, did not show myoclonus or myoclonus epilepsy in the juvenile forms, although generalized epilepsy was seen. European families showed a similar lack of myoclonus with the exception of one family of Maltese origin.[96] Average duration of the disease was 11 years, with death frequently occurring suddenly in association with seizures.

### LABORATORY AND PATHOLOGICAL FINDINGS

Computed tomography and MRI scans have shown diffuse cerebral and cerebellar atrophy, marked atrophy of the midbrain tegmentum, prominent lateral ventricles (with preserved caudate heads), a large cisterna magna, and deep white matter changes in adult forms of the illness. A high signal intensity on $T_2$-weighted MRIs was reported in a patient in the early stages of DRPLA of the myoclonic epilepsy type.[98] Patients with late-onset may show high signal intensities in subcortical white matter and thalamus.[99]

Electroencephalographic studies have shown focal and generalized epileptiform activity, paroxysmal and generalized slow wave activity, and photosensitivity, while BAERs and EMG/NCV studies have been normal.[100] No definitive blood, urine, or cerebrospinal fluid abnormalities have been found.

Neuropathologically, neuronal loss and

reactive gliosis are seen in the dentate nucleus and its projections to the red nucleus and the lateral segment of the globus pallidus and its projection to the subthalamic nucleus, as well as in Purkinje cells, brain stem tegmentum, and lateral corticospinal tract.[101] The cell loss in the lateral segment of the pallidum contrasts with changes in the medial segment in MJD.[59] The Haw River pedigrees have shown, in addition, microcalcifications of the globus pallidus, neuroaxonal dystrophy of the nucleus gracilis, and demyelination of the centrum semiovale.[100]

Somatic mosaicism has been detected in brains affected by DRPLA.[102,103] Repeats in cerebral and cerebellar cortical areas are smaller than in associated white matter regions. Repeat sizes did not correlate with the severity of neuropathological lesions.

## THE *DRPLA* GENE

A CAG repeat in a gene previously mapped to 12p was shown to be expanded in Japanese patients with DRPLA.[91,104] On normal alleles, the repeat ranges from 7 to 25 CAGs with a heterozygosity of 0.9. Expanded alleles in DRPLA patients range from 54 to 68 repeats. Expanded alleles of more than 80 have been observed.[94,99] Age of onset showed a strong inverse correlation with the number of repeats.

The *DRPLA* gene is predicted to encode a 1184 amino acid protein with the polyglutamine tract starting after 484 amino acids.[92,104,105] Northern blot analysis showed a widely expressed 4.5kb transcript.[104] Both normal and expanded alleles were transcribed.[105] Immunohistochemically, the DRPLA protein is found in the neuronal cytoplasm.[106] *In vitro,* the DRPLA protein interacts with the enzyme glyceraldehyde-phosphate dehydrogenase.[106a] The rat DRPLA gene is 92% homologous at the amino acid level, but the polyglutamine stretch is reduced to seven glutamines. Northern blot analysis showed embryonic expression, suggesting that the protein may be important during embryogenesis.[108]

Remarkable meiotic instability in the CAG repeat has been found, with changes in repeat length in nearly every transmission (−4 to +4 in maternal transmissions, 0 to +28 in paternal). This results in earlier onsets in children of affected mothers by approximately 20 years and of affected fathers by approximately 30 years. Anticipation was not completely explained by increasing CAG repeat length.[94]

When truncated DRPLA proteins containing expanded polyglutamine stretches are overexpressed in COS-7 cells, filamentous peri- and intranuclear aggregates are detected.[109] This was not seen with full-length proteins, pointing to the importance of processing of these proteins, to smaller fragments. Apoptotic cell death was inhibited by cystamine and monodansyl cadaverine, suggesting that inhibition of transglutaminase activity may provide a therapeutic basis for polyglutamine disorders.

## GENOTYPE–PHENOTYPE CORRELATIONS

Inverse correlation of repeat length with age of onset has been observed in all studies. Juvenile disease is found with repeats of 62 or larger, late adult disease with less than 64 repeats, and intermediate disease with 54 to 57 repeats. Patients with more than 70 repeats had the earliest onset and worst prognosis, such as onset at 1 year of age with 88 repeats and death before the age of 12 years.[94] More than 75% of juvenile cases had paternally transmitted DRPLA, and affected fathers seemed to preferentially transmit the abnormal allele to offspring.[94,95] One reported homozygote with two alleles of 57 repeats each had juvenile onset disease.

The absence of myoclonus was a distinguishing feature of DRPLA in an African American family from rural North Carolina, which had been called the Haw River syndrome. Progressive ataxia was followed by development of personality changes, chorea, and tonic–clonic seizures. Ultimately dementia and death ensued after 15 to 25 years of illness.[100,107] Despite the different phenotype, the Haw River syndrome is caused by expansion of the DRPLA repeat with a repeat size range from 63 to 68 repeat units.[107]

## Inherited Prion Diseases

The transmissible spongiform encephalopathies (or prion diseases) are discussed in detail in Chapter 10. Clinically, ataxic Gerstmann-Straussler syndrome (GSS) might be distinguishable from other dominant ataxic syndromes by its associated dementia and relatively short course for adults. Age of onset varies (even within the same pedigree) from 24 to 66 years (average, 43 years), beginning with mild (almost intermittent) symptoms of gait ataxia and leg pains or parasthesias. Clinical progression includes pancerebellar ataxia, hyporeflexia or areflexia in the lower extremities with extensor plantar responses, and mild wasting or weakness in the legs. Impaired proprioception occurs occasionally. Computed tomography or MRIs reveal cerebellar and brain stem atrophy. Electroencephalographic studies may be normal or show diffuse, nonspecific changes. The periodic complexes characteristic of Creutzfeld-Jacob disease have been seen in some GSS patients with dementia and myoclonus. An Australian pedigree with the D178N (cis-129M) mutation has been described in which the phenotypes ranged from Creutzfeld-Jacob disease to fatal familial insomnia to an autosomal dominant cerebellar ataxia–like presentation.[110]

## Dominant Episodic Ataxias

Episodic ataxias are rare disorders, causing attacks of generalized ataxia with normal or near-normal neurologic functioning in between. Although a number of recessive metabolic and X-linked causes of episodic ataxia have been found (Table 12–5), the majority of cases are autosomal dominant. Autosomal-based partial pyruvate dehydrogenase complex deficiencies present with a phenotype of episodic weakness and ataxia with altered pyruvate/lactate ratio, often triggered by febrile illness.

Two dominant forms have been mapped to discrete chromosome loci. The first, episodic ataxia type 1 (with interictal myokymia; EA-1) localizes to the voltage-gated potassium channel gene *(KCNA-1)* on chromosome 12p13. In four families four

Table 12–5. **Inherited Ataxic Syndromes with Known Metabolic Defects**

| Intermittent Ataxias | Progressive Ataxias | Disorders Associated with Defective DNA Repair |
|---|---|---|
| With hyperammonemia | Hexosaminidase deficiency* | Ataxia telangiectasia |
| Argininosuccinase deficiency (argininosuccinic aciduria) | Sphingomyelin storage disorders (Niemann-Pick type C)* | Xeroderma pigmentosum* |
| Arginase deficiency | Cholestanolosis* | Cockayne's syndrome |
| Hyperornithinemia, Ornithine transcarbamylase deficiency (citrullinemia) | Leukodystrophies* (metachromatic, late onset globoid cell adrenoleukomyeloneuropathy) | |
| Aminoacidurias | Mitochondrial encephalomyopathies* | |
| Hartnup's disease | Abetalipoproteinemia | |
| Isovaleric acidemia | Hypobetalipoproteinemia | |
| Intermittent branched chain ketoaciduria | Isolated vitamin E deficiency | |
| Disorders of pyruvate and lactate metabolism | Partial HGPRT deficiency* | |
| Pyruvate dehydrogenase deficiency | Wilson's disease* | |
| Pyruvate carboxylase deficiency | Ceroid lipofuscinosis* | |
| Leigh's syndrom | Sialidosis X-linked ataxia | |
| Multiple carboxylase deficiencies | Ichthyosis and tapetoretinal dystrophy (arylsulfatase C deficiency) | |

*Ataxia may not be prominent feature.

different point mutations have been found in the heterozygous state.[111]

Episodic ataxia type 2 with interictal nystagmus and mild ataxia (EA-2) localizes to chromosome 19p13[112] and is allelic to FHM and SCA6. In contrast to FHM, which is caused by missense mutations in the human $\alpha_{1A}$ voltage-dependent calcium channel subunit gene *(CACNL1A4)*, EA-2 is caused by mutations predicted to truncate the protein. A missense mutation in the *CACN4a* gene resulting in a glycine to arginine substitution has been described in a family with a progressive cerebellar degeneration.[113] In families with FHM, the presence of a progressive cerebellar ataxia is associated with the T666M missense mutation.[114] These ataxias are further discussed with the channelopathies in Chapter 3.

## Periodic Vestibulocerebellar Ataxia

Dominantly inherited periodic vestibulocerebellar ataxia (PATX) does not link to EA1 or EA2[115] loci and appears to be a genetically distinct disease.[115] Age of onset is from the third to sixth decades. Attacks last minutes to hours and consist of horizontal diplopia, oscillopsia, ataxia, nausea, vertigo, and tinnitus. Attacks occur with greater frequency over time and may eventually become constant. Symptoms are exacerbated by sudden changes in head position, fatigue, or opticokinetic stimuli and may be alleviated by lying quietly for 15 to 30 minutes with the eyes closed. Acetazolamide does not modify the symptoms.[116] The earliest clinical signs are abnormal smooth pursuit, decreased opticokinetic nystagmus, lack of suppression of the vestibulo-ocular reflex, and the presence of gaze-evoked nystagmus and esophoria. Ataxia gradually increases and leads to motor disability.

Computed tomographic and MRI scans, EEGs, and BAERs are reported to be normal. Pathology has not been reported.

## Animal Models of Dominant SCAs

Several animal models have been generated by overexpressing polyglutamine-containing proteins either in their entirety or as fragments (reviewed by Burright and colleagues[117]). The only transgenic animal with a phenotype when a full-length protein is overexpressed are transgenic lines overexpressing the human *SCA1* gene with 82 repeats under the control of the Purkinje cell–specific Pcp-2 (L7) promoter. The first pathological abnormalities are the formation of cytoplasmic vacuoles within Purkinje cells at postnatal day 25 (P25). At 5 weeks of age, animals show reduced motor learning and become visibly ataxic at 12 weeks.[118] At this time there is only minimal Purkinje cell loss, but simplification of dendritic arborization. At 24 weeks, Purkinje cell numbers are reduced by about one third. Thus, in these mice dysfunction precedes cell death. Nuclear localization of ataxin-1, but not nuclear aggregation, is important for pathogenesis in this animal model.[119]

In contrast, when full-length MJD constructs containing 79 repeats are introduced into mice under the control of the PcP-2 promoter, no phenotype is seen.[55] When truncated proteins or a fragment consisting purely of $(CAG)_{79}$ are overexpressed, however, posture and gait abnormalities are seen beginning at 4 weeks of age. These findings may indicate that ataxin-3 is not properly processed in Purkinje cells (which are not the site of major abnormality in MJD) with the result that only the "processed" polyglutamine tract is pathogenic.

In mice expressing ataxin-2 under the control of the PcP-2 promoter, Purkinje cell degeneration is seen with full-length proteins and relatively short repeat numbers of 58 glutamines. In contrast to other animal models, intranuclear localization of the gene product does not appear to be necessary.[120]

The tottering mutation *(tg)* and the tottering leaner *($tg^{la}$)* mutation occur in the mouse *CACNL1A4* homologue. Homozygosity for tg leads to ataxia and absence-like seizures in mice, whereas the *$tg^{la}$* mutation leads to a recessive chronic ataxia and degeneration of Purkinje and granule cells.[121]

# THE RECESSIVE FRIEDREICH-LIKE ATAXIAS

The Friedreich-like ataxias are a group of sporadic or recessively inherited, SCAs.[3,122] Their usual onset is before age 20 to 25 years, with progressive spinal tract degeneration. Central cerebellar and brain stem changes are seen later in the course. There may be associated peripheral systems deterioration and, in classic Friedreich's ataxia (FRDA), dysfunction in non-neurologic systems. Mutations in the gene causing FA are the most common cause. Other FA-like ataxias caused by mutations in other genes include familial ataxia with vitamin E deficiency and abetalipoproteinemia. Certain recessively inherited inborn errors of metabolism, which typically present in infancy or early childhood, have adult forms that may resemble FRDA. Some X-linked metabolic diseases or maternally transmitted mitochondrial disorders have also shown phenotypes similar to FA.

## Friedreich's Ataxia

Friedreich's ataxia is the most common of the hereditary ataxias. Its prevalence of about 2 in 100,000 is equal to the prevalence of all the dominant ataxias combined. Carrier frequency is estimated at 1 in 120 in European populations. The most common mutation causing FRDA is expansion of an intronic GAA repeat in the frataxin gene.[123] It is now well established that classic FRDA phenotypes as well as late onset FRDA (LOFA) and FRDA with retained reflexes (FARR) can all be caused by mutations in the frataxin gene, although some patients with these phenotypes appear not to have mutations in the frataxin gene.

### RANGE OF CLINICAL FINDINGS

Age of onset of symptoms is usually between 8 and 15 years, but later onset occurs.[122,124] After identification of the FRDA gene, late onset apparent sporadic ataxic patients have been shown to have frataxin mutations (see below). Essential criteria for diagnosis of "classic" FRDA are onset before the age of 25 years and within 5 years after onset the development of the following signs: progressive limb and gait ataxia, absent tendon reflexes in the legs, extensor plantar responses, and motor nerve conduction velocity of more than 40 m/sec in upper limbs with small or absent sensory action potential. Five years after onset, dysarthria should develop.[3] The criteria of Geoffrey and associates[125] are more restrictive and require onset before age 20 years and the presence of decreased position and/or vibration sense as well as muscle weakness. Ataxia of gait is the typical presenting feature, but can be occasionally preceded by scoliosis or cardiomyopathy. Children may show a motor restlessness early in the course of the illness.

Dysarthria, scoliosis, abnormal echocardiogram, areflexia of the upper limbs, pyramidal weakness of the legs, extensor plantar responses, and distal loss of joint position and vibration sense are not found in all patients at the time of presentation or within 5 years of onset, but are eventually seen in two-thirds of patients. The presence of some of these signs correlates with increasing repeat length (see below). Most patients have abnormal ocular pursuit. Other less common features include optic atrophy, mild sensorineural deafness, distal wasting, diabetes, and pes cavus. Scoliosis is associated with increased cardiopulmonary morbidity. Evidence of heart muscle disease is found in at least two-thirds of patients with FRDA.[126] Cardiac symptoms, however, are relatively rare, and heart failure occurs late in the disease. Glucose intolerance is seen in 20% of patients, with insulin-dependent diabetes in 10%.

The prognosis of FRDA is variable. More than 95% of patients are chairbound by the age of 45 years. On average, they lose the ability to walk 15 years after the onset of symptoms. Reported mean ages at death have been in the mid-30s, but survival into the sixth and seventh decades can occur, particularly if there is no heart disease or diabetes.[3]

### LABORATORY AND PATHOLOGICAL FINDINGS

Magnetic resonance imaging scans show atrophy of the spinal cord in FRDA and LOFA.[127] Cerebellar atrophy is only seen in the later stages of disease and is usually mild (Fig. 12–2). Positron emission tomographic scanning has shown early diffuse cerebral hypermetabolism, with a later decline in activity except in basal ganglia regions. Electroencephalograms are normal. Evoked potential studies[128] have shown symmetrical, severe, and early changes in SSEPs and abnormal central motor conduction. There may be late changes in VERs, BAERs, and audiometry.

Nerve conduction velocity studies confirm early loss of sensory action potentials, but only mild to moderate reductions in motor NCVs. One-third of patients have EMG evidence of denervation. This axonal feature serves to differentiate FRDA from the demyelinating neuropathies (Charcot-Marie-Tooth disease type 1). Electronystagmography can be diagnostic and shows a prolonged Vestibulo-occular reflex phase with low Vestibulo-occular reflex gain, ocular flutter, and normal optokinetic responses. These findings correlate well with known sites of pathology in FRDA, which differentiate FRDA from the primary cerebellar ataxias and olivo pontocerebellar ataxias.[129] Detailed neuropsychological testing has shown changes in processing of auditory information, but no progressive cognitive decline.

About 65% of patients with FRDA have an abnormal electrocardiogram (ECG). Widespread T-wave inversion is the most common finding, particularly in the inferior standard and lateral chest leads, along with ventricular hypertrophy. The most frequent echocardiographic abnormality is symmetrical, concentric ventricular hypertrophy, although some have asymmetrical septal hypertrophy.[130]

Neuropathology shows changes primarily in the spinal cord, with degeneration of posterior columns and spinocerebellar tracts, which is most severe in the cervical region. Extensive loss of larger cells is seen in the dorsal root ganglia. Degeneration of pyramidal tracts is most severe in the lumbar region.[131] Brain stem, cerebellum, and cerebrum are relatively spared, with patchy loss of Purkinje cells in the cerebellum and mild degenerative changes in the pontine and medullary nuclei and optic tracts. Loss of large myelinated axons in peripheral nerves is seen even in very young patients.[132]

## THE FRIEDREICH'S ATAXIA GENE

Linkage studies mapped the FRDA locus to chromosome 9q13–21.1. All families meeting strict diagnostic criteria mapped to this locus.[133] This was confirmed in several populations and in patients with LOFA.[134–136]

The FRDA gene, initially designated χ25 and now called the *frataxin gene,* was recently identified with a positional cloning strategy.[137] It has five exons spread over 40 kb that encode a 210 amino acid protein designated *frataxin.* There is an alternatively spliced exon 5b located 40 kb downstream of exon 5a. The alternatively spliced transcript is predicted to result in a shorter protein of 171 amino acids.

Although the most common disease-causing mutation was subsequently shown to be the expansion of a GAA trinucleotide repeat in intron 1 of the χ25 gene, the χ25 gene became a candidate for FRDA when three point mutations were detected by screening all five exons in 184 patients with FRDA. A T–G transversion in exon 3 changed a leucine to a stop codon, an A to G transition disrupted the acceptor splice site at the end of the third intron, and five patients from three Southern Italian families had an isoleucine to phenylalanine substitution in exon 4. For all three mutations, carriers were heterozygous for the point mutation.

Screening of genomic DNAs by Southern blot analysis for major rearrangements revealed that most FRDA patients had an enlarged *Eco*RI fragment containing intron 1. Direct sequence analysis proved that the size difference was attributable to expansion of a GAA repeat. GAA expansion accounted for more than 98% of the FRDA chromosomes, and expansion varied from 200 to more than 900 repeat units. In normal individuals the repeat was polymorphic, varying from 7 to 22 repeat units. The identification of point mutations in the frataxin gene clearly demonstrated that no other genes in the region cause FRDA, although they could in principle be affected by the GAA expansion.

With cDNA probes containing exons 1 to 5b, a 1.3 kb transcript was detected on Northern blots. Expression was most marked in spinal cord and heart, the primary sites of pathology in FRDA, with intermediate levels in liver, skeletal muscle, and pancreas. Little expression was found in other tissues, including the brain, in contrast to gene expression of SCA genes, which is more widespread.

The molecular mechanism by which GAA expansion causes FRDA is likely related to the formation of an abnormal DNA structure that interferes with transcription.[138] Patients with FRDA have very low levels of FRDA gene expression, consistent with recessive inheritance.[137] The effect of the GAA trinucleotide expansion (especially more than 700 repeats) may be to reduce mRNA to undetectable or very low amounts compared with carriers or controls, possibly due to interference with RNA transcription or processing. By homology with the yeast *YFH1* gene, which is involved in iron homeostasis, it was discovered that human frataxin is also a mitochondrial protein.[139]

## GENOTYPE–PHENOTYPE CORRELATIONS

Durr and coworkers[139a] studied 187 patients with autosomal recessive ataxia, including patients with atypical phenotypes. Expansions ranged from 120 to 1700 repeats, and 140 patients were homozygous for the expansion. Only six patients were heterozygous for GAA expansion and presumably carried a different mutation on the second allele. The repeat showed meiotic instability, and variable repeat numbers were found in siblings.

Larger expansions correlated with earlier disease onset and more rapid progression. The best correlation was detected with the size of the smaller allele, indicating that smaller expansions are consistent with some residual function. The frequencies of cardiomyopathy, flexor plantar responses, and skeletal deformities increased with increasing GAA repeat number.

All patients who met the strict FRDA criteria[3] were homozygous (94%) or heterozygous (6%) for the expansion. Even 46% of patients who did not meet the strict criteria, however, had expansion of the repeat. About one-fourth of patients with homozygous expansion had atypical features. Atypical features included onset after 25 years of age in 19 patients, retained reflexes in 13, and absence of plantar responses in 21. In four patients reflexes were brisk. Ten patients with early onset cerebellar ataxia with retained reflexes had small GAA expansions. About one-fourth of the ataxia patients tested did not show GAA expansion.

Filla and associates,[140] in a study of 67 patients from 48 families, found an inverse correlation of the lengths of both the larger and smaller alleles with age of onset, the smaller alleles showing the best correlation, accounting for about 50% of the variation in age of onset. Expanded alleles were also seen in patients with the LOFA and FARR phenotypes, as well as in one patient with both late onset and retained reflexes. Onset of disease at age 21 years or later had an average repeat length of the smaller allele of 462 compared with 755 to 856 for earlier onset cases. Age of becoming wheelchair bound showed an inverse correlation with GAA repeat lengths. In contrast to the findings of Duerr and coworkers,[46] rate of progression did not correlate with repeat length. There was meiotic instability with a median variation of 150 repeats.

Five compound heterozygous patients with one expanded allele and one allele carrying the I154F mutation had a phenotype that was indistinguishable from those of patients with two expanded alleles. Three patients with progressive ataxia, dysarthria, absence of lower limb reflexes, and onset at ages 3, 11, and 29 years did not have expanded alleles. The I154F mutation was excluded as well. None of the patients had extensor plantar responses, diabetes, or cardiomyopathy, and two had atypical findings such as head tremor or marked distal muscle wasting.

Geschwind and colleagues[141] examined 39 patients with classic FRDA, LOFA, and FARR and other recessive or sporadic ataxias of early onset. Two of 15 families with typical FRDA did not show GAA expansion. In the LOFA and FARR group, only 4 of 11 patients showed GAA expansion, and in the last group only 1 of 11 patients carried a small GAA expansion. The lower rate of positive FRDA tests compared with other studies[46,140] may lie in the fact that this group of patients was not preselected to fit FRDA criteria as part of an ongoing effort to identify the FRDA gene.

Schols and associates[142] confirmed these findings and identified homozygous repeat expansions ranging form 66 to 1360 repeats in 36 of 102 patients with idiopathic ataxia. Although 27 patients had a typical FRDA phenotype, 9 did not. One patient with a typical FRDA phenotype did not have any GAA expansion, suggesting either the presence of point mutations in both alleles or locus heterogeneity.

### DIFFERENTIAL DIAGNOSIS AND WORK-UP

The diagnosis of FRDA is essentially a clinical one, but can now be confirmed by a direct genetic test for GAA expansion that will detect abnormality in at least one allele in 95% of patients meeting strict clinical criteria. The condition most frequently confused with FRDA is the demyelinating form of hereditary motor and sensory neuropathy (Charcot-Marie-Tooth neuropathy type 1 [CMT1], see Chapter 4), as some patients with the latter present in childhood with clumsiness and areflexia and minimal distal muscle weakness. Differentiation between the two conditions may be difficult if a child with FRDA has not developed dysarthria or extensor plantar responses. This distinction, which is important because the prognosis in CMT1 is much better than in FRDA and inheritance is dominant, can be made by DNA analysis and by performing NCV studies. Upper limb motor nerve conduction velocity is always greater than 40 m/sec in FRDA and slower than this in hereditary motor-sensory neuropathy type I.

Abetalipoproteinemia and isolated vitamin E deficiency should also be excluded in patients presenting with the clinical features of FRDA. Friedriech's ataxia is distinguished from other early onset ataxias by virtue of their clinical features (see later). The ECG is a useful investigative study for possible cases of FRDA as the changes seen are virtually diagnostic in the setting of an ataxic patient. Computed tomography or MRI scanning is either normal or shows mild cerebellar atrophy (Fig. 12–2). Friedreich's ataxia should also be considered for patients with late onset sporadic cerebellar ataxia.[142]

## Friedreich-Like Ataxias Due to Treatable or Common Metabolic Abnormalities

### VITAMIN E DEFICIENCY ATAXIAS

A mutation in the α-tocopherol transfer protein (α-TTP) on chromosome 8q13 causes a familial ataxia (AVED) with a neurologic phenotype indistinguishable from that of FRDA.[143,144] AVED patients cannot incorporate α-tocopherol into lipoproteins secreted by the liver, a function putatively attributable to the α-TTP. Ouahchi and associates[144] reported the identification of three frameshift mutations in the α-TTP gene. A 744delA mutation accounted for 68% of the mutant alleles in 17 families from North Africa and Italy. Cavalier and coworkers[145] recently summarized the findings in 27 AVED families with 13 different mutations. They identified a decreased incidence of cardiomyopathy, but increased incidence of head titubation and dystonia in AVED as differentiating features from FRDA. Benomar and associates[146] confirmed the increased head titubation in Moroccan families with AVED. An FRDA-like ataxia with retinitis pigmentosa was described in four unrelated individuals with a His101GLN missense mutation.[147]

AVED can be diagnosed through low plasma vitamin E levels and treated with continuing supplementation of vitamin E (600 IU or 5 to 10 mg/kg twice daily), which corrects the plasma values and appears to have beneficial effects on neurologic function.[148] Tamaru and coworkers,[149] however, described a patient with a splice site mutation resulting in protein truncation with resistance to vitamin E supplementation.

### ABETALIPOPROTEINEMIA AND HYPOBETALIPOPROTEINEMIA

Abetalipoproteinemia (Bassen-Kornzweig disease), a recessive disorder due to a defect in apolipoprotein B-100 (chromosome 2p24), results in fat malabsorption and low levels of the fat-soluble vitamins A, D, E, and K. The initial presentation may be visual loss. By the second decade of life, neurologic abnormalities develop that include a progressive, FRDA-like peripheral neuropathy and SCA, as well as retinitis pigmentosa and, occasionally, ptosis and external ophthalmoplegia. Electrophysiologic studies (EEG, EMG/NCV, ECG) show changes similar to those of FRDA, as do sural nerve biopsy and cardiac pathology at autopsy. Central nervous system pathology is also similar, but shows more loss of anterior horn cells and Purkinje cells than is described in FRDA. Acanthocytes are present on fresh blood smears. Plasma studies show low levels of the fat-soluble vitamins, cholesterol and other plasma lipids, and apolipoprotein B. Treatment has been successful at ameliorating or preventing the retinal and neurologic disease by supplementing vitamins E, A, and K and restricting intake of long-chain fatty acids.[3]

Hypobetalipoproteinemia, a genetically distinct disorder, causes reduced low-density lipoprotein and cholesterol in plasma of heterozygotes compared with normal values in abetalipoproteinemia heterozygotes. Homozygotes manifest clinical and laboratory findings similar to those of patients homozygous for abetalipoproteinemia.[3] Abetalipoproteinemia and hypobetalipoproteinemia are most easily differentiated by examining plasma lipid levels in the parents of the affected individual.

#### ATYPICAL HEXOSAMINIDASES A AND AB DEFICIENCY SYNDROMES

Milder deficiencies of hexosaminidase A (Tay-Sachs disease) or hexosaminidase AB can present in the same age range as FRDA, with slowly progressive ataxia with retained reflexes, early dysarthria and intention tremor, neurogenic proximal weakness resembling spinal muscular atrophy, and later dementia or psychiatric features.[150,151] The phenotype is not as close to that of FRDA as it is to that of vitamin E deficiency ataxia, due to lack of sensory involvement, but patients may be misdiagnosed.

Hexosaminidase A screening with artificial substrates typically shows the same absence of activity as seen in infantile Tay-Sachs disease, although some residual activity is suspected. Hund and associates[152] described a sibship with four individuals who were compound heterozygotes for the infantile and adult mutation with some residual enzyme activity using fluorogenic substrates. Rectal biopsy material showed lamellar inclusions in neurons of the myenteric plexus. Brain specimens showed excess ganglioside in neurons and severe parenchymatous degeneration of the cerebellum.[3] Magnetic resonance imaging confirms the presence of severe cerebellar atrophy during life.[152] There is as yet no specific treatment for this syndrome, although inhibition of glycosphingolipid biosynthesis has shown promise in animal models.[153] Premarital and prenatal screening are in wide usage.

## THE NON-FRIEDREICH-LIKE ATAXIAS

The non-FA–like ataxias are a heterogeneous group of sporadic, recessive, or maternally inherited SCAs that lack some of the essential features of FA or prominently display features not usually seen. Many of the conditions are so rare that a genetic classification may never be achieved. From this group two recessive diseases are discussed in greater detail: ataxia telangiectasia and early onset cerebellar ataxia with retained reflexes.

### Ataxia Telangiectasia

In contrast to Cockayne's syndrome and xeroderma pigmentosum, which may also be associated with ataxia, ataxia telangiectasia (A-T) does not demonstrate severe cognitive changes or seizures. Ataxia telangiectasia is the most common cause of recessively inherited ataxia with onset before age 5 years with a prevalence of 1/40,000 to 1/100,000 live births. It has a well-defined phenotype, making diagnosis relatively easy, and shows complete penetrance. The early presence of basal ganglia features, the intact sensation, and downgoing toes help differentiate this syndrome from FRDA. The gene on chromosome 11q, designated *ATM,* that is mutated in AT has been identified.[154]

#### RANGE OF CLINICAL FINDINGS

Onset can be in the first year of life, with gait ataxia being noted when the child begins to walk, or as late as the second decade. Titubation of the head, intention tremor, myoclonic jerks, and choreoathetosis follow. Dystonia is seen in postadolescent patients.

Speech is slow and slurred. Patients have hypotonic facies and posture, with a tendency to drool. Characteristic eye movements show oculomotor apraxia, with the use of compensatory head thrusting and overshoot to look at objects. Saccades are slowly initiated and of long latency. Ocular telangiectases usually present later than the ataxia (from 3 to 5 years of age) and are followed by cutaneous telangiectases along with other progeric hair and skin changes. As the disease progresses, generalized or distal weakness, neurogenic atrophy, and axonal sensory loss may appear. Delayed sexual development with associated growth retardation is frequent. The child usually needs a wheelchair by age 10 or 11 years.

Associated non-neurologic features include recurrent sinopulmonary disease, lymphoreticular malignancies and leukemia in preadolescents and epithelial or other solid tumors in postadolescents. Death is usually due to infection or neoplasia.

## LABORATORY AND PATHOLOGICAL FINDINGS

Non-radiographic–based imaging techniques are preferred for diagnostic purposes. They typically show early cerebellar atrophy, thymic and adenoidal hypoplasia or absence, and chronic sinus and pulmonary changes. Electronystagmography reveals the diagnostic changes in saccade initiation combining cerebellar and basal ganglia dysfunction. In older patients, denervation, as well as reduced motor velocities and sensory potentials, can be seen.

Serologic markers include elevated levels of α-fetoprotein and carcinoembryonic antigen and changes in humoral or cellular immunity in two-thirds of patients with absent or low IgG2, IgA, and IgE; normal or low IgG; normal or elevated IgM; decreased responsiveness to skin test antigens; decreased T cells and T cell mitogenic response, and increased natural killer cells. A particular IgM antibody may be directed against insulin receptors, leading to mild glucose intolerance. Cytogenetic studies for chromosomal breaks ideally show t(7;14) translocations.

Neuropathological studies confirm primary changes in cerebellum and its connections in brain stem and rostral centers. Cerebellar cortical atrophy predominates, with thinning of molecular and granular cell layers and decreased numbers of Purkinje cells. In spinal cord, demyelination of long tracts and loss of anterior horn cells may be noted.

## THE *ATM* GENE

The gene mutated in A-T has been localized to chromosome 11q23.1[155] and cloned.[154] The gene, designated *ATM* for "mutated in A-T," is large and extends over 180 kb. A 12 kb transcript is predicted to encode a protein of 3056 amino acids.[156,157] In its C-terminal half, it shares homology with phosphatidylinositol-3 kinase and a family of other genes, some involved with DNA double-strand break repair, cell cycle checkpoint control, and control of telomere length.

The majority of *ATM* mutations are predicted to result in truncated proteins due to deletions and splice mutations. Missense mutations producing an altered full-length protein are associated with milder phenotypes in compound heterozygotes or patients homozygous for the milder alleles.[158–160]

Heterozygote carriers of the *ATM* mutations gene also have increased clinical sensitivity to radiation, and females may have an increased risk of breast cancer.[161]

Although the functions of the ATM protein in cell cycle control are beginning to be understood, the mechanisms underlying neuronal degeneration are less well defined. *Atm* knock-out mice did not show any light microscopic abnormalities, but synaptic abnormalities were visible by electron microscopy.[162]

The large number of different mutations that have been found in the *ATM* gene make direct DNA testing impractical for the isolated patient, although linkage analysis has been helpful in prenatal testing for couples who already have one or more affected children. Radiation sensitivity can be demonstrated in transformed lymphocyte colonies (colony-stimulating assay), which is performed in a few A-T-dedicated research laboratories and thought to be the most specific diagnostic test in the appropriate clinical setting.

## Early Onset Cerebellar Ataxia with Retained Reflexes

Early onset cerebellar ataxia with retained reflexes occurs at a frequency about one-fourth of that of FRDA and is often confused with FRDA. Inheritance is autosomal recessive in most cases.[163,164] The distinction is of value because the prognosis is better than for FRDA, with patients losing the ability to walk approximately 13 years later. The age of onset of symptoms ranges between 2 and 20 years. The upper limb and knee reflexes are normal or increased, but the ankle jerks may be absent. Optic atrophy, severe skeletal deformity, and cardiac involvement do not occur. Cerebellar atrophy is frequently found on CT or MRI scanning.[127] The pathology is that of olivopontocerebellar atrophy in some cases. Some patients may be cases of FARR.

In the experience of our group and others,[141] early onset ataxias with retained reflexes and variable other criteria are not likely to represent frataxin mutations unless they show the typical eye movement findings, abnormal SSERs, severe axonal sensory loss, or cardiomyopathy.[165] The presence of dementia, seizures, retinal degeneration, ophthalmoplegia, basal ganglia dysfunction, early onset severe weakness or atrophy, diabetes insipidus, or early cerebellar atrophy make the presence of a mutation in the FRDA gene unlikely.

## Other Autosomal Recessive Ataxias

Other autosomal recessive ataxias are rare (Table 12–5) and are defined by their associated features.[3] Autosomal recessive inheritance of late onset cerebellar ataxia is very unusual other than those cases associated with short GAA expansions in the frataxin gene.[142,166]

### INFANTILE ONSET SCA

Koskinen and associates[167] reported the clinical findings in 19 Finnish patients, including 6 pairs of sibs, with onset between 1 and 2 years of age. The first manifestation was clumsiness and loss of ability to walk. Ataxia, athetosis, and muscle hypotonia with loss of deep tendon reflexes were discovered on clinical examination. By school age, ophthalmoplegia and hearing loss were found, and sensory neuropathy developed by adolescence. The main finding in neuroradiologic studies was cerebellar atrophy. Infantile onset SCA has been mapped to 10q24.[87]

### OTHER RECESSIVE ATAXIAS

An autosomal recessive ataxia with hypogonadism was first described by Gordon Holmes. Abnormal sexual development is caused by hypogonadotrophic hypogonadism. Age of onset of neurologic symptoms ranges from 1 to 30 years, but is usually in the third decade. The disorder comprises dysarthria, nystagmus, and progressive limb and gait ataxia. Cerebello-olivary atrophy is found at autopsy.[168]

The autosomal recessive spastic ataxia of Charlevoix-Saguenay (ARSACS) presents with spasticity and shows ataxia only later. ARSACS was recently mapped to 13q12.[169]

## X-Linked Ataxias

X-linked inheritance is rare in hereditary ataxias and is associated with a variety of phenotypes. In five generations of one family, the neurologic syndrome had onset in childhood or adolescence with a mild spastic paraparesis, followed by the development of upper limb ataxia and dysarthria.[170] Another X-linked spastic-ataxic syndrome with dementia has been described.[171] Recently, a syndrome of mental retardation, ataxia, and hearing impairment was localized to Xq21.33–q24.[172] Of known metabolic causes, the adult form of adrenoleukodystrophy (adrenomyeloneuropathy; chromosome Xq28) presents with this phenotype, with the addition of peripheral neuropathy, sphincter disturbances, and cognitive or psychiatric features.

Pyruvate dehydrogenase complex, the mitochondrial matrix enzyme that catalyzes the conversion of pyruvate to acetyl coenzyme A, has three subunit enzymes and two or three regulatory components, synthesized by a total of nine genes. One of these genes, for the E1a subunit, is on the X chromosome (Xp22.1). Point mutations can produce severe congenital lactic acidosis and seizures in males, but milder symptoms of intermittent lactic acidosis, trunkal ataxia, dysarthria, and mental retardation in heterozygous females due to variable X-inactivation patterns in different organs.[173] These patients may fall into the differential diagnosis of early onset episodic ataxias and may show a phenotypic overlap with FA.

### Mitochondrial Ataxias

Cerebellar ataxia occurring in combination with myoclonus is often called the Ramsay-Hunt syndrome. This is a heterogeneous syndrome and includes mitochondrial encephalomyopathy (myoclonic epilepsy with ragged red fibers) sialidosis, and Baltic myoclonus epilepsy (Unverricht-Lundborg disease). Cerebellar ataxia is a late feature in Baltic myoclonus epilepsy (see Chapter 17).

Clinical features that suggest a mitochondrial cause of a SCA include onset of myoclonus or generalized seizures after onset of the ataxia, concomitant myopathy, progressive external ophthalmoplegia, retinopathy or optic atrophy, hearing loss, heart block or cardiomyopathy, diabetes, intestinal pseudo-obstruction, stroke-like episodes, dementia, or "buffalo hump" fat pad. Fasting, postprandial, or exercise studies of serum pyruvate/lactate ratios, DNA analysis, muscle biopsy, and muscle biochemistry may help confirm the diagnosis of a mitochondrial-based oxidative disorder. Mitochondrial disorders are further discussed in Chapter 15.

## CEREBELLAR SYNDROMES OF UNCERTAIN INHERITANCE

Harding[3] divided 36 reported cases of sporadic ataxia into three groups depending on the prominence of ataxia and the presence of pyramidal signs and dementia. These categories were described before the availability of genetic tests for the SCAs and FA, however, and did not examine the neuropathological features of the multiple system atrophy syndromes (see later).

An infantile or juvenile onset progressive cerebellar syndrome might represent a recessive metabolic or X-linked/mitochondrial condition. A syndrome of early onset cerebellar ataxia, areflexia, pes cavus, optic atrophy, and sensorineural hearing loss (CAPOS) has been described by Nicolaides and colleagues.[174] Three family members presented with a relapsing, early onset cerebellar ataxia associated with progressive optic atrophy and sensorineural deafness. All three patients had a pes cavus deformity and areflexia in the absence of a peripheral neuropathy. An autosomal dominant or maternal mitochondrial pattern of inheritance was suggested.

Relatively early onset in the third or fourth decade without a family history could still suggest a familial cerebellar syndrome rather than a sporadic olivopontocerebellar atrophy if accompanied by signs of optic atrophy, retinal degeneration, ophthalmoplegia, nonpyramidal spinal involvement, or involuntary movements (choreoathetosis, myoclonus).[168] Progressive supranuclear palsy, although it may begin in this age group with gait instability, usually develops its characteristic vertical supranuclear gaze palsy and axial extension posture within 2 years.[175] Progressive supranuclear palsy is rarely familial. A dominant pedigree has been described,[176] and an association with alleles of the tau gene have been observed in other studies.[177,178] The genetics of progressive supranuclear palsy are discussed in Chapter 18.

In the multiple system atrophy syndromes, with involvement of cerebellar, basal ganglia, and autonomic systems, some patients may present with ataxia. Cerebellar symptoms and signs were the initial feature in only 5% of patients, but developed in half during the course of the disease.[179] All these phenotypes have been shown to have similar PET scan patterns. With fluorodopa and diprenorphine scanning, decreased activity is seen in cerebellum, but also in cortex, thalamus, and putamen. Neuropathologically, the multiple syndrome atrophy syndromes also share the characteristic changes of argyrophilic cytoplasmic inclusion bodies in oligodendroglia and neurons, which seem to be tangles of microtubules different from those seen in Alzheimer's disease or progressive supranuclear palsy.[180–182]

## WORK-UP FOR CHRONIC ATAXIAS

As outlined in Table 12–6, it is important to characterize the phenotype to guide additional diagnostic procedures for the patient with a cerebellar syndrome of uncertain inheritance pattern. The clinical examination can often determine whether the phenotype is a purely cerebellar, brain stem–cerebellar, or spinal–long tract phenotype. The MRI scan of the brain and upper cervical cord can confirm which anatomic structures are predominantly involved and can rule out demyelinating diseases and leukodystrophies.

Although ataxia patients harboring mutations in the SCA genes in the absence of a positive family history are relatively rare, testing is warranted. A family history that is noncontributory (parents cannot be evaluated or died early, small number of first-degree relatives) should not be equated with a negative family history. A predominant spinocerebellar presentation should prompt testing for a mutation in the frataxin gene even when reflexes are retained.[183] It is now well established that small GAA expansions are associated with later onset and variant phenotypes. Friedreich's ataxia testing of patients with typical olivopontocerebellar atrophy/multiple syndrome atrophy syndrome features is unlikely to be helpful.

Screening of sporadic ataxia patients for the presence of antigliadin and antiendo-

Table 12–6. **Workup of the Patient with Progressive Ataxia**

| | Primary | Secondary |
|---|---|---|
| Phenotype assessment | History and Physical examination<br>Family history<br>MRI of brain | Imaging of remaining neuraxis<br>NCV, SSER, BAER, ENG, VER |
| Basic workup | Genetic testing<br>Anticerebellar antibodies<br>TSH, T4<br>Vitamins B12, E<br>CSF for infection, demyelination, neoplasm | Cu/ceruloplasmin<br>Urine heavy metals<br>VDRL/FTA<br>Lyme, EBV titers<br>Anti-HTLV1 |
| Onset before age 20 years or spinal phenotype | Testing for frataxin GAA expansion<br>α-fetoprotein<br>Quantitative immunoglobulins | 2 hr post-prandial glucose, lactate pyruvate, ammonia, amino acids lysosomal hydrolases, Tay-Sachs test<br>Very long chain fatty acids (if spastic)<br>Cholestanol (if cataracts) |
| With mitochondrial features | Fasting and 2 hr post-prandial glucose<br>Lactate, pyruvate<br>Muscle biopsy<br>Specific mt DNA studies | serum carnitine |
| With dementia, seizures or abnormal EEG or ERG | Prion protein DNA testing (GSS)<br>Conjunctival biopsy (NCL)<br>Bone marrow biopsy (Niemann-Pick type C)<br>Jejunal biopsy (Whipple's disease) | brain biopsy |

NCL: Neuronal ceroid lipofuscinosis.

mysium antibodies resulted in positive findings in 3 of 24 patients, whereas none out of 23 patients with hereditary ataxias were positive.[184] The positive patients did not have distinguishing features. These results need to be reproduced in a separate group of ataxia patients before testing for celiac disease can be universally recommended.

## GENETIC COUNSELING

General issues regarding genetic counseling and use of DNA testing are discussed in Chapter 22. The ataxias present some additional challenges. Similar phenotypes can be caused by mutations in one of a number of genes. In addition, identical mutations in the same gene can be associated with very different phenotypes, as best exemplified by SCA3 and MJD or by DRPLA and the Haw River syndrome. Different types of mutations in the same gene may cause different, but partially overlapping phenotypes as seen in SCA6 and EA-2.

The new direct gene tests are highly accurate and specific and can greatly reduce the cost of diagnostic evaluation of the symptomatic patient. Tests for the SCAs should be offered to patients with a dominant family history or a late onset, progressive, cerebellar syndrome. Tests for recessive or metabolic ataxias should be reserved for those without a dominant family history unless features suggestive of mitochondrial disease are present.

Most genetic testing centers adhere to strict pretest and post-test counseling protocols to identify individuals who may not handle the genetic information well and to help ameliorate these effects. Presymptomatic testing has been traditionally restricted to adults (over age 18 years), when informed decision-making and psychological counseling can be more effectively employed and the risks of stigmatization are lessened. Surprisingly, predictive and prenatal tests for the hereditary ataxias represent only 8 of almost 6000 tests that are performed in U.S. laboratories.[185]

Maintaining confidentiality of the asymptomatic patient's DNA test results is important to minimize subtle discrimination on the part of relatives and friends and less-than-subtle discrimination on the part of employers and the health, life, and disability insurance industries. Anonymous genetic counseling and testing protocols have been proposed to avoid these pitfalls.[186]

## SUMMARY

The classification and phenotypic definitions of the inherited ataxias have undergone a significant change in the 1990s. A phenotype-based classification has been largely replaced by a system based on the genotype. The genes for several dominant ataxias have been identified, and a common disease mutational mechanism based on expansion of CAG DNA trinucleotide repeats has been demonstrated. The CAG repeats are in the coding region of genes and encode polyglutamine-containing proteins. Identification of the gene for FRDA has shown that mutations in this gene cause a more diverse phenotype than initially suspected. The mutations for other rare ataxias have also been identified.

## REFERENCES


1. Greenfield JG: The Spinocerebellar Degenerations. Charles C Thomas, Springfield, IL, 1954.
2. Konigsmark BS, Weiner LP: The olivopontocerebellar atrophies. A review. Medicine 49:227–241, 1970.
3. Harding AE: The Hereditary Ataxias and Related Disorders. Churchill Livingston, New York, 1984.

3a. Becker PE: Enfermedades de localizacion preferente en al sisterna espinocerebeloso. In S.A. Toray (ed.), *Genetica Humana*, Vol. V/I, Barcelona, pp.233–320, 1969.

3b. Eadie MJ. Olivo-ponto-cerebellar atrophy (variant 1). In P.J. Vinken and G.W. Bruyn (eds.) Handbook of Clinical Neurology, Vol. 21, System Disorders and Atrophies, Part 1. North Holland Publishing Company, Amsterdam, pp.451–457, 1975.

4. Gudmundsson K: The prevalence and occurrence of some rare neurological diseases in Iceland. Acta Neurol Scand 45:114–118, 1969.
5. Yakura H, Wakisaka A, Fujimoto S, Itakur K: Hereditary ataxia and HLA genotypes. N Engl J Med 291:154–155, 1974.
6. Orr HT, Chung M, Banti S, et al.: Expansion of an unstable trinucleotide CAG repeat in spinocerebellar ataxia type 1. Nat Genet 4:221–226, 1994.
7. Ranum LP, Chung M, Banfi S, et al.: Molecular and clinical correlations in spinocerebellar ataxia type 1: Evidence for familial effects on the age at onset. Am J Hum Genet 55:244–252, 1994.

8. Dubourg O, Durr A, Canul G, et al.: Analysis of the SCA1 CAG repeat in a large number of families with dominant ataxia: Clinical and molecular correlations. Ann Neurol 37:176–180, 1995.
9. Genis D, Matilla T, Jolpini V: Clinical neuropathologic, and genetic studies of a large spinocerebellar ataxia type 1 (SCA1) kindred: $(CAG)_n$ expansion and early premonitory signs and symptoms. Neurology 45:24–30, 1995.
10. Kameya T, Abe K, Aoki M, et al.: Analysis of spinocerebellar ataxia type 1 (SCA1) related CAG trinucleotide expansion in Japan. Neurology 45: 1587–1594, 1995.
11. Ranum LPW, Lundgren JK, Schut LJ, et al.: Spinocerebellar ataxia type 1 and Machado-Joseph disease: Incidence of CAG expansions among adult-onset ataxia patients from 311 families with dominant recessive, or sporadic ataxia. Am J Hum Genet 57:603–608, 1995.
12. Goldfarb LG, Vasconcelos O, Platonov FA, et al.: Unstable triplet repeat and phenotypic variability of spinocerebellar ataxia type 1. Ann Neurol 39: 500–506, 1996.
13. Gilman S, St Laurent RT, Kreppe RA, et al.: A comparison of cerebral blood flow and glucose metabolism in olivopontocerebellar atrophy using PET. Neurology 45:1345–1352, 1995.
14. Tedeschi G, Bertolino A, Massaquoi SG, et al.: Proton magnetic resonance spectroscopic imaging in patients with cerebellar degeneration. Ann Neurol 39:71–78, 1996.
15. Gilman S, Sima AAF, Junck L, et al.: Spinocerebellar ataxia type 1 with multiple system degeneration and glial cytoplasmic inclusions. Ann Neurol 39: 241–255, 1996.
16. Lopes-Cendes I, Maciel P, Kish S, et al.: Somatic mosaicism in the central nervous system in spinocerebellar ataxia type 1 and Machado-Joseph disease. Ann Neurol 40:199–206, 1996.
17. Servadio A, Koshy B, Armstrong D, et al.: Expression analysis of the ataxia-1 protein in tissues from normal and spinocerebellar ataxia type 1 individuals. Nat Genet 10:94–98, 1995.
18. Matilla A, Koshy BT, Cummings CJ, Isobe T, Orr HT: The cerebellar leucine-rich acidic nuclear protein interacts with ataxin-1. Nature 389:974–978, 1997.
19. Skinner PJ, Koshy BT, Cummings CJ, et al.: Ataxin-1 with an expanded glutamine tract alters nuclear matrix-associated structures. Nature 389:971–974, 1997.
20. Gispert S, Twells R, Orozio G, et al.: Chromosomal assignment of the second (Cuban) locus for autosomal dominant cerebellar ataxia (SCA2) to chromosome 12q23–24.1. Nat Genet 4:295–299, 1993.
21. Pulst SM, Starkman S, Nechiporuk A: Anticipation in spinocerebellar ataxia type 2. Nat Genet 5:8–10, 1993.
22. Filla A, DeMichele G, Banfi S, et al.: Has spinocerebellar ataxia type 2 a distinct phenotype? Genetic and clinical study of an Italian family. Neurology 45:793–796, 1995.
23. Belal S, Cancel G, Stevanin G, et al.: Clinical and genetic analysis of a Tunesian family with autosomal dominant cerebellar ataxia type 1 linked to the SCA2 locus. Neurology 44:1423–1426, 1994.
24. Lopes-Cendes I, Andermann E, Attig E: Confirmation of the SCA-2 locus as an alternative locus for dominantly inherited spinocerebellar ataxia and refinement of the candidate region. Am J Hum Genet 54:774–781, 1994.
25. Nechiporuk A, Lopes-Cendes I, Nechiporuk T, et al.: Genetic mapping of spinocerebellar ataxia type 2 gene on human chromosome 12. Neurology 46: 1731–1735, 1996.
26. Pulst SM, Nechiporuk A, Nechiporuk T, et al.: Moderate expansion of a normally biallelic trinucleotide repeat in spinocerebellar ataxia type 2. Nat Genet 14:269–276, 1996.
27. Sanpei K, Takano H, Igarashi S, et al.: Identification of the spinocerebellar ataxia type 2 gene using a direct identification of repeat expansion and cloning technique, DIRECT. Nat Genet 14:277–284, 1996.
28. Imbert G, Saudou F, Yvert G, et al.: Cloning of the gene for spinocerebellar ataxia 2 reveals a locus with high sensitivity to expanded CAG glutamine repeats. Nat Genet 14:285–291, 1996.
29. Orozco G, Nodarse A, Cordoves R, Auburger G: Autosomal dominant cerebellar ataxia: Clinical analysis of 263 patients from a homogeneous population in Holguin, Cuba. Neurology 40:1369–1375, 1990.
30. Cancel G, Durr A, Didierjean O, et al.: Molecular and clinical correlations in spinocerebellar ataxia 2: A study of 32 families. Hum Mol Genet 6:709–715, 1997.
31. Geschwind D, Perlman S, Figueroa P, Treiman L, Pulst SM: The prevalence and wide clinical spectrum of the spinocerebellar ataxia type 2 trinucleotide repeat in patients with autosomal dominant cerebellar ataxia. Am J Hum Genet 60:842–850, 1997.
32. Adams C, Pulst SM: Clinical and molecular analysis of a pedigree of southern Italian ancestry with spinocerebellar ataxia type 2. Neurology 49:1163–1166, 1997.
33. Huynh DH, Del Bigio MR, Sahba SD, Ho DH, Pulst SM: Expression of ataxin-2 in brains from normal individuals and patients with Alzheimer disease and spinocerebellar ataxia 2 (SCA2). Ann Neurol 45:232–241, 1999.
34. Riess O, Laccone F, Gispert S, et al.: SCA2 trinucleotide expansion in German SCA patients. Neurogenetics 1:59–64, 1997.
35. Schols S, Gispert S, Vorgert, et al.: Spinocerebellar ataxia type 2: Genotype and phenotype in German kindred. Arch Neurol 54:1073–1080, 1997.
36. Burk K, Abele M, Fetter M, et al.: Autosomal dominant cerebellar ataxia type 1: Clinical features and magnetic resonance imaging in families with SCA1, SCA2 and SCA3. Brain 119:1497–1505, 1996.
37. Buttner N, Geschwind D, Jen JC, Perlman S, Pulst SM: Oculomotor phenotypes in the SCA syndromes. Arch Neurol 55:1353–1357, 1998.
38. Storey E, Forrest SM, Shaw JH, Mitchell P, McKinley Gardner RJ: Spinocerebellar ataxia type 2: Clinical features of a pedigree displaying prominent frontal-executive dysfunction. Arch Neurol 56:43–50, 1999.
39. Romanul FCA, Fowler HL, Radvany J, et al.: Azo-

rean disease of the nervous system. N Engl J Med 296:1505–1508, 1977.
40. Kawaguchi Y, Okamoto T, Taniwaki M, et al.: CAG expansions in a novel gene for Machado-Joseph disease at chromosome 14q32.1. Nat Genet 8:221–228, 1994.
41. Matilla T, McCall A, Subramony SH, Zoghbi HY, et al.: Molecular and clinical correlations in spinocerebellar ataxia type 3 and Machado-Joseph disease Ann Neurol 38:68–72, 1995.
42. Tuite PJ, Rogneva EA, St. George-Hyslop PH, et al.: Dopa-responsive parkinsonism phenotype of Machado-Joseph disease: Confirmation of 14q CAG expansion. Ann Neurol 38:684–687, 1995.
43. Sutton JP, Pulst SM: Atypical parkinsonism in a family of Portuguese ancestry: Absence of CAG repeat expansion in the *MJD1* gene. Neurology 48: 1285–1290, 1997.
44. Cancel G, Abbas N, Stevanin G, et al.: Marked phenotypic heterogeneity associated with expansion of a CAG repeat sequence at the spinocerebellar ataxia 3/Machado-Joseph disease locus. Am J Hum Genet 57:809–816, 1995.
45. Kitamura J, Kubyki Y, Tsuruta T, et al.: A new family with Machado-Joseph disease in Japan: Homovanillic acid, magenetic resonance, and sleep apnea studies. Arch Neurol 46:425–428, 1989.
46. Durr A, Stevanin G, Cancel G, et al.: Spinocerebellar ataxia 3 and Machado Joseph disease: Clinical, molecular and neuropathological features. Ann Neurol 39:490–499, 1996.
47. Takiyama Y, Oyanagi S, Kawashima S, et al.: A clinical and pathologic study of a large Japanese family with Machado-Joseph disease tightly linked to the DNA markers on chromosome 14q. Neurology 44: 1302–1308, 1994.
48. Lopes-Cendes I, Silveira I, Maciel P, et al.: Limits of clinical assessment in the accurate diagnosis of Machado-Joseph disease. Arch Neurol 53:1168–1174, 1996
49. Takiyama Y, Oyanagi S, Kawashima S, et al.: A clinical and pathologic study of a large Japanese family with Machado-Joseph disease tightly linked to the DNA markers on chromosome 14Q. Neurology 44: 1298–1301, 1993.
50. Maciel P, Garaspar C, DeStefano AL, et al.: Correlation between CAG repeat length and clinical features in Machado-Joseph disease. Am J Hum Genet 57:54–61, 1995.
51. Maruyama H, Nakamura S, Matsuyaina Z, et al.: Molecular features of the CAG repeats and clinical manifestations of Machado-Joseph disease. Hum Mol Genet 4:807–812, 1995.
52. Schols L, Vieira-Saecker AM, Schols S, et al.: Trinucleotide expansion within the *MJD1* gene presents clinically as spinocerebellar ataxia and occurs most frequently in German SCA patients. Hum Mol Genet 4:1001–1005, 1995.
53. Takiyama Igamshi S, Rogaeva EA, et al.: Evidence for intergenerational instability in the CAG repeat in the *MJD1* gene and for continual haplotypes and flanking markers amongst Japanese and Caucasian subjects with Machado-Joseph disease. Hum Mol Genet 4:1137–1146, 1995.
54. Takiyama Y, Sakoe K, Nakano I Nishizawa M: Machado-Joseph disease: Cerebellar ataxia and autonomic dysfunction in a patient with the shortest known expanded allele (56 CAG repeat units) of the *MJD1* gene. Neurology 40:604–606, 1997.
55. Ikeda H, Yamaguchi M, Sugai SS, et al.: Expanded polyglutamine in the Machado-Joseph disease protein induces cell death *in vitro* and *in vivo*. Nat Genet 13:196–202, 1996.
56. Paulson HL, Perez MK, Trottier Y, et al.: Intranuclear inclusions of expanded polyglutamine protein in spinocerebellar ataxia type 3. Neuron 19: 333–344, 1997.
57. DeStefano AL, Cupples LA Maciel P, et al.: A familial factor independent of CAG repeat length influences age of onset of Machado-Joseph disease. Am J Hum Genet 59:119–127, 1996.
58. Ikeuchi T, Igamshi S, Takiyama Y, et al.: Nonmendelian transmission in dentatorubral-pallidoluysian atrophy and Machado-Joseph disease and the mutant allele is preferentially transmitted in male meiosis. Am J Hum Genet 58:730–733, 1996.
59. Sakai T, Kawakaini H: Machado-Joseph disease: A proposal of spastic paraplegic subtype. Neurology 46:846–847, 1996.
60. Ishikawa K, Mizusawa H, Igamshi S, et al.: Pure cerebellar ataxia phenotype in Machado-Joseph disease. Neurology 46:1776–1777, 1996.
61. Lang EE, Rogaura SA, Tsuda T, et al.: Homozygous inheritance of the Machado-Joseph disease gene. Ann Neurol 36:443–447, 1994.
62. Gadoth N, Slotogora J, Merims D: Correlation between clinical and molecular genetic analysis in Machado-Joseph disease. Neurology (Suppl) 46: A329, 1996.
63. Flanigan K, Gardner K, Alderson K, Galster B, et al.: Autosomal dominant spinocerebellar ataxia with sensory axonal neuropathy (SCA4): Clinical description and genetic localization to chromosome 16q22.1. Am J Hum Genet 59:392–399, 1996.
64. Nachmanoff DB, Segal RA, Dawson DM, Brown RB, De Girolami U: Hereditary ataxia with sensory neuronopathy: Biemond's ataxia. Neurology 48: 273–275, 1997.
65. Ranum LPW, Schut LJ, Lundgren JK, Orr HT: Spinocerebellar ataxia type 5 in a family descended from the grandparents of president Lincoln maps to chromosome. Nat Genet 8:280:284, 1994.
66. Zhuchenko O, Bailey J, Bonnen P, et al.: Autosomal dominant cerebellar ataxia (SCA6) associated with small polyglutamine expansions in the $\alpha$ 1 A–voltage-dependent calcium channel. Nat Genet 15: 62–69, 1997.
67. Subramony SH, Fratkin JD, Manyam BV, Currier RD: Dominantly inherited cerebello-olivary atrophy is not due to a mutation at the spinocerebellar ataxia-I, Machado-Joseph disease, or dentato-rubro-pallido-luysian atrophy locus. Mov Disord 11:174–180, 1996.
68. Matsumura R, Futamura N, Fujimoto Y, et al.: Spinocerebellar ataxia type 6. Neurology 49:1238–1242, 1997.
69. Stevanin G, Durr A, David G, Didierjean O, et al.: Clinical and molecular features of spinocerebellar ataxia type 6. Neurology 49:1243–1246, 1997.
70. Geschwind DH, Perlman S, Figueroa KP, et al.: Spinocerebellar ataxia type 6 frequency of the muta-

tion and genotype–phenotype correlations. Neurology 49:1247–1251, 1997.
71. Schols L, Gispert S, Vorgerd M, et al.: Spinocerebellar ataxia type 2. Genotype and phenotype in German kindreds. Arch Neurol 54:1073–1080, 1997.
72. Lorenzetti D, Bohlega S, Zoghbi HY: The expansion of the CAG repeat in ataxin-2 is a frequent cause of autosomal dominant spinocerebellar ataxia. Neurology 49:1009–1013, 1997.
73. Schols L, Kruger R, Amoiriddis G, et al.: Spinocerebellar ataxia type 6: Geneotype and phenotype in German kindreds. J Neurol Neurosurg Psychiatry 64:67–73, 1998.
74. David G, Giunti P, Abbas N, et al.: The gene for autosomal dominant cerebellar ataxia type II is located in a 5-cM region in 3p12–p13: Genetic and physical mapping of the SCA7 locus. Am J Hum Genet 59:1328–1336, 1996.
75. Benomar A, Krols L, Stevanin G, et al.: The gene for autosomal dominant cerebellar ataxia with pigmentary macular dystrophy maps to chromosome 3p12–p21.1. Nat Genet 10:84–88, 1995.
76. Gouw LG, Kaplan CD, Haines JH, et al.: Retinal degeneration characterizes a spinocerebellar ataxia mapping to chromosome 3p. Nat Genet 10:89–93, 1995.
77. David G, Abbas N, Stevanin G, et al.: Cloning of the SCA7 gene reveals a highly unstable CAG repeat expansion. Nat Genet 17:65–70, 1997.
78. Enevoldson TP, Sanders MD: Autosomal dominant cerebellar ataxia with pigmentary macular dystrophy. A clinical and genetic study of eight families. Brain 117:445–460, 1994.
79. Benomar A, Le Guern E, Durr A, Ouhabi H, et al.: Autosomal-dominant cerebellar ataxia with retinal degeneration (ADCA type II) is genetically different from ADCA type I. Ann Neurol 35:439–444, 1994.
80. Gouw LG, Digre KB, Harris CP, et al.: Autosomal dominant cerebellar ataxia with retinal degeneration: Clinical neuropathologic and genetic analysis of a large kindred. Neurology 44:1441–1447, 1994.
81. Del-Favero J, Korls L, Michalik A, et al.: Molecular genetic analysis of autosomal dominant cerebellar ataxia with retinal degeneration (ADCA type II) caused by CAG triplet repeat expansion. Hum Mol Genet 7:177–186, 1998.
82. Koob MD, Benzow KA, Bird TD, Day JW, Moseley ML, Ranum LP: Rapid cloning of expanded trinucleotide repeat sequences from genomic DNA. Nat Genet 18:72–75, 1998.
83. David G, Durr A, Stevanin G, et al.: Molecular and clinical correlations in autosomal dominant cerebellar ataxia with progressive macular dystrophy. Hum Mol Genet 7:165–170, 1998.
84. Johansson J, Forsgren L, Sandgren O, Brice A, Holmgren G, Holmberg M: Expanded CAG repeats in Swedish spinocerebellar ataxia type 7 (SCA7) patients: Effect of CAG repeat length on the clinical manifestation. Hum Mol Genet 7:171–176, 1998.
85. Gouw LG, Castaneda MA, McKenna CK, et al.: Analysis of the dynamic mutation in the SCA7 gene shows marked parental effects on CAG repeat transmission. Hum Mol Genet 7:525–532, 1998.
86. Koob DM, Moseley ML, Benzow KA, et al.: A 3' untranslated CTG repeat causes spinocerebellar ataxia type 8 (SCA8). Nat Genet 21:379–389, 1999.
87. Nikali K, Isosomppi J, Lonnqvist T, Mao JI, Suomalainen A, Peltonen L: Toward cloning of a novel ataxia gene: Refined assignment and physical map of the IOSCA locus (SCA8) on 10q24. Genomics 39:185–191, 1997.
88. Grewal R, Tayag E, Figueroa KP, et al.: Clinical and genetic analysis of a new autosomal dominant spinocerebellar ataxia. Neurology 51:1423–1426, 1998.
89. Zu L, Figueroa KP, Grewal R, Pulst SM: Mapping of a new autosomal dominant spinocerebellar ataxia (SCA10) to chromosome 22. Am J Hum Genet 64:594–599, 1999.
90. Matsuura T, Achari M, Khajavi M, et al.: Mapping of the gene for a novel spinocerebellar ataxia with pure cerebellar signs and epilepsy. Ann Neurol (in press), 1999.
91. Koide R, Ikeuchi T, Onodega O, et al.: Unstable expansion of CAG repeat in hereditary dentatorubral-pallidoluysian atrophy (DRPLA). Nat Genet 6:9–13, 1994.
92. Nagafuchi S, Yanagisawa H, Sato K, et al.: Dentatorubral and pallidoluysian atrophy expansion of an unstable CAG trinucleotide on chromsome 12p. Nat Genet 6:14–18, 1994.
93. Potter NT, Meyer MA, Zimmerman AW, et al.: Molecular and clinical findings in a family with dentatorubral-pallidoluysian atrophy. Ann Neurol 37:273–277, 1995.
94. Komure O, Sano A, Nishino N, et al.: DNA analysis in hereditary dentatorubral-pallidoluysian atrophy: Correlation between CAG repeat length and phenotypic variation and the molecular basis of anticipation Neurology 4:143–149, 1995.
95. Ikeuchi, T, Koide R, Tanka H, et al.: Dentatorubral-pallidoluysian atrophy: Clinical features are closely related to unstable expansions of trinucleotide (CAG) repeat. Ann Neurol 37:769–775, 1995.
96. Warner TT, Williams LD, Walker RWH, et al.: A clinical and molecular genetic study of dentatorubral-pallidoluysian atrophy in four European families Ann Neurol 47:452–259, 1995.
97. Nielsen JE, Sorensen SA, Hasholt L, Norremolle A: Dentatorubral-pallidoluysian atrophy. Clinical features of a five-generation Danish family. Mov Disord 11:533–541, 1996.
98. Imamura A, Sugai K, Watanabe S, Hamada F, Kurashige T, Takashima S, et al.: High intensity in the globus pallidus on proton and $T_2$-weighted MRI in case of dentato-ruburo-pallido-luysian atrophy of myoclonus epilepsy type. Acta Paediatr 36:527–530, 1994.
99. Uyama E, Kondo I, Uchino M, et al.: Dentatorubral-pallidoluysian atrophy (DRPLA): clinical genetic, and neuroradiologic studies in a family. J Neurol Sci 130:146–153, 1995.
100. Farmer TW, Wingfield MS, Lynch SA, et al.: Ataxia, chorea, seizures and dementia: Pathologic features of a newly defined familial disorder. Arch Neurol 46:774–779, 1989.
101. Takahashi H, Ohama E, Naito H, et al.:

Hereditary dentatorubral-pallidoluysian atrophy: Clinical and pathologic variants in a family. Neurology 38:1065–1070, 1988.
102. Takano H, Onodera O, Takahashi H, et al.: Somatic mosaicism of expanded CAG reports in brains of patients with dentatorubral-pallidoluysian atrophy: Cellular population dependent dynamics of mitotic instability. Am J Hum Genet 58:1212–1222, 1996.
103. Ueno S, Kondoh K, Kotani Y, et al.: Somatic mosaicism of CAG repeat in dentatorubral-pallidoluysian atrophy (DRPLA). Hum Mol Genet 4:663–666, 1995.
104. Nagafuchi S, Yanagisawa H, Ohsaki E, et al.: Structure and expression of the gene responsible for the triplet repeat disorder, dentatorubral and pallidoluysian atrophy (DRPLA). Nat Genet 8:177–182, 1994.
105. Onodera O, Oyake M, Takano H, Ikeuchi T, Igarashi S, Tsuji S: Molecular cloning of a full-length cDNA for dentatorubral-pallidoluysian atrophy and regional expressions of the expanded alleles in the CNS. Am J Hum Genet 57:1050–1060, 1995.
106. Yazawa I, Nukina N, Hashida H, Goto J, Yamada M, Kanazawa I: Abnormal gene product identified in hereditary dentatorubral-pallidoluysian atrophy (DRPLA) brain. Nat Genet 10:99–103, 1995.
106a. Burke JR, Enghild JJ, Martin ME, et al.: Huntingtin and DRPLA proteins selectively interact with the enzyme GAPDH. Nat Med 2:347–350, 1996.
107. Burke JR, Wingfield MS, Lewis KE, et al.: The Haw River syndrome: Dentatorubral-pallidoluysian atrophy (DRPLA) in an African-American family. Nat Genet 7:521–524, 1994.
108. Schmitt I, Epplen JT, Riess O: Predominant neuronal expression of the gene responsible for dentatorubral-pallidoluysian atrophy (DRPLA) in rat. Hum Mol Genet 4:1619–1624, 1995.
109. Igarashi S, Koide R, Shimohata T, et al.: Suppression of aggregate formation and apoptosis transglutaminase inhibitors in cells expressing truncated DRPLA protein with an expanded polyglutamine stretch. Nat Genet 18:111–117, 1998.
110. McLean CA, Storey E, Gardner RJ, Tannenberg AE, Cervenakova L, Brown P: The D178N (cis-129M) "fatal familial insomnia" mutation associated with diverse clinicopathologic phenotypes in an Australian kindred. Neurology 49:552–558, 1997.
111. Browne DL, Gancher ST, Nutt JG, et al.: Episodic ataxia/myokymia syndrome is associated with point mutations in the human potassium channel gene, *KCNA1*. Nat Genet 8:136–140. 1994.
112. Vahedi F, Joutel A, Van Bogaert P, et al.: A gene for hereditary paroxysmal cerebellar ataxia maps to chromosome 19p. Ann Neurol 37:289–293, 1995.
113. Yue Q, Jen JC, Nelson SF, Baloh RW: Progressive ataxia due to a missense mutation in a calcium-channel gene. Am J Hum Genet 61:1078–1087, 1997.
114. Ducros, A, Denier, C, Joutel A, et al.: Recurrence of the T666M calcium channel *CACNA1A* gene mutation in familial hemiplegic migraine with progressive cerebellar ataxia. Am J Hum Genet 64:89–98, 1999.
115. Damji KF, Allingham RR, Pollock SC, et al.: Periodic vestibulocerebellar ataxia, an autosomal dominant ataxia with defective smooth pursuit, is genetically distinct from other autosomal dominant ataxia. Arch Neurol 53:338–344, 1996.
116. Griggs RC, Nutt JG: Episodic ataxias as channelopathies. Ann Neurol 37:285–287, 1995.
117. Burright EN, Orr HT, Clark HB: Mouse models of human CAG repeat disorders. Brain Pathol 7: 965–977, 1997.
118. Burright EN, Clark HB, Servadio A, et al.: SCA transgenic mice: A model for neurodegeneration caused by an expanded CAG trinucleotide repat. Cell 82:937–948, 1995.
119. Klement IA, Skinner PJ, Kaytor MD, et al.: Ataxin-1 nuclear localization and aggregation: Role in polyglutamine-induced disease in SCA1 transgenic mice. Cell 95:41–53, 1998.
120. Huynh DP, Koeppen AH, Shibata H, et al.: SCA2, absence of intranuclear aggregates and animal model. Neurology (suppl) (in press), 1999.
121. Fletcher CF, Lutz CM, O'Sullivan TN, et al.: Absence epilepsy in tottering mutant mice is associated with calcium channel defects. Cell 15:607–617, 1996.
122. Harding AE: Friedreich's ataxia: A clinical and genetic study of 90 families with an analysis of early diagnostic criteria and intrafamilial clustering of clinical features. Brain 104:589–620, 1981.
123. Campuzano V, Montermini L, Molto MD, et al.: Friedreich's ataxia: Autosomal recessive disease caused by an intronic GAA triplet repeat expansion. Science 271:1423–1427, 1996.
124. De Michele G, Filla A, Cavalcanti F, et al.: Late onset Friedreich's disease. Clinical features and mapping of mutation to the FRDA locus. J Neurol Neurosurg Psychiatry 57:977–979, 1994.
125. Geoffrey G, Barbeau A, Greton A, et al.: Clinical description and roentgenologic evaluation of patients with Friedreich's ataxia. Can J Neurol Sci 3: 27–286, 1976.
126. Harding AE, Hewer RL: The heart disease of Friedreich's ataxia: A clinical and electrocardiographic study of 115 patients, with an analysis of serial electrocardiographic changes in 30 cases. Q J Med 52:489–502, 1983.
127. Klockgether T, Wullner V, Dichgans J, et al.: Clinical and imaging correlations in inherited ataxias. Adv Neurol 61:77–96, 1993.
128. Nuwer MR, Perlman SL, Packwood JW, et al.: Evoked potential abnormalities in the various inherited ataxias. Ann Neurol 13:20–27, 1983.
129. Moschner C, Perlman S, Baloh RW: Comparison of oculomotor findings in the progressive ataxia syndromes. Brain 117:15–25, 1994.
130. Child JS, Perloff JK, Bach PM, et al.: Cardiac involvement in Friedreich's ataxia: A clinical study of 75 patients. J Am Coll Cardiol 7:1370–1378, 1986.
131. Lamarche JB, Lemieux B, Lieu HB: The neuropathology of "typical" Fredreich's ataxia in Quebec. Can J Neurol Sci 11:592–600, 1984.
132. Ouvrier RA, McLeod JG, Conchin TE: Friedreich's ataxia. Early detection and progression of peripheral nerve abnormalities. J Neurol Sci 55(2):137–145, 1982.

133. Chamberlain S, Shaw J, Rowland S, et al.: Mapping of the mutation causing Friedreich's ataxia to human chromosome 9. Nature 334:248–250, 1988.
134. Pandolfo M, Sirugo G, Antonelli A, et al.: Friedreich ataxia in Italian familes: Genetic homogeneity and linkage disequilibrium with the marker loci D9S5 and D9S15. Am J Hum Genet 47:228–235, 1990.
135. Keats B, Ward LJ, Shaw, et al.: Acadian and classical forms of Friedreich's ataxia are most probably caused by mutation at the same locus. Am J Med Genet 35:266–268, 1989.
136. Klockgether T, Chamberlain S, Wullner U, et al.: Late-onset Friedreich ataxia. Molecular genetics, clinical neurophysiology, and magnetic resonance imaging. Arch Neurol 50:803–806, 1993.
137. Campuzano V, Montermini L, Molto MD, et al.: Friedreich's ataxia: Autosomal recessive disease caused by an intronic GAA triplet repeat expansion. Science 271:1423–1427, 1996.
138. Bidichandani SI, Ashizawa T, Patel PI: The GAA triplet-repeat expansion in Friedreich ataxia interferes with transcription and may be associated with an unusual DNA. Am J Hum Genet 62:111–121, 1998.
139. Babcock M, de Silva D, Oaks R, et al.: Regulation of mitochondrial iron accumulation by Yfh1p, a putative homolog of frataxin. Science 276:1709–1712, 1997.
139a. Durr A, Cossee M, Agid Y, Campuzano V, Mignard C, Penet C, Mandel JL, Brice A, Koenig M: Clinical and genetic abnormalities in patients with Friedreich's ataxia. N Engl 1.5 Med 335:1169–1175, 1996.
140. Filla A, DeMichele G, Cavalcanti F, et al.: The relationship between trinucleotide (GAA) repeat length and clinical features in Friedreich's ataxia. Am J Hum Genet 59:554–460, 1996.
141. Geschwind DH, Perlman S, Grody WW, et al.: Friedreich's ataxia GAA repeat expansion in patients with recessive or sporadic ataxia. Neurology 49:1004–1009, 1997.
142. Schols L, Amoiridis G, Przuntek H, Frank G, Epplen JT, Epplen C: Friedreich's ataxia. Revision of the phenotype according to molecular genetics. Brain 120:2131–2140, 1997.
143. Ben Hamida C, Doerflinger N, et al.: Localization of Friedreich ataxia phenotype with selective vitamin E deficiency to chromosome 8q by homozygosity mapping. Nat Genet 5(2):195–200, 1993.
144. Ouahchi K, Arita M, Kayden H, et al.: Ataxia with isolated vitamin E deficiency is caused by mutations in the alpha-tocopherol transfer protein. Nat Genet 9(2):141–145, 1995.
145. Cavalier L, Ouahchi K, Kayden HJ, et al.: Ataxia with isolated vitamin E deficiency: Heterogeneity of mutations and phenotype variability in a large number of families. Am J Hum Genet 62:301–310, 1998.
146. Benomar A, Yahyaoui M, Meggouh F, et al.: Clinical differences between AVED patients and Friedreich ataxia with GAA expansion in 15 Moroccan families. Arch Neurol (in press).
147. Yokota T, Shiojiri T, Gotoda T, et al.: Friedreich-like ataxia with retinitis pigmentosa caused by the His 101 Gin mutation of the alpha-tocopherol transfer protein gene. Ann Neurol 41:826–832, 1997.
148. Belal S, Hentati F, Ben Hamida C, Ben Hamida M: Friedreich's ataxia–vitamin E responsive type. The chromosome 8 locus. Clin Neurosci 3 :39–42, 1995.
149. Tamaru Y, Hirano M, Kusaka H, Ito H, Imai T, Ueno S: alpha-Tocopherol transfer protein gene: Exon skipping of all transcripts causes ataxia. Neurology 49(2):584–588, 1997.
150. Johnson WG: The clinical spectrum of hexosaminidase deficiency diseases. Neurology 31:1453–1456, 1981.
151. Navon R, Argov Z, Frisch A: Hexosaminidase a deficiency in adults. Am J Med Genet 24:179–196, 1986.
152. Hund E, Grau A, Fogel W, et al.: Progressive cerebellar ataxia, proximal neurogenic weakness and ocular motor disturbances: Hexosaminidase a deficiency with late clinical onset in four siblings. J Neurol Sci 145:25–31, 1997.
153. Kolter T, Sandhoff K: Recent advances in the biochemistry of sphingolipidoses. Brain Pathol 8:79–100, 1998.
154. Savitsky K, Bar-Shira A, Gilad S, et al.: A single ataxia telangiectasia gene with a product similar to PI-3 kinase. Science 268:1749–1753, 1995.
155. Gatti RA, Berkei I, Boder E, et al.: Localization of an ataxia-telangiectasia gene to chromosome 11q22–23. Nature 336:577–580, 1988.
156. Savitsky K, Sjez S, Tagle DA, et al.: The complete sequence of the coding region of the ATM gene reveals similarity to cell cycle regulators in different species. Hum Mol Genet 4:2025–2032, 1995.
157. Byrd PJ, McConville CM, Cooper P, et al.: Mutations revealed by sequencing the 5' half of the gene for ataxia telangietaxia. Hum Mol Genet 5: 145–149, 1996.
158. Gilad S, Khosravi R, Shkedy D, et al.: Predominance of null mutations in ataxia-telangiectasia. Hum Mol Genet 5:433–439, 1996.
159. Stankovic T, Kidd Am Sutcliffe A, et al.: ATM mutations and phenotypes in ataxia-telangiectasia families in the British Isles: Expression of mutant ATM and the risk of leukemia, lymphoma, and breast cancer. Am J Hum Genet 62:334–345, 1998.
160. Telatar M, Teraoka S, Wang Z, et al.: Ataxia-telangiectasia: Identification and detection of founder-effect mutations in the ATM gene in ethnic populations. Am J Hum Genet 62:86–97, 1998.
161. Vorechovsky I, Luo L, Lindblom A, et al.: ATM mutations in cancer families. Cancer Res 56 (18): 4130–4133, 1996.
162. Kuljis RO, Xu Y, Aguila MC, Baltimore D: Degeneration of neurons, synapses, and neuropil and glial activation in a murine Atm knockout model of ataxia-telangiectasia. Proc Natl Acad Sci USA 94(23):12688–12693, 1997.
163. Harding AE: Hereditary "pure" spastic paraplegia: A clinical and genetic study of 22 families. J Neurol Neurosurg Psychiatry 44:871–883, 1981.

164. Filla A, DeMichele G, Marconi R, et al.: Prevalence of hereditary ataxias and spastic paraplegias in Molise, a region of Italy. J Neurol 239:351–353, 1990.
165. Klockgether T, Zuhlke C, Schulz JB, et al.: Friedreich's ataxia with retained tendon reflexes: Molecular genetics, clinical neurophysiology, and magnetic resonance imaging. Neurology 46:118–121, 1996.
166. Ragno M, De Michele G, Cavalcanti F, et al.: Broadened Friedreich's ataxia phenotype after gene cloning. Minimal GAA expansion causes late-onset spastic ataxia. Neurology 49:1617–1620, 1997.
167. Koskinen T, Santavuori P, Sainio K, Lappi M, Kallio AK, Pihko H: Infantile onset spinocerebellar ataxia with sensory neuropathy: A new inherited disease. J Neurol Sci 121:50–56, 1994.
168. Berciano J: Olivopontocerebellar atrophy. A review of 117 cases. J Neurol Sci 53:253–272, 1982.
169. Richter A, Rioux JD, Bouchard JP, Mercier J, Mathieu J, Ge B, Poirier J, Julien D, Gyapay G, Weissenbach J, Hudson TJ, Melancon SB, Morgan K: Location score and haplotype analyses of the locus for autosomal recessive spastic ataxia of Charlevoix-Saguenay, in chromosome region 13q11. Am J Hum Genet 64:768–775, 1999.
170. Spira PJ, McLeod JG, Evans WA: A spinocerebellar degeneration with X-linked inheritance. Brain 102:27–41, 1979.
171. Farlow MR, DeMyer W, Dlouhy SR, Hodes ME: X-linked recessive inheritance of ataxia and adult-onset dementia: Clinical features and preliminary linkage analysis. Neurology 37(4):602–607, 1987.
172. Kremer H, Hamel BC, van den Helm B, et al.: Localization of the gene (or genes) for a syndrome with X-linked mental retardation, ataxia, weakness, hearing impairment, loss of vision and a fatal course in early childhood. Hum Genet 98: 513–517, 1996.
173. Fujii T, Van Coster RN, Old SE, et al.: Pyruvate dehydrogenase deficiency: Molecular basis for intrafamilial heterogeneity. Ann Neurol 36:83–89, 1994.
174. Nicolaides P, Appeton RE, Fryer A: Cerebellar ataxia, areflexia, pes cavus, optic atrophy, and sensorineural hearing loss (CAPOS): A new syndrome. J Med Genet 33:419–421, 1996.
175. Litvan I, Agid Y, Jankovic J, et al.: Accuracy of clinical criteria for the diagnosis of progressive supranuclear palsy (Steele-Richardson-Olszewski syndrome). Neurology 46:922–930, 1996.
176. de Yebenes JG, Sarasa JL, Daniel SE, Lees AJ: Familial progressive supranuclear palsy. Description of a pedigree and review of the literature. Brain 118:1095–1103, 1995.
177. Conrad C, Andreadis A, Trojanowski JQ, et al.: Genetic evidence for the involvement of tau in progressive supranuclear palsy. Ann Neurol 41: 277–281, 1997.
178. Higgins JJ, Litvan I, Pho LI, Li W, Nee LE: Progressive supranuclear gaze palsy is in linkage disequilibrium with the tau and not the alpha-synuclein gene. Neurology 50:270–273, 1998.
179. Wenning GK, Ben Shlomo Y, Maglhaes M, Daniel SE, Quinn NP: Clinical features and natural history of multiple system atrophy. An analysis of 100 cases. Brain 117:835–845, 1994.
180. Penney JB: Multiple systems atrophy and nonfamilial olivopontocerebellar atrophy are the same disease. Ann Neurol 37:553–554, 1995.
181. Rinne JO, Burn DJ, Mathias CJ, Quinn NP, Marsden CD, Brooks DJ: Positron emission tomography studies on the dopaminergic system and striatal opioid binding in the olivopontocerebellar atrophy variant of multiple system atrophy. Ann Neurol 37:568–573, 1995.
182. Takeda A, Arai N, Komori T, Iseki E, Kato S, Oda M: Tau immunoreactivity in glial cytoplasmic inclusions in multiple system atrophy. Neurosci Lett 234:63–66, 1997.
183. Moseley ML, Benzow KA, Schut LJ, Bird TD, Gomez CM, Barkhaus PE, Blindauer KA, Labuda M, Pandolfo M, Koob MD, Ranum LP: Incidence of dominant spinocerebellar and Friedreich triplet repeats among 361 ataxia families. Neurology 51:1666–1671, 1998.
184. Pellecchia MT, Scala R, Filla A, De Michele G, Ciacci C, Barone P: Idiopathic cerebellar ataxia associated with celiac disease: Lack of distinctive neurological features. J Neurol Neurosurg Psychiatry 66:32–35, 1999.
185. Sequeiros J, Nance MA: Offer and utilization of genetic testing in the dominant ataxias: Towards guidelines. Am J Hum Genet 61:A227, 1997.
186. Mehlman MJ, Kodish ED, Whitehouse P, et al.: The need for anonymous genetic counseling and testing. Am J Hum Genet 58:393–397, 1996.

# Chapter 13

# HUNTINGTON'S DISEASE

Michael R. Hayden, MB, ChB, DCh, PhD



Huntington's disease (HD) is part of a growing family of disorders caused by CAG expansion in the coding region of novel genes. The genes code for proteins that are expressed ubiquitously but are associated with selective neuropathology. Patients with HD have CAG lengths of 36 or greater. The age of onset of HD shows a significant association with CAG length. New mutations for HD are more common than previously recognized and occur on expansion of an intermediate allele through the male germline.

## FREQUENCY

Many different epidemiological surveys have been performed worldwide. Although recorded rates differ, there is general agreement that the frequencies of HD in populations of Western European descent are between 3 and 7 affected individuals per 100,000 population. The disease is less frequent in Japan, China, and Finland and in African blacks.[1,2]

## CLINICAL PRESENTATION

A broad definition of age of onset is the age when the first neurologic or psychiatric symptoms appear that represent a permanent change from the normal state. The age when signs and symptoms for HD occur has a mean of around 40 years.[1–3] The earliest age of onset has been approximately 2 years, and patients with onset of the disorder in their 70s and early 80s have been noted.

In the earliest phases of HD, there is an insidious and slow deterioration with clumsiness as well as mild personality change.[4,5] This zone of onset during which the diagnosis of HD cannot be made unequivocally is frequently witnessed by changes in caudate metabolic rates of glucose as determined with positron emission tomography (PET).[6,7] The mean age of death in different studies varies from 51.4 to 62.9 years.[8,9]

The duration of HD is around 15 years, with no differences between the sexes.[2] Length of survival with HD has not significantly changed over the past 50 years, which reflects the failure of medical therapy to delay progression of the disease. It appears that in some families HD follows a milder course with longer survival.

## DIAGNOSIS

A definite diagnosis of HD can be made in the presence of *(1)* a positive family history consistent with autosomal dominant inheritance; *(2)* progressive motor disability involving both involuntary and voluntary movements, and *(3)* mental disturbances, including cognitive decline and affective disturbances with or without changes in personality.

The diagnosis of HD is made primarily on clinical examination. Demonstration of atrophy of the caudate nucleus and the putamen by computed to tomography (CT) or magnetic resonance imagining (MRI) provides additional support for the diagnosis. A decrease in the uptake and metabolism of glucose may be detected with PET in the caudate nucleus before structural tissue loss becomes evident. DNA analysis allows the conclusion that the patient has the DNA changes associated with the disease, but the diagnosis depends on the clinical examination.

## EARLY SIGNS

Most individuals will initially display minor motor abnormalities.[5] These include general restlessness, abnormal eye movements or optokinetic nystagmus, hyperreflexia, impaired finger tapping or rapid alternating hand movements, and excessive and inappropriate movements of the fingers, hands, or toes during emotional stress,[5] as well as mild dysarthria. Minor motor abnormalities usually precede the obvious signs of extrapyramidal dysfunction by at least 3 years. Persons with a completely normal neurologic examination have a 3% chance of being diagnosed with HD within the next 3 years.[5] The clinical onset of HD is gradual, with patients passing from an asymptomatic period through a transitional phase during which diagnosis is still difficult, to a stage when overt signs and symptoms allow a definitive diagnosis to be made.

## MAJOR NEUROLOGIC FINDINGS

Chorea is the major motor sign of HD. These involuntary movements are continuously present during waking hours, cannot be voluntarily suppressed by the patient, and worsen during stress. With advancing duration, features of bradykinesia, rigidity, and dystonia become more obvious. Chorea is seen less frequently in patients with juvenile onset[2,10] and may rarely be absent in adult onset cases.[11]

Bradykinesia and rigidity are infrequent in the early phases of adult onset HD. They gradually appear, however, and often dominate the final stages of the illness in which the patient becomes severely rigid and grossly akinetic.[12] Early in the illness, bradykinesia alone may contribute to an impairment in voluntary motor performance.[13] Dystonia, characterized by slow abnormal movements and abnormal posturing, is infrequent in the early symptomatic period but worsens and becomes a prominent feature toward the later stages of the illness.[14]

Oculomotor disturbances, apart from being among the earliest signs in the transitional phase, are present in most affected patients.[11,15] Slowing of saccades may be seen in up to 75% of symptomatic individuals,[15,16] especially in early onset cases[17] and more particularly affecting the vertical rather than horizontal movements.[11,16–18]

An early sign is impairment of voluntary motor function.[19,20] Patients and their family describe clumsiness in common daily activities. Disturbances in motor speed, fine motor control, and gait correlate with disease progression and appear to be better measures of duration of illness than chorea.[21] Clumsiness may increase with deterioration of functional capacity.[5]

Gait disturbances ultimately result in severe disability.[5,12] Subtle changes in gait may be observed early in the illness, including difficulty with tandem walking, sudden stopping on command, and turning.[22] With more advanced disease, walking difficulties are more pronounced.

Most patients have speech abnormalities,[2] which develop early in the illness.[5,23,24] Initially a mild disturbance of clarity appears, which is aggravated by changes in rate and rhythm of speech as the disease progresses.

Disturbances in swallowing generally occur later with progression of the illness. Initially this may primarily affect intake of fluids but later also affects intake of solids. Choking with aspiration secondary to dysphagia is a common cause of morbidity.

## COGNITIVE DISTURBANCES

A global decline in cognitive capabilities is ultimately present in all HD patients.[12] Although global measurements of cognitive function may be preserved,[25–28] a typical pattern of decline becomes apparent very early in the disease, including slowness of thought, altered personality, affective changes, and impaired ability to integrate new knowledge.

Memory impairment is common early in the disease and is often one of the patient's presenting symptoms.[25] Visuospatial memory involving visual retention is particularly affected,[28] whereas verbal memory remains fairly preserved until late.[29,30] For example, patients have difficulty reproducing geometric designs but may remember facts, words, or stories.

Retrieval of information is impaired,[31,32] but verbal cues, priming, and sufficient time may lead to partial or total recall.[26,33–35] Recall of recent events and remote events is equally impaired.[19,26]

The learning and acquiring of new motor skills (procedural memory) is also affected in HD patients. In contrast to other amnestic syndromes, orientation in both time and place remains intact until late in the illness.[36]

Attention and concentration are affected early,[28] resulting in easy distractability by interfering stimuli. Difficulties in performing sustained simple motor tasks such as gazing laterally, sticking out the tongue, or tightly closing the eyelids may be manifestations of this distractability rather than of motor disturbances, Problems with organizing, sequencing, and planning, inability to coordinate and initiate complex actions, and inability to maintain a mental set or organize cognitive strategies constitute other early impairments.[25,26,37]

Dysarthria, slowness, and lack of initiative interfere significantly with fluency and spontaneous speech,[38] but semantic and syntactic structure, word finding, and speech comprehension remain intact until the final stages of the disease.[10,23] Difficulties in writing and recognizing objects have been ascribed to defective nonlinguistic modalities such as visuoperceptual analysis, attention and concentration, and overall cognition.[23,25,38–40] In contrast, simple naming of daily objects, as tested by the Mini-Mental State Examination, may remain intact until the latest stages of the disease.[36]

## PSYCHIATRIC DISTURBANCES

Although psychiatric disturbances are as characteristic for the disease as are motor and cognitive abnormalities, these appear less consistently[25] and are not necessarily related to the severity of chorea or dementia.[41] Changes in mood and affect are common, ranging from anxiety and ill-defined irritability to prolonged periods of depression.[13,42] Suicide is more common in HD patients than in the affected population.[43] Manic or hypomanic episodes also occur with increased frequency. Affective syndromes may precede the first signs of motor impairment by many years[10] and do not usually manifest for the first time late in the illness.[44]

Apathy, aggressive behavior, sexual disinhibition, and alcohol abuse are other symptoms seen in HD patients.[42] These symptoms may be either manifestations of the progressive cognitive decline or, alternatively, manifestations of the mood disturbances, especially if they are reversible and related to the premorbid personality.[45]

Delusions are common[42] and may be seen in depressive or manic episodes, or they may be isolated and are frequently paranoid in nature. In contrast, hallucinations are much less common.[2]

## OTHER ABNORMALITIES

Weight loss is one of the features of late HD.[12] Clinical follow-up,[46] anthropometric studies,[47] and dietary assessment[48] show that the vast majority of HD patients lose weight in the course of the disease. Intriguingly, a relationship has been found between weight at initial examination and rate of disease progress.[49]

Sleep may be disturbed in advanced disease, with frequent nocturnal sleeplessness and reversal of the day–night pattern of sleep.[50] Choreic movements disappear during sleep.

Approximately 20% of all patients are incontinent of urine and feces in the terminal phases of the illness, whereas in early symptomatic persons incontinence rarely occurs.[2] Choreatic contractions have been electromyographically recorded from perineal musculature in affected patients.[51]

## JUVENILE ONSET

Approximately 10% of all patients with HD have onset before age 20 years. The youngest patient described had onset at age 2 years.[2] In contrast to adult cases, in juvenile cases bradykinesia and rigidity are conspicuous, dominating the neurologic findings in about 50% of the cases. [2,12,52–54] Chorea is present in almost all cases but is often of short duration and is superseded by rigidity.[2] Frequent falls, dysarthria, clumsiness, hyperreflexia, and oculomotor disturbances are frequent in children with HD and occur early. Although difficult to assess in HD,[55] cerebellar dysfunction is more prominent than seen in adult patients.[2,5]

Mental deterioration is first manifested by declining school performance. Over the years a severe progressive dementia develops. Epileptic seizures, occurring with a similar frequency in adult HD patients as in the general adult population (1%),[2] are common in early onset cases, with an estimated 30% to 50% of the juvenile patients affected.[2,54,56] Partial or generalized, tonic-clonic, or absence seizures may all appear. Seizures should be differentiated from myoclonic jerks, which also rarely occur in adult cases.[57] The epilepsy of juvenile HD patients is often difficult to control.

## LATE ONSET

In contrast, the manifestations in late onset disease are less severe. Approximately 25% of all patients will display first signs and symptoms after age 50 years, and in these patients the disease will progress slower than usual.[58] Chorea is the presenting motor disorder, and gait disturbances and dysphagia are common, though not severe. Cognitive impairment, although invariably present, may be less debilitating than in younger patients.[58] An older onset is associated with a slower disease progression, as measured by functional disability.[59]

## LABORATORY INVESTIGATIONS

### Computed Tomography and Magnetic Resonance Imaging

Computed tomography and MRI scanning can demonstrate caudate atrophy in affected patients, but appreciable atrophy usually appears after the chorea.[60] Measurements of the area of the head of the caudate neclues,[61] or standardized measurements such as the ratio of the distance of the caudate heads and the inner tables of the skull,[62] or the ratio of the bicaudate diameter and distances between the frontal heads[63] will achieve up to 90% discrimination between patients with established disease and controls.[64] A number of other conditions may also be associated with caudate atrophy, such as normal aging, multiple infarcts, obstructive hydrocephalus, and neuroacanthocytosis.[65,66] A CT or MRI scan is also useful to detect basal ganglia calcifications. Obviously, a scan showing caudate atrophy supports a diagnosis, but a normal scan does not exclude the diagnosis.

### Positron Emission Tomography

Positron emission tomography with 18F-deoxyglucose demonstrates decreased glucose metabolism in the caudate nucleus that appears normal on CT or MRI scan in affected persons and some persons at risk.[6,7,67–69] This later finding has not been replicated in all studies.[70] Particularly during the transitional clinical phase when definitive diagnosis cannot yet be made, PET scanning may be a sensitive method to detect early HD-related changes. The finding of caudate hypometabolism, however, lacks specificity. Significantly decreased caudate glucose metabolism has been demonstrated in neuroacanthocytosis, dentato-rubral-pallido-luysian atrophy,[71] and Wilson's disease,[72] while chorea due to systemic lupus erythematosus[73] seems associated with normal glucose metabolism. Both abnormal[74] and normal[75] results have been found in patients with benign hereditary chorea. It has been claimed that single-photon emission computed tomography may yield equivalent results, but the method is not yet sufficiently validated.[76–79]

### DNA Testing

Approximately 98% of all patients (686/700 affected persons in one series) with the clinical phenotype of HD have expansion of the (CAG) repeat. Therefore, in patients with signs and symptoms suggestive of HD, DNA assessment is helpful to confirm that the patient has the DNA changes associated with HD.

## NEUROPATHOLOGY

Atrophy of the caudate nucleus and the putamen (the neostriatum) is the most characteristic pathological feature of the disease.[12] The severity of neostriatal abnormalities, however, is highly variable. In a series of 163 clinically diagnosed cases, 13 lacked macroscopically visible atrophy, while in 18 cases the caudate was extremely shrunken and the putamen markedly atrophic.[12,80]

Microscopically the neostriatal atrophy is characterized by neuronal loss and gliosis,[12,80] which again may be highly variable. Full appreciation of neuronal loss, however, can only be obtained by cell counting. In these instances, even in the absence of caudate abnormalities macroscopically, regional loss of up to 40% of the normal neurons may be found.[49] Medium- and small-sized neurons, which are the most abundant class in human striatum,[81] disappear, while larger neurons appear relatively preserved.[12,82–84]

Gross cerebellar atrophy is rare,[85] but some cerebellar changes are well established.[12,82] Even in adult cases, the density of cortical Purkinje cells may often be decreased to, on average, half the value of age-matched controls.[86]

## NEUROCHEMISTRY

The earliest and most Extensively affected neurons are the medium-sized spiny neurons that express gamma-aminobutyric acid (GABA) and enkephalin or GABA and substance P as their neurotransmitter.[87] A decreased number of fibers immunoreactive for enkephalin and substance P in the globus pallidus and substantia nigra, respectively, was already observable in the brain of an asymptomatic individual at high risk for having inherited the HD.[88]

Medium-sized and large neurons containing the enzyme NADPH-diaphorase[89] remain intact.[90] These neurons contain somatostatin and neuropeptide Y as their neurotransmitter and are localized in the striatal matrix, [91,92] probably serving as interneurons. Another relatively spared group are large aspiny acetylcholine esterase (AChE)–containing and locally arborizing interneurons,[93] which are not localized in any particular compartment.

## GENETICS

Huntington's disease is inherited as an autosomal dominant trait. It is assumed that all heterozygotes for HD show signs and symptoms if they live long enough.

A novel gene containing a trinucleotide repeat (CAG) that is expanded on HD chromosomes was recently described.[94] This highly polymorphic CAG repeat, located in the 5' region of the *HD* gene, has been shown to range from 10 to 35 copies on normal chromosomes, while it is expanded beyond 36 repeats in HD, with the largest expansion observed of 121 trinucleotides.

Two mRNA species were observed to originate from a single gene and were accounted for by 3' differential polyadenylation leading to transcripts of different sizes.[95] Currently there is no obvious homology for this gene, and detailed sequence analysis has provided no clues to its function.

## RELATIONSHIP BETWEEN TRINUCLEOTIDE (CAG) REPEAT LENGTH AND CLINICAL FEATURES

A significant correlation between the number of CAG repeats and the age of onset of HD has been demonstrated.[96–99] This association was present irrespective of the mode of clinical presentation at time of onset. The number of trinucleotide repeats accounted for about 50% of the variation in the age of onset.[96] Repeat length, however, is not indicative of any other particular clinical phenotype as there is no independent association between any particular clinical feature of the illness and the number of repeats.

Curves for age of onset of offspring have been constructed previously that gave estimations of age of onset in offspring based on age of onset in the parent.[100] In earlier counseling programs, persons at risk have been informed that there is in general an aggregation of age of onset among siblings with less correlation of the age of onset between parent and child.

Prior studies of the relationship between age at onset and CAG repeat size have not included asymptomatic, at-risk individuals with CAG length in the affected range. This makes it impossible to account for the number of asymptomatic persons with a particular CAG at a specific age, and thus it prevents a complete understanding of the relationship between CAG size and age at onset of HD. To further explore the relationship between CAG repeat size and the age at onset of clinical manifestations of HD and to determine the risk of developing HD by a certain age in a patient with a particular CAG repeat size, we analyzed CAG size in large numbers of affected and asymptomatic at-risk individuals.

Inclusion of the asymptomatic at-risk individuals with expanded CAG repeat lengths, along with use of the more accurate CAG repeat measurement, allowed us to develop estimates of the probability of developing HD, by a particular age, with a given CAG size. The large numbers of individuals in our database also enabled us to clarify the ranges of normal and HD-associated CAG repeat sizes.

This study[101] has clearly shown that CAG repeat length is the major determinant of age of onset of HD. By assessing the CAG size alone, we were able to predict the likelihood that an individual would be affected by a particular age, with a relatively narrow 95% (±10%) confidence interval for most persons being tested. This study confirms the prior assessments of ranges of CAG repeat length in affected persons and clearly shows that reduced penetrance for HD may occur only for a CAG repeat length less than 42.

Furthermore, it is apparent that reduced penetrance may occur with the range of 36 to 41 CAG repeats (Table 13-1). Clearly, this data needs validation in other independently ascertained large groups of patients because the numbers are too small to allow for meaningful penetrance estimates for each specific repeat size. It is obvious, however, that there is a trend toward increasing penetrance with increasing repeat length in the 36 to 41 repeat range: less than 90% for 39 CAG repeats and 99% for 41 CAG repeats.

## MOLECULAR ANALYSIS OF NEW MUTATIONS

New mutations causing HD have been proposed to be exceedingly rare, with the mutation rate estimated as the lowest for any

Table 13–1. **Estimation of Penetrance of CAG Expansion in the *HD* Gene by CAG Repeat Size**

| CAG Repeat Size | No. of Affected Individuals | No. of Unaffected Individuals | No. of Unaffected Individuals, Age >75 Years (Males) or >80 Years (Females) |
|---|---|---|---|
| <29–35 | 0 | 86 | 9 |
| 36 | 1 | 12 | 2 |
| 37 | 4 | 4 | 0 |
| 38 | 2 | 9 | 1 |
| 39 | 8 | 13 | 1 |
| 40 | 64 | 47 | 1 |
| 41 | 74 | 24 | 1 |
| >41 | 575 | 126 | 0 |

**Source:** Adapted from Brinkman et al.[101]

human genetic disease.[98,102] This may reflect that proof of a new mutation in HD is difficult, as previous criteria for identification of a new mutation have stipulated that parents of the sporadic case must have lived beyond the expected age of onset of HD without any manifestations of the disease, paternity of the sporadic case must be confirmed, and the disease should be transmitted to the offspring of the sporadic case.[103]

Recently the CAG repeat length in sporadic cases of HD and the families were assessed to learn more about the molecular events underlying new mutations for HD. In these families the sporadic HD patient had an upper allele that was in the size range seen in patients with this disorder. In all families where DNA was available from parents, one parental allele was found to be significantly greater than that seen in the general population (>29), but below the range seen in patients with HD (an intermediate allele [IA]).[104]

The sex of origin of the IA was determined by examining DNA from parents. In all families (16/16) thus far studied, preferential origin of the new mutation from the paternally derived allele was demonstrated. This would suggest that the paternal allele in the IA range is more likely to undergo significant expansion to a repeat length in the range seen in patients affected with HD.

These findings have implications for family members of sporadic patients, in particular for siblings and second-degree relatives of such affected persons. There is a small but increased risk for such relatives to manifest with HD.[104]

## THE GENE PRODUCT FOR HUNTINGTON'S DISEASE

The mRNA contains a long open reading free that codes for a protein of approximately 350 kDa that has not shown any homology to other genes. This protein product is expressed in many different cells throughout the central nervous system, as well as in cell lines from different somatic tissues.[105–107] There is no particular enrichment of the protein product in the basal ganglia. Furthermore, there is no altered expression of the protein with the expanded repeat in HD patients.[105,106,108] Thus, the patterns of expression of both the mRNA and the protein do not provide any clues to the causes of selective neuronal death in HD.

## ANIMAL STUDIES IN HUNTINGTON'S DISEASE: INSIGHTS INTO PATHOGENESIS

The finding of early embryolethality and the evidence that the clinical phenotype of heterozygotes with CAG expansion is not obviously different from that of persons homozygous for CAG expansion suggest that HD is not caused by complete loss-of-function of huntingtin associated with CAG expansion. Furthermore, the embryolethality in the HD knock-out mice also indicates that the disease cannot be explained by a simple dominant-negative effect whereby the mutant protein interacts with and inactivates the normal gene product leading to a complete loss-of-function. The absence of any phenotype in animals with a highly expressed transcript containing CAG expansion but not expressing a protein translation is crucial for the pathogenesis of HD.[109]

Recent studies have provided some insights into the normal function of the HD gene. Gene targeting strategies resulting in deletion of this gene from mice reveals that offspring are not viable. Furthermore, timed pregnancies studies revealed that these mice die before 8.5 days of age, showing that this protein is crucial for normal development and particularly for normal gastrulation.[109–112] Studies of animals with heterozygous deletion of this gene have revealed in one report[110] that they have abnormal behavior characterized by increased locomotor activity, as well as some changes in cognitive ability. Furthermore, detailed morphometric studies have revealed that these animals have significant reduction of neurons in the subthalamic nucleus.[110]

Increasing evidence supports the idea that CAG expansion contributes a gain-of-function to the gene product for HD (huntingtin).[113] Whether this gain-of-function is completely novel or whether it represents an enhancement of a normal function is unknown.

Polyglutamine length modulates several functions of the gene product for HD. These include the susceptibility of huntingtin to cleavage by a crucial pro-apoptotic enzyme caspase 3)[114] and the interaction of huntingtin with different cellular proteins.[115–116a]

Recently we have generated transgenic mice that replicate the disease causing genetic mutation within the context of the full-length HD gene expressed in the appropriate developmental, tissue, and cell specific manner seen in patients with the disease. To this end, yeast artificial chromosomes (YACs) containing human genomic DNA spanning the full-length gene, including all regulatory elements, were used. The HD clones were engineered to contain CAG sizes similar to these seen in either adult onset (YAC46 containing 46 CAG) or juvenile onset HD (YAC72 containing 72 CAG repeats).[117]

We found that YAC46 and 72 mice develop progressive electrophysiological abnormalities that preceed nuclear translocation and aggregation of huntingtin. YAC72 mice have behavioural abnormalities with onset influenced by the level of mutant protein. A mouse expressing mutant huntingtin with 72 glutamines at higher levels presented with an early onset behavioural phenotype (~ 6 weeks) and had intranuclear aggregates and neurodegeneration specifically in the striatum. Other YAC72 mice expressing lower levels of mutant protein had progressive electrophysiologic abnormalities at 6 and 10 months, followed by selective striatal neurodegeneration first seen at 12 months of age. No aggregates were visible by light or electron microscopy, clearly indicating that aggregates are not necessary for initiation of selective neuronal loss. On the other hand, translocation of N-terminal fragments of htt into the nucleus is seen, providing *in vivo* evidence for cleavage of htt and the toxic gain of function of these fragments as first proposed by Goldberg and colleagues.[117a]

*In vitro* evidence has suggested that proteolytic cleavage of huntingtin plays an important role in the pathogenesis of huntingtin.[117b,117c] The studies in the YAC transgenic mice now provide direct evidence of cleavage of huntingtin by demonstration of N-terminal fragments in the nucleus and C-terminal fragments in the cytoplasm. Furthermore, immunogold-labeled EM has revealed gold-labeled htt fragments traversing the nuclear pore to the nucleus from the cytosol. It is important to note that the N-terminal translocation of htt appears to be evident only in those neurons that are susceptible to subsequent neurodegeneration, namely the medium spiny neurons. The striatal interneurons that are largely spared in HD did not show presence of htt in the nucleus. This suggests that one reason for selective neuronal degeneration in HD might be the generation of proteolytic cleavage of htt in specific cells with resultant N-terminal translocation of htt into the nucleus specifically in those cells.

Recently, there have been reports of other transgenic mice expressing different portions of huntingtin[117d–117g] under control of varying promoters. These mice display a significant neurological phenotype associated with development of intranuclear aggregates and, in some cases, neurodegeneration, but as yet they display no evidence for the selective neurodegeneration seen in HD. This suggests that expression of full-length huntingtin and/or expression in a cell specific and developmental manner as seen with its own promoter may be important to accurately recapitulate the disease phenotype.

## APOPTOSIS IN HUNTINGTON'S DISEASE

Neuronal cell death associated with HD appears to involve apoptosis. *In situ* DNA fragmentation studies (TUNEL) suggest that the cell death in HD as well as in the excitatory quinolinic acid model of HD involves apoptosis.[118–120] In addition, nullizygous embryos for the murine HD gene show increased apoptosis in regions where the gene is known to be expressed, suggesting that normal huntingtin may play a role in cell survival by deferring apoptosis.[112]

Proteolytic cleavage of key cellular substrates by cysteine proteases related to mammalian interleukin-1b–converting enzyme (ICE) and CED-3, the product of a gene that is absolutely required for programmed cell death in *Caenorhabditis elegans,* is an important central mechanism in apoptotic cell death. Caspase 3 is a human counterpart to the nematode death-gene product CED-3 and is at or near the apex of a cascade of proteolytic events that culminate in apoptotic cell death.[121] Caspase 3 is specifically responsible for the proteolytic cleavage and functional disabiling of key homeostatic nuclear proteins at the onset of apoptosis, including poly(ADP-ribose)polymerase (PARP), an enzyme involved in genome surveillance and DNA repair in stressed cells.

Apoptotic extracts known to cleave PARP are also able to cleave huntingtin *in vitro.* This cleavage is preventable with an apopain-specific tetrapeptide inhibitor.[114]

Susceptibility of huntingtin to cleavage by caspase 3 is influenced by polyglutamine length, with increased CAG length associated with increased cleavage. How proteolytic cleavage of huntingtin may be associated with selective neuronal loss is not known. This could, however, be due to selective vulnerability of certain cells such as neurons to the toxic effects of truncated fragments of huntingtin, particularly when these fragments contain polyglutamine stretches.

## INTERACTING PROTEINS

Huntingtin directly interacts with other proteins that may have restricted patterns of expression, which could confer selective vulnerability to particular cells. To date, three such interacting proteins have been identified. In two instances, polyglutamine length influences this interaction.

Using the yeast two-hybrid system, Li and colleagues[122] have identified a protein (HAP1) that is expressed predominantly in brain. The binding of HAP1 to huntingtin was enhanced by an expanded polyglutamine tract. HAP1 is localized to neurons in a pattern similar to that of neuronal nitric oxide synthase.[109] Although HAP1 is expressed in the cortex and striatum, regions selectively involved in HD, it is also expressed in regions of the brain relatively spared in HD such as the cerebellum and the brain stem. Therefore, other factors besides the expression of HAP1, such as increased vulnerability of affected cells, must be invoked to account for the selective neuronal death in HD.

It has also been shown that huntingtin interacts with an enzyme (GAPDH) critical to cellular glycolysis.[116] Defective energy metabolism may play a role in neurodegenerative disorders, including HD.

The huntingtin–GAPDH interaction is intriguing because GAPDH has also been shown to bind to other polyglutamine-containing proteins, including the gene product in dentato-rubral-pallido-luysian atrophy and ataxin in spinocerebellar ataxia type 1.[116]

With the yeast two-hybrid system, another protein interacting with huntingtin, namely, human ubiquitin conjugating enzyme (hE2-25K), has been identified.[117] Huntingtin represents the first identified substrate for this protein. This conjugating enzyme is highly expressed in brain, and a slightly larger protein recognized by an anti-E2-25K polyclonal antibody is selectively expressed in brain regions affected in HD. The huntingtin–E2-25K interaction, however, is not obviously modulated by CAG length. Huntingtin not only interacts with a specific ubiquitin-conjugating enzyme but is itself ubiquitinated.[117]

The precise role of each of these interactive proteins in the pathogenesis of HD and how they might interact with each other is unclear at this time.

In addition to these direct interactions, huntingtin, in the presence of calcium, also interacts indirectly with calmodulin,[122] and this also appears to be influenced by polyglutamine length.

## GENETIC COUNSELING

The geneticist and genetic counselor commonly encounter a healthy person at risk for HD who wants to know his or her risk for having inherited the illness. For a person in early adult life with an affected parent, the risk is very close to 50%. By the time the person has reached beyond the age of 60 years, however, the risk will have decreased considerably.

Familial aggregation of age of onset can also be taken into account in assessing the risk for an asymptomatic individual who has a parent affected with HD. This has been thoroughly investigated for siblings of persons with juvenile HD.[123]

There is a significant correlation between CAG length and age of onset. Studies of this subject, however, have been confounded by different measures of CAG length, inaccurate sizing, and failure to include asymptomatic persons with CAG in the expanded range.[96–99] For patients being informed that they have DNA changes associated with HD, the next question is when the disease will manifest.

## PREDICTIVE TESTING

Recent findings from different studies have indicated that no patients have been reported who have manifest with HD with a CAG length less than 36 repeats.[101,124] All patients affected with HD have a CAG size of 36 repeats and greater. Between a CAG length of 36 and 41, however, there is reduced penetrance, and only a proportion of those individuals with a CAG size in this range would be expected to manifest with HD in their lifetime.[101] Although the exact numbers are not known, clearly as the CAG size increases to 41, the likelihood of manifesting with HD within an expected life span increases. With a CAG size of 41 and greater, the mutation for HD is fully penetrant.

The intermediate range is defined as that from which new mutations have been proven to arise. These include persons with a CAG size between 29 and 35 repeats. Although these individuals will never manifest with HD based on all data currently ascertained, there may be some small risk for HD to their offspring, though this risk would appear only to be for offspring of men with IAs. At the present time there are no reports of females with IAs that have led to expansion and new mutations in their offspring. The normal range for CAG size is below 29 repeats.

There is clearly value in distinguishing between these different ranges as they each have different clinical significance. Below 29 such individuals will never manifest with HD, and there are no reports of such individuals transmitting this disease to their offspring. Between 29 and 35 repeats, the individuals, again, will not manifest with HD, but there is a slightly increased risk for manifesting with CAG expansion and signs and symptoms of this illness for offspring of males with IAs. Between 36 and 41 is the range of reduced penetrance. CAG size modulates the likelihood of manifesting with this disease. This is clearly still within the clinical range, but not everyone will manifest with HD within their lifetime. Above 41 repeats, all persons are expected to manifest with signs and symptoms of HD within their lifetime. This is based on the expected lifespan of 75 years for males and 80 years for females.[101]

Predictive testing for HD has been offered in different parts of the world for several years. Before the introduction of predictive testing, research protocols were developed to evaluate the psychological impact of receiving either an increased or a decreased risk result.[125–125] There was major concern that an increased risk result would precipitate catastrophic reactions such as emotional breakdown or suicide.

Short-term follow-up studies of participants in the Canadian Predictive Testing Program have revealed that predictive testing for HD may maintain or even improve the psychological well-being of at-risk individuals.[129] Most individuals who receive a decreased risk result have shown improvement in psychological health whereas the individuals who have received an increased risk result have not responded to predictive testing in the negative manner feared when predictive testing programs for HD were first developed.[129] Despite the fact that both groups as a whole responded well to predictive testing programs, several individuals did have difficulties in adjusting to their new status. For those who received an increased risk, there has been a new focus on physical symptoms with a request for a physical examination and the need for continued support and reassurance that DNA testing is not synonymous with diagnosis of illness.[129] Although it was expected that some individuals might have difficulty coping with an increased risk result, a similar frequency of problems was not expected among those receiving a decreased risk.[130] About 10% of the decreased risk group have had serious difficulties adapting to their new status. The major hurdle for these individuals appears to be the realization that they are facing an unplanned future.

The demand for predictive testing has been found to be lower than expected in studies conducted before the advent of predictive testing.[126,131,132] In addition, prenatal testing for HD is not a frequently chosen option.[133] The reason most frequently cited by patients for declining prenatal testing was the hope for the development of a cure in time for their children.[134]

Cloning of the gene for HD has had impact on the attitudes of at-risk individuals toward both predictive and prenatal testing. The demand for predictive testing has increased significantly. The possibility of hope for an effective therapy that may arise as a result of the cloning of the gene for HD, however, is likely to further reduce the demand for prenatal testing. Termination of a pregnancy for a curable or potentially treatable adult onset illness is likely to be even less acceptable. The medium-term and long-term effects of predictive testing for HD are not known, and there is a continued need for longitudinal investment to examine the psychological and social effects of testing and to collect data that best predicts responses to change in risk status.

Prior to the implementation of predictive-testing programs for HD, there was significant concern about the likelihood of catastrophic events (CEs), particularly in those persons receiving an increased-risk result. We have investigated the frequency of CEs—namely, suicide, suicide attempt, and psychiatric hospitalization—after an HD predictive-testing result, through questionnaires sent to predictive-testing centers worldwide. A total of 44 persons (0.97%) in a cohort of 4,527 test participants had a CE: 5 successful suicides, 21 suicide attempts, and 18 hospitalizations for psychiatric reasons. All persons committing suicide had signs of HD, whereas 11 (52.4%) of 21 persons attempting suicide and 8 (44.4%) of 18 who had a psychiatric hospitalization were symptomatic. A total of 11 (84.6%) of 13 asymptomatic persons who experienced a CE during the first year after HD predictive testing received an increased-risk result. Factors associated with an increased risk of a CE included a psychiatric history five years or less prior to testing and unemployment. Among persons receiving results of predictive testing through linkage analysis, the frequency of CEs did not differ between those in whom there were changes only in direction of risk and those receiving definitive results after analysis for the mutation underlying HD. These findings provide insights into the frequency, associated factors, and timing of CEs in a worldwide cohort of persons receiving predictive-testing result and, as such, highlight persons for whom ongoing support may be beneficial.[135]

## SUMMARY

Recently, new insights concerning the function of the HD gene and the mechanism by which CAG expansion causes HD have been derived. The gene product for HD, huntingtin, is crucial for normal mammalian development, and its absence is associated with increasing apoptosis, which is also a feature of HD. Huntingtin is a substrate for a crucial pro-apoptotic cystein protease, apopain. The extent of cleavage of huntingtin is influenced by length of the polyglutamine tract. The identification of novel interacting proteins specific to the central nervous system may explain in part the selective neuropathology of this illness.

## ACKNOWLEDGEMENTS

This work was supported by the National Centre of Excellence (Genetics), the Medical Research Council (MRC) (Canada) (to M.R.H.). Dr. Hayden is an established investigator of the British Columbia Children's Hospital.

## REFERENCES

1. Harper PS: Huntington's Disease. WB, Saunders, London, 1991.
2. Hayden MR: Huntington's Chorea. Springer-Verlag, Heidelberg, 1981.
3. Adams P, Falek A, Arnold J: Huntington disease in Georgia: Age at onset. Am J Hum Genet 43:695–704, 1988.
4. Zolliker A: Die Chorea Huntington in der Schweiz. Schweiz Arch Neurol Psychiatr 64:448–457, 1949.
5. Young AB, Shoulson I, Penney JB, et al.: Huntington's disease in Venezuela: Neurologic features and functional decline. Neurology 36:244–249, 1986.
6. Hayden MR, Hewitt J, Stoessel AJ, Clark C, Moennich D, Martin WR: The combined use of positron emission tomography and DNA polymorphisms for preclinical detection of Huntington's disease. Neurology 37:1441–1447, 1987.
7. Grafton ST, Mazziotta JC, Pahl JJ, et al.: A comparison of neurological, metabolic, structural, and genetic evaluations in persons at risk for Huntington's disease. Ann Neurol 28:614–621, 1990.
8. Brothers CRD: Huntington's chorea in Victoria and Tasmania. J Neurol Sci i:405–420, 1964.
9. Pridmore SA: The prevalence of Huntington's disease in Tasmania. Med J Aust 153:133–134, 1990.
10. Folstein SE: Huntington's Disease: A Disorder of Families. Johns Hopkins University Press, Baltimore, 1989.
11. Folstein SE, Leigh RJ, Parhad IM, Folstein MF: The diagnosis of Huntington's disease. Neurology 36: 1279–1283, 1986.
12. Bruyn GW: Huntington's chorea. Historical, clinical and laboratory synopsis. In Vinken PJ, Bruyn GW (eds.): Diseases of the Basal Ganglia. Handbook of Clinical Neurology, Vol 6. North Holland, Amsterdam, 1968, pp298–378.
13. Thompson PD, Berardelli A, Rothwell JC, et al.: The coexistence of bradykinesia and chorea in Huntington's disease and its implications for theories of basal ganglia control of movement. Brain 111:223–244, 1988.
14. Bittenbender JB, Quadfasel FA: Rigid and akinetic forms of Huntington's chorea. Arch Neurol 7:275–288, 1962.
15. Beenen N, Buttner U, Lange HW: The diagnostic value of eye movement recordings in patients with Huntington's disease and their offspring. Electroencephalogr Clin Neurophysiol 63:119–127, 1986.
16. Oepen G, Clarenbach P, Thoden U: Disturbance of eye movements in Huntington's chorea. Arch Psychiatrie Nervenkr 229:205–213, 1981.
17. Lasker AG, Zee DS, Hain TC, Folstein SE, Singer HS: Saccades in Huntington's disease: Slowing and dysmetria. Neurology 38:427–431, 1988.
18. Tian JR, Zee DS, Lasker AG, Folstein SE: Saccades in Huntington's disease: Predictive tracking and interaction between release of fixation and initiation of saccades. Neurology 41:875–881, 1991.
19. Beatty WW, Salmon DP, Butters N, Heindel WC, Granholm EL: Retrograde amnesia in patients with Alzheimer's disease or Huntington's disease. Neurobiol Aging 9:181–186, 1988.
20. Hefter H, Hömberg V, Lange HW, Freund HJ: Impairment of rapid movement in Huntington's disease. Brain 110:585–612, 1987.
21. Folstein SE, Jensen B, Leigh RJ, Folstein MF: The measurement of abnormal movement: Methods developed for Huntington's disease. Neurobehav Toxicol Teratol 5:605–609, 1983.
22. Koller WC, Trimble J: The gait abnormality of Huntington's disease. Neurology 35:1450–1454, 1985.
23. Podoll K, Caspary P, Lange HW, Noth J: Language functions in Huntington's disease. Brain 111:1475–1503, 1988.
24. Coleman R, Anderson D, Lovrien E: Oral motor dysfunction in individuals at risk of Huntington disease. Am J Med Genet 37:36–39, 1990.
25. Caine ED, Fisher JM: Dementia in Huntington's disease. In Vinken PJ, Bruyn GW, Klawans HL, Frederiks JAM (eds): Handbook of Clinical Neurology, Vol 46, Rev. Series 2, Neurobehavioural Disorders. Elsevier, Amsterdam, 1985, pp305–310.

26. Brandt J, Butters N: The neuropsychology of Huntington's disease. Trends Neurosci 9:118–120, 1986.
27. Jason GW, Pajurkova EM, Suchowersky O, et al.: Presymptomatic neuropsychological impairment in Huntington's disease. Arch Neurol 45:769–773, 1988.
28. Pillon B, Dubois B, Ploska A, Agid Y: Severity and specificity of cognitive impairment in Alzheimer's, Huntington's, and Parkinson's diseases and progressive supranuclear palsy. Neurology 41:634–643, 1991.
29. Choi DW, Rothman SM: The role of glutamate neurotoxicity in hypoxic-ischemic neuronal death. Annu Rev Neurosci 13:171–182, 1990.
30. Pritchard CA, Casher D, Uglum E, Cox DR, Myers RM: Isolation and field-inversion gel electrophoresis analysis of DNA markers located close to the Huntington disease gene. Genomics 4:408–418, 1989.
31. Wilson RS, Como PG, Garron DC, Klawans HL, Barr A, Klawans D: Memory failure in Huntington's disease. J Clin Exp Neuropsychol 9:147–154, 1987.
32. Massman PJ, Delis DC, Butters N, Levin BE, Salmon DP: Are all subcortical dementias alike? Verbal learning and memory in Parkinson's and Huntington's disease patients. J Clin Exp Neuropsychol 12:729–744, 1990.
33. Folstein SE: Appendix 1. The documentation of clinical features of Huntington's disease: Clinical assessment instruments. In Folstein SE (ed): Huntington's Disease: A Disorder of Families. Johns Hopkins University Press, Baltimore, 1989, pp189–195.
34. Scholz OB, Berlemann C: Memory performance in Huntington's disease. Int J Neurosci 35:155–162, 1987.
35. Randolph C: Implicit, explicit, and semantic memory functions in Alzheimer's disease and Huntington's disease. J Clin Exp Neuropsychol 13:479–494, 1991.
36. Brandt J, Folstein SE, Folstein MF: Differential cognitive impairment in Alzheimer's disease and Huntington's disease. Ann Neurol 23:555–561, 1988.
37. Starkstein SE, Brandt J, Folstein S, et al.: Neuropsychological and neuroradiological correlates in Huntington's disease. J Neurol Neurosurg Psychiatry 51:1259–1263, 1988.
38. Wallesch CW, Fehrenbach RA: On the neurolinguistic nature of language abnormalities in Huntington's disease. J Neurol Neurosurg Psychiatry 51:367–373, 1988.
39. Hodges JR, Salmon DP, Butters N: The nature of the naming deficit in Alzheimer's and Huntington's disease. Brain 114:1547–1558, 1991.
40. Speedie LJ, Brake N, Folstein SE, Bowers D, Heilman KM: Comprehension of prosody in Huntington's disease. J Neurol Neurosurg Psychiatry 53:607–610, 1990.
41. Caine ED, Shoulson I: Psychiatric syndromes in Huntington's disease. Am J Psychiatry 140:728–733, 1983.
42. Morris M, Tyler A. Management and therapy. In Harper PS (ed): Huntington's Disease. WB Saunders, London, 1991, pp205–250.
43. Farrer LA: Suicide and attempted suicide in Huntington disease: Implications for preclinical testing of persons at risk. Am J Med Genet 24:305–311, 1986.
44. Folstein SE: The psychopathology of Huntington's disease. Res Publ Assoc Res Nerv Ment Dis 69:181–191, 1991.
45. Burns A, Folstein S, Brandt J, Folstein M: Clinical assessment of irritability, aggression, and apathy in Huntington and Alzheimer disease. J Nerv Ment Dis 178:20–26, 1990.
46. Sanberg PR, Fibiger HC, Mark RF: Body weight and dietary factors in Huntington's disease patients compared with matched controls. Med J Aust 1:407–409, 1981.
47. Farrer LA, Yu PL: Anthropometric discrimination among affected, at-risk, and not-at-risk individuals in families with Huntington disease. Am J Med Genet 21:307–316, 1985.
48. Morales LM, Estēvez J, Suarez H, Villalobos R, Chacin de Bonilla L, Bonilla E: Nutritional evaluation of Huntington disease patients. Am J Clin Nutr 50:145–150, 1989.
49. Myers RH, Vonsattel JP, Paskevich PA, et al.: Decreased neuronal and increased oligodendroglial densities in Huntington's disease caudate nucleus. J Neuropathol Exp Neurol 50:729–742, 1991.
50. Hansotia el al.: 1985.
51. Wheeler JS, Sax DS, Krane RJ, Siroky MB: Vesicourethral function in Huntington's chorea. Br J Urol 57:63–66, 1985.
52. Markham CH, Knox JW: Observations on Huntington's chorea in childhood. J Pediatr 67:46–57, 1965.
53. Oliver J, Dewhurst K: Childhood and adolescent forms of Huntington's disease. J Neurol Neurosurg Psychiatry 32:455–459, 1969.
54. Osborne JP, Munson P, Burman D: Huntington's chorea. Report of 3 cases and review of the literature. Arch Dis Child 57:99–103, 1982.
55. Paulson GW: Lioresal in Huntington's disease. Dis Nerv Syst 37:465–467, 1976.
56. Jervis GA: Huntington's chorea in childhood. Arch Neurol 9:244–257, 1963.
57. Vogel CM, Drury I, Terry LC, Young AB: Myoclonus in adult Huntington's disease. Ann Neurol 29:213–215, 1991.
58. Myers RH, Sax DS, Schoenfeld M, et al.: Late onset of Huntington's disease. J Neurol Neurosurg Psychiatry 48:530–534, 1985.
59. Davies DD: Abnormal response to anesthesia in a case of Huntington's chorea. Br J Anaesth 38:490–491, 1966.
60. Terrence CF, Delaney JF, Alberts MC: Computed tomography for Huntington's disease. Neuroradiology 13:173–175, 1977.
61. Wardlaw JM, Sellar RJ, Abernethy LJ: Measurement of caudate nucleus area—A more accurate measurement for Huntington's disease? Neuroradiology 33:316–319, 1991.
62. Starkstein SE, Folstein SE, Brandt J, Pearlson GD, McDonnell A, Folstein M: Brain atrophy in Huntington's disease. A CT-scan study. Neuroradiology 31:156–159, 1989.
63. Clark C, Hayden M, Hollenberg S, Li D, Stoessl AJ: Controlling for cerebral atrophy in positron emis-

sion tomography data. J Cereb Blood Flow Metab 7:510–512, 1987.
64. Simmons JT, Pastakia B, Chase TN, Shults CW: Magnetic resonance imaging in Huntington disease. AJNR. 7:25–28, 1986.
65. Hardie RJ, Pullon HWH, Harding AE, et al.: Neuroacanthocytosis. A clinical, haematologic and pathological study of 19 cases. Brain 114:12–48, 1991.
66. Serra S, Xerra A, Scribano E, Meduri M, Di Perri R: Computerized tomography in amyotrophic choreo-acanthocytosis. Neuroradiology 29:480–482, 1987.
67. Kuhl DE, Phelps ME, Markham CH, Metter EJ, Riege WH, Winter J: Cerebral metabolism and atrophy in Huntington's disease determined by 18FDG and computed tomographic scan. Ann Neurol 12:425–434, 1982.
68. Hayden MR, Martin WR, Stoessl AJ, et al.: Position emission tomography in the early diagnosis of Huntington's disease. Neurology 36:888–894, 1986.
69. Mazziotta JC, Phelps ME, Pahl JJ, et al.: Reduced cerebral glucose metabolism in asymptomatic subjects at risk for Huntington's disease. N Engl J Med 316:357–362, 1987.
70. Young AB, Penney JB, Starosta-Rubinstein S, et al.: Normal caudate glucose metabolism in persons at risk for Huntington's disease. Arch Neurol 44:254–257, 1987.
71. Hosokawa S, Ichiya Y, Kuwabara Y, et al.: Position emission tomography in cases of chorea with different underlying diseases. J Neurol Neurosurg Psychiatry 50:1284–1287, 1987.
72. Hawkins RA, Mazziotta JC, Phelps ME: Wilson's disease studies with FDG and position emission tomography. Neurology 37:1707–1711, 1987.
73. Lang AE, Garnett ES: Position emission tomography in cases of chorea with different underlying diseases [Letter]. J Neurol Neurosurg Psychiatry 1988.
74. Suchowersky O, Hayden MR, Martin WR, Stoessl AJ, Hildebrand AM, Pate BD: Cerebral metabolism of glucose in benign hereditary chorea. Mov Discord 1:33–44, 1986.
75. Kuwert T, Lange HW, Langen KJ, et al.: Normal striatal glucose consumption in two patients with benign hereditary chorea as measured by positron emission tomography. J Neurol 237:80–84, 1990.
76. Reid IC, Besson JA, Best PV, Sharp PF, Gemmell HG, Smith FW: Imaging of cerebral blood flow markers in Huntington's disease using single photon emission computed tomography. J Neurol Neurosurg Psychiatry 51:1264–1268, 1988.
77. Nagel JS, Johnson KA, Ichise M, et al.: Decreased iodine-123 IMP caudate nucleus uptake in patients with Huntington's disease. Clin Nucl Med 13:486–490, 1988.
78. Smith FW, Gemmell HG, Sharp P F, Besson JA: Technetium-99m HMPAO imaging in patients with basal ganglia disease. Br J Radiol 61:914–920, 1988.
79. Botsch H, Oepen G, Deuschl G, Wolff G: [SPECT studies with 9mmTc-Tc-HMPAO in Huntington's chorea patients]. ROFO. Fortschr Geb Rontgenstr Nuklearmed 147:666–668, 1987.
80. Vonsattel JP, Myers RH, Stevens TJ, Ferrante RJ, Bird ED, Richardson EP Jr: Neuropathological classification of Huntington's disease. J Neuropathol Exp Neurol 44:559–577, 1985.
81. Graveland GA, Williams RS, DiFiglia M: Evidence for degenerative and regenerative changes in neostriatal spiny neurons in Huntington's disease. Science 227:770–773, 1985.
82. McCaughey WTE: The pathologic spectrum of Huntington's chorea. J Nerv Ment Dis 133:91–103, 1961.
83. Dom R, Baro F, Brucher JM. A cytometric study of the putamen in different types of Huntington's chorea. Adv Neurol 1:369–385, 1973.
84. Lange H, Thorner G, Hopf A, Schroder KF: Morphometric studies of the neuropathological changes in choreatic diseases. J Neurol Sci 28:401–425, 1976.
85. Rodda RA: Cerebellar atrophy in Huntington's disease. J Neurol Sci 50:147–157, 1981.
86. Jeste DV, Barban L, Parisi J: Reduced Purkinje cell density in Huntington's disease. Exp Neurol 85:78–86, 1984.
87. Kowall NW, Ferrante RJ, Martin JB: Patterns of cell loss in Huntington's disease. Trends Neurosci 10: 24–29, 1987.
88. Albin RL, Qin Y, Young AB, Penney JB, Chesselet MF: Preproenkephalin messenger RNA-containing neurons in striatum of patients with symptomatic and presymptomatic Huntington's disease: An *in situ* hybridization study. Ann Neurol 30:542–549, 1991.
89. Hope BT, Michael GJ, Knigge KM, Vincent SR: Neuronal NADPH-diaphorase is a nitric oxide synthase. Proc Natl Acad Sci USA 88:2811–2814, 1991.
90. Ferrante RJ, Kowall NW, Beal MF, Richardson EP Jr, Bird ED, Martin JB: Selective sparing of a class of striatal neurons in Huntington's disease. Science 230:561–563, 1985.
91. Dawbarn D, De Quidt ME, Emson PC: Survival of basal ganglia neuropeptide Y–somatostatin neurones in Huntington's disease. Brain Res 340:251–260, 1985.
92. Ferrante RJ, Kowall NW, Beal MF, Martin JB, Bird ED, Richardson EP Jr: Morphologic and histochemical characteristics of a spared subset of striatal neurons in Huntington's disease. J Neuropathol Exp Neurol 46:12–27, 1987.
93. Ferrante RJ, Beal MF, Kowall NW, Richardson EP Jr, Martin JB: Sparing of acetylcholinesterase-containing striatal neurons in Huntington's disease. Brain Res 411:162–166, 1987.
94. Huntington's Disease Collaborate Research Group: A novel gene containing a trinucleotide repeat that is expanded and unstable on Huntington's disease chromosomes. Cell 72:971–983, 1993.
95. Lin B-Y, Rommens JM, Graham RK, et al.: Differential 3' polyadenylation of the Huntington disease gene results in two mRNA species with variable tissue expression. Hum Mol Genet 2:1541–1545, 1993.
96. Andrew SE, Goldberg YP, Kremer B, et al.: The relationship between trinucleotide repeat length (CAG) and clinical features of Huntington disease. Nat Genet 4:398–403, 1993.
97. Norremolle A, Riess O, Epplen JT, Fenger K, Hasholt L, Sorenson SA: Trinucleotide repeat elongation in the Huntington gene in Huntington disease

patients from 71 Danish families. Hum Mol Genet 2:1475–1476, 1993.
98. Snell RG, MacMillan JC, Cheadle JP, et al.: Relationship between trinucleotide repeat expansion and phenotypic variation in Huntington's disease. Nat Genet 4(4):329–330, 1993.
99. Duyao M, Ambrose C, Myers R, et al.: Trinucleotide repeat length instability in Huntington disease. Nat Genet 4:387–392, 1993.
100. Telenius H, et al.: Molecular analysis of juvenile Huntington disease: The major influence on (CAG)n repeat length is the sex of the affected parent. Hum Mol Genet 2:1535–1540, 1993.
101. Brinkman RR, Mezei MM, Thielmann J, et al.: The likelihood of being affected with Huntington disease by a particular age for a specific CAG size. Am J Hum Genet 60:1202–1210, 1997.
102. Vogel F, Motuksky AG. Human Genetics, ed 2. Springer Verlag, New York, 1986.
103. Stevens D, Parsonage M: Mutation in Huntington's chorea. J Neurol Neurosurg Psychiatry 32: 140–143, 1969.
104. Goldberg YP, McMurray CT, Zeisler J, et al.: Increased instability of intermediate alleles in families with sporadic Huntingtoin disease compared to similar sized intermediate alleles in the general population. Nat Genet 4(10):1911–1918, 1995.
105. Sharp A, Loev SJ, Schilling G, et al.: Widespread expression of Huntington's disease gene (IT-15) protein product. Neuron 14:1065–1074, 1995.
106. Trottier Y, Devys D, Imberg G, et al.: Cellular localization of the Huntington's disease protein and discrimination of the normal and mutated form. Nat Genet 10:104–110, 1995.
107. DiFiglia M, Sapp E, Chase K, et al.: Huntingtin is a cytoplasmic protein associated with vesicles in human and rat brain neurons. Neuron 14:1075–1081, 1995.
108. Schilling G, Sharp AH, Loev SJ, et al.: Expression of the HD gene (IT15) protein product in HD patients. Hum Mol Genet 1995.
109. Goldberg YP, Kalchman MA, Zeisler J, et al.: Absence of disease phenotype and intergenerational stability of the CAG repeat in transgenic mice expressing the Huntington disease transcript. Hum Mol Genet 5(2):177–185, 1996.
110. Nasir J, Floresco SB, O'Kusky JR, et al.: Targeted disruption of the Huntington's disease gene results in embryonic lethality and behavioral and morphological changes in heterozygotes. Cell 81: 811–823, 1995.
111. Duyao MP, Auerbach AB, Ryan A, et al.: Inactivation of the mouse Huntington's disease gene homolog *Hdh*. Science 269:407–410, 1995.
112. Zeitlin S, Liu J-P, Chapman DL, Papaioannou VE, Efstratiadis A: Increased apoptosis and early embryonic lethality in mice nullizygous for the Huntington's disease gene homologue. Nat Genet 11: 155–162, 1995.
113. Housman D: Gain of glutamines, gain of fuction? Nat Genet 10:3–4, 1995.
114. Goldberg YP, Nicholson DW, Rasper DM, et al.: Cleavage of huntingtin by apopain, a proapoptotic cystein protease, is modulated by the polyglutamine tract. Nat Genet 13:442–449, 1996.
115. Li X-J, Li S-H, Sharp AH, et al.: A huntingtin-associated protein enriched in brain with implications for pathology. Nature 378:398–402, 1995.
116. Burke JR, Enghild JJ, Margin ME, et al.: Huntingtin and DRPLA proteins selectively interact with the enzyme GAPDH. Nat Med 2(3):347–350, 1996.
116a. Kalchman MA, Graham RK, Xia G, et al.: Huntingtin is ubiquitinated and interacts with a specific ubiquitin conjugated enzyme. J Biol Chem. 271(32):19385–19394, 1996.
117. Hodgson JG, Agopyan N, Gutekunst C-A, et al.: A YAC mouse model for Huntington's disease with full-length mutant huntingtin (http) cytoplasmic toxicity, nuclear translocation of htt, and selective striatal neurodegeneration. Neuron 23:181–192, 1999.
117a. Goldberg YP, Nicholson DW, Rasper DM, Kalchman MA, Koide HB, Graham RK, Bromm M, Kazemi-Esfarjani P, Thornberry NA, Vaillancourt JP, Hayden MR: Cleavage of huntingtin by apopain, a proapoptotic cysteine protease, is modulated by the polyglutamine tract. Nat Genet 13: 442–449, 1996.
117b. Martindale D, Hackam AS, Wieczorek A, Ellerby L, Wellington CL, McCutcheon K, Singaraja R, Kazemi-Esfarjani P, Devon R, Bredesen DE, Tufaro F, Hayden MR: Length of the protein and polyglutamine tract influence localization and frequency of intracellular aggregates of huntingtin. Nat Genet 18:150–154, 1998.
117c. Hackam AS, Singaraja R, Wellington CL, Metzler M, McCutcheon K, Zhang T, Kalchman M, Hayden MR: The influence of huntingtin protein size on nuclear localization and cellular toxicity. J Cell Biol 141:1097–1105, 1998.
117d. Mangiarini L, Sathasivam K, Seller M, Cozens B, Harper A, Hetherington C, Lawton M, Trottier Y, Lehrach H, Davies SW, Bates GP: Exon 1 of the *HD* Gene with an Expanded CAG Repeat Is Sufficient to Cause a Progressive Neurological Phenotype in Transgenic Mice. Cell 87:493–506, 1996.
117e. White JK, Augood SJ, Duyao MP, Vonsattel J-P, Gusella JF, Joyner AL, MacDonald ME: Huntingtin is required for neurogenesis and is not impaired by the Huntington's disease CAG expansion. Nat Genet 17:404–410, 1997.
117f. Reddy PH, Williams M, Charles V, Garrett L, Pike-Buchanan L, Whetsell WO Jr, Miller G, Tagle DA: Behavioral abnormalities and selective neuronal loss in HD transgenic mice expressing mutated full-length HD cDNA. Nat Genet 20:198–202, 1998.
117g. Schilling G, Becher MW, Sharp AH, Jinnah HA, Duan K, Kotzuk JA, Slunt HH, Ratovitski T, Cooper JK, Jenkins NA, Copeland NG, Price DL, Ross CA, Borchelt DR: Intranuclear inclusions and neuritic aggregates in transgenic mice expressing a mutant N-terminal fragment of huntingtin. Hum Mol Genet 8:397–407, 1999.
118. Thomas LB, Gates DJ, Richfield EK, O'Brien TF, Schweitzer JB, Steindler DA: DNA end labeling (TUNEL) in Huntington's disease and other neuropathological conditions. Exp Neurol 133:265–272, 1995.
119. Dragunow M, Faull RLM, Lawlor P, et al.: *In situ*

evidence for DNA fragmentation in Huntington's disease striatum and Alzheimer's disease temporal lobes. Clin Neurosci Neuropathol 6:1053–1057, 1995.

120. Protera-Cailliau C, Hedreen JC, Price DL, Koliatsos VE: Evidence for apoptotic cell death in Huntington disease and excitotoxic animal models. J Neurosci 15(5):3775–3787, 1995.

121. Nicholson DW, Ali A, Thornberry NA, et al.: Identification and inhibition of the ICE/CED-3 protease necessary for mammalian apoptosis. Nature 376:37–43, 1995.

122. Li X-J, Sharp AH, Li S-H, Dawson TM, Snyder SH, Ross CA: Huntingtin-associated protein (HAP1): Discrete neuronal localization resemble those of neuronal nitric oxide synthase. Proc Natl Acad Sci USA 93:4839–4844, 1996.

123. Hayden MR, Soles JA, Ward RH: Age of onset in siblings of persons with juvenile Huntington disease. Clin Genet 28:100–105, 1985.

124. Rubinsztein DC, Leggo J, Coles R, et al.: Phenotypic characterisation of individuals with 30–40 CAG repeats in the Huntington's disease gene reveals HD cases with 36 repeats and apparently normal elderly individuals with 36–39 repeats. Am J Hum Genet 59:16–22, 1996.

125. Skraastad MI, Verwest A, Bakker E, et al.: Presymptomatic, prenatal, and exclusion testing for Huntington disease using seven closely linked DNA markers. Am J Med Genet 39:217–222, 1991.

126. Craufurd D, Dodge A, Kerzin-Storrar L, Harris R: Uptake of presymptomatic predictive testing for Huntington's disease. Lancet 2:603–605, 1989.

127. Brandt J, Quaid KA, Folstein SE, et al.: Presymptomatic diagnosis of delayed-onset disease with linked DNA markers. The experience in Huntington's disease [see comments]. JAMA 261:3108–3114, 1989.

128. Wiggins S, Whyte P, Huggins M, et al.: The psychological consequences of predictive testing for Huntington disease. N Engl J Med 327:20:1401–1405, 1992.

129. Bloch M, Adam S, Wiggins S, Huggins M, Hayden MR: Predictive testing for Huntington disease in Canada: The experience of those receiving an increased risk. Am J Med Genet 42:499–507, 1992.

130. Huggins M, Bloch M, Wiggins S, et al.: Predictive testing for Huntington disease in Canada: Adverse effects and unexpected results in those receiving a decreased risk. Am J Med Genet 42:508–515, 1992.

131. Meissen GJ, Berchek RL: Intended use of predictive testing by those at risk for Huntington disease. Am J Med Genet 26:283–293, 1987.

132. Mastromauro C, Myers RH, Berkman B: Attitudes toward presymptomatic testing in Huntington disease. Am J Med Genet 26:271–282, 1987.

133. Tyler A, Quarrell OW, Lazarou LP, Meredith AL, Harper PS: Exclusion testing in pregnancy for Huntington's disease. J Med Genet 27:488–495, 1990.

134. Adam S, Wiggins S, Whyte P, et al.: Five year study of prenatal testing for Huntington disease: Demand, attitudes and psychological assessment. J Med Genet 30:549–556, 1993.

135. Almqivst EW, Bloch M, Brinkman R, Craufurd D, Hayden MR, on behalf of an international Huntington disease collaborative group: A worldwide assessment of the frequency of suicide, suicide attempts, or psychiatric hospitalization after predictive testing for Huntington disease. Am J Hum Genet 64:1293–1304, 1999.

Chapter 14

# INHERITED MOTOR NEURON DISEASES

Robert H. Brown, Jr, D Phil, MD



In recent years there has been substantial progress in delineating the molecular bases of several inherited diseases of the motor neuron. For many of the major familial motor neuron diseases, genetic loci for the underlying defects have been described, and, in some instances, the primary lesion and defective protein(s) have been identified (Table 14–1). Understanding the diversity of molecular lesions that trigger motor neuron cell death helps to define the pathophysiology of inherited and sporadic motor neuron diseases and also provides insight into basic neurobiological properties of the motor neuron. In the long term, this will be the basis for new strategies to treat these disorders. This chapter provides an overview of inherited motor neuron disorders, focusing on the more common variants. It is helpful to subdivide these disorders anatomically, depending on whether they involve the corticospinal (upper) motor neurons or brain stem and spinal (lower) motor neurons or both.

## DISORDERS OF THE UPPER AND LOWER MOTOR NEURONS

### Dominantly Inherited, Adult Onset Amyotrophic Lateral Sclerosis

Amyotrophic lateral sclerosis (ALS) is a rapidly advancing, lethal, paralytic disorder caused by death of motor neurons in the brain, brain stem, and spinal cord (reviewed by Tandan and Bradley[1,2]). This is an age-dependent disease, with onset in the mid-50s. Survival is 3 to 5 years; rare cases of prolonged survival are documented. The incidence and prevalence of ALS, respectively, are 1 to 3/100,000 and 3 to 5/100,000. There are, however, scattered endemic foci of higher prevalence in the Western Pacific (e.g., regions of Guam or Papua New Guinea). Males are somewhat more frequently affected. Approximately 5% to 10% of cases are inherited as an autosomal dominant trait (familial ALS [FALS]).

Amyotrophic lateral sclerosis usually starts focally and then disseminates, frequently in an anatomic pattern suggesting that the disease is somehow spread between contiguously located groups of motor neu-

Table 14–1. **Inherited Motor Neuron Disorders**

| Disease | Defect | Locus | Senior Author |
|---|---|---|---|
| *Upper and Lower Motor Neurons* | | | |
| Amyotrophic lateral sclerosis (ALS) | | | |
| Dominant, adult onset | Superoxide dismutase 1 | 21q | Rosen[9] |
| | Neurofilament subunit H | 11 | Figlewicz[46] |
| Dominant, juvenile onset | | 9q | Chance[101] |
| Recessive, juvenile onset | | 2q33–35 | Hentati[50] |
| ALS with Pick's disease | | ? | Constantinidis[100] |
| *Lower Motor Neurons* | | | |
| Spinal muscular atrophy (SMA) | Survival motor neuron (? NAIP) | 5q11.2–13.3 | Brzustowicz[52] |
| SMA I, onset <6 months (Werdnig-Hoffmann disease) | | | |
| SMA II, onset <18 months | | | |
| SMA III, onset >18 months (Kugelberg-Welander disease) | | | |
| SMA IV, onset >30 years | | | |
| $GM_2$-gangliosidoses | | | |
| Tay-Sach's disease | Hex A deficiency (α-subunit) | 15q23–24 | Takeda[96] |
| Sandhoff's disease | Hex A+B deficiency (β-subunit) | 5q11.2–13.6 | Takeda[96] |
| AB variant | $GM_2$-activator protein | 5q | Burg[97] |
| Scapuloperoneal muscular atrophy | | ? | Kaeser,[92] DeLong[93] |
| Progressive juvenile bulbar paralysis Fazio-Londe | | ? | McShane[87] |
| Arthrogryposis | | 9 | Bamshad[90] |
| X-linked | | | |
| Spinal muscular atrophy | | Xp | |
| Spino-bulbar muscular atrophy | Androgen receptor | Xq11 | LaSpada[68] |
| Arthrogryposis | | Xp11–q11 | Kobayashi[98] |
| | | | Hall[99] |
| Scapuloperoneal muscular atrophy | | | Skre[95] |
| *Upper Motor Neurons (Hereditary Spastic Paraplegia)* | | | |
| Dominant | | | Fink[81] |
| | | 2p | Hazan[79] |
| | | 14q | Hazan[75] |
| | | 15q | Fink[77] |
| | Other | ? | |
| Recessive | | 8q | Hentati[82] |
| X-linked | Proteolipid protein | Xq22 | Saugier-Veber[83] |
| | L1CAM | Xq28 | Jouet[84] |

rons. Regardless of the site of onset, in 2 to 3 years all of the limbs and the bulbar muscles are affected, and there is evidence that both the lower and upper motor neurons are deteriorating. In ALS there is no involvement of sensory and sphincteric function, cognition, or memory.

When lower motor neurons are predominantly involved at onset, patients present with weakness and muscle atrophy ("amyotrophy"). This early denervation begins insidiously, causing asymmetric weakness that is usually distal. This is often associated with muscle cramping caused by volitional movements, especially in the early hours of the morning (e.g., while turning or stretching in bed). These symptoms are also often accompanied by the spontaneous twitching of motor units, or fasciculations. In the forearms, weakness is often most pronounced in the extensor muscles. When the initial denervation involves bulbar muscles, the initial complaint is difficulty with chewing, swallowing, and speech. Rarely, ALS presents as primary respiratory disease due to initial involvement of motor neurons that innervate the diaphragm.

When corticospinal (upper) motor neurons are afflicted first, the clinical picture is one of weakness with spasticity (exaggerated stretch reflexes, increased limb tone, and scissoring of the gait). Muscle-stretch reflexes and spastic resistance to passive movements of the affected limbs are also enhanced.

Bilateral involvement of the corticobulbar motor neurons to the brain stem cause dysarthria and exaggeration of the motor expressions of emotional reflexes. The hallmark of this "pseudo-bulbar" disturbance is inappropriate intensification of behavioral responses to emotional stimuli.

The pathological hallmark of ALS is a loss of motor neurons, which appear to shrink. There usually is little evidence of any cellular reaction other than a subtle gliosis (but see Appel and coworkers[3]). The degenerating corticospinal tracts acquire a grayish hue ("lateral sclerosis"). Within ALS motor neurons, there are distinctive cytoskeletal aberrations, including axonal "spheroids" of neurofilaments[4,5] and filamentous aggregations within the cell bodies. The latter sometimes show immunostaining for ubiquitin, sometimes in thread-like "skein" structure.[6] This indicates that one or more proteins labeled by ubiquitin have adopted an abnormal conformation and thus are marked by the cell for destruction. Insight into the identity of these proteins, and the process by which they are induced to fold abnormally, might provide an understanding of the early stages of cell toxicity in motor neurons in ALS.

Clinically, FALS is essentially indistinguishable from sporadic ALS (SALS).[7] Pathologically, the diseases are also similar, although findings in FALS may be more widespread than in SALS.[8] The high degree of similarity between FALS and SALS prompts the hypothesis that these diseases involve similar pathogenetic mechanisms. Thus, insights into FALS may also be pertinent to SALS. Motivated in part by this premise, a consortium undertook linkage analysis in FALS. In 1993, mutations in the gene for cytosolic, copper/zinc superoxide dismutase *(SOD1)* on 21q[9] were identified in a subset of FALS pedigrees. At present, more than 50 *SOD1* mutations have been detected in such families.[10]

SOD1 is a homodimeric enzyme of 153 amino acids. This protein has been highly conserved during evolution; it belongs to a small family of related proteins, including a manganese-dependent SOD expressed in mitochondria (SOD2) and an extracellular form (Cu/Zn dependent, SOD3). The function of the protein is to convert superoxide anion $O_2^{\cdot}$ to hydrogen peroxide $H_2O_2$. In turn, $H_2O_2$ is converted to $H_2O$ by either catalase or glutathione peroxidase[11] (Fig. 14–1). A copper ion within the active site of the molecule is the actual catalyst of the SOD1 reaction. The protein also binds zinc, which may be important in protein folding. That SOD1 thus plays an important role in free radical homeostasis[11] prompted the hypothesis that FALS, and potentially SALS, might be a disorder of free radical metabolism.

A first approach to assessing this free radical hypothesis is to evaluate the biochemical properties of the mutant SOD1 proteins and to directly assess ALS tissues for evidence of free radical–mediated oxidative injury. There is some reduction in total brain SOD1 activity in FALS patients with SOD1

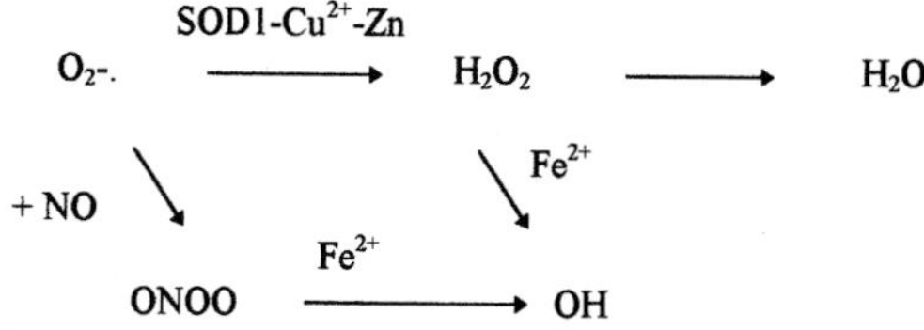


**Figure 14–1.** Selected reactions of cytosolic Cu/Zn superoxide dismutase (SOD1). SOD1 converts superoxide anion (O2−·) to hydrogen peroxide ($H_2O_2$). In turn, $H_2O_2$ is converted to water by catalase and glutathione peroxidase. Superoxide anion can combine with nitric oxide (NO) to form peroxynitrite (ONOO−). Both peroxynitrite and hydrogen peroxide can interact with reduced metals such as $Fe^{2+}$ or $Cu^{1+}$ to hydroxl radicals.

mutations, but not in SALS patients or FALS patients without SOD1 mutations.[12] Some, but by no means all, *SOD1* mutations reduce SOD1 activity in red blood cells and lymphoblastoid lines ions.[13–18] When expressed in COS cells, different SOD1 mutations vary in enzyme activity.[19] In addition, the stability of many of the mutant SOD1 proteins are reduced.[19]

The hypothesis that there is oxidative injury in neurons bearing mutant SOD1 molecules is supported by reports that levels of carbonyl proteins, markers of oxidative injury to proteins, are elevated in brain[12] and spinal cord[20] in SALS but not FALS patients. Moreover, levels of 8-OH-2-deoxy-guanine, a marker of oxidative DNA damage, are also elevated in ALS brain tissues.[21] By contrast, selected markers of oxidative stress were not elevated in spinal fluid in ALS patients.[22]

These reports documenting that SOD1 activity is decreased in tissues of patients with SOD1-associated FALS raise the possibility that motor neuron death is a direct consequence of this loss of SOD1 function. Studies of motor neurons *in vitro* demonstrate unequivocally that diminished dismutation of superoxide anion triggers programmed cell death of neurons.[23–25] Nonetheless, several considerations favor the alternative possibility that the mutant SOD1 protein has acquired adverse properties that are lethal for the motor neuron. Perhaps the strongest are the observations that mice with targeted inactivation of SOD1 and neither SOD1 proteins nor its activity show motor neuron cell death in the first few months of life.[26] In contrast, overexpression of SOD1 protein with FALS mutations causes a lethal, paralytic disorder in mice beginning at 3 to 5 months of age.[27–29]

These considerations indicate that the mutant SOD1 molecule is cytotoxic, activating a cascade of events causing motor neuron death. Although the novel activity is not yet well established, several hypothetical adverse functions for the mutant molecule have been proposed (Fig. 14–2). One possibility is that metal binding properties of some mutants (e.g., G85R and G93A) are abnormal and that either copper or zinc metal ions act as a toxin for motor neurons.[30,31] A second hypothesis is that nitration of critical tyrosine residues is a key event. Superoxide anion, $O_2^{\cdot}$, can normally combine with nitric oxide (NO) to form peroxynitrite (ONOO). The formation of ONOO may be enhanced if SOD1 activity is lost, as levels of $O_2^{\cdot}$ then increase secondarily. ONOO can act as a nitrogen donor, nitrating tyrosine residues, possibly through an interaction with the active channel of the SOD1 molecule, which can catalyze nitration by accepting ONOO as a substrate, forming a nitronium ion with enhanced ability to nitrate tyrosines.[32] By relaxing the conformation of the SOD1 molecule, the SOD1 mutations may enhance this nitration process.[33] If the tyrosines are in critical cellular proteins, such as neurofilaments or tyrosine kinase receptors, their nitration may be injurious to the motor neuron. Data from high-performance liquid chromatography and immunochemical studies

$$\text{(1)}\quad \text{SOD1-Cu}^{2+}\text{-Zn}^{*} \longrightarrow \text{SOD1} + \text{Cu}^{2+} + \text{Zn}$$

$$\text{(2)}\quad \text{ONOO} + \text{H-tyr} \xrightarrow{\text{SOD1-Cu}^{2+}\text{-Zn}^{*}} \text{NO}_{2}\text{-tyr} + \text{OH}^{-}$$

$$\text{(3)}\quad \text{H}_2\text{O}_2 + \text{SOD1-Cu}^{1+}\text{-Zn}^{**} + \text{R} \longrightarrow \text{R-}(^{\cdot}\text{OH}) + \text{SOD1-Cu}^{2+}\text{-Zn}^{*} + \text{OH}^{-}$$

**Figure 14–2.** Possible reactions of mutant Cu/Zn SOD1. Mutant SOD1 may have a diminished affinity for copper and zinc (Reaction 1). The mutations may also enhance the reaction of SOD1 with ONOO− (Reaction 2), increasing the generation of nitronium anions and thereby accelerating transfer of nitrate groups to tyrosines. Some FALS-associated mutations increase the ability of SOD1 with reduced copper ($Cu^1$) to act as a peroxidase, reducing substrates such as $H_2O_2$ and forming hydroxy adducts of interacting substances (Reaction 3). * and ** indicate mutant SOD1 molecules with $Cu^{2+}$ and $Cu^{1+}$, respectively.

strongly suggests that levels of nitrotyrosine are augmented in ALS brains both in humans[34] and in mice.[35,36]

Another hypothesis is that the mutant SOD1 protein has an enhanced ability to accept $H_2O_2$ as a substrate, generating hydroxyl radicals. That wild-type SOD1 can thus act as a peroxidase was reported several years ago.[37] In recent months, it has been reported that mutant SOD1 has an enhanced peroxidation capacity.[38–40] Other hypotheses have been proposed. SOD1 is abundant, accounting for as much as 0.5% of intracellular proteins.[13] Possibly the accumulation of large quantities of unstable, mutant protein as insoluble aggregates is toxic, perhaps by taxing normal endogenous mechanisms for protein reutilization.

Although the precise neurotoxic biochemical properties of the mutant SOD1 protein are not well defined, it is apparent that the molecule can activate one or more cell death cascades. In a neural cell line of nigral origin, expression of mutant SOD1 is pro-apoptotic,[41] while the wild-type protein is clearly anti-apoptotic. Similar activation of apoptosis by mutant SOD1 protein has been documented in primary neurons in culture.[42,43,43a] Strikingly, in one model the pro-apoptotic mutant SOD1 protein, but not its wild-type counterpart, is prone to aggregation and precipitation from within the cytosol of motor neurons.[42]

It remains to be established how fully these studies in cell culture relate to ALS *in vivo.* It is striking that inactivation of the cell death gene caspase 1 (also known as interleukin-1 β converting enzyme [ICE]) produces a subtle prolongation of survival in ALS mice bearing the glycine 93 to alanine mutation.[44] Analogously, overexpression of the anti-apoptotic protein bcl-2 slows the onset of the disease in these mice.[45]

Unfortunately, only about 20% of ALS families have mutations in the gene for SOD1. Evidently there are other ALS genes yet to be identified. Intriguingly, it has also recently been reported that mutations in the gene encoding the heavy subunit of neurofilament (NF-H) are present infrequently in some individuals with apparently sporadic ALS[46]; in a large follow-up study, these mutations were not detected in either SALS or FALS.[47] The importance of the NF-H mutations as primary defects causing motor neuron disease has not been fully defined at this time.

### Dominantly Inherited, Juvenile Onset Amyotrophic Lateral Sclerosis

A single large family has been described with a slowly evolving disorder of both upper and lower motor neurons. Symptoms develop in middle to late childhood, and patients typically have long-term survival. Recent studies have established genetic linkage from a large pedigree with this disease to chromosome 9q34.[48,101]

### Recessively Inherited, Juvenile Onset Amyotrophic Lateral Sclerosis

An unusual type of motor neuron disease that begins in early childhood was described by Ben Hamida and associates.[49] In this disorder, there is degeneration of both upper and lower motor neurons with a very protracted time course, compatible with survival of several decades. This ''juvenile ALS'' arises in inbred families and thus appears to be recessively inherited. Most affected individuals have limb atrophy reminiscent of a severe motor neuropathy. This is concurrent with severe spasticity and, at times, a pronounced pseudobulbar disturbance of affect. Cognition and sensation are spared. In some families the disorder is genetically linked to chromosome 2q33; however, the identity of the defective gene is unknown.[50]

## DISORDERS OF THE LOWER MOTOR NEURON

### Spinal Muscular Atrophy

Spinal muscular atrophy (SMA) is inherited as an autosomal recessive trait leading to the progressive death of motor neurons in the brain stem and spinal cord. The hallmark of SMA is symmetrical weakness denervational atrophy. Type I SMA, or Werdnig-Hoffmann disease, begins before 6 months of age, possibly even prenatally. Mothers of SMA I babies sometimes describe diminished fetal movements in the final week or two before delivery. Babies with Werdnig-Hoffmann disease are feeble at sucking and crying and severely weak and floppy. They lack the ability to sit up and usually survive less than 2 years. This form of SMA affects as many as 1/20,000 babies; its carrier frequency is about 1/80.[51] Type II SMA is clinically evident before 18 months of age and is compatible with long-term survival. These patients can sit, but do not stand or walk. Type III SMA begins after age 18 months; these patients do walk. In late-onset SMA III (also designated Kugelberg-Welander disease), denervation affects proximal more than distal power, and involves legs more than the arms.

Pathologically, SMA disease is characterized by death of lower motor neurons. Early in the death process in SMA, the motor neurons appear swollen and chromatolytic.

The gene defect in most cases of SMA I, II, and III is genetically linked to chromosome 5.[52,53] This locus has two candidate genes: a novel protein of 294 amino acids designated "survival motor neuron" (SMN)[54] and a protein of 1232 amino acids labeled "neuronal apoptosis inhibitory protein" (NAIP). The chromosomal region encoding SMN and NAIP is complex, with a duplication such that there are at least two copies each of SMN and NAIP (telomeric or centromeric). Survival motor neuron has been localized to both the nucleus and cytoplasm in cells *in vitro*.[55] It complexes tightly with an SMN-interacting protein (SIP1). At least in frog oocytes, the SMN–SIP1 proteins associate with ribonucleoproteins (snRNP) in the cytoplasm, presumably playing a role in the formation of premRNA spliceosomes. This suggests that the fundamental defect in SMA may, in some manner, involve aberrant splicing and trafficking of mRNA species.[56,57]

The centromeric and telomeric copies of SMN are both expressed; both undergo alternate splicing in some tissues.[58] The telomeric copy of SMN is deleted in 98% of SMA patients; in many of the rest, it has undergone gene conversion such that it has the sequence of the centromeric copy of the protein.[59] At least one study has shown that the severity of SMA is determined in part by the levels of the SMN protein. More than 90% of the full-length SMN transcript is derived from the telomeric copy of SMN. Far less of the protein expressed from the centromeric copy is full length; instead, protein from the centromeric locus includes isoforms lacking exon 5 or 7. Thus, centromeric SMN cannot fully rescue the phenotype that arises from loss of the telomeric SMN. In this context, it is striking that in mice, which have only a single copy of SMN, genetic deletion of SMN is embryonically lethal.[60]

These considerations suggest a model for the severity of SMA.[61] In the model, the null SMN state is lethal; individuals with only centromeric SMN have some minimal capacity to compensate for the loss of telomeric SMN, developing SMA type I. Individuals with gene-converted SMN, composed of telomeric and centromeric SMN, are better compensated for loss of telomeric SMN and thus develop SMN types II and III. Individuals with normal telomeric SMN are normal. SMA may also be determined by levels of the NAIP protein.[62–64]

## Adult Onset Tay-Sach's Disease

Patients with $GM_2$-gangliosidosis may clinically resemble SMA patients.[65] These individuals have life-long motor incoordination accompanied by progressive proximal muscle weakness and other manifestations of denervation, such as cramps and fasciculations. Some individuals also show behavioral manifestations (e.g., shortened attention span and rare psychotic episodes[66]). Dysphagia, spasticity, and even positive Babinski responses are possible as the illness advances. Brain imaging may show cerebellar atrophy indicating that some cerebellar neurons, like spinal moles neurons, undergo neurodegenerition in this disease. The primary biochemical defect in Tay-Sach's disease is an accumulation of $GM_2$-ganglioside. This ganglioside is normally metabolized by *N*-acetyl-hexosaminidases A and B. These dimeric enzymes consist of an α-subunit and a β-subunit (hexosaminidase A) or two β-subunits (hexosaminidase B). Each dimer is complexed with a third protein, $GM_2$ activator, which modulates the activity of both enzymes.

### X-Linked Spinal Bulbar Muscular Atrophy

X-linked spinal bulbar muscular atrophy (XSBMA) is an insidiously progressive, male-specific, lower motor neuropathy.[67] Like SMA, XSBMA is a disease of lower motor neurons. In XSBMA, variable gynecomastia and testicular atrophy suggest androgen insensitivity. The molecular defect in XSBMA is an expansion of a coding CAG repeat in exon 1 of the androgen receptor gene.[68] This is predicted to produce an expanded polyglutamine tract within the receptor. In general, the longer the tract of repeated CAGs, the more severe the illness.[69,70] The mechanism of neurotoxicity of the CAGs is not known, although recent data suggests that the expanded polyglutamine tract may aggregate to form nuclear inclusions in these CAG-expansion diseases.[71]

## DISORDERS OF THE UPPER MOTOR NEURON

### Primary Lateral Sclerosis

Primary lateral sclerosis (PLS) arises sporadically in adults. Clinically it presents with stiffness and weakness of the limbs without amyotrophy or sensory changes. Electromyography and muscle biopsy do not show denervation. The course of PLS is variable; although long-term survival is documented, the course may be as aggressive as in ALS, with an approximately 3-year survival from onset to death. Early in the course of PLS, it may be difficult to exclude the possibility that the patient has multiple sclerosis or another type of demyelinating disease. Autopsy reveals loss of the large pyramidal cells in the precentral gyrus and degeneration of the corticospinal and corticobulbar projections.

### Hereditary Familial Spastic Paraplegia

Hereditary familial spastic paraplegia (HSP) is typically inherited as an autosomal dominant trait with a distinctive clinical picture marked by spastic weakness beginning in the distal legs. It is reviewed in detail in Chapter 11. The major neuropathological finding is corticospinal tract degeneration, which is more pronounced caudally.[72,73] Cases of HSP may be "pure" or "uncomplicated" or, less commonly, "complicated"; in the latter form of HSP, pathological findings are not confined to the corticospinal tracts. There may also be amyotrophy, mental retardation, optic atrophy, and sensory neuropathy (superbly reviewed by Harding[74]). These complex types of HSP underscore the difficulties in classifying some degenerative neurologic disorders. Fortunately, gene linkage analyses are now clarifying these clinical distinctions.

At least five loci for HSP are known (Table 14–1). In 1993, an early onset pedigree with spastic gait, relatively little weakness, and a very slow disease course was mapped to chromosome 14q.[75] Like the type I families described by Harding,[76] this family included individuals who were asymptomatic but clinically affected. Two clinically similar families were not linked to chromosome 14q. A second large family with uncomplicated HSP type I was linked to chromosome 15q.[77] The 15q family had more variability in age of onset and a more aggressive course than the 14q family.[78] Both early and late onset families map to a third HSP locus on chromosome 2p.[79,80] A recent summary estimated that uncomplicated HSP is distributed among these loci as follows: 2p, 45%; 14q, 6%; 15q, 3%; other, 45%.[81] Thus, it is abundantly clear that there is extensive genetic heterogeneity in dominantly inherited, uncomplicated HSP and that other HSP loci remain to be identified.

There has also been progress in genetically mapping recessively inherited, uncomplicated HSP. One locus has been identified on chromosome 8q.[82] X-linked recessive forms are also encountered. One arises from mutations in the gene encoding proteolipid protein; interestingly, other mutations within this gene cause the more fulminant Pelizaeus-Merzbacher disease.[83] Another type of complicated, infantile onset HSP is caused by mutations in the gene encoding the adhesion molecule L1CAM.[84]

## OTHER INHERITED MOTOR NEURON DISEASES

Several other inherited motor neuron diseases are recognized.[85] Although some are purely motor diseases, others, like HSP, are complex disorders with multisytem degenerations. These include such entities as *Fazio-Londe disease* (progressive juvenile bulbar palsy), a neuronopathy of bulbar motor nerves beginning before the third year[86,87]; the *arthrogryposes,* a complex set of disorders with contractures at birth from motor neuron cell loss (these are apparently sporadic but may be inherited as autosomal recessive,[88] autosomal dominant,[89,90] or X-linked[91] traits); and the *scapuloperoneal muscular atrophies,* which are characterized by focal distribution of neuropathic weakness in the shoulders muscles and in the peroneal groups. This disease also shows considerable diversity with dominantly inherited (midlife onset[92] and early onset[93,94] and possible X-linked[95]) forms.

## SUMMARY

The inherited motor neuron diseases are a diverse group of disorders characterized by degeneration or abnormal development of subsets of motor nerves. Foremost among these is familial amyotrophic lateral sclerosis, a dominantly inherited disease characterized by mid-life onset. Some cases arise from genetic defects in a gene that encodes the protein cytosolic superoxide dismutase. Although the mechanisms whereby the defects trigger motor neuron cell death are not fully defined, it is clear that protein aggregation and ultimate activation of cell death genes are involved in the pathogenesis of this disease. Another important, recessively inherited motor neuron disease is spinal muscular atrophy. This is caused by loss of a critical spliceosome factor known as the survival motor neuron protein. A third disorder, X-linked spinal bulbar muscular atrophy, arises because of an expanded exonic CAG-repeat in the gene for the androgen receptor. For many other inherited motor neuron diseases, such as the hereditary spastic paraplegias, the chromosomal location of the defective genes have been identified, although the precise gene defects are unknown. We hope these genetic insights will ultimately lead to improved therapeutic strategies for these disabling diseases.

## REFERENCES


1. Tandan R, Bradley WG: Amyotrophic lateral sclerosis: Part 1. Clinical features, pathology and ethical issues in management. Ann Neurol 18:271–280, 1985.
2. Tandan R, Bradley WG: Amyotrophic lateral sclerosis: Part 2. Etiopathogenesis. Ann Neurol 18:419–431, 1985.
3. Appel S, Smith R, Engelhardt J, Stefani E: Evidence of autoimmunity in amyotrophic lateral sclerosis (Review). J Neurol Sci 124 (suppl):14–19, 1994.
4. Leigh PN, Swash M: Cytoskeletal pathology in motor neuron diseases. In Rowland LP (ed): Amyotrophic Lateral Sclerosis and Other Motor Neuron Diseases, Vol 56. Raven Press, New York, 1991, pp3–23.
5. Griffin J, Clark A, Parhad I, Watson D, Hoffman P: The neuronal cytoskeleton in disorders of the motor neuron. Adv Neurol 56:103–113, 1991.
6. Leigh PN, Anderton BH, Dodson A, et al.: Ubiquitin deposits in anterior horn cells in motor neurone disease. Neurosci Lett 93:197–203, 1988.
7. Mulder D, Kurland L, Offord K, Beard C: Familial adult motor neuron disease: Amyotrophic lateral sclerosis. Neurology 36:511–517, 1986.
8. Hirano A, Kurland L, Sayre G: Familial amyotrophic lateral sclerosis. A subgroup characterized by posterior and spinocerebellar tract involvement and hyaline inclusions in the anterior horn cells. Arch Neurol 16:232–243, 1967.
9. Rosen DR, Siddique T, Patterson D, et al.: Mutations in Cu/Zn superoxide dismutase gene are associated with familial amyotrophic lateral sclerosis. Nature 362:59–62, 1993.
10. Sapp P, Rosen D, Hosler B, et al.: Identification of three novel mutations in the gene for Cu/Zn superoxide dismutase in patients with familial amyotrophic lateral sclerosis. Neuromusc Disord 5: 353–357, 1995.

11. Fridovich I: Superoxide dismutases. Adv Enzymol 58: 61–97, 1986.
12. Bowling AC, Schulz JB, Brown RHJ, Beal MF: Superoxide dismutase activity, oxidative damage and mitochondrial energy metabolism in familial and sporadic amyotrophic lateral sclerosis. J Neurochem 61: 2322–2325, 1993.
13. Bowling A, Barkowski E, McKenna-Yasek D, et al.: Superoxide dismutase concentration and activity in familial amyotrophic lateral sclerosis. J Neurochem 64: 2366–2369, 1995.
14. Deng H-X, Hentati A, Tainer JA, et al.: Amyotrophic lateral sclerosis and structural defects in Cu,Zn superoxide dismutase. Science 261: 1047–1051, 1993.
15. Robberecht W, Sapp P, Viaene MK, et al.: Cu/Zn superoxide dismutase activity in familial and sporadic amyotrophic lateral sclerosis. J Neurochem 62: 384–387, 1993.
16. Puymirat J, Cossette L, Gosselin F, Bouchard J-P: Red blood cell Cu/Zn superoxide dismutase activity in sporadic amyotrophic lateral sclerosis. J Neurol Sci 127: 121–123, 1994.
17. Pramatarova A, Goto J, Nanba E, et al.: A two base pair deletion in the SOD1 gene causes familial amyotrophic lateral sclerosis. Hum Mol Genet 3: 2061–2062, 1994.
18. Pramatarova A, Figlewicz D, Krizus A, et al.: Identification of new mutations in the CuZn superoxide dismutase gene of patients with familial amyotrophic lateral sclerosis. Hum Mol Genet 56: 592–596, 1995.
19. Borchelt DR, Lee MK, Slunt HS, et al.: Superoxide dismutase 1 with mutations linked to familial amyotrophic lateral sclerosis possesses significant activity. Proc Nat Acad Sci USA 91: 8292–8296, 1994.
20. Shaw P, Ince P, Falkous G, Mantle D: Oxidative damage to protein in sporadic motor neurone disease spinal cord. Ann Neurol 38: 691–695, 1995.
21. Ferrante R, Browne S, Shinobu L, et al.: Evidence of increased oxidative damage in both sporadic and familial amyotrophic lateral sclerosis. J Neurochem 69: 2064–2074, 1997.
22. Mitchell JD, Jackson MJ, Pentland B: Indices of free radical activity in the cerebrospinal fluid of motor neuron disease. J Neurol Neurosurg. Psychiatry 50: 919–912, 1987.
23. Rothstein JD, Bristol LA, Hosler BA, Brown RHJ, Kuncl RW: Chronic inhibition of superoxide dismutase produces apoptotic death of spinal neurons. Proc Nat Acad Sci USA 91: 4155–4159, 1994.
24. Troy CM, Shelanski M: Down-regulation of copper/zinc superoxide dismutase causes apoptotic death in PC12 neuronal cells. Proc Nat Acad Sci USA 91: 6384–6387, 1994.
25. Greenlund L, Deckwerth T, Johnson E: Superoxide dismutase delays neuronal apoptosis: A role for reactive oxygen species in programmed neuronal death. Neuron 14: 303–315, 1995.
26. Reaume A, Elliott J, Hoffman E, et al.: Motor neurons in Cu/Zn superoxide dismutase-deficient mice develop normally but exhibit enhanced cell death after axonal injury. Nat Genet 13: 43–47, 1996.
27. Ripps ME, Huntley GW, Hof PR, Morrison JH, Gordon JW: Transgenic mice expressing an altered murine superoxide dismutase gene provide an animal model of amyotrophic lateral sclerosis. Proc Nat Acad Sci USA 92: 689–693, 1995.
28. Gurney ME, Pu H, Chiu AY, et al.: Motor neuron degeneration in mice that express a human Cu,Zn superoxide dismutase mutation. Science 264: 1772–1775, 1994.
29. Wong P, Pardo C, Borchelt D, et al.: An adverse property of a familial ALS-linked SOD1 mutation causes motor neuron disease characterized by vacuolar degeneration of mitochondria. Neuron 14: 1105–1116, 1995.
30. Nishida C, Gralla E, Valentine J: Characterization of three yeast copper–zinc superoxide dismutase mutants analogous to those coded for in familial amyotrophic lateral sclerosis. Proc Natl Acad Sci USA 91: 9906–9910, 1994.
31. Carri M, Battistoni A, Polizio F, Desideri A, Rotillo G: Impaired copper binding by H46R mutant of human Cu,Zn superoxide dismutase, involved in amyotrophic lateral sclerosis. FEBS Lett 356: 314–316, 1994.
32. Ischiropoulos H, Zhu L, Chen J, et al.: Peroxynitrite-mediated tyrosine nitration catalyzed by superoxide dismutase. Arch Biochem Biophys 298: 431–437, 1992.
33. Beckman JS, Carson M, Smith CD, Kuppenol WH: ALS, SOD, and peroxynitrite. Nature 364: 584, 1993.
34. Beal M, Ferrante R, Browne S, et al.: Increased 3-nitrotyrosine in both sporadic and familial amyotrophic lateral sclerosis. Ann Neurol 42: 644–654 1997.
35. Ferrante R, Shinobu L, Schultz J, et al.: Increased 3-nitrotyrosine and oxidative damage in mice with human copper zinc superoxide dismutase mutations. Ann Neurol 42:326–334, 1997.
36. Bruijn L, Beal M, Becher M, et al.: Elevated free nitrotyrosine levels but not protein-bound nitrotyrosine or hydroxyl radicals, throughout amyotrophic lateral sclerosis (ALS)–like disease implicate tyrosine nitration as an aberrant *in vivo* property of one familial ALS-linked superoxide dismutase 1 mutant. Proc Natl Acad of Sci USA 94: 7606–7611, 1997.
37. Hodgson E, Fridovich I: The interaction of bovine erythrocyte superoxide dismutase with hydrogen peroxide: Inactivation of the enzyme. Biochemistry 14: 5294–5299, 1975.
38. Wiedau-Pazos M, Goto J, Rabizadeh S, et al.: Altered reactivity of superoxide dismutase in familial amyotrophic lateral sclerosis. Science 271: 515–518, 1996.
39. Yim M, Kang J, Yim H, et al.: A gain-of-function mutation of an amyotrophic lateral sclerosis–associated Cu,Zn-superoxide dismutase mutant: An enhancement of free radical formation due to a decrease in Km for hydrogen peroxide. Proc Natl Acad Sci USA 93: 5709–5714, 1996.
40. Yim H, Kang J, Chock P, Stadtman E, Yim M: A familial amyotrophic lateral sclerosis–associated A4V Cu,Zn superoxide dismutase mutant has a lower Km for hydrogen peroxide. Correlation between severity and the Km value. J Biol Chem 272: 8861–8863, 1997.
41. Rabizadeh S, Gralla E, Borchelt D, et al.: Mutations

associated with amyotrophic lateral sclerosis convert superoxide dismutase from an antiapoptotic gene to a proapoptotic gene: Studies in yeast and neural cells. Proc Natl Acad Sci USA 92:3024–3028, 1995.
42. Durham H, Roy J, Dong L, Figlewicz D: Aggregation of mutant Cu/Zn superoxide dismutase proteins in a culture model of ALS. J Neuropathol Exp Neurol 56:523–530, 1997.
43. Ghadge G, Lee J, Bindokas V, et al.: Mutant superoxide dismutase-1–linked familial amyotrophic lateral sclerosis: Molecular mechanisms of neuronal death and protection. J Neurosci 17:8756–8766, 1997.
43a. Pasinelli P, Borchelt DR, Houseweart MK, Cleveland DW, Brown RH, Jr. Caspase-1 is activated in neural cells and tissues with amyotrophic lateral sclerosis-associated mutations in copper-zinc superoxide dismutase. Proc Natl Acad Sci 95:15763–15768.
44. Friedlander R, RH Brown J, Gagliardini V, Wang J, Wang J: Inhibition of ICE slows ALS in mice. Nature 388:31, 1997.
45. Kostic V, Jackson-Lewis V, Bilbao FD, Dubois-Dauphin M, Przedborski S. Bcl-2: Prolonging life in a transgenic mouse model of familial amyotrophic lateral sclerosis. Science 277:559–562, 1997.
46. Figlewicz DA, Krizus A, Martinoli MG, et al.: Variants of the heavy neurofilament subunit are associated with the development of amyotrophic lateral sclerosis. Hum Mol Genet 3:1757–1761, 1994.
47. Vechio J, Bruijn L, Xu Z, Jr RB, Cleveland D: Sequence variants in human neurofilament proteins: Absence of linkage to familial ALS. Ann Neurol 40: 603–610, 1996.
48. Chance P: Linkage of autosomal recessive ALS of childhood onset to chromosome 9. Personal communication, 1996.
49. Ben Hamida M, Hentati F, Ben Hamida C: Hereditary motor system diseases (chronic juvenile amyotrophic lateral sclerosis). Conditions combining a bilateral pyramidal syndrome with limb and bulbar atrophy. Brain 113:347–363, 1990.
50. Hentati A, Bejaoui K, Pericak-Vance MA, et al.: Linkage of recessive familial amyotrophic lateral sclerosis to chromosome 2q33–35. Nat Genet 7: 425–428, 1994.
51. Pern JH, Carter CO: The genetic identity of acute infantile spinal muscular atrophy. Brain 96:463–470, 1973.
52. Brzustowicz L, Lehner T, Castilla L, et al.: Genetic mapping of chronic childhood-onset spinal muscular atrophy to chromosome 5q11.2–13.3. Nature 344:540–541, 1990.
53. Gilliam TC, Brzustowicz LM, Castilla LH. Genetic homogeneity between acute and chronic forms of spinal muscular atrophy. Nature 345:823–825, 1990.
54. Lefebvre S, Bürglen L, Reboullet S, et al.: Identification and characterization of a spinal muscular atrophy–determining gene. Cell 80:155–165, 1995.
55. Francis J, Sandrock A, Bhide P, Vonsattel J-P, Brown R: Heterogeneity of subcellular localization and electrophoretic mobility of survival motor neuron (SMN) protein in mammalian neural cells and tissues. Proc Natl Acad Sci USA 95:6492–6497, 1998.
56. Fischer U, Liu Q, Dreyfuss G: The SMN–SIP1 complex has an essential role in spliceosomal snRNP biogenesis. Cell 90:1023–1029, 1997.
57. Liu Q, Fischer U, Wang F, Dreyfuss G: The spinal muscular atrophy disease gene product, SMN, and its associated protein SIP-1 are in a complex with spliceosomal snRNP proteins. Cell 90:1013–1021, 1997.
58. Gennarelli M, Lucarelli M, Capon F, et al.: Survival motor neuron gene transcript analysis in muscles from spinal muscular atrophy patients. Biochem Biophys Res Commun 213:342–348, 1995.
59. DiDonato C, Ingraham S, Mendell J, et al.: Deletion and conversion in spinal muscular atrophy patients: Is there a relationship to severity? Ann Neurol 41:230–237, 1997.
60. Shrank B, Gotz R, Gunnerson J, et al.: Inactivation of the survival motor neuron gene, a candidate gene for human spinal muscular atrophy, leads to massive cell death in early mouse embyos. Proc Natl Acad Sci USA 94:9920–9925, 1997.
61. Burghes A: When is a deletion not a deletion? When it is converted. Am J Hum Genet 61:9–15, 1997.
62. Lefebvre W, Burlet P, Liu Q, et al.: Correlation between severity and SMN protein level in spinal muscular atrophy. Nat Genet 16:265–269, 1997.
63. Somerville M, Hunter A, Aubry H, et al.: Clinical application of the molecular diagnosis of spinal muscular atrophy: Deletions of neuronal apoptosis inhibitor protein and survival motor neuron genes. Am J Med Genet 69:159–165, 1997.
64. Morrison K: Advances in SMA research: Review of gene deletions. Neuromusc Disord 6:397–408, 1996.
65. Jellinger K, Anzil AP, Seeman D, Bernheimer H: Adult GM2 gangliosidosis masquerading as a slowly progressive muscular atrophy: Motor neuron disease phenotype. Clini Neuropathol 1:31–44, 1982.
66. Streifler H, Golomb M, Gadoth N: Psychiatric features of adult GM2 gangliosidosis. Br J Psychiatry 155:410–413, 1989.
67. Kennedy WB, Alter M, Sung JG: Report of an X-linked form of spinal muscular atrophy. Neurology 18:671–680, 1968.
68. LaSpada AR, Wilson EM, Lubahn DB, Harding AE, Fischbeck KH: Androgen receptor gene mutations in X-linked spinal and bulbar muscular atrophy. Nature 352:77–79, 1991.
69. LaSpada AR, Roling DB, Harding AE, et al.: Meiotic instability and genotype–phenotype correlation of the trinucleotide repeat in X-linked spinal and bulbar muscular atrophy. Nat Genet 2:301–304, 1992.
70. Doyu M, Sobue G, Mukai, E, et al.: Severity of X-linked recessive bulbospinal neuronopathy correlates with size of the tandem CAG repeat in androgen receptor gene. Ann Neurol 32:707–710, 1992.
71. Davies S, Turmaine M, Cozens B, et al.: Formation of neuronal intranuclear inclusions underlies the neurological dysfunction in mice transgenic for the HD mutation. Cell 90:537–548, 1997.
72. Schwartz GA, Liu CN. Hereditary (familial) spas-

tic paraplegia: Further clinical and pathological observations. Arch Neurol Psychiatry 75:144–162, 1956.
73. Behan WMH, Maia M: Strumpell's familial spastic paraplegia: Genetics and neuropathology. J Neurol Neurosurg Psychiatry 37:8–20, 1974.
74. Harding AE: Complicated Forms of Hereditary Spastic Paraplegia: The Hereditary Ataxias and Related Disorders. Churchill Livingstone, London, 1984, pp191–213.
75. Hazan J, Lamy C, Melki J, et al.: Autosomal dominant familial spastic paraplegia is genetically heterogeneous and one locus maps to chromosome 14q. Nat Genet 5:163–167, 1993.
76. Harding AE: Hereditary "pure" spastic paraplegia: A clinical and genetic study of 22 families. J Neurol Neurosurg Psychiatry 44:871–883, 1981.
77. Fink JK, Wu CT, Jones SM, et al.: Autosomal dominant familial spastic paraplegia: Tight linkage to chromosome 15q. Am J Hum Genet 56:188–192, 1995.
78. Fink JK, Sharp GB, Lange BM, et al.: Autosomal dominant, familial spastic paraplegia, type I: Clinical and genetic analysis of a large North American family. Neurology 45:325–331, 1995.
79. Hazan J, Fontaine B, Bruyn R, et al.: Linkage to a new locus for autosomal dominant familial spastic paraplegia to chromosome 2p. Hum Mol Genet 3: 1569–1573, 1994.
80. Hentati A, Pericak-Vance M, Lennon F, et al.: Linkage of a locus for autosomal dominant familial spastic paraplegia to chromosome 2p markers. Hum Mol Genet 3:1867–1871, 1994.
81. Fink J, Heiman-Patterson T, Bird T, et al.: Hereditary spastic paraplegia: Advances in genetic research. Neurology 46:1507–1514, 1996.
82. Hentati A, Pericak-Vance MA, Hung WY, et al.: Linkage of "pure" autosomal recessive familial spastic paraplegia to chromosome 8 markers and evidence of genetic locus heterogeneity. Hum Mol Genet 3:1263–1267, 1994.
83. Saugier-Veber P, Munnich A, Bonneau D, et al.: X-linked spastic paraplegia and Pelizaeus-Merzbacher disease are allelic disorders at the proteolipid protein locus. Nat Genet 6:257–262, 1994.
84. Jouet M, Rosenthal A, Armstrong G, et al.: X-linked spastic paraplegia (SPG1), MASA syndrome, and X-linked hydrocephalus result from mutations in the L1 gene. Nat Genet 7:402–407, 1994.
85. deJong J: The World Federation of Neurology classification of spinal muscular atrophies and other disorders of motor neurons. In Vinken P, Bruyn G, Klawans H (eds): Diseases of the Motor System, Handbook of Clinical Neurology, Vol 59. Elsevier, New York, 1991, pp1–12.
86. Gomez M: Progressive bulbar paralysis of childhood. In deJong J (ed): Diseases of the Motor System, Handbook of Neurology, Vol 59. Elsevier, New York, 1991, pp121–131.
87. McShane M, Boyd S, Harding B, Brett E, Wilson J: Progressive bulbar paralysis of childhood: A reappraisal of Fazio-Londe disease. Brain 115:1889–1900, 1992.
88. Vuopala K, Ignatius J, Herva R: Lethal arthrogryposis with anterior horn cell disease. Hum Pathol 26:12–19, 1995.
89. Frins C, Deutekom JV, Frants R, Jennekens F: Dominant congenital benign spinal muscular atrophy. Muscle Nerve 17: 192–197, 1994.
90. Bamshad M, Watkins W, Zenger R, et al.: A gene for distal arthrogryposis type I maps to the pericentromeric region of chromosome 9. Am J Hum Genet 55: 1153–1158, 1994.
91. Osawa M, Shishikura K: Werdnig-Hoffmann disease and variants. In deJong J (ed): Diseases of the Motor Neuron, Handbook of Clinical Neurology, Vol 59. Elsevier, New York, 1991, pp.51–80.
92. Kaeser H: Scapuloperoneal muscular atrophy. Brain 88: 407–418, 1965.
93. DeLong R, Siddique T: A large New England kindred with autosomal dominant neurogenic scapuloperoneal amytrophy with unique features. Arch Neurol 49: 905–908, 1992.
94. BenAyed G, Samoud A, Dridi MB: Amyotrophie scapulo-peroniere d'origine type Kaeser-Stark. Etude d'une observation familiale. Arch Franc Pediatrie 50: 135–137, 1993.
95. Skre H, Mellgren S, Bergsholm P, Slagsvold J: Unusual type of neural muscular atrophy with a possible X-chromosomal inheritance pattern. Acta Neurol Scand 58: 249–260, 1978.
96. Takeda K, Nakai H, Hagiwara H, et al.: Fine assignment of beta-hexosaminidase A alpha subunit on 15q23–24 by high resolution *in situ* hybridization. Tohoku J Exp Med 160: 203–211, 1990.
97. Burg J, Conzelmann E, Sandhoff K, Solomon E, Swallow D: Mapping of the gene coding for the human GM2-activator protein to chromosome 5. Ann Hum Genet 49: 41–45, 1985.
98. Kobayashi H, Baumbach L, Matise T, et al.: A gene for a severe, lethal form of X-linked arthrogryposis (X-linked infantile spinal muscular atrophy) maps to human chromosome Xp11.3–q11.2. Hum Mol Genet 4: 1213–1216, 1995.
99. Hall J, Reed S, Scott C, et al.: Three distinct types of X-linked arthrogryposis seen in 6 families. Clin Genet 21: 81–97, 1982.
100. Constantinidis J: A familial syndrome: A combination of Pick's disease and amyotrophic lateral sclerosis. Encephale 13: 285–293, 1987.
101. Chance P, Rabin BA, Ryan SG, et al.: Linkage of the gene for an autosomal dominant form of juvenile amyotrophic lateral sclerosis to chromosome 9q34. Am J Hum Genet 62: 633–640, 1998.

Chapter 15

# MITOCHONDRIAL DNA AND THE GENETICS OF MITOCHONDRIAL DISEASE

Ricardo Fadic, MD
Donald R. Johns, MD



Mitochondria are the intracellular organelles that produce most of a cell's energy via the production of adenosine triphosphate (ATP). The respiratory chain, located in the inner mitochondrial membrane, is a series of multisubunit protein complexes that capture energy from the transfer of electrons and utilize it to produce ATP. Energy failure can potentially affect any organ system, and this is reflected in the heterogeneity of mitochondrial disorders. The respiratory chain enzymes are genetically unique as they are encoded by two genomes, the nuclear and the mitochondrial. Heritable errors leading to mitochondrial dysfunction can arise from either one, and both mendelian and maternal modes of inheritance are possible for these disorders. The discovery in 1988 of large deletions of mitochondrial DNA (mtDNA) in Kearns-Sayre syndrome[1,2] and a missense mutation at nucleotide 11,778 of mtDNA in Leber's hereditary optic neuropathy[3] initiated our understanding of the correlation between clinical syndromes and mtDNA molecular biology. The number of known pathogenic mtDNA mutations has increased dramatically in the last 11 years. This chapter examines recent advances in mitochondrial genetics, with particular focus on mitochondrial disorders due to defects in oxidative phosphorylation. Mitochondrial disorders due to defects in intermediary metabolism are covered in recent comprehensive reviews.[4–6]

## MITOCHONDRIAL DNA

Mitochondrial DNA is a closed, circular, double-stranded molecule of 16,569 nucleotides that contains only 37 genes (Fig. 15–1). The guanosine-rich heavy strand codes for two ribosomal RNAs (12s and 16s), 14 transfer RNAs, and 12 polypeptides. The cytosine-rich light strand codes for one

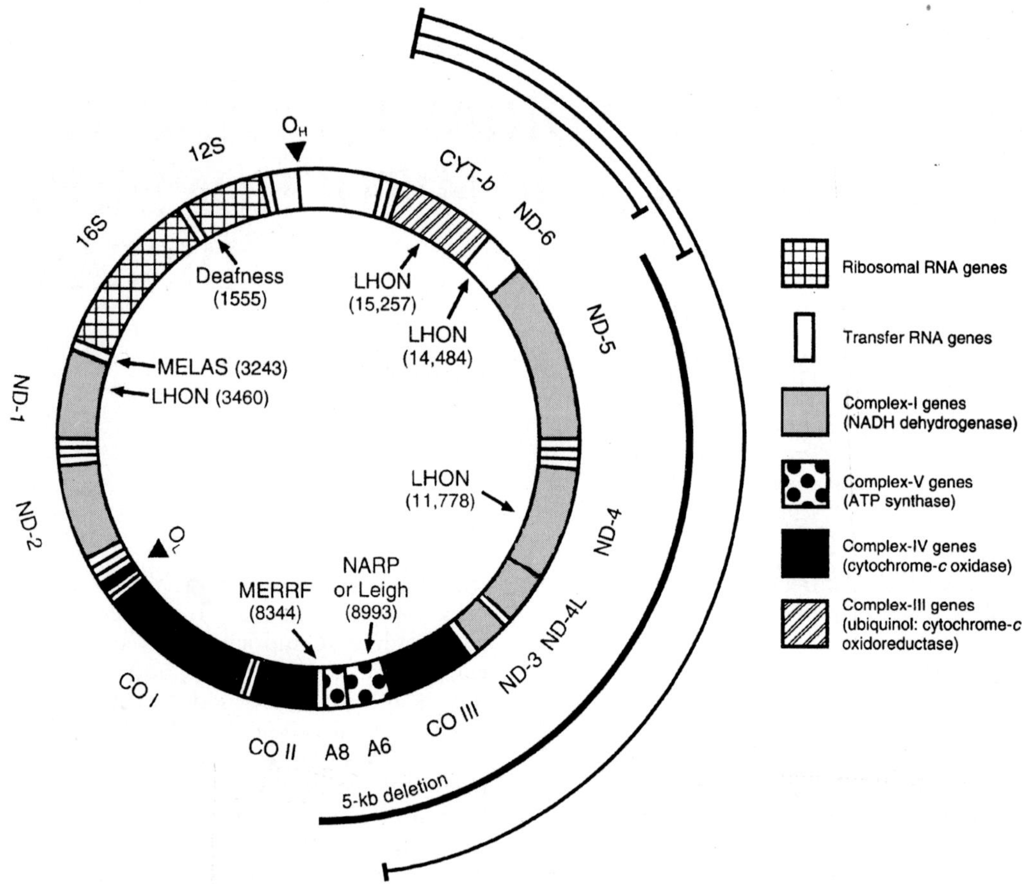


**Figure 15–1.** Schematic diagram of the human mitochondrial DNA molecule. Examples of point mutations with their associated clinical phenotype are indicated inside the circle. The position of the most common single deletion and multiple deletions are represented by arcs outside the circle.

polypeptide (ND6 subunit of complex I) and 8 transfer RNAs. Of the 13 polypeptides coded in mtDNA, 7 are subunits of complex I, one subunit of complex III, 3 subunits of complex IV, and 2 subunits of complex V. All four subunits of complex II (succinate-ubiquinone oxidoreductase) are encoded in the nuclear DNA. The mitochondrion has independent replication, transcription, and translation systems, which have both prokaryotic and eukaryotic features.[7] There are two origins of replication, one for each strand. The heavy strand origin is located in the displacement loop (D-loop), which is the major mtDNA control region. Heavy strand synthesis extends clockwise around the mtDNA. After traversing two-thirds of the genome, the light strand origin of replication is exposed, and its replication proceeds back along the free parental heavy strand in a counterclockwise fashion.[7] Interestingly, most mtDNA deletions occur in the segment limited by the replication origins.

Mitochondrial DNA transcription starts from two promoters, one for each strand, located in the displacement loop. Both transcripts include the entire genome, and they are polycystronic, that is, they contain multiple messenger RNAs (mRNAs) resembling prokaryotic transcription. As the transfer RNAs (tRNAs) are read, they fold into their three-dimensional structures and are excised as free tRNAs, thereby also releasing the intervening mRNAs and rRNAs.[7] These mRNAs are then polyadenylated and translated on mitochondrial ribosomes.

The transcription of the heavy strand, which contains the rRNAs, occurs in two versions: the full-length polycystronic and the shorter transcript extending from the heavy strand promoter to the end of the 16s rRNA gene. The shorter transcript is produced at a higher rate than the full-length transcript, maintaining the stoichiometry between the mRNAs and rRNAs. The transcription of the shorter segment is terminated at a site within the tRNA$^{Leu}$ gene by a specific terminator protein.[8] Interestingly, the tRNA$^{Leu}$ gene is a hot spot for mtDNA mutations for unknown reasons. Like bacterial protein synthesis, mitochondrial protein synthesis is initiated with formylmethionine and is sensitive to the bacterial ribosome inhibitor chloramphenicol.[7] Mitochondrial DNA has a unique genetic code, with AUA read as methionine instead of isoleucine, UGA as tryptophan instead of "stop," and both AGA and AGG as "stop" instead of arginine.[9] Therefore, mtDNA cannot be translated in the cytoplasmic compartment, and nuclear DNA cannot be translated within the mitochondria.

## MITOCHONDRIAL DNA GENETICS

Genetic diseases arising from mutations in the mtDNA are influenced in their manifestation by several distinctive features of mtDNA: maternal inheritance, polyplasmy, heteroplasmy, mitotic segregation, and threshold effect.

### Maternal Inheritance

Mitochondrial DNA is almost exclusively maternally inherited in humans; however, spermatozoa do contain a few mitochondria, and there is evidence that they can be inherited at an insignificant level.[10,11] Mitochondrial DNA does not recombine and has a poorly developed repair systems so that mutations accumulate sequentially along maternal lines.[12,13] Mothers can transmit an error to both sons and daughters, but only daughters will pass the mutation to their descendants. Due to the variability of the phenotypic manifestation associated with mtDNA mutations, analysis of large pedigrees is necessary to prove maternal transmission.

### Polyplasmy

Every cell contains multiple mitochondria, and each mitochondrion contains several mtDNAs. The exceptions are unfertilized eggs[14] and platelets,[15] which contain on average one mtDNA copy per mitochondrion. At mitosis, mitochondria distribute at random between daughter cells. Therefore, population genetics represent a better approximation to mitochondrial genetics than mendelian.

### Heteroplasmy

In normal cells, all mtDNA molecules are identical, a condition known as *homoplasmy*. When a mutation arises in mtDNA, an intracellular mixture of mutant and wild-type molecules known as *heteroplasmy* is created. In general, nondeleterious polymorphisms of mtDNA are homoplasmic. In contrast, all deletions and most of the pathogenic point mutations, especially in tRNAs, are heteroplasmic. Over many cell generations, heteroplasmic mtDNA genotypes drift toward either pure mutant or normal mtDNA populations.[16,17]

### Mitotic Segregation

As heteroplasmic cells undergo mitotic or meiotic division, the proportions of mutant and normal mtDNA allocated to daughter cells shift. This phenomenon can partially explain the different phenotypic expressions of an mtDNA mutation between different tissues and through time. Patients with a single common deletion (see later) may help to illustrate this concept. For example, children with Pearson's syndrome exhibiting sideroblastic anemia and exocrine pancreatic failure who survive into the second decade develop Kearns-Sayre syndrome.[18,19] The improvement of the anemia is likely due to the selection of blood cells without the deletion during cell division. The opposite occurs in muscle, a postmitotic tissue, where it has been shown that the proportion of deleted mtDNA increases in sequential muscle biopsies.[18] Mitotic segregation also explains the markedly different levels of mutated mtDNA in various members of the same family[20], and among different tissues within an individual.[21]

### Threshold Effect

The onset and severity of clinical manifestations depend on a delicate balance between the energy supply (determined in part by the proportion of mutant and normal mtDNA) and oxidative demands of different organ systems. *In vitro* studies show that a certain level of mutant mtDNA must be surpassed before a cell expresses an oxidative phosphorylation defect.[22] Organs more dependent on oxidative metabolism, such as the brain, retina, heart, and skeletal muscle, are frequently more affected.

## MITOCHONDRIAL ENCEPHALOMYOPATHIES

Mitochondrial disorders involve virtually all levels of the central and peripheral nervous system. These neurologic manifestations are collectively referred to as *mitochondrial encephalomyopathies* to indicate the breadth of nervous system involvement. The term *mitochondrial cytopathies* has been employed by some authors to indicate broader clinical manifestations beyond the nervous system, including somatic organ manifestations.

### Pathophysiology

The pathogenesis of mitochondrial diseases involves a progressive decline in mitochondrial ATP-generating capacity, leading to energetic failure and eventual cell death in affected tissues. A human cell line depleted of mtDNA by exposure to ethidium bromide (which inhibits mtDNA replication) was created by King and Attardi.[23] With this cell line it has been possible to produce mitochondria with known proportions of mutant and wild-type mtDNA. These constructs have defective mitochondrial protein synthesis, impairment of oxidative phosphorylation, or both.[24–26]

The enzymes of the respiratory chain and ATP synthase are assembled in the lipid bilayer of the inner mitochondrial membrane. Electrons are transmitted successively through the different enzymatic complexes to molecular oxygen to form water. The energy generated is used to pump protons across the mitochondrial inner membrane. Dissipation of the electrochemical gradient by transport back through the ATP synthase–proton channel releases energy used to condense ADP and inorganic phosphate to make ATP. Most of the oxygen consumed by the mitochondrion is converted to water. About 1%–4% of the oxygen molecules pick up electrons directly from reduced Coenzyme Q (CoQ) and flavin dehydrogenases to generate superoxide anion.[27,28] Superoxide anion is converted to $H_2O_2$ by superoxide dismutase and the highly reactive hydroxyl anion in the presence of transition metals. Inhibition of mitochondrial electron transport increases the electronegativity of the electron transport chain and accentuates the production of reactive oxygen species.[7,29] Mitochondrial DNA is particularly susceptible to the mutagenic effects of free radicals due to its proximity to the respiratory chain, few noncoding sequences,[9] lack of protective histones,[30] and limited DNA repair mechanisms.[12,13,31] The accumulation of mtDNA mutations might result in decreased activity of the oxidative phosphorylation enzymatic complexes that contain mtDNA-encoded subunits. This produces a self-perpetuating and amplifying cycle of respiratory chain dysfunction and free radical production. Other mechanisms of damage are possible, as mtDNA is also particularly susceptible to the effect of genotoxins.[32,33] Mitochondrial DNA has a mutation rate that is at least ten times greater than that of the nuclear genome.[7]

Aging in humans is associated with an increase in the number of cytochrome *c* oxidase–deficient fibers in skeletal muscle[34] and a decline in both the respiratory rate and oxidative phosphorylation enzyme activities.[35] Evidence for cumulative mtDNA oxidative damage with aging comes from the observed increased frequency of deletions,[36,37] point mutations,[38] and oxidized forms of mtDNA.[39,40]

There is an increased proportion of mtDNA deletions in human ischemic hearts, postulated to be secondary to increased oxygen radical production.[41] Quantification of the deletions that accumulate in various organs with age show that they represent a minimal amount compared with the total mtDNA.[42,43] The low level of individual mutations is unlikely to produce the respiratory defects observed in those tissues. It is possible that several different mutations accumulate simultaneously and explain the functional defect. Doxorubicin induces free radical formation, and in the animal model of doxorubicin-induced cardiotoxicity a deletion of mtDNA has been detected. The incidence of the deletion increases with the duration and dosage of doxorubicin; however, the administration of CoQ prevents the mtDNA damage.[44]

## Muscle Pathology

Mitochondrial DNA mutations involving the respiratory chain are typically but not invariably associated with mitochondrial proliferation in skeletal muscle. The morphological hallmark of these diseases is the ragged red muscle fibers[45], that contain large collections of mitochondria immediately beneath the sarcolemma and between the myofibers. They appear as red deposits with the modified Gomori trichrome stain and generally react strongly with succinate dehydrogenase, which is exclusively an intramitochondrial enzyme ("ragged blue fibers"). Collections of lipids and glycogen are also seen under the sarcolemma and between the myofibers.

Ragged red fibers are not specific for mitochondrial diseases as they can also be seen in acid maltase deficiency, as a nonspecific isolated finding in various myopathies, and in normal muscle.[46] In normal muscle their frequency increases with age and reaches a maximum of about 0.4% by the eighth decade.[34] In mitochondrial myopathies, the frequency of ragged red fibers varies between 1% anf 30% of all fibers.[46]

The mitochondria accumulating in ragged red fibers are frequently morphologically abnormal and biochemically defective.[46] The trigger for ragged red fiber formation is not known. In general, ragged red fibers are present in patients with defects in mitochondrial protein synthesis (mutations in tRNA genes and mtDNA deletions) but not in patients with missense mutation in the protein-coding genes[47] such as Leber's hereditary optic neuropathy (see later). As oxidative phosphorylation is affected in both types of disorders, it has been postulated that the signal for mitochondrial proliferation may be impaired protein synthesis.[48] Decreased or absent cytochrome *c* oxidase staining appears to be a more sensitive histochemical indicator of mitochondrial dysfunction and may be the only detectable pathologic abnormality.[5]

## Clinical Phenotypes

Mitochondrial dysfunction can affect virtually all organ systems, individually or in different combinations (Fig. 15–2). We discuss briefly the clinical features of the most common mitochondrial encephalomyopathy syndromes and their molecular genetic bases. The diversity of genetic errors responsible for these disorders reflects the dual genetic control (nuclear and mtDNA-encoded subunits of oxidation phosphorylation) and the complexity of the intergenomic communication between the nuclear and mitochondrial genomes.

### DEFECTS OF MITOCHONDRIAL DNA

A wide array of mtDNA mutations have now been demonstrated in patients with a variety of clinical phenotypes. Large-scale single deletions of mtDNA were the first type of mutation linked to human disease, but duplications and multiple mtDNA deletions have also been discovered. Point mutations

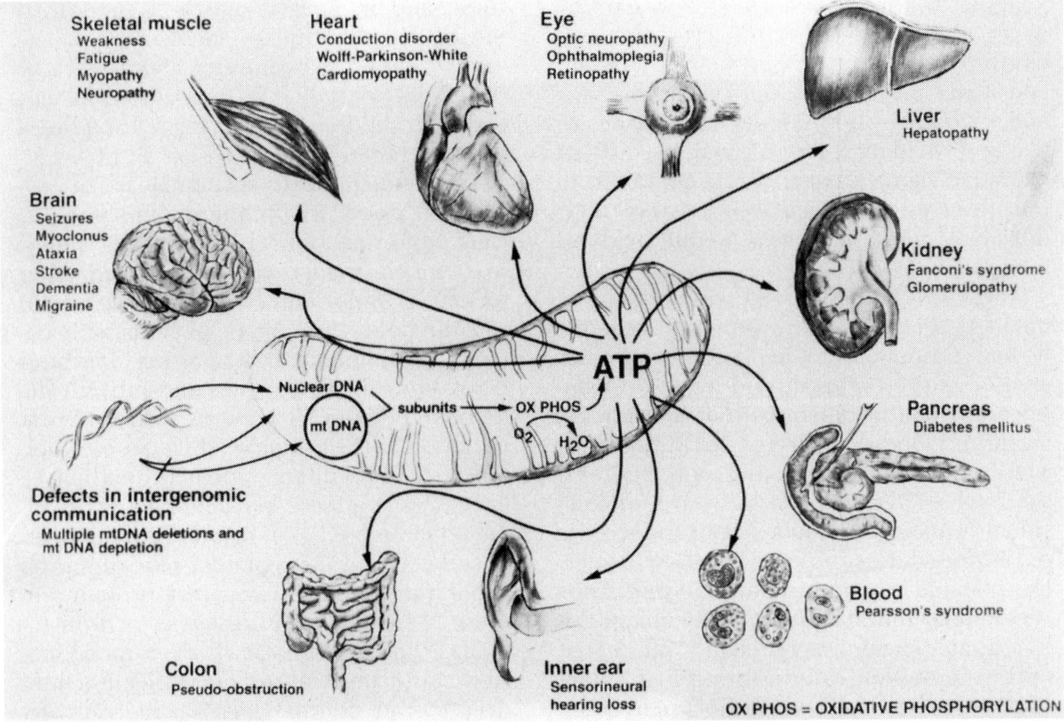


**Figure 15–2.** Pathogenesis of multisystemic involvement in mitochondrial dysfunction. Defects in the mtDNA, nuclear DNA, or the intergenomic communication between them disrupt the mitochondrial energy production, affecting multiple organ systems.

have been demonstrated in each of the three major types of mtDNA-encoded genes: protein-coding genes, transfer RNA genes, and ribosomal RNA genes. We discuss each of these types of mtDNA mutations and the phenotypes associated with them.

## POINT MUTATIONS IN PROTEIN-CODING GENES

Leber's hereditary optic neuropathy (LHON) is a maternally inherited form of severe, subacute, painless loss of central vision, predominantly affecting young men.[49,50] The acute phase of LHON is associated with swelling of the optic disc and adjacent nerve fiber layer. Visual field loss initially consists of an enlarged blind spot progressing to involve central vision as a large centrocecal scotoma. Symptoms generally start in one eye followed by the other within weeks or months; however, they may remain unilateral for more than 10 years.[51] Although most patients have only optic nerve involvement, associated features seen in rare pedigrees include dystonia, ataxia, athetosis, spasticity, peripheral neuropathy, and cardiac conduction abnormalities. There are no major differences in the clinical presentations of men and women other than a later onset in women in the same pedigree[52] and LHON's association with a multiple sclerosis–like illness in women from families with the 11,778 mtDNA mutation.[53]

LHON was the first mitochondrial disease to be defined at the molecular level, when a point mutation at position 11,778 of mtDNA that changes a highly conserved arginine to a histidine in the ND4 subunit of complex I was discovered.[3] This mutation generates a restriction site loss for *Sfa*NI 3 and a site gain for *Mae*III.[54] The mutation is homoplasmic in most families and heteroplasmic in others.[55] LHON has been associated with at least 10 other point mutations in eight genes that encode subunits of complexes I, III, and IV.[55] Four mutations at nucleotide positions 11,778, 3460, 15,257, and 14,484 may have primary pathogenic importance.[55] The others seem to act only in concert with additional mutations.[56]

Although clearly, associated with LHON, mtDNA mutations are not the sole determinants of the phenotype. In particular, they do not explain the excess of affected males. There is no convincing evidence of an X-linked modifying nuclear gene to explain this discrepancy.[55,57,58] Exposure to alcohol and tobacco may be important epigenetic factors.[59,60] The variety of primary mtDNA mutations in LHON has clinical significance, as the different mutations are associated with different prognoses for visual recovery.

Neurogenic weakness, ataxia, and retinitis pigmentosa (NARP) syndrome and maternally inherited Leigh's syndrome (MILS): are closely related. NARP is maternally inherited and characterized as a multisystem disorder involving developmental delay, dementia, retinitis pigmentosa, ataxia, seizures, sensory neuropathy, and proximal weakness. It is associated with two mutations at base pair 8993 in the ATPase 6 gene (complex V subunit): a T to G transversion,[16] and a T to C transition.[61] The mutations are always heteroplasmic, and there is a correlation between the proportion of mutated mtDNA and the severity of the clinical manifestation, as shown by different individuals in the same family.[62,63] Moreover, when the proportion of the mutation is high (>90%), it produces a fatal infantile encephalopathy with the neuropathologic and neuroradiologic features of Leigh's syndrome.[64–66] Leigh's syndrome is also inherited as a mendelian trait. A retrospective analysis of 50 Leigh's patients without cytochrome *c* oxidase or pyruvate dehydrogenase deficiency showed that 12 had the NARP mutation.[67] Patients with NARP and MILS may coexist in the same pedigree, representing different degrees of severity of the same disease.

## POINT MUTATION IN TRANSFER AND RIBOSOMAL RNA GENES

Mutations in the structural (tRNA and rRNA) mtDNA-encoded genes are very important in mitochondrial disease and differ in many ways from mutations in protein-coding genes. Transfer RNA mutations generally occur in diseases with severe, multisystemic manifestations and are invariably heteroplasmic. Given the relatively small proportion of the mitochondrial genome occupied by the 22 tRNAs, these genes harbor a disproportionate number of pathogenetic mutations. The only well-documented rRNA mutation is heteroplasmic and is associated with the phenotype of spontaneous and aminoglycoside-induced deafness.

The hallmarks of mitochondrial encephalomyopathy, lactic acidosis, and stroke-like episodes (MELAS) syndrome are recurrent focal neurologic deficits that resemble strokes.[68] Patients with MELAS syndrome usually have a normal early development, followed by focal or generalized seizures, growth retardation, dementia, recurrent headaches and vomiting, and the stroke-like episodes, which are frequently preceded by seizures. The cerebral lesions have a definite posterior predominance and thus tend to produce cortical blindness or hemianopia rather than hemiparesis. Strokes may be followed by a complete recovery, but residual symptoms or a progressive encephalopathy usually occur and have been increasingly recognized. Many patients with MELAS present before age 15 years, but onset later in life also occurs. Most patients harbor a point mutation at nucleotide position (np) 3243 in the $tRNA^{Leu(UUR)}$ gene (Fig. 15–3),[69,70] and a minority have a mutation at np 3771 in the same gene.[71] There is a correlation between the proportion of mutated mtDNA and the severity of symptoms in families with the np 3243 mutation.[72,73] Other mutations in the same gene at np 3251,[74] 3252,[75] 3256,[47] and 3291[76] require further cases to determine their significance. One patient with the MELAS phenotype had a heteroplasmic missense mutation at np 9957 in the Cytochrome *c* oxidase III gene.[77] The muscle biopsy from this patient was unusual, as there were few ragged red fibers, a feature typical of mtDNA peptide-coding genes.[77] The 3243 mutation is the most pleiotropic of all pathogenetic mtDNA mutations and is associated with a

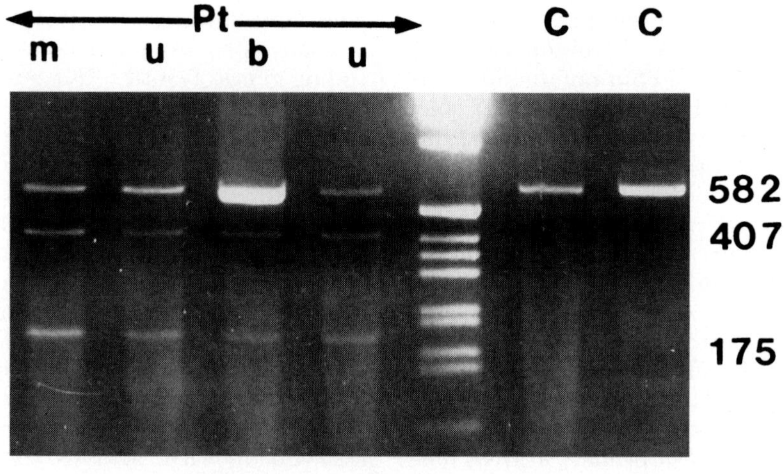


**Figure 15–3.** Molecular diagnosis of the MELAS mutation. The G to A transition at the mtDNA np 3243 creates a restriction site for the enzyme *Apa*I. The image shows a DNA electrophoresis of PCR products in an agarose gel stained with ethidium bromide. In the controls, the enzyme does not cut the 582 bp PCR product. In the MELAS patient, two new bands of 407 and 175 bp are created. Notice the different proportions between wild-type and mutated mtDNA in the patient's tissues (muscle, urine, and blood).

broad collection of clinical syndromes. These include chronic progressive external ophthalmophlegia,[78] myopathy with exercise intolerance,[79] cardiomyopathy,[80] and diabetes and deafness.[81,82] The tRNA$^{Leu(UUR)}$ gene appears to be a "hot spot" for pathogenetic mutations.[47]

Myoclonic epilepsy and ragged red fibers (MERRF) is characterized by myoclonus, cerebellar ataxia, and seizures. Associated features include myopathy, deafness, dementia, vascular headache, peripheral neuropathy, cervical lipomas, and pyramidal signs.[83] Myoclonus is often the initial symptom, and it may be induced by noise, action, or photic stimulation. A variety of seizure types occur in MERRF patients, including focal seizures, atypical absence, drop attacks, and photosensitive tonic-clonic seizures.[84,85] There is marked variability in the clinical course and prognosis. Some patients have onset of symptoms in early childhood with a severe course leading to death during the second decade, whereas other family members are asymptomatic or have a milder, later onset. The mutation most commonly associated with MERRF is an A to G transition at np 8344 in the tRNA$^{Lys}$ gene.[86,87] A second mutation in the same gene at np 8356 has been described in a few pedigrees.[88,89] There is some correlation between the proportion of mutated mtDNA at the np 8344 and the severity of the clinical manifestations.[85,90] Other clinical phenotypes associated with the np 8344 mutation include Leigh's syndrome,[79,91–93] spinocerebellar degeneration,[93] and Ekbom's syndrome.[94] The two mtDNA point mutations at np 8344 and 8356 in the tRNA$^{Lys}$ gene associated with MERRF are readily detectable in blood.

Maternally inherited cardiomyopathy, alone or as a predominant component of multisystemic disorders, has been increasingly associated with mtDNA mutations, primarily point mutation affecting tRNA genes. Two of those tRNAs appear to be hot spots for mutations associated with cardiomyopathy: tRNA$^{Ile}$ with mutations at np 4269,[95] 4300,[96] 4317,[97] and 4320[98] and tRNA$^{Leu(UUR)}$ with mutations at np 3243,[99] 3260,[100] and 3303.[101] Hypertrophic cardiomyopathy has also been described in association with MELAS.[102] Other possible mutations in tRNA genes are at np 9997 in the $tRNA^{Gly}$ gene[103] and at np 8344 in the $tRNA^{Lys}$ gene (MERRF mutation).[83] There is one pedigree with the NARP/MILS mutation in the ATPase 6 gene in which hypertrophic cardiomyopathy was part of the clinical expression.[92] The association between multiple mtDNA deletions and cardiomyopathy is discussed below.

Sensorineural hearing loss is common in patients with mitochondrial encephalomyopathies and in the proper clinical context should be thought of as a clinical marker of these disorders. A specific mutation in the 12s rRNA gene of mtDNA has been found in association with both aminoglycoside and spontaneous deafness.[104] Two mutations in the $tRNA^{Ser(UCN)}$ gene have been described. A family with maternally inherited pure sensorineural hearing loss harbored a mutation at np 7445.[105,106] A second family, with an insertion point mutation at np 7472, had a syndrome characterized by a combination of deafness, ataxia, and myoclonus.[107] The combination of diabetes and deafness is one of the manifestations of the nt 3243 mutation.[81,82]

## REARRANGEMENTS OF MITOCHONDRIAL DNA

Complex rearrangements of mtDNA are also associated with mitochondrial disease and differ significantly from point mutations. Large-scale deletions are the most common of these pathogenetic rearrangements. Multiple mtDNA deletions differ in molecular structure and inheritance pattern from single deletions. Deletions occur only in heteroplasmic form and are likely lethal in homoplasmic mutant form. Duplications of mtDNA may also be associated with mitochondrial disease, or they may act as intermediates in mtDNA deletion formation.

Patients with chronic progressive external ophthalmoplegia (CPEO) present with ptosis and symmetrical weakness of the extraocular muscles, usually in association with a proximal limb myopathy. CPEO is insidious in onset, and ptosis is usually the initial, but rarely the only, manifestation. Dysfunction of extraocular movement begins with a slowing of saccadic eye movements.[108] The term *CPEO-plus* designates the association of other neurologic or somatic manifestations.[109] Kearns-Sayre syndrome is a subset of CPEO-plus that is defined as CPEO with onset before age 20 years and pigmentary retinopathy plus heart block, ataxia, or elevated cerebrospinal fluid protein.[110]

Most CPEO patients harbor a heteroplasmic, large, single mtDNA deletion that occurs clinically sporadically (Fig. 15–4).[1,2,111,112] The size and location of the deletions and the proportions of deleted and wild-type mtDNA genomes do not correlate with the severity of the clinical presentation.[2,111–114] The junction of most deletions contains directly repeated sequences, including a molecular hot spot that accounts for about one-third of the cases. This "common deletion" is a 5.0 kb segment between the ATPase 8 and ND5 genes. Homologous recombination and a "slipped mispairing" mechanism have been suggested to explain the generation of mtDNA deletions.[115–120] Mitochondrial genomes with deletions are transcribed but not translated, including genes not involved by the deletion.[121,122] The deleted genomes have been shown to be dominant over the wild type.[123]

A single species of deleted mtDNA molecule appears to be present in all tissues of the body in patients with Kearns-Sayre syndrome (Fig. 15–5),[124,125] and the fraction of deleted molecules increases during the lifespan of the patient.[18,19] These facts, plus the sporadic nature of the Kearns-Sayre syndrome suggest that the deletions are new mutations occurring in the oocytes, zygote, or early embryo. Alternatively, oocytes containing mtDNA deletions may not be functional. It is uncertain if a woman with Kearns-Sayre syndrome can transmit the disease to her progeny,[126,127] although one family with diabetes and deafness has been associated with a large maternally inherited mtDNA deletion.[128] Rarely, patients with sporadic CPEO/Kearns-Sayre syndrome have partial duplications of the mtDNA.[129,130]

CPEO can display other modes of inheritance. Maternally inherited CPEO occurs in association with the point mutation at np 3243 in the $tRNA^{Leu(URR)}$ gene.[78] Autosomal dominant CPEO associated with multiple mtDNA deletions is reviewed later.

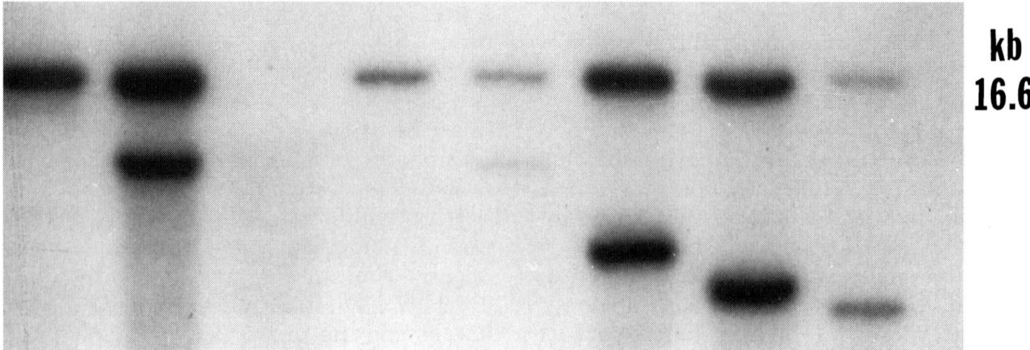


**Figure 15–4.** Molecular diagnosis of single mtDNA deletions. Southern blot analysis of total DNA extracted from the muscle of different CPEO patients, digested with *Pvu*II, and hybridized with radiolabeled human mtDNA. The 16.6 kb band represents the normal mtDNA molecule. Different patients with deletions of diverse size are shown.

Patients with Pearson's syndrome present in infancy with refractory sideroblastic anemia, thrombocytopenia, neutropenia, and pancreatic exocrine dysfunction.[131,132] Single mtDNA deletions have also been identified in patients with Pearson's syndrome. Those who survive into adolescence develop Kearns-Sayre syndrome as deleted mtDNA accummulates.[18,19]

Neither the clinical nor the molecular diagnosis of mitochondrial disease is specific. A single mtDNA mutation can be associated with different clinical syndromes, and a clinical syndrome may be due to diverse mutations. Also, mitochondrial diseases are multisystemic syndromes with very protean manifestations. Patients do not neatly classify into discrete subcategories of syndromes and may fall into multiple groups. There are examples of patients with features of both MELAS and MERRF,[133–136] MELAS and Kearns-Sayre Syndrome,[1,137] and MERRF and CPEO.[79,138,139]

## DEFECTS OF NUCLEAR DNA

Defects of nuclear DNA (nDNA) that are responsible for mitochondrial disorders show mendelian inheritance. We discuss defects of intergenomic communication between the nuclear and mitochondrial genomes.

Multiple mtDNA deletions were reported originally as an autosomal dominant disorder in an Italian family.[140] CPEO in this family typically presented in the third decade, ac-

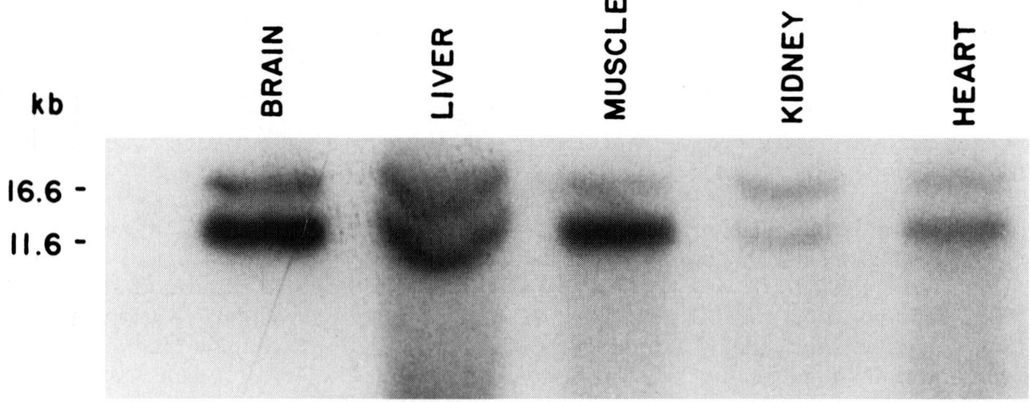


**Figure 15–5.** Southern blot analysis of a patient with Kearns-Sayre syndrome. The common deletion (~5 kb) is present in different proportions in all the tissues examined.

companied by slowly progressive proximal myopathy. Other reported accompanying symptoms in the large pedigrees have been depression,[141] sensorineural hearing loss, cataracts, ataxia, tremor, and peripheral neuropathy.[140,142] Multiple mtDNA deletions were found in both the cardiac and skeletal muscle of a mother and a son with idiopathic dilated cardiomyopathy.[143] Two unrelated families from Saudi Arabia were recently described with childhood onset CPEO associated with severe cardiomyopathy, suggesting autosomal recessive inheritance.[144] The myoneurogastrointestinal encephalopathy (MNGIE) syndrome has also been associated with multiple mtDNA deletions.[145–149] It is characterized by recurrent vomiting, pseudo-obstruction, intermittent diarrhea, peripheral neuropathy, myopathy, and encephalopathy. The molecular genetic basis of the MNGIE syndrome was recently demonstrated to be due to mutations in a nuclear gene involved in nucleotide biosynthesis, thymidine phosphorylase.[150] This mutation is the first defect to be demonstrated in the intergenomic communication between the nuclear and mitochondrial genomes.

The pathogenic role of multiple mtDNA deletions for a variety of conditions is unclear. These conditions include sideroblastic anemia with pancreatic failure and myopathy,[151] recurrent myoglobinuria,[152] inclusion body myositis,[153] late-onset mitochondrial myopathy,[154] multiple symmetrical lipomatosis,[155] periodic attacks of paralysis,[156] and the Wolfram's syndrome (diabetes insipidus, diabetes mellitus, optic atrophy, and deafness).[157] In the mendelian-inherited CPEO syndromes, mutations in nuclear genes that control mtDNA integrity may be responsible. The nuclear gene for a Finnish autosomal dominant CPEO Pedigree is located in the long arm of chromosome 10,[158] and in one of the Italian families the putative gene is located on the short arm of chromosome 3.[159]

### DEPLETION OF MITOCHONDRIAL DNA

Disorders involving depletion of mtDNA are characterized by quantitative defects in the mtDNA in specific tissues. Both mendelian-inherited genetic defects and environmental causes have been described in association with mtDNA depletion. Severe depletion of mtDNA has been reported in infants in association with different organ-specific syndromes such as nephropathy, hepatopathy, or myopathy. These patients have a rapidly progressive fatal course as mtDNA depletion reaches 98% in affected tissues. A milder form has been described in a few patients, in whom the level of depleted mtDNA was approximately 70% to 90%. Those children were normal until about 1 year of age, when they developed a progressive myopathy. Death due to respiratory failure occurred a few years later.[160] Besides muscle, no other tissue was affected in this milder form.

Deficiencies in mtDNA levels have been associated with reductions in mtDNA gene products, but not to nuclear oxidative phosphorylation gene products. This demonstrates an association between the copy number defect and the biochemical defect.[161–165]

An environmental cause of mtDNA depletion is zidovudine or (azidothymidine; AZT). Azidothymidine causes a myopathy with structural and biochemical abnormalities similar to those of the mitochondrial encephalomyopathies not only in patients with acquired immunodeficiency syndrome[166,167] but also in healthy rats and in cultured human myotubes.[168] Azidothymidine inhibits the gamma DNA polymerase, disrupts the replication of mtDNA, and causes mtDNA depletion.[169] L-carnitine prevents the structural changes caused by AZT toxicity in cultured human myotubes.[170]

## MITOCHONDRIAL DEFECTS IN COMMON CHRONIC DISEASES

We next outline the evidence that a defect in mitochondrial function may contribute to common chronic diseases, such as diabetes mellitus and neurodegenerative disorders.

### Mitochondrial DNA and Diabetes Mellitus

Diabetes mellitus (DM) is one of the most common chronic disorders. Clues that mtDNA mutations might contribute to the development of DM came from two different observations. First, DM is frequently associated with a variety of mitochondrial encephalomyopathies.[83,108,129,171–176] Also, epidemiological studies have shown a predominance of maternal transmission of non-insulin-dependent DM (NIDDM).[177–180] Two large families whose primary clinical manifestations were DM and deafness were reported in 1992. One of the pedigrees was associated with a 10.4 kb deletion in the mtDNA,[128] and the other with the np 3243 point mutation in the $tRNA^{Leu(UUR)}$ gene (MELAS mutation).[81] Several other reports confirmed an association between the np 3243 mutation and diabetes, including families without evidence of severe neurologic deficit.[82,181–185]

In a recent review of 199 affected members of 45 families with diabetes and the $tRNA^{Leu(UUR)}$ mutation, 48% suffered from DM and deafness, 13% had DM and deafness with other neurologic symptoms including MELAS, 21% had only DM, 15% had deafness alone, and 3% had deafness plus other neurologic deficits.[186] The combination of DM and deafness should raise the possibility of an mtDNA mutation.

Three other mutations in the $t\text{-}RNA^{Leu(UUR)}$ gene that produce multisystemic disease have DM as an associated manifestation.[47,75,100] Overall the $t\text{-}RNA^{Leu(UUR)}$ −3243 mutation has been estimated to be found in 1.5% in all diabetics, and the prevalence is about 2- to 5-fold higher in cases with a family history of DM.[186] This number may be an underestimation, as the mutation was measured in blood samples and not the affected tissue. The prevalence of DM in association with other mtDNA mutations is currently unknown.

Wolfram's syndrome was originally described as a combination of familial juvenile-onset DM and optic atrophy. Other neurologic features subsequently emerged, and the acronym DIDMOAD (diabetes insipidus, DM, optic atrophy, and deafness) became commonly accepted. There is extensive phenotypic variability and multisystemic involvement in these patients, suggesting mtDNA involvement. Indeed, mitochondrial morphological[187] and biochemical[187,188] abnormalities have been reported in patients with Wolfram's syndrome. Sporadic cases have been associated with a single 7.6 kb mtDNA deletion[188] and a point mutation at np 11,778, also seen in patients with LHON.[189] Two pedigrees with the syndrome have multiple mtDNA deletions; with a disease locus linked to 4p16.[157]

Impaired insulin secretion by the β cells of the pancreas has been shown in patients with DM associated with the np 3243 mutation[185,190,191] and the 10.4 kb mtDNA deletion.[192] In contrast to NIDDM, in which only the β cell function is affected, DM related to mtDNA mutations is also characterized by a defect in the glucagon-secreting α-cell function.[190,192] The linkage of DM to a heterogeneous group of mitochondrial syndromes due to both mtDNA and nDNA mutations suggests that defects in oxidative phosphorylation and ATP production may be a common cause of diabetes.

## Mitochondrial DNA and Neurodegenerative Disorders

As we discussed in the section on pathophysiology, aging in humans is associated with an increase in mtDNA mutations and a decline in mitochondrial respiratory function.[34–40] The percentage change of age-associated increases in the level of mtDNA deletions is significant, but the absolute level of these deletions is low.[42,43] Although the effect of this small level of individual mutation may not be significant, it is possible that several different mutations accummulate simultaneously and contribute to the functional defect. Keeping this in mind, we review the evidence that mitochondrial dysfunction is associated with neurodegenerative disorders.

### PARKINSON'S DISEASE

There is evidence for a defect of mitochondrial respiratory function in Parkinson's disease (PD). A decrease in complex I activity[193–195] and in complex I subunits by immunohistochemistry[196] have been shown in the substantia nigra of patients with PD. 1-Methyl-4-phenyl-1,2,3,6-tetrahydropyridine (MPTP), which produces a model of PD, is converted to 1-methyl-4-phenylpyridinium MPP+), an inhibitor of complex I.[197,198] Complex I activity is also decreased in platelets of patients with PD,[199–201] but, as enzyme activities vary considerably among individuals, a single value cannot be used as a diagnostic measure.

Studies of oxidative phosphorylation enzymes in skeletal muscle produced conflicting results.[194,202–205] No significant mutation of mtDNA has been reported in association with PD. Despite an initial report of an increase in the "common" mtDNA deletion in striatum from PD brain,[205] subsequent reports showed no increase in this deletion in the substantia nigra compared with age-matched controls.[204,206] Three mtDNA point mutations were reported, with a small increased frequency in patients with Alzheimer's disease and PD.[207]

### ALZHEIMER'S DISEASE

Mitochondrial defects may be involved in Alzheimer's disease (AD) by lowering the oxidative efficiency of critical neuronal population, at an earlier age. A defect in pyruvate dehydrogenase has been reported in AD brain material,[208,209] and abnormalities in brain positron emission tomography scans have been consistently described in AD patients.[210,211] A threefold increase in oxidative damage to mtDNA in AD brain material was recently reported.[212] Analysis of the respiratory chain enzyme activities have shown decreased cytochrome *c* oxidase activity (complex IV) in AD brain material.[213–215] A reduction in mRNA for cytochrome *c* oxidase subunits was found in the temporal lobe of AD patients.[216,217] A reduction in cytochrome *c* oxidase activity has also been reported in platelets of AD patients.[218] Interestingly, cytochrome *c* oxidase inhibition resulted in an increased production of potentially amyloidogenic fragments due to abnormal processing of the amyloid precursor protein in cultured neurons.[219] Evidence that mtDNA mutations may play a role in AD pathophysiology comes from an increased level of the common mtDNA deletion in AD patients younger than 75 years[220] and from the higher frequency of np 4336 mutations in AD patients compared with age-matched controls.[221]

### HUNTINGTON'S DISEASE

Although a Huntington's disease (HD) gene defect has been identified, the structure of the abnormal gene product and the mechanism of cell death are not understood. Defects in complex II, III, and IV activities of the mitochondrial respiratory chain function were found in the caudate nucleus from HD patients, suggesting that a abnormal energy metabolism contributes to the pathophysiology of HD.[222] Contradictory results have been reported regarding the level of the common mtDNA deletion in HD patients brain.[223,224]

## CLINICAL ASSESSMENT AND INVESTIGATION

Detailed personal and family histories are the basis of diagnosis for mitochondrial disorders. The association of apparently unrelated symptoms from several different organ systems may be a helpful clue in considering mitochondrial disease as a possible diagnosis (Table 15–1). Mitochondrial disorders express prominent symptoms in the peripheral and central nervous systems, often simultaneously. On physical examination, signs of subtle organ involvement such as mild ptosis, muscle fatigue on sustained contraction, and retinopathy should be vigilantly pursued. Examination of purportedly asymptomatic relatives may provide valuable information. A maternal pattern of inheritance strongly implicates an mtDNA etiology; however, the lack of maternal inheritance does not preclude a mitochondrial disorder, which can also be sporadic or autosomally inherited.

A number of laboratory studies aid in the diagnosis of mitochondrial disorders. Resting serum lactate level is one screening test for mitochondrial disease, but the level is not consistently increased in all patients with mitochondrial disorders. In a large series of patients with mitochondrial disease, two-thirds had a significantly elevated lactate level after aerobic exercise in compar-

Table 15–1. **Systemic and Neurologic Manifestation of Mitochondrial Encephalomyopathies**

| Neurologic | Systemic |
|---|---|
| Ophthalmoplegia | Cardiomyopathy |
| Optic neuropathy | Cardiac conduction defects |
| Pigmentary retinopathy | Corneal opacities and cataracts |
| Nystagmus | Adrenocorticotrophin deficiency |
| Seizures | Diabetes mellitus |
| Myoclonus | Hypothyroidism |
| Stroke-like episodes (commonly cortical blindness, hemianopia, hemiparesis) | Hypoparathyroidism |
| Dementia | Hypogonadism |
| Depression | Hyperaldosteronism |
| Vascular headache | Primary ovarian failure |
| Central hypoventilation | Short stature |
| Sensorineural hearing loss | Exocrine pancreas dysfunction |
| Dystonia | Hepatopathy |
| Ataxia | Intestinal pseudo-obstruction |
| Myelopathy | Renal tubulopathies |
| Myopathy | Pancytopenia |
| Exercise intolerance | Sideroblastic anemia |
| Recurrent myoglobinuria | Lactic acidosis |
| Neuropathy | |

ison with normal and disease controls.[108] Serum creatine kinase level is usually normal or slightly elevated and is not very helpful diagnostically.

Phosphorous magnetic resonance spectroscopy allows a noninvasive assessment of energy metabolism *in vivo*. The inorganic phosphate/phosphocreatine (Pi/PCr) ratio has proved the most useful parameter and an increased Pi/PCr ratio has been found in the muscle of most patients with mitochondrial encephalomyopathy. MR spectroscopy is not widely available, and the abnormalities found are not specific for mitochondrial disorders.

Clinical neurophysiologic procedures can provide supportive evidence of mitochondrial disease. Audiometry can detect subclinical hearing loss. Electromyography (EMG) and nerve conduction studies can detect sublinical myopathy, peripheral neuropathy, or both.

Neuroimaging of the central nervous system with either computerized tomography (CT) or magnetic resonance imaging (MRI) may be useful to diagnose mitochondrial disease. Basal ganglia calcification is seen in association with a number of different mitochondrial phenotypes (Fig. 15–6). The stroke-like lesions of MELAS syndrome appear hypodense on CT scan, and serial studies demonstrate multiple ''migrating infarcts'' in various stages of evolution, involving primarily the posterior temporal and occipital regions. Specific MRI findings in MELAS syndrome are described by Mathews and colleagues[225] as multifocal areas of hyperintense signal confined to the cortex of the cerebrum, cerebellum, and immediately adjacent white matter on $T_2$-weighted images. This pattern is distinct from the wedge-shaped lesions seen in thromboembolic stroke, as the white matter is less involved and is not confined to a single vascular territory. The stroke-like lesions of MELAS syndrome have been confused radiographically with stroke, tumor, and encephalitis. Subcortical white matter involve-

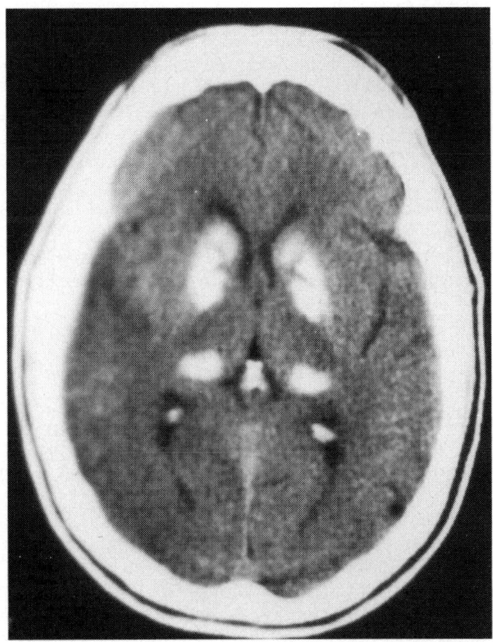

**Figure 15–6.** Computerized tomographic scan from a patient with MELAS syndrome. The patient is a 42-year-old man with an 11-year history of deafness, seizures, and stroke-like episodes. The CT shows extensive calcification affecting the basal ganglia and thalami.

ment has been reported as the only radiologic manifestation in MELAS, MERRF, and MNGIE syndromes. Bilateral symmetrical lesions in the basal ganglia have been described in LHON-plus dystonia and in maternally inherited Leigh's disease. Positron emission tomography and single-photon emission computed tomography have shown focal reductions in metabolism and blood flow in patients with mitochondrial disease with normal MRI studies.

Muscle biopsy is the most helpful diagnostic procedure for the comprehensive evaluation of a mitochondrial encephalomyopathy. An open biopsy is preferred, to obtain adequate tissue for histologic, biochemical, and molecular genetic studies. A comprehensive battery of histologic, histochemical, and ultrastructural studies improves the diagnostic yield. Histopathologic findings were reviewed earlier.

Molecular genetic tests are commercially available for the most common mtDNA point mutations, and most are readily detectable in blood. The absence of the known point mutations in leukocyte DNA does not preclude a diagnosis, and the yield can be improved by testing muscle mtDNA. Indeed, muscle mtDNA is required for molecular genetic detection of single and multiple mtDNA deletions.

Predictions about the prognosis and recurrence risk of the mitochondrial diseases are difficult to make with any degree of confidence. The classic mitochondrial syndromes are rare conditions that have a notoriously variable natural history. The molecular genetic basis of these disorders has been established only recently, and very limited follow-up data of confirmed cases is available. The reliable estimation of recurrence risk is complicated by the different patterns of inheritance (sporadic, maternal, autosomal dominant, autosomal recessive), the clinical overlap between syndromes, the clinical variability within and between families, and the influence of environmental factors on the disease (e.g., influence of alcohol and tobacco use on visual loss in LHON).

Optimally, the definitive demonstration of a pathogenetic mtDNA mutation will facilitate genetic counseling. For instance, single mtDNA deletions are virtually always sporadic, and the recurrence risk to family members is very low. Perhaps the most robust genetic counseling can be given to affected males with an mtDNA point mutation, to reassure that they will not pass the disease to their offspring.

## SUMMARY

Mitochondrial disorders are clinically diverse and are defined by structural or functional abnormalities in mitochondria or mitochondrial DNA (mtDNA). An increasing number of mtDNA mutations have been described in a variety of known and novel mitochondrial diseases over the last decade. This chapter reviews the characteristics of mtDNA and some of its unique genetic features: maternal inheritance, heteroplasmy, mitotic segregation, and the threshold effect.

The clinical phenotype and causative mtDNA mutations are reviewed for each of the classic mitochondrial diseases. Mitochondrial diseases have protean clinical manifestations with prominent involvement of both the peripheral and central nervous systems. Mitochondrial DNA mutations may also be implicated in prevalent neurodegenerative diseases and in aging itself. An integrated diagnostic approach to the perplexing disorders is outlined.

## REFERENCES


1. Holt IJ, Harding AE, Morghan-Hughes JA: Deletions of muscle mitochondrial DNA in patients with mitochondrial myopathies. Nature 331:717–719, 1988.
2. Zeviani M, Moraes CT, DiMauro S, et al.: Deletions of mitochondrial DNA in Kearns-Sayre syndrome. Neurology 38:1339–1346, 1988.
3. Wallace DC, Singh G, Lott MT, et al.: Mitochondrial DNA mutation associated with Leber's hereditary optic neuropathy. Science 242:1427–1430, 1988.
4. Di Donato S: Disorders of lipid metabolism affecting skeletal muscle: carnitine deficiency syndromes, defects in the catabolic pathway, and chanarin disease. In Engel AG, Franzini-Armstrong C (eds): Myology, ed 2. McGraw-Hill, New York, 1994, pp1587–1586.
5. Morgan-Hughes JA: Mitochondrial diseases. In Engel AG, Franzini-Armstrong C (eds): Myology, ed 2. Mc Graw-Hill, New York, 1994, pp1610–1659.
6. Zierz S: Carnitine palmitoyl transferase deficiency. In Engel AG, Franzini-Armstrong C (eds): Myology, ed 2. McGraw-Hill, New York, 1994, pp1577–1586.
7. Wallace DC: Diseases of the mitochondrial DNA. Annu Rev Biochem 61:1175–1212, 1992.
8. Kruse B, Narasinham N, Attardi G: Termination of transcription in human mitochondria: Identification and purification of a DNA binding protein factor that promotes termination. Cell 58:391–397, 1989.
9. Anderson S, Bankier AT, Barrell BG, et al.: Sequence and organization of the human mitochondrial genome. Nature 290:457–465, 1981.
10. Giles RE, Blanc H, Cann HM, Wallace DC: Maternal inheritance of human mitochondrial DNA. Proc Natl Acad Sci USA 77:6715–6719, 1980.
11. Gillensten U, Wharton D, Josefsson A, Wilson AC: Paternal inheritance of mitochondrial DNA in mice. Nature 352:255–257, 1991.
12. Clayton DA, Doda JN, Friedberg EC: The absence of a pyrimidine dimer repair mechanism in mammalian mitochondria. Proc Natl Acad Sci USA 71: 2777–2781, 1975.
13. Pettepher CC, LeDoux SP, Bohr VA, Wilson GL: Repair of alkali-labile sites within the mitochondrial DNA of RINr 38 cells after exposure to the nitrosourea streptozotocin. J Biol Chem 266:3113–3117, 1991.
14. Michaels GS, Hauswirth WW, Laipis PJ: Mitochondrial DNA copy number in bovine oocytes and somatic cells. Dev Biol 94:246–251, 1982.
15. Shuster RC, Rubenstein AJ, Wallace DC: Mitochondrial DNA in anucleated human blood cells. Biochem Biophys Res Commun 155:1360–1365, 1988.
16. Holt IJ, Harding AE, Petty RKH, Morgan-Hughes JA: A new mitochondrial disease associated with mitochondrial DNA heteroplasmy. Am J Hum Genet 46:428–433, 1990.
17. Lott MT, Voljavec AS, Wallace DC: Variable genotype of Leber's hereditary optic neuropathy patients. Am J Ophthalmol 109:625–631, 1990.
18. Larsson NG, Holme B, Kristiansson B: Progressive increase of the mutated mitochondrial DNA fraction in Kearns-Sayre syndrome. Pediatr Res 28:131–136, 1990.
19. McShane MA, Hammans SR, Sweeney M, et al.: Pearson syndrome and mitochondrial encephalopathy in a patient with a deletion of mtDNA. Am J Hum Genet 48:39–42, 1991.
20. Ciafaloni E, Ricci E, Shanske S, et al.: MELAS: Clinical features, biochemistry, and molecular genetics. Ann Neurol 31:391–398, 1992.
21. MacMillan C, Lach B, Shoubridge EA: Variable distribution of mutant mitochondrial DNAs (t-RNALeu[3243]) in tissues of symptomatic relatives with MELAS: The role of mitotic segregation. Neurology 43:1686–1590, 1993.
22. Attardi G, Yoneda M, Chomyn A: Complementation and segregation behavior of disease causing mitochondrial DNA mutations in cellular model systems. Biochim Biophys Acta 1271:241–248, 1995.
23. King MP, Attardi G: Injection of mitochondria into human cells leads to a rapid replacement of the endogenous mitochondrial DNA. Cell 52:811–819, 1988.
24. Chomyn A, Meola G, Bresolin N, et al.: *In vitro* genetic transfer of protein synthesis and respiration defects to mitochondrial DNA-less cells with myopathy-patient mitochondria. Mol Cell Biol 11: 2236–2244, 1991.
25. Hayashi J-I, Ohta S, Kikuchi A, et al.: Introduction of disease related mitochondrial DNA deletions into Hela cells lacking mitochondrial DNA results in mitochondrial dysfunction. Proc Natl Acad Sci USA 88:10614–10618, 1991.
26. Chomyn A, Martinuzzi A, Yoneda, et al.: MELAS mutation in mtDNA binding site for transcription termination factor causes defects in protein synthesis and in respiration but not changes in levels of upstream and downstream mature transcrips. Proc Natl Acad Sci USA 89:4221–4225, 1992.
27. Cardenas E, Boveris A, Ragan CI, Stoppani AOM: Production of $O_2$ radicals and $H_2O_2$ by NADH-ubiquinone reductase and ubiquinol-cytochrome *c* reductase from beef heart mitochondria. Arch Biochem Biophys 180:248–257, 1977.??
28. Bandy B, Davidson AJ: Mitochondria mutations may increase oxidative stress: Implications for carcinogenesis and aging. Free Radical Biol Med 8: 523–539, 1990.
29. Wallace DC, Shoffner JM, Trounce I, et al.: Mitochondrial DNA mutations in human degenerative diseases and aging. Biochim Biophys Acta 1271: 141–151, 1995.

30. Caron F, Jacq C, Rouviere-Yaniv J: Characterization of a histone-like protein extracted from yeast mitochondria. Proc Natl Acad Sci USA 76:4265–4269, 1979.
31. Ames BN: Endogenous DNA damage as related to cancer and aging. Mutat Res 214:41–46, 1989.
32. Backer JM, Weinstein IB: Mitochondrial DNA is a major cellular target for a dihydrodiol-epoxide derivative of benzo(α)pyrene. Science 209:297–299, 1980.
33. Niranjan BG, Bhat NK, Avadhani NG: Preferential attack of mitochondrial DNA by aflotoxin B1 during hepatocarcinogenesis. Science 215:73–75, 1981.
34. Muller-Hocker J: Cytochrome *c* oxidase deficient fibers in the limb muscles and diaphragm of man without muscular disease: An age related alteration. J Neurol Sci 100:14–21, 1990.
35. Trounce I, Byrne E, Marzuki S: Decline in skeletal muscle mitochondrial respiratory function: Possible factor in ageing. Lancet 1 (8639):637–639, 1989.
36. Cortopassi GA, Arnheim N: Detection of a specific mitochondrial DNA deletion in tissues of older humans. Nucleic Acids Res 18:6927–6933, 1990.
37. Simonetti S, Chen X, DiMauro S, Schon EA: Accumulation of deletions in human mitochondrial DNA during normal aging: Analysis by quantitative PCR. Biochim Byophis Acta 1180:113–122, 1992.
38. Zhang C, Linnane AW, Nagley P: Occurrence of a particular base substitution (3243 A to G) in mitochondrial DNA of tissues of ageing humans. Biochem Biophys Res Commun 195:1104–1110, 1993.
39. Hayakawa M, Torii K, Sugiyama S, Tanaka M, Ozawa T: Age associated accumulation of 8-hydroxydeoxyguanosine in mitochondrial DNA of human diaphragm. Biochem Biophys Res Commun 179:1023–1029, 1991.
40. Mecocci P, Mac Garvey U, Kaufman AE, et al.: Oxidative damage to mitochondrial DNA shows marked age-dependent increases in human brain. Ann Neurol 34:609–616, 1993.
41. Corral-Debrinski M, Stepien G, Shoffner JM, Lott MT, Kanter K, Wallace DC: Hypoxemia is associated with mitochondrial DNA damage and gene induction. JAMA 266:1812–1816, 1991.
42. Cooper JM, Mann VM, Schapira AHV: Analyses of mitochondrial respiratory chain dysfunction and mitochondrial DNA deletion in human skeletal muscle. J Neurol Sci 113:91–98, 1992.
43. Corral-Debrinski M, Horton T, Lott MT, et al.: Mitochondrial DNA deletions in human brain: Regional variability and increase with advance age. Nat Genet 2:324–329, 1992.
44. Adachi K, Fujiura Y, Mayumi F, et al.: A deletion of mitochondrial DNA in murine doxorubicin-induced cardiotoxicity. Biochem Biophys Res Commun 195:945–951, 1993.
45. Olson W, Engel WK, Walsh GO, Einaugler R.: Oculocraniosomatic neuromuscular disease with "ragged-red" fibers: Histochemical and ultrastructural changes in limb muscles of a group of patients with idiopathic progressive external ophthalmoplegia. Arch Neurol 26:193–211, 1972.
46. Banker BQ, Engel AE: Basic reactions of muscle. In Engel AG, Franzini-Armstrong C (eds): Myology, (ed 2.) Mc Graw-Hill, New York, 1994, pp832–888.
47. Moraes CT, Ciacci F, Bonilla E, et al.: Two novel pathogenic mitochondrial DNA mutations affecting organelle number and protein synthesis. Is the tRNALeu(UUR) gene an etiologic hot spot? J Clin Invest 92:2906–2915, 1993.
48. Moraes CT, Ricci E, Petruzella V, et al.: Molecular analysis of the muscle pathology associated with mitochondrial DNA deletions. Nat Genet 1:359–367, 1992.
49. Nikoskeilainen EK, Savontaus M-L, Wanne OP, Katila MJ, Nummelin KU: Leber's hereditary optic neuroretinopathy, a maternally inherited disease. A genealogic study in four pedigrees. Arch Ophthalmol 105:665–671, 1987.
50. Johns DR. Genotype-specific phenotypes in Leber hereditary optic neuropathy. Clin Neurosci 2:146–150, 1994.
51. Carroll WM, Mastaglia FL: Leber's optic neuropathy. A clinical and visual evoked potential study of affected and asymptomatic members of a six generation family. Brain 102:559–580, 1979.
52. Nikoskelainen E, Hoyt WF, Nummelin K. Ophthalmoscopic findings in Leber's hereditary optic neuropathy. The fundus findings in the affected family members. Arch Ophthalmol 101:1059–1068, 1983.
53. Harding AE, Sweeney MG, Miller DH, et al.: Occurrence of a multiple sclerosis–like illness in women who have a Leber's hereditary optic neuropathy mitochondrial DNA mutation. Brain 115: 979–989, 1992.
54. Johns DR. Improved molecular genetic of Leber's hereditary optic neuropathy. N Engl J Med 323: 1488–1489, 1990.
55. Newman NJ. Leber's hereditary optic neuropathy: New genetic considerations. Arch Neurol 50:540–548, 1993.
56. Johns DR, Neufeld MJ: Cytochrome *b* mutation in Leber hereditary optic neuropathy. Biochem Biophys Res Commun 181:1358–1364, 1992.
57. Vilkki J, Ott J, Savontaus ML, Aula P, Nikoskelainen EK. Optic atrophy in Leber hereditary optic neuroretinopathy is probably determined by an X-chromosome gene closely linked to DXS7. Am J Hum Genet 48:486–491, 1991.
58. Bu X, Rotter JI: X chromosome-linked and mitochondrial gene control of Leber hereditary optic neuropathy: Evidence from segregation analysis for dependence on X chromosome inactivation. Proc Natl Acad Sci USA 88:8198–8202, 1991.
59. Cullom ME, Heher KL, Savino PJ, Miller NR, Johns DR: Leber's hereditary optic neuropathy masquerading as tobacco–alcohol amblyopia. Arch Ophthalmol 111:1482–1485, 1993.
60. Tsao K, Aitken PA, Johns DR. Smoking as an aetiological factor in a pedigree with Leber's hereditary optic neuropathy. Br J Ophthalmol 1999;83: 577–581.
61. de Vries DD, van Engelen BGM, Gabreels FJM, Ruitenbeek W, van Oost BA: A second missense mutation in the mitochondrial ATPase gene in Leigh's syndrome. Ann Neurol 34:410–412, 1993.
62. Tatuch Y, Pagon RA, Vlcek B, Roberts R, Korson

M, Robinson BR. The 8993 mtDNA mutation: Heteroplasmy and clinical presentation in three families. Eur J Hum Genet 2:35–43, 1994.
63. Fryer A, Appleton R, Sweeney MG, Rosenbloom L, Harding AE. Mitochondrial DNA 8993 (NARP) mutation presenting with a heterogeneous phenotype including "cerebral palsy." Arch Dis Child 71:419–422, 1994.
64. Tatuch Y, Christodoulou J, Feigenbaum A, et al.: Heteroplasmic mtDNA mutation (T → G) at 8993 can cause Leigh disease when the percentage of abnormal mtDNA is high. Am J Hum Genet 50: 852–858, 1992.
65. Shoffner JM, Fernhoff PM, Krawiecki NS, et al.: Subacute necrotizing encephalopathy: oxidative phosphorylation defects and the ATPase 6 point mutation. Neurology 42:2168–2174, 1992.
66. Sakuta R, Goto Y, Horai S, et al.: Mitochondrial DNA mutation and Leigh's syndrome. Ann Neurol 32:597–598, 1992.
67. Santorelli FM, Shanske S, Macaya A, DeVivo D, DiMauro S: The mutation at nt8993 is a common cause of Leigh's syndrome. Ann Neurol 34:827–834, 1993.
68. Pavlakis SG, Phillips PC, DiMauro S, De Vivo DC, Rowland L: Mitochondrial myopathy, encephalopathy, lactic acidosis and stroke-like episodes: A distinctive clinical syndrome. Ann Neurol 16:481–488, 1984.
69. Goto Y, Nonaka I, Horai S: A mutation in the t-RNA$^{Leu(UUR)}$ gene associated with MELAS subgroup of mitochondrial encephalomyopathies. Nature 348:651–653, 1990.
70. Kobayashi Y, Momoi MY, Tominaga K, et al.: A point mutation in the mitochondrial t-RNALeu(UUR) gene in MELAS (mitochondrial myopathy, encephalopathy, lactic acidosis and stroke-like episodes). Biochem Biophys Res Commun 173:816–822, 1990.
71. Goto Y, Nonaka I, Horai S: A new mtDNA mutation associated with mitochondrial myopathy, encephalopathy, lactic acidosis and stroke-like episodes (MELAS). Biochim Biophys Acta 1097:238–240, 1991.
72. Goto Y, Horai S, Matsuoka T, et al.: Mitochondrial myopathy, encephalopathy, lactic acidosis and stroke-like episodes (MELAS): A correlative study of the clinical features and mitochondrial DNA mutation. Neurology 42:545–550, 1992.
73. Ciafaloni E, Ricci E, Shanske S, et al.: MELAS: Clinical features, biochemistry and molecular genetics. Ann Neurol 31:391–398, 1992.
74. Sweeney MG, Bundey S, Brockington M, Poulton JR, Winer JB, Harding AE: Mitochondrial myopathy associated with sudden death in young adults and a novel transfer RNA[Leu(UUR)] gene. Q J Med 86:709–713, 1993.
75. Morten KJ, Cooper JM, Brown GK, Lake BD, Pike D, Poulton J: A new point mutation associated with mitochondrial encephalopathy. Hum Mol Genet 2: 2081–2087, 1993.
76. Goto Y, Tsugane K, Tanabe Y, Nonaka I, Horai S: A point mutation at nucleotide pair 3291 of the mitochondrial tRNALeu(UUR) gene in a patient with mitochondrial myopathy, encephalopathy, lactic acidosis and stroke-like episodes (MELAS). Biochem Biophys Res Commun 202:1624–1630, 1994.
77. Manfredi G, Schon EA, Moraes CT, et al.: A new mutation associated with MELAS is located in a mitochondrial DNA polypeptide-coding gene. Neuromusc Disord 5:391–398, 1995.
78. Moraes CT, Ciacci F, Silvestri G, et al.: Atypical clinical presentations associated with the MELAS mutation at position 3243 of human mitochondrial DNA. Neuromusc Disord 3:43–50, 1993.
79. Hammans SR, Sweeney MG, Brockington M, et al.: Mitochondrial encephalomyopathies: Molecular genetic diagnosis from blood samples. Lancet 337: 1311–1313, 1991.
80. Obayashi T, Hattori K, Sugiyama S, et al.: Point mutations in mitochondrial DNA in patients with hypertrophic cardiomyopathy. Am Heart J 124: 1263–1269, 1992.
81. Van den Ouweland JMW, Lemkes HHPJ, Ruitenbeek W, et al.: Mutation in the mitochondrial t-RNALeu(UUR) gene in a large pedigree with maternally transmitted type II diabetes and deafness. Nat Genet 1:368–371, 1992.
82. Reardon W, Ross RJM, Sweeney MG, et al.: Diabetes mellitus associated with a pathogenic point mutation in mitochondrial DNA. Lancet 340:1376–1379, 1992.
83. Silvestri G, Ciafaloni E, Santorelli FM, et al.: Clinical features associated with the A > G transition at nucleotide 8344 of mtDNA ("MERRF mutation"). Neurology 43:1200–1206, 1993.
84. Berkovic SF, Carpenter S, Evans A, et al.: Myoclonus epilepsy and ragged-red fibers (MERRF). 1. A clinical, pathological, biochemical, magnetic resonance spectrographic and positron emission tomographic study. Brain 112:1231–1260, 1989.
85. Hammans SR, Sweeney MG, Brockingham M, et al.: The mitochondrial DNA transfer RNA Lys A > G(8344) mutation and the syndrome of myoclonic epilepsy with ragged red fibers (MERRF). Brain 116:617–632, 1993.
86. Shoffner JM, Lott MT, Lezza AM, Seibel P, Ballinger SW, Wallace DC: Myoclonic epilepsy and ragged red fiber disease (MERRF) is associated with a mitochondrial DNA tRNA-Lys mutation. Cell 61: 931–937, 1990.
87. Yoneda M, Tanno Y, Horai S, Ozawa T, Miyataki T, Tsuji S: A common mitochondrial DNA mutation in the t-RNA Lys of patients with myoclonic epilepsy and ragged-red fibers. Biochem Int 21:789–796, 1990.
88. Silvestri G, Moraes CT, Shanske S, Oh SJ, DiMauro S: A new mtDNA mutation in the tRNALys gene associated with myoclonic epilepsy and ragged-red fibers (MERRF). Am J Hum Genet 51:1213–1217, 1992.
89. Zeviani M, Muntoni F, Savarese N, et al.: A MERRF/MELAS overlap syndrome with a new point mutation in the mitochondrial DNA t-RNALys gene. Eur J Hum Genet 1:80–87, 1993.
90. Shoffner JM, Lott MT, Wallace DC. MERRF: A model disease for understanding the principles of mitochondrial genetics. Rev Neurol 147:431–435, 1991.
91. Sweeney MG, Hammans SR, Duchen LW, et al.: Mitochondrial DNA mutation underlying Leigh's

syndrome: Clinical, pathological, biochemical, and genetic studies of a patient presenting with progressive myoclonic epilepsy. J Neurol Sci 121: 57–65, 1994.
92. Pastores GM, Santorelli FM, Shanske S, et al.: Leigh syndrome and hypertrophic cardiomyopathy in an infant with a mitochondrial DNA point mutation (T8993G). Am J Med Genet 50:265–271, 1994.
93. Howell N, Kubacka I, Smith R, Frerman F, Parks JK, Parker WD.: Association of the mitochondrial 8344 MERRF mutation with maternally inherited spinocerebellar degeneration and Leigh disease. Neurology 46:219–222, 1996.
94. Calabresi PA, Silvestri G, DiMauro S, Griggs RC.: Ekbom's syndrome: Lipomas, ataxia, and neuropathy with MERRF. Muscle Nerve 17:943–945, 1994.
95. Taniike M, Fukushima H, Yanagihara I, et al.: Mitochondrial tRNA Ile mutation in fatal cardiomyopathy. Biochem Biophys Res Commun 186:47–53, 1992.
96. Casali C, Santorelli FM, D'Amati G, Bernucci P, DeBiase L, DiMauro S: A novel mtDNA point mutation in maternally inherited cardiomyopathy. Biochem Biophys Res Commun 213:588–593, 1995.
97. Tanaka M, Ino H, Ohno K, et al.: Mitochondrial mutation in fatal infantile cardiomyopathy. Lancet 336:1452, 1990.
98. Santorelli FM, Mak SH, Vazquez-Acevedo M, et al.: A novel mitochondrial DNA point mutation associated with mitochondrial encephalocardiomyopathy. Biochem Biophys Res Commun 216:835–840, 1995.
99. Obayashi T, Hattori K, Sugiyama S, et al.: Point mutations in mitochondrial DNA in patients with hypertrophic cardiomyopathy. Am Heart J 124: 1263–1269, 1992.
100. Zeviani M, Gellera C, Antozzi C, et al.: Maternally inherited myopathy and cardiomyopathy: Association with mutation in mitochondrial DNA tRNA Leu (UUR). Lancet 338:143–147, 1991.
101. Silvestri G, Santorelli FM, Shanske S, et al.: A new mtDNA mutation in the tRNALeu (UUR) gene associated with maternally inherited cardiomyopathy. Hum Mutat 3:37–43, 1994.
102. Yoneda M, Tanaka M, Nishikimi M, et al.: Pleiotrophic molecular defects in energy-transducing complexes in mitochondrial encephalomyopathy. J Neurol Sci 92:143–158, 1989.
103. Merante F, Tein I, Benson L, Robinson BH: Maternally inherited hypertrophic cardiomyopathy due to a novel T-to-C transition at nucleotide 9997 in the mitochondrial tRNA glycine gene. Am J Human Genet 55:437–446, 1994.
104. Prezant TR, Agapian JV, Bohlman MC, et al.: Mitochondrial ribosomal RNA mutation associated with both antibiotic-induced and non-syndromic deafness. Nat Genet 4:289–294, 1993.
105. Reid FM, Vernham GA, Jacobs HT: A novel mitochondrial point mutation in a maternal pedigree with sensorineural deafness. Hum Mutat 3: 243–247, 1994.
106. Vernham GA, Reid FM, Rundle PA, Jacobs HT: Bilateral sensorineural hearing loss in members of a maternal lineage with a mitochondrial point mutation. Clin Otolaryngol 19:314–319, 1994.
107. Tiranti V, Chariot P, Carella F, et al.: Maternally inherited hearing loss, ataxia and myoclonus associated with a novel point mutation in mitochondrial tRNA Ser(UCN) gene. Hum Mol Genet 4: 1421–1427, 1995.
108. Petty RKH, Harding AH, Morgan-Hughes JA. The clinical features of mitochondrial myopathy. Brain 109:915–938, 1986.
109. Berenberg BA, Pellock JM, DiMauro S, et al.: Lumping or splitting? "ophthalmoplegia-plus" or Kearns-Sayre syndrome? Ann Neurol 1:37–54, 1977.
110. Drachman DA: Ophthalmoplegia plus; classification of disorders associated with progressive external ophthalmoplegia. Handbk Clin Neurol 22: 203–216, 1975.
111. Holt IJ, Harding AE, Cooper JM, et al.: Mitochondrial myopathies: Clinical and biochemical features of 30 patients with major deletions of muscle mitochondrial DNA. Ann Neurol 26:699–708, 1989.
112. Moraes CT, DiMauro S, Zeviani M, et al.: Mitochondrial DNA deletions in progressive external ophthalmoplegia and Kearns-Sayre syndrome. N Engl J Med 320:1293–1299, 1989.
113. Goto Y-i, Koga Y, Horai S, Nonaka I: Chronic progressive external opthalmoplegia: A correlative study of mitochondrial DNA deletions and their phenotypic expression in muscle biopsies. J Neurol Sci 100:63–69, 1990.
114. Gerbitz K-D, Obermaier-Kusser B, Zierz S, et al.: Mitochondrial myopathies: Divergence of genetic deletions, biochemical defects and the clinical syndromes. J Neurol 237:5–10, 1990.
115. Johns DR, Rutledge SL, Stine OC, Hurko O: Directly repeated sequences associated with pathogenic mitochondrial DNA deletions. Proc Natl Acad Sci USA 86:8059–8062, 1989.
116. Johns DR, Hurko O: Preferential amplification and molecular characterization of junction sequences of pathogenetic deletion in human mitochondrial DNA. Genomics 5:623–628, 1989.
117. Schon EA, Rizzuto R, Moraes CT, Nakase H, Zeviani M, DiMauro S: A direct repeat is a hot spot for large-scale deletions of human mitochondrial DNA. Science 244:346–349, 1989.
118. Shoffner JM, Lott MT, Voljavec AS, Soueidan SA, Costigan DA, Wallace DC: Spontaneous Kearns-Sayre? Chronic external ophthalmoplegia plus syndrome associated with a mitochondrial DNA deletion: A slip-replication model and metabolic therapy. Proc Natl Acad Sci USA 86:7952–7956, 1989.
119. Tanaka M, Sato W, Ohno K, Yamamoto T, Ozawa T: Direct sequencing of deleted mitochondrial DNA in myopathic patients. Biochem Biophys Res Commun 164:156–163, 1989.
120. Mita S, Rizzuto R, Moraes CT, et al.: Recombination via flanking direct repeats is a major cause of large-scale deletions of human mitochondrial DNA. Nucleic Acids Res 18:561–567, 1990.
121. Mita S, Schmidt B, Schon EA, DiMauro S, Bonilla E: Detection of "deleted" mitochondrial genomes in cytochrome *c* oxidase–deficient muscle

fibers of a patient with Kearns-Sayre syndrome. Proc Natl Acad Sci USA 86:9509–9513, 1989.

122. Nakase H, Moraes CT, Rizzuto R, Lombes A, DiMauro S, Schon EA: Transcription and translation of deleted mitochondrial genomes in Kearns-Sayre syndrome: Implications for pathogenesis. Am J Hum Genet 46:418–427, 1990.
123. Shoubridge EA, Karpati G, Hastings KEM: Deletion mutants are functionally dominant over wild-type mitochondrial genomes in skeletal muscle fiber segments in mitochondrial disease. Cell 62: 43–49, 1990.
124. Obermaier-Kusser B, Muller-Hocker J, Nelson I, et al.: Different copy numbers of apparently identical deleted mitochondrial DNA in tissue from a patient with Kearns-Sayre syndrome. Biochem Biophys Res Commun 169:1001–1015, 1990.
125. Shanske S, Moraes CT, Lombes A, et al.: Widespread tissue distribution of mitochondrial DNA deletions in Kearns-Sayre syndrome. Neurology 40:24–28, 1990.
126. Poulton J, Deadman ME, Ramacharan S, Gardiner RM: Germ-line deletions of mitochondrial DNA in mitochondrial myopathy. Am J Hum Genet 48:649–653, 1991.
127. Larsson N-G, Eiken HG, Holme E, Oldfors A, Tulinius MH: Lack of transmission of deleted mtDNA from a woman with Kearns-Sayre syndrome to her child. Am J Hum Genet 50:360–363, 1992.
128. Ballinger SW, Shoffner JM, Hedaya EV, et al.: Maternally transmitted diabetes and deafness associated with a 10.4 kb mitochondrial DNA deletion. Nat Genet 1:11–15, 1992.
129. Poulton J, Deadman ME, Gardiner RM: Duplications of mitochondrial DNA in mitochondrial myopathy. Lancet 1:236–240, 1989.
130. Poulton J: Duplications of mitochondrial DNA: Implications for pathogenesis. J Inherit Metab Dis 15: 487–498, 1992.
131. Pearson HA, Lobel JS, Kocoshis SA, et al.: A new syndrome of refractory sideroblastic anemia with vacuolization of bone marrow precursors and exocrine pancreas dysfunction. J Pediatr 95:976–984, 1975.
132. Rotig A, Cormier V, Blanche S, et al.: Pearson's marrow-pancreas syndrome: A multisystem mitochondrial disorder in infancy. J Clin Invest 86: 1601–1608, 1990.
133. Byrne E, Trounce I, DennetT X, et al.: Progression from MERRF to MELAS phenotype in a patient with combined respiratory complex I and IV deficiencies. J Neurol Sci 88:327–338, 1988.
134. Zeviani M, Muntoni F, Savarese N, et al.: A MERRF/MELAS overlap syndrome associated with a new point mutation of mitochondrial DNA tRNALys gene. Eur J Hum Genet 1:25–29, 1993.
135. Campos Y, Martin MA, Lorenzo G, Aparicio M, Cabello A, Arenas J.: Sporadic MERRF/MELAS overlap syndrome associated with the 3243 tRNA Leu(UUR) mutation of mitochondrial DNA. Muscle Nerve 19:187–190, 1996.
136. Nakamura M, Nakano S, Goto Y, et al.: A novel point mutation in the mitochondrial t-RNASer(UCN) gene detected in a family with MERRF/MELAS overlap syndrome. Biochem Biophys Res Commun 214:86–93, 1995.??
137. Zupanc ML, Moraes CT, Shanske S, et al.: Deletion of mitochondrial DNA in patients with combined features of Kearns-Sayre and MELAS syndromes. Ann Neurol 29:680–683, 1991.
138. Truong DD, Harding AE, Scaravilli F, et al.: Movement disorders in mitochondrial myopathies. Mov Disord 5:109–117, 1990.
139. Verma A, Moraes CT, Shebert RT, Bradley WG: A MERRF/PEO overlap syndrome associated with the mitochondrial DNA 3243 mutation. Neurology 46:1334–1336, 1996.
140. Zeviani M, Servidei S, Gerella C, Bertini E, DiMauro S, DiDonato S: An autosomal dominant disorder with multiple deletions of mitochondrial DNA starting at the D-loop region. Nature 339: 309–311, 1989.
141. Suomalainen A, Majander A, Haltia M, et al.: Multiple deletions in mitochondrial DNA in several tissues of a patient with severe retarded depression and familial progressive external ophthalmoplegia. J Clin Invest 90:61–66, 1992.
142. Servidei S, Zeviani M, Manfredi G, et al.: Dominantly inherited mitochondrial myopathy with multiple deletions of mitochondrial DNA: Clinical, morphological and biochemical studies. Neurology 41:1053–1059, 1991.
143. Suomalainen A, Paetau A, Leinonen H, et al.: Inherited idiopathic dilated cardiomyopathy with multiple deletions of mitochondrial DNA. Lancet 340:1319–1320, 1992.
144. Bohlega S, Tanji K, Santorelli SM, et al.: Multiple mitochondrial DNA deletions associated with autosomal recessive ophthalmoplegia and severe cardiomyopathy. Neurology 46:1329–1334, 1996.
145. Bardosi A, Creutzfeldt W, DiMauro S, et al.: Myo-, neuro-, gastrointestinal encephalopathy (MNGIE) syndrome due to partial deficiency of cytochrome-*c*-oxidase. Acta Neuropathol 748:248–258, 1987.
146. Cervera R, Bruix J, Bayes A, et al.: Chronic intestinal pseudo-obstruction and ophthalmoplegia in a patient with mitochondrial myopathy. Gut 29: 544–547, 1988.
147. Johns DR, Threlkeld AB, Miller NR, Hurko O: Multiple mitochondrial DNA deletions in myoneuro-gastrointestinal encephalopathy syndrome. Am J Ophthalmol 115:108–109, 1993.
148. Hirano M, Silvestri G, Blake DM, et al.: Mitochondrial gastrointestinal encephalomyopathy (MNGIE): Clinical, biochemical, and genetic features of an autosomal recessive mitochondrial disorder. Neurology 44: 721–727, 1994.
149. Uncini A, Servidei S, Silvestri G, et al.: Ophthalmoplegia, demyelinating neuropathy, leukoencephalopathy, myopathy and gastrointestinal dysfunction with multiple deletions of mitochondrial DNA: A mitochondrial multisystem disorder in search of a name. Muscle Nerve 17: 667–664, 1994.
150. Nishino I, Spinazzola A, Hirano M: Thymidine phosphorylase gene mutations in MNGIE, a human mitochondrial disorder. Science 283: 689–692, 1999.
151. Casademont J, Barrientos A, Cardellach F, et al.:

Multiple deletions of mtDNA in two brothers with sideroblastic anemia and mitochondrial myopathy and in their asymptomatic mother. Hum Mol Genet 3: 1945–1949, 1994.
152. Ohno K, Tanaka M, Sahashi K, et al.: Mitochondrial DNA deletions in inherited recurrent myoglobinuria. Ann Neurol 29: 364–369, 1991.
153. Oldfors A, Larsson NG, Lindberg C, Holme E: Mitochondrial DNA deletions in inclusion body myositis. Brain 116: 325–336, 1993.
154. Johnston W, Karpati G, Carpenter S, et al.: Late-onset mitochondrial myopathy. Ann Neurol 37: 16–23, 1995.
155. Klopstock T, Naumman M, Schalke B, et al.: Multiple symmetric lipomatosis: Abnormalities in complex IV and multiple deletions in mitochondrial DNA. Neurology 44: 862–866, 1994.
156. Prelle A, Moggio M, Checarelli N, et al.: Multiple deletions of mitochondrial DNA in a patient with periodic attacks of paralysis. J Neurol Sci 117: 24–27, 1993.
157. Barrientos A, Volpini V, Casademont J, et al.: A nuclear defect in the 4p16 region predisposes to multiple mitochondrial DNA deletions in families with Wolfram syndrome. J Clin Invest 97: 1570–1576, 1996.
158. Suomalainen A, Kaukonen J, Amati P, et al.: An autosomal locus predisposing to deletions of mitochondrial DNA. Nat Genet 9: 146–151, 1995.
159. Kaukonen JA, Amati P, Suomalainen A, et al.: An autosomal locus predisposing to multiple deletions of mtDNA on chromosome 3p. Am J Hum Genet 58: 763–769, 1996.
160. Tritschler HJ, Andreetta F, Moraes CT, et al.: Mitochondrial myopathy of childhood associated with depletion of mitochondrial DNA. Neurology 42: 209–217, 1992.
161. Moraes CT, Shanske S, Tritschler H-J, et al.: Mitochondrial DNA deletion with variable tissue expression: A novel genetic abnormality in mitochondrial diseases. Am J Hum Genet 48: 492–501, 1991.
162. Telerman-Toppet N, Biarent D, Bouton J-M, et al.: Fatal cytochrome *c* oxidase–deficient myopathy of infancy associated with mtDNA depletion. Differential involvement of skeletal muscle and cultured fibroblasts. J Inherit Metab Dis 15: 323–326, 1992.
163. Mazziota E, Ricci E, Bertini E, et al.: Fatal liver failure associated with mitochondrial DNA depletion. J Pediatr 121: 896–901, 1992.
164. Bodnar AG, Cooper JM, Holt IJ, Leonard JV, Schapira AHV: Nuclear complementation restores mtDNA levels in cultured cells from a patient with mtDNA deletion. Am J Hum Genet 53: 663–669, 1993.
165. Mariotti C, Uziel G, Carrara F, et al.: Early-onset encephalomyopathy associated with tissue-specific mitochondrial DNA depletion : A morphological, biochemical and molecular-genetic study. J Neurol 242: 547–556, 1996.
166. Dalakas MC, Illa I, Pezeshkpour GH, Laukaitis JP, Cohen B, Griffin JL: Mitochondrial myopathy caused by a long-term zidovudine (AZT) therapy. N Engl J Med 322: 1098–1105, 1990.
167. Mhiri C, Baudrimont M, Bonne G, et al.: Zidovudine myopathy: A distinctive disorder associated with mitochondrial dysfunction. Ann Neurol 29: 606–614, 1991.
168. Lamperth L, Dalakas MC, Dagani F, Anderson J, Ferrari R: Abnormal skeletal and cardiac muscle mitochondria induced by zidovudine (AZT) in human muscle *in vitro* and in animal model. Lab Invest 65: 742–751, 1991.
169. Arnaudo E, Dalakas MC, Shanske S, Moraes CT, DiMauro S, Schon EA: Depletion of muscle mitochondrial DNA in AIDS patients with zidovudine-induced myopathy. Lancet 337: 508–510, 1991.
170. Semino-Mora MC, Leon-Monzon ME, Dalakas MC: Effect of L-carnitine on the zidovudine-induced destruction of human myotubes. Part I: L-carnitine prevents the myotoxicity of AZT *in vitro*. Lab Invest 71: 102–112, 1994
171. Kamieniecka Z: Myopathies with abnormal mitochondria. A clinical, histological, and electrophysiological study. Acta Neurol Scand 55: 57–75, 1977.
172. McLeod JG, Baker W, Shorey CD, et al.: Mitochondrial myopathy with multisystem abnormalities and normal ocular movements. J Neurol Sci 24: 39–52, 1975.
173. Egger J, Lake BD, Wilson J: Mytochondrial cytopathy. A multisystem disorder with ragged red fiber in muscle biopsy. Arch Dis Child 56: 741–752, 1981.
174. Tanabe Y, Miyamoto S, Kinoshita Y, et al.: Diabetes mellitus in Kearns-Sayre syndrome. Eur Neurol 28: 34–38, 1988.
175. Gerbitz K-D: Does the mitochondrial DNA play a role in the pathogenesis of diabetes? Diabetologia 35: 1181–1186, 1992.
176. Quade A, Zierz S, Klingmuller D: Endocrine abnormalities in mitochondrial myopathy with external ophthalmoplegia. Clin Invest 70: 396–702, 1992.
177. Dorner G, Mohnike A: Further evidence for predominantly maternal transmission of maturity-onset type diabetes. Endokrinologie 68: 121–124, 1976.
178. Martin AO, Simpson JL, Ober C, Freinkel N: Frequency of diabetes mellitus in mothers of probands with gestational diabetes: A possible maternal influence on the predisposition to gestational diabetes. Am J Obstet Gynecol 151: 471–475, 1985.
179. Alcolado JC, Alcolado R: Importance of maternal history of non-insulin dependent diabetic patients. Br Med J 302: 1178–1180, 1991.
180. Thomas F, Balkau B, Vauzelle-Kervroedan F, Papoz L: The CODIAB-INSERM-ZENECA group. Maternal effect and familial aggregation in NIDDM. Diabetes 43: 63–67, 1994.
181. Onishi H, Inoue K, Osaka H, et al.: Mitochondrial myopathy, encephalopathy, lactic acidosis and stroke-like episodes (MELAS) and diabetes mellitus: Molecular genetic analysis and family study. J Neurol Sci 114: 205–208, 1993.
182. Gerbitz KD, Paprotta A, Jaksch M, Zierz S, Dreschel J: Diabetes mellitus is one of the heterogeneous phenotypic features of a mitochondrial

DNA point mutation within the tRNALeu(UUR) gene. FEBS Lett 321: 194–198, 1993.
183. Sue CM, Holmes Walker DJ, Morris JG, Boyages SC, Crimmins DS, Byrne E: Mitochondrial gene mutation and diabetes mellitus. Lancet 341:347–348, 1993.
184. Schulz JB, Klockgether T, Dichgans J, Seibel P, Reichmann H: Mitochondrial gene mutation and diabetes mellitus. Lancet 341:348–349, 1993.
185. Kadowaki T, Kadowaki H, Mori Y, et al.: A subtype of diabetes mellitus associated with a mutation of mitochondrial DNA. N Engl J Med 330:962–968, 1994.
186. Gerbitz K-D, van den Ouweland JMW, Maassen JA, Jaksch M: Mitochondrial diabetes mellitus: A review. Biochim Biophys Acta 1271:253–260, 1995.
187. Bundey S, Poulton K, Whitwell H, Curtis E, Brown IAR, Fielder AR: Mitochondrial abnormalities in the DIDMOAD syndrome. J Inherit Metab Dis 15: 315–319, 1992.
188. Rotig A, Cormier V, Chatelain P, et al.: Deletion of mitochondrial DNA in a case of early-onset diabetes mellitus, optic atrophy, and deafness (Wolfram syndrome, MIM 222300). J Clin Invest 91: 1095–1098, 1993.
189. Pilz D, Quarell OWJ, Jones EW: Mitochondrial mutation commonly associated with Leber's hereditary optic neuropathy in a patient with Wolfram syndrome (DIDMOAD). J Med Genet 31:328–330, 1994.
190. Kishimoto M, Hashiramoto M, Araki S, et al.: Diabetes mellitus carrying a mutation in the mitochondrial tRNA(Leu(UUR)) gene. Diabetologia 38:193–200, 1995.
191. Velho G, Byrne MM, Clement K, et al.: Clinical phenotypes, insulin secretion, and insulin sensitivity in kindreds with maternally inherited diabetes and deafness due to mitochondrial t-RNALeu (UUR) gene mutation. Diabetes 45:478–487, 1996.
192. Ballinger SW, Shoffner JM, Gebhart S, Koontz DA, Wallace DC: Mitochondrial diabetes revisited. Nat Genet 7:458–459, 1994.
193. Schapira AHV, Mann VM, Cooper JM, et al.: Anatomic and disease specificity of NADH CoQ1 reductase (complex I) deficiency in Parkinson's disease. J Neurochem 55:2142–2145, 1990.
194. Mann VM, Cooper JM, Krige D, Daniel SE, Shapira AHV, Marsden CD: Brain, skeletal muscle and platelet homogenate mitochondrial function in Parkinson's disease. Brain 115:333–342, 1992.
195. Janetnky B, Hauck S, Youdim MBH, et al.: Unaltered aconitase, but decreased complex I activity in subtantia nigra pars compacta of patients with Parkinson's disease. Neurosci Lett 169:126–128, 1994.
196. Hattori N, Tanaka M, Ozawa T, Mizuno Y: Immunohistochemical studies on complexes I, II, III, and IV of mitochondria in Parkinson's disease. Ann Neurol 30:563–571, 1991.
197. Nicklas WJ, Vyas I, Heikkila RE: Inhibition of NADH-linked oxidation in brain mitochondria by MPP+, a metabolite of neurotoxin MTPT. Life Sci 36:2503–2508, 1985.
198. Mizuno Y, Suzuki K, Sone N, Saitoh T: Inhibition of mitochondrial respiration by MPTP in mouse brain *in vivo*. Neurosci Lett 91:349–353, 1988.
199. Parker WD, Boyson SJ, Parks JK: Abnormalities of the electron transport chain in idiopathic Parkinson's disease. Ann Neurol 26:719–723, 1989.
200. Krige D, Carroll MT, Cooper JM, Marsden CD, Schapira AHV: Platelet mitochondrial function in Parkinson's disease. Ann Neurol 32:782–788, 1992.
201. Benecke R, Strumper P, Weiss H: Electron transfer complexes I and IV of platelets are abnormal in Parkinson's disease but normal in Parkinson-plus syndromes. Brain 116:1451–1463, 1993.
202. Wallace DC, Schoffner JM, Watts RL, Juncos JL, Torrino A: Mitochondrial oxidative phosphorylation defects in Parkinson's disease. Ann Neurol 32:113–114, 1992.
203. Hattori YN, Yoshino H, Kondo T, Mizuno Y, Horai S: Is Parkinson's disease a mitochondrial disorder? J Neurol Sci 10:29–33, 1992.
204. DiDonato S, Zeviani M, Giovannini P, et al.: Respiratory chain and mitochondrial DNA in muscle and brain in Parkinson's disease patients. Neurology 43:2262–2268, 1993.
205. Ozawa T, Tanaka M, Ikebe S, Ohno K, Kondo T, Mizuno Y: Quantitative determination of deleted mitochondrial DNA relative to normal DNA in parkinsonian striatum by a kinetic PCR analysis. Biochem Biophys Res Commun 172:483–489, 1990.
206. Mann VM, Cooper JM, Schapira AHV: Quantitation of a mitochondrial DNA deletion in Parkinson's disease. FEBS Lett 299:218–222, 1992.
207. Shoffner JM, Brown MD, Torroni A, et al.: Mitochondrial DNA mutations associated with Alzheimer's and Parkinson's disease. Genomics 17:171–184, 1993.
208. Perry EK, Perry RH, Tomlinson BE: Coenzyme-A acetylating enzymes in Alzheimer disease: Possible cholinergic "compartment" of pyruvate dehydrogenase. Neurosci Lett 18:105–110, 1980.
209. Sorbi S, Bird ED, Blass JP: Decreased pyruvate dehydrogenase complex activity in Huntington and Alzheimer brain. Ann Neurol 13:72–78, 1983.
210. Haxby JV, Grady CL, Duara R, Schlageter N, Berg G, Rapoport SI: Neocortical metabolic abnormalities precede non-memory cognitive deficits in early Alzheimer-type dementia. Arch Neurol 43: 882–885, 1986.
211. Duara R, Grady C, Haxby J, et al.: Positron emission tomography in Alzheimer's disease. Neurology 36:879–887, 1986.
212. Mecocci P, MacGarvey U, Beal MF: Oxidative damage to mitochondrial DNA is increased in Alzheimer's disease. Ann Neurol 36:747–751, 1994.
213. Kish SJ, Bergeron C, Rajput A, et al.: Brain cytochrome oxidase in Alzheimer's disease. J Neurochem 59:776–779, 1992.
214. Parker WD, Parks J, Filley CM, Kleinschmidt-DeMasters BK: Electron transport chain defects in Alzheimer's disease brain. Neurology 44:1090–1096, 1994.
215. Mutisya EM, Bowling AC, Beal MF: Cortical cytochrome oxidase activity is reduced in Alzheimer's disease. J Neurochem 63:2179–2184, 1994.
216. Simonian NA, Hyman BT: Functional alterations

in Alzheimer's disease: Diminution of cytochrome oxidase in hippocampal formation. J Neuropathol Exp Neurol 52:580–585, 1993.

217. Chandrasekaran K, Giordano T, Brady DR, Stoll J, Martin LJ, Rapoport SI: Impairment in mitochondrial cytochrome oxidase gene expression in Alzheimer disease. Mol Brain Res 24:336–340, 1994.

218. Parker WDJr, Filley CM, Parks JK: Cytochrome oxidase deficiency in Alzheimer's disease. Neurology 40:1302–1303, 1990.

219. Gabuzda D, Busciglio J, Chen LB, Matsudaira P, Yankner BA: Inhibition of energy metabolism alters the processing of amyloid precursor protein and induces a potentially amyloidogenic derivative. J Biol Chem 269:13623–13628, 1994.

220. Corral-Debrinski M, Horton T, Lott MT, et al.: Marked changes in mitochondrial DNA deletion levels in Alzheimer brains. Genomics 23:471–476, 1994.

221. Hutchin T, Cortopassi G: A mitochondrial DNA clone is associated with increased risk for Alzheimer disease. Proc Natl Acad Sci USA 92:6892–6895, 1995.

222. Gu M, Gash MT, Mann VM, Javoy-Agid F, Cooper JM, Schapira AH: Mitochondrial defect in Huntington's disease caudate nucleus. Ann Neurol 39:385–389, 1996.

223. Horton TM, Graham BH, Corral-Debrinski M, et al.: Marked increase in mitochondrial DNA deletion levels in the cerebral cortex of Huntington's disease patients. Neurology 45: 1879–1883, 1995.

224. Chen X, Bonilla E, Sciacco M, Schon EA: Paucity of deleted mitochondrial DNAs in brain regions of Huntington's disease patients. Biochim Biophys Acta 1271:229–233, 1995.

225. Matthews PM, Tampieri D, Berkovic SF, Andermann F, Silver K, Chityat D, Arnold DL: Magnetic resonance imaging shows specific abnormalities in the MELAS syndrome. Neurology 41:1043–1046, 1991.

Chapter 16

# ALZHEIMER'S DISEASE: GENETIC FACTORS

Ephrat Levy-Lahad, MD
Thomas D. Bird, MD



Alzheimer's disease (AD) is a clinicopathological entity. Clinically, there is a slowly progressive dementia with memory loss lasting a period of several years. Pathologically, there is diffuse cerebral atrophy associated microscopically with Aβ amyloid neuritic plaques, silver-staining neurofibrillary tangles (NFTs), and amyloid angiopathy of cerebral blood vessels (Fig. 16–1). The most important risk factor for AD is age. Approximately 10% of the U.S. and European population over the age of 70 years has dementia, and more than half of these cases are AD. Perhaps 20% to 40% of the population over the age of 85 years has clinically significant dementia.[1,2]

The second most important risk factor for AD is family history. This observation led to a more detailed study of genetic factors in AD and the following three phenomena became apparent: First, epidemiological studies revealed that the presence of an affected first-degree relative with AD is associated with an approximately fourfold increased risk for the disease and a total lifetime risk of 23% to 48%.[3–5] In some studies the lifetime risk for first-degree relatives of AD patients approached 50%. This is especially true if more than one generation is affected and there is early onset of disease (before age 60 to 65 years).[6,7] Second, in rare families AD has occurred in numerous persons over multiple generations, compatible with a single-gene autosomal dominant trait (Fig. 16–2).[8–14] Third, essentially all persons with trisomy 21 (Down syndrome) who survive beyond the age of 40 years invariably show the neuropathological characteristics of AD.[15,16] These three findings led to the hypotheses that genetic factors were important in AD, that AD might be caused by a single dominant gene in some families, and an important genetic factor for AD lies on chromosomes 21. All three of these hypotheses have proven to be true and are reviewed in this chapter.

## FAMILIAL ALZHEIMER'S DISEASE

There is no universally accepted definition of familial Alzheimer's disease (FAD).[17] A typical working definition of FAD is the

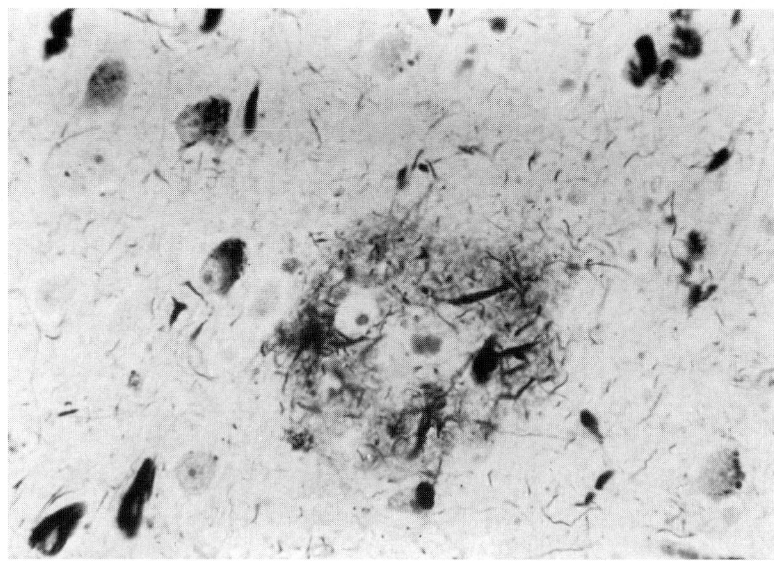

Figure 16–1. Neuritic plaque and neurofibrillary tangle formation in the cerebral cortex of a 73-year-old woman dying with late onset familial Alzheimer's disease. There were four affected individuals in her family, with a mean age of onset of 69 years and mean age at death of 81 years. Bielshowsky stain. (Courtesy S. M. Sumi.)

presence of three or more affected persons in more than one generation with autopsy-documented features in at least one individual. Some families have a dozen or more persons with dementia in three or more generations, and more than 100 such families have been reported (Fig. 16–2).[8–14] Clinically the affected individuals have progressive dementia that is indistinguishable from typical nonfamilial or sporadic AD. In addition to memory loss, the dementing illness may or may not include language disturbance, rigidity and parkinsonian features, seizures, and myoclonus.

Disease duration is usually 6 to 10 years, with a broad range of 2 to more than 20 years. Familial AD is frequently divided into early and late onset categories with 60 to 65 years

**L Family**

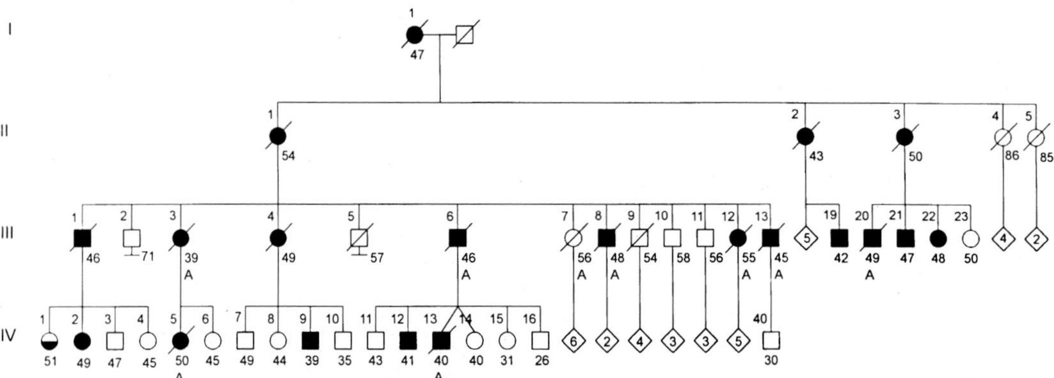


Figure 16–2. Pedigree of a family with autosomal dominant, early onset, familial Alzheimer's disease. The disease is autopsy documented (A). This family has a mutation in the presenilin 1 gene on chromosome 14. Mean age of onset is 41 years, and mean age at death is 47 years. Ages in the figure are present age or age at death. The family is described in greater detail by Lampe et al.[60] (From Bird et al.[157])

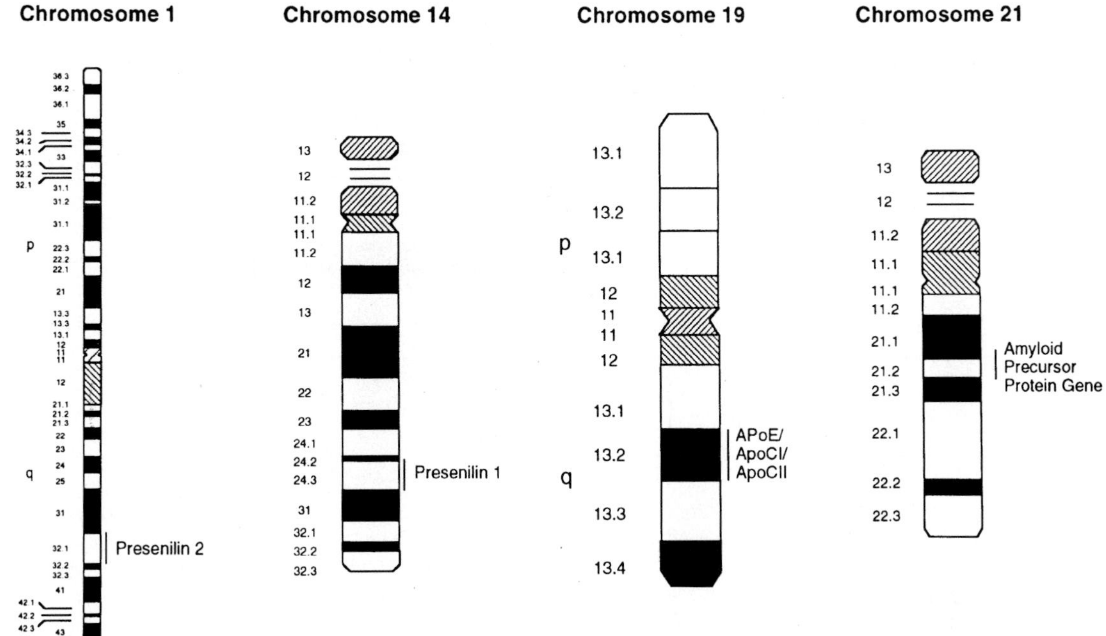


**Figure 16–3.** Four different genes have been documented to play a role in various types of Alzheimer's disease. They are the presenilin 2 gene on chromosome 1, the presenilin 1 gene on chromosome 14, the Apolipoprotein E gene on chromosome 19, and the amyloid precursor protein gene on chromosome 21. (From Levy-Lahad and Bird.[158])

somewhat arbitrarily as the dividing line. This age of onset phenomenon has proven to have some biologic relevance. Thus far, FAD has been shown to be caused by three different genes and influenced by a specific genetic risk factor. The three genes are the amyloid precursor protein gene *(APP)* on chromosome 21, the presenilin 1 *(PS-1)* gene on chromosome 14, and the presenilin 2 *(PS-2)* gene on chromosome 1 (Fig. 16–3). The risk factor is the Apolipoprotein E *(Apoe)* gene on chromosome 19.

## AMYLOID PRECURSOR PROTEIN GENE

The *APP* gene maps to the long arm of chromosome 21. This suggests that overexpression of APP plays a role in the association of AD neuropathology with trisomy 21 (Fig. 16–3). The *APP* gene encodes for a 695 to 770 amino acid precursor protein that is proteolytically cleaved to form Aβ amyloid. Aβ is a 39 to 43 amino acid peptide that is the major component of the amyloid neuritic plaque, one of the neuropathological hallmarks of AD. The *APP* gene has 19 exons, and Aβ is encoded by parts of exons 16 and 17.[18–20]

In 1990, it was discovered that a substitution of glutamine for glutamic acid at codon 693 of *APP* causes the rare condition of cerebral hemorrhagic amyloidosis of the Dutch type.[21] This finding led to a concerted effort to search for *APP* mutations in FAD. In 1991, two such families were discovered with isoleucine substituted for valine at codon 717 (Fig. 16–4).[22] Subsequently more than 20 different families have been discovered to have *APP* gene mutations as the cause of FAD.[23–27] The valine/isoleucine substitution at codon 717 is the most common mutation, but phenylalanine and glycine substitutions at the same position have been reported, as has a double mutation at codon 670 to 671 (the Swedish mutation).[28–30] Figure 16–4 demonstrates that early onset FAD can be caused by *APP* mutations flanking the Aβ sequence,

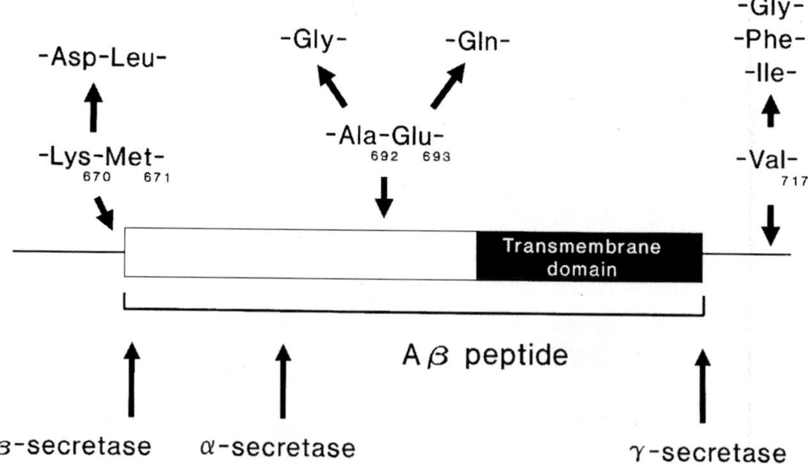


**Figure 16–4.** Schematic diagram of a portion of the amyloid precursor protein (coded by the APP gene on chromosome 21) showing the region of the Aβ peptide and the sites of action of α-, β-, and γ-secretases. Sites of mutations resulting in early onset FAD are also indicated. The most common mutation is substitution of isoleucine for valine at position 717. (From Levy-Lahad and Bird.[157])

whereas mutations within the Aβ sequence result in cerebral hemorrhage with vascular amyloidosis with or without dementia. A mutation at codon 716 has also been reported in a single family.[30a]

*APP* mutations are a very rare cause of early onset FAD (in itself quite rare), accounting for probably not more than 5% of published early onset FAD pedigrees. There is no evidence of linkage of late onset FAD to chromosome 21 markers, and *APP* mutations have not been found in late onset FAD or truly sporadic AD cases.[31,32] It is assumed that the extra copy of chromosome 21 containing the *APP* gene is the cause of AD neuropathology in Down syndrome resulting from the slow cerebral accumulation of Aβ peptide over a period of decades (Fig. 16–5 and 32a).

Clinically, *APP* mutations result in early onset AD. The inheritance pattern is autosomal dominant, and penetrance is essentially complete by the early 60s. The oldest reported unaffected carrier of an *APP* mutation is 67 years old. In the Val717Ile mutation, age of onset ranges from 41 to 64 years, with a typical mean age of onset of about 50 years.[22–27] Mean age of onset is 59 years in the Val717Gly kindred,[29] 43 years in the Val717Phe kindred,[28] and 55 years in the Swedish double mutation family.[30] Furthermore, persons with Down syndrome may develop a progressive dementing illness after the age of 40 years in addition to their baseline mental retardation.[33,34]

The fact that *APP* mutations are sufficient to cause AD implicates the Aβ peptide as a critical pathogenetic factor in at least some forms of AD. Furthermore, a mouse model that mimics the neuropathology of AD has been produced by overexpression of an *APP* construct with or without the Val717Phe mutation.[35,36] The location of the known *APP* mutations underlying FAD suggest that aberrant APP processing may underlie AD in these families.

Two proteolytic pathways for APP processing have been shown to occur normally (Fig. 16–4). The first is cleavage within the Aβ sequence by an unidentified protease referred as α-secretase.[37] Aβ is destroyed by this cleavage, meaning that this pathway does not contribute to Aβ formation. The second is cleavage on either side of the Aβ sequence by unidentified proteases referred to as β- and γ-secretase. These two cleavages result in production of the full Aβ peptide. Cleavage by the β- and γ-secretases occurs normally and not just in the disease state.[38,39]

Because *APP* mutations flank or occur within the Aβ sequence, they are assumed to influence APP proteolysis. Support for this hypothesis comes from the finding that

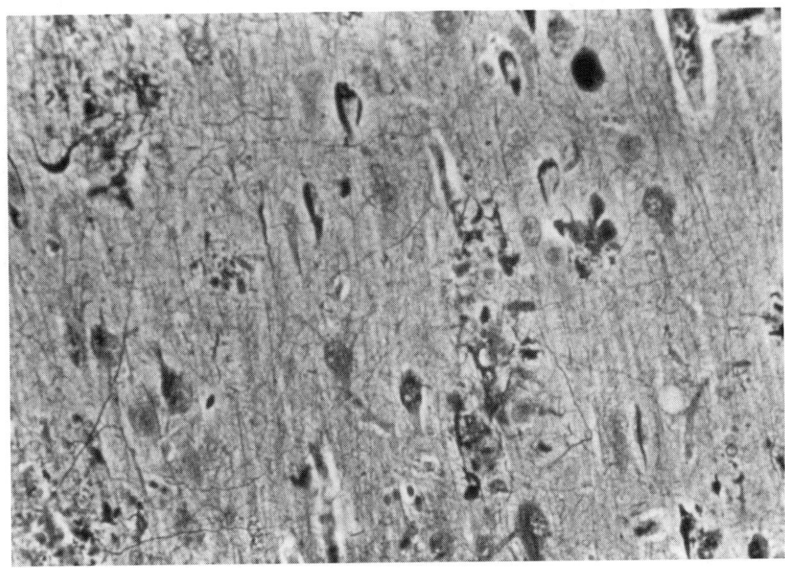

**Figure 16–5.** Neuritic plaques and neurofibrillary tangles in the cortex of a 49-year-old female with trisomy 21 Down syndrome dying after a 2-year course of severe progressive dementia. Bielskowsky stain. (Courtesy S. M. Sumi.)

cultured fibroblasts from both affected and presymptomatic carriers of the Swedish mutation also secrete an increased amount of Aβ peptide.[40] In transfection experiments with *APP* having the Val717Ile and Val717Phe mutations, total Aβ production was not increased, but there was a relative increase of long (42 amino acid) versus short (40 amino acid) Aβ.[41,42] The longer Aβ peptides form fibrils more rapidly than the shorter form and are assumed to be more deleterious.[43]

## THE PRESENILIN 1 GENE ON CHROMOSOME 14

Genetic linkage of early onset FAD to a chromosome 14 locus was established in 1992 and quickly confirmed in many of the previously published early onset FAD kindreds.[44–47] The gene (also designated *S182*) was subsequently identified, cloned, and named presenilin 1 (*PS-1*)[48] This gene is predicted to encode a 467 amino acid protein with 7 to 10 hydrophobic transmembrane domains (Fig. 16–6). The coding region of *PS-1* is composed of 10 exons numbered 3 through 12. Alternative splicing may result in shorter isoforms of the protein.

More than 40 separate mutations in more than 50 families have been described. The families are from a variety of ethnic backgrounds, including Caucasian, Japanese, Jewish, and Hispanic.[49–59,71] Thus far, most mutations are missense, that is, they result in a single amino acid substitution rather than in premature termination of the code and a truncated protein. This suggests that *PS-1* mutations may cause AD by a change or gain in protein function rather than by a loss of function. More than nine mutations have been found in the last hydrophilic loop. The relative frequency of mutations in the sixth hydrophilic domain/loop, which is encoded by the alternatively spliced exon 8, suggests that this region of the protein is functionally important.

Of the three genes known to cause FAD, the *PS-1* mutations are associated with the earliest age of onset and most progressive disease (Fig. 16–2).[9,10,12–14, 49–61] Mean ages of onset in *PS-1* FAD pedigrees range from 35 to 55 years. Within each kindred, the age of onset is relatively narrow, for example, 44.8 ± 4.8 years in our series. Onset as early as age 26 years has occurred in one family.[14] The *PS-1* clinical phenotype is usually char-

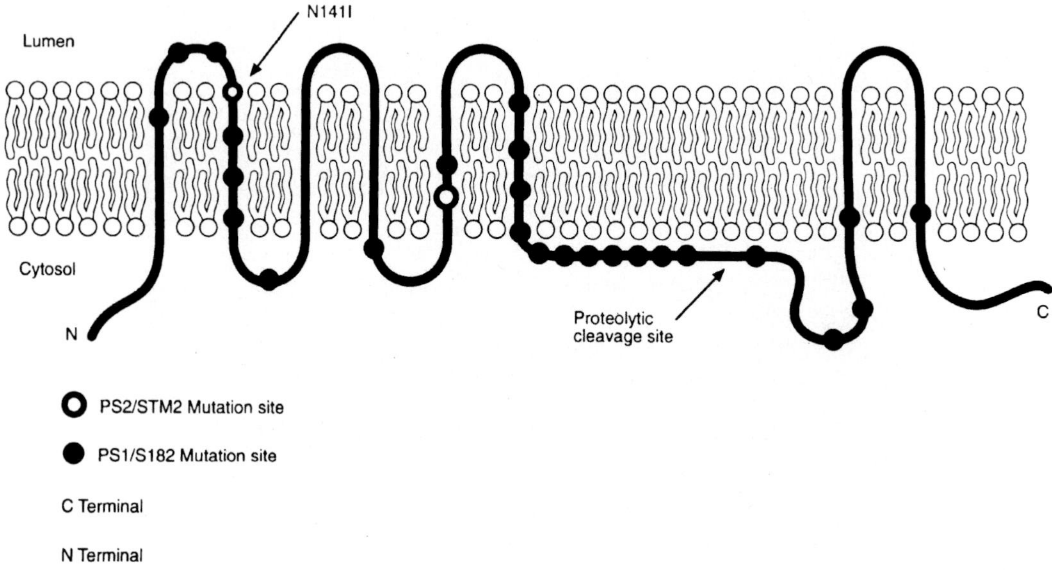


**Figure 16–6.** Schematic diagram of the proteins encoded by the presenilin 1 and presenilin 2 genes. The putative eight-transmembrane domains are indicated. Also shown are locations of many of the known mutations associated with early onset familial Alzheimer's disease. Closed circles are presenilin 1 mutations (chromosome 14 gene), and open circles are presenilin 2 mutations (chromosome 1 gene). The N141I mutation occurs in the Volga German families with FAD.

acterized by severe dementia associated with language disturbance and myoclonus that appear relatively early in the disease course as well as a high frequency of generalized seizures and extrapyramidal signs.[60] Disease duration is usually short (5.8 to 6.8 years). Penetrance appears to be nearly complete by age 65 years.

Neuropathologic characteristics include Aβ plaques, NFTs, and amyloid angiopathy typical of sporadic AD (Fig. 16–5).[9,10,12–14,58] There is increased deposition of $A\beta_{1-42}$ amyloid in the brains of patients with *PS-1* mutations.[62] A few families with *PS-1* mutations have been described with initial spastic paraparesis associated with large "cotton wool" amyloid plaques.[63]

## THE PRESENILIN 2/ CHROMOSOME 1 GENE

The third AD gene was discovered by evaluating a group of FAD families with Volga German (VG) ancestry.[64,65] The VG are ethnic Germans who migrated to Russia in the 1760s during the reign of Catherine the Great and remained distinct from the surrounding Russian population. Many of this group subsequently immigrated to the United States between 1880 and 1920, settling in the Great Plains and the Far West. Eight families originating from the same two VG villages were found to have FAD presumably on the basis of a genetic founder effect (a single common affected ancestor).

Linkage analysis demonstrated that AD in these kindreds was linked to a region on the long arm of chromosome 1.[66] The analysis was complicated by the occurrence of phenocopies in these families, that is, persons with the AD phenotype who actually had sporadic AD rather than the inherited genetic mutation. The chromosome 1 FAD gene was cloned by virtue of its homology to *PS-1* and has been named *PS-2*.[67,68] It was also called *STM-2* for seven-transmembrane domains, although the exact number of transmembrane domains remains uncertain. *PS-2* is predicted to encode a 448 amino acid protein that is 67% identical to *PS-1* (Fig. 16–4). The greatest identity (84%) is within the hydrophobic/transmembrane domains. The *PS-2* gene is composed of 12 exons (two are noncoding).

The genomic organizations of *PS-1* and *PS-2* are strikingly similar, suggesting that they arose by duplication.[69] The regions of greatest divergence between the two genes are the two largest hydrophilic loops (the first N-terminal loop and the loop between the sixth and seventh transmembrane domains). These regions probably define functional specificity.[69,70]

Thus far, only four FAD mutations in the *PS-2* gene have been discovered. One of these mutations was found in the VG pedigrees, one in an Italian family, and one each in a Belgian and a Spanish patient.[67,68,71 71a] A single mutation (N141I) occurs in all the VG pedigrees, consistent with the founder effect hypothesis. Similar to *PS-1, PS-2* mutations are also missense.

Clinical features associated with *PS-2* mutations have been reported primarily in the VG. Mean age of onset in the N141 I mutation carriers is 54.9 ± 8.5 years, significantly greater than in most *PS-1* pedigrees.[64,65,72] Mean disease duration in the VG *PS-2* individuals is 7.6 ± 3.2 years, significantly longer than that in most *PS-1* families, which reflects a somewhat less malignant character of *PS-2*–associated FAD. The VG *PS-2* families show a strikingly wide variation in age of onset (40 to 75 years) in individuals who carry an identical mutation (N141I). There have also been a few cases of nonpenetrance over the age of 80 years (Fig. 16–7).[65] Thus, although penetrance is high (>95%), it is not complete and is quite variable in terms of age of onset. *PS-2* mutations seem to be unique among early onset FAD mutations in that they can result in disease onset over the age of 70 years. The dementia in the VG families is not different from that in sporadic AD, and the neuropathological characteristics include Aβ neuritic plaques, NFTs, and amyloid angiopathy.[72,73] One instance of late onset dementia associated primarily with cerebral amyloid angiopathy has been noted in a VG patient.[74]

## FREQUENCY OF PS-1 AND PS-2 MUTATIONS

Early onset autosomal dominant FAD accounts for only a small proportion of all AD (<5%). Thus, *PS-1* and *PS-2* FAD mutations are a very rare cause of AD in the general population. *PS-1* mutations are thought to be responsible for about 20% to 70% of early onset FAD. *PS-2* mutations have been discovered thus far in only four families. *PS-1* and *PS-2* mutations have not been reported in persons with documented sporadic AD, but it is possible that less deleterious mutations or polymorphisms in these genes are relevant to late onset AD.[67,72,73,75] A possible example is the reported association between an intronic polymorphism in the *PS-1* gene and late onset AD.[76] In a series of late onset AD cases (about half with a family history of AD), homozygosity for allele 1 of this polymorphism was associated with a doubling of the risk for AD. In contrast to the dominant inheritance of other AD mutations, this polymorphism is a recessive risk factor. Its exact role in AD remains to be determined and confirmed.[76a]

## *PS-1* AND *PS-2* GENES IN THE PATHOGENESIS OF ALZHEIMER'S DISEASE

The PS-1 and PS-2 presenilin proteins are assumed to have similar functions because of their high homology. Both genes are expressed ubiquitously and, within the brain, expression is almost entirely neuronal.[48,67,73] By *in situ* hybridization both presenilins have been localized to intracellular membranes, presumably Golgi and endoplasmic reticulum.[77] The presenilins may be involved in intracellular trafficking of APP which is normally processed in the Golgi apparatus. PS-1 and PS-2 are homologous to two *Caenorhabditis elegans* genes: *Sel-12* and *Spe-4*. *Sel-12* is a modulator of a notch-like pathway involved in cell–cell recognition, possibly by influencing receptor localization.[78] *Spe-4* is involved in cytoplasmic protein partitioning during spermatogenesis.[79] Knock-out of the *PS-1* gene in mice produces an embryonic lethal with skeletal deformaties.[80] Neuronal cultures derived from PS-1 knock-out mouse embryos show lack of cleavage of APP by γ-secretase and a decrease in Aβ amyloid production, suggest-

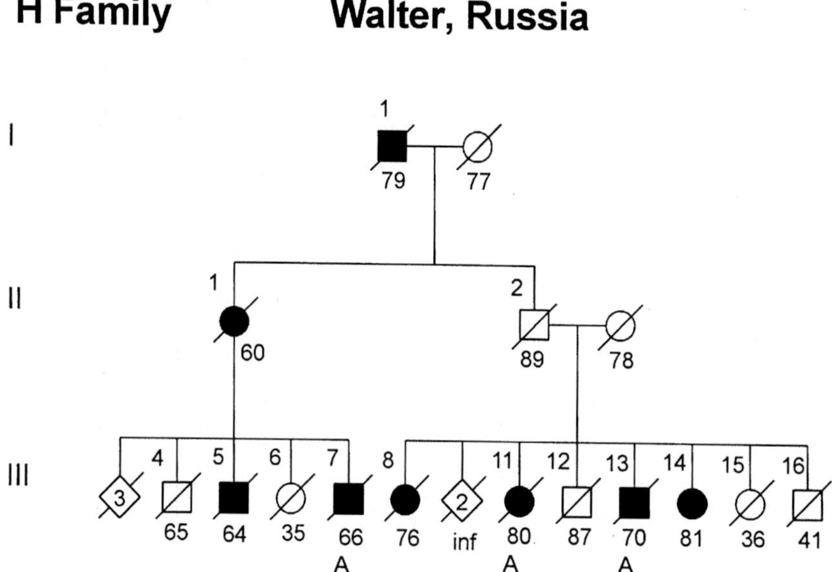


**Figure 16–7.** Pedigree of a Volga German family with familial Alzheimer's disease and a known mutation in the presenilin 2 gene (N141 I). Mean age of onset in this family is 59 years, and mean age at death is 71 years. Individual II-2 survived to age 89 without dementia but must have been a carrier of the PS2 gene mutation. This is an uncommon example of lack of penetrance of this gene over the age of 80 years. This family also demonstrates that both early (III-7, 56 years) and late (III-14, 68 years) onset of AD can be found with PS2 mutations. Ages in the figure are present age or age at death.

ing that the normal function of PS-1 is to promote cleavage of the membrane domain of APP, and *PS-1* mutations may result in a gain of this function.[81] There is evidence that PS1 may function as the gamma secretase that cleaves APP.[81a,81b] Also, accelerated brain amyloid deposition occurs in mice coexpressing mutant *PS-1* and *APP* genes.[82] Subjects with *PS-1* or *PS-2* mutations have an increase in fibroblast production and plasma levels of $A\beta_{1-42,1-43}$, the long amyloidogenic form of Aβ.[83,84] FAD mutations in both *PS-1* and *PS-2* do not seem to grossly alter their subcellular localization.

In a murine cellular model of apoptosis, the murine homologue of *PS-2* was identified as a gene that inhibits apoptosis.[85] It is possible that the alteration of the normal function of *PS-2* and possibly *PS-1* may result in increased neuronal apoptosis. Because all known FAD mutations are inherited as autosomal dominant conditions and all but one are missense mutations, AD may result from an alteration in the functions encoded by these genes rather than from a loss of their normal function.

## GENETIC COUNSELING OF AUTOSOMAL DOMINANT FAD KINDREDS

Genetic counseling of families with *APP,PS-1*, and *PS-2* mutations is similar to that for other severe, autosomal dominant, neurogenetic disorders such as Huntington's disease, familial amyotrophic lateral sclerosis, and the hereditary ataxias.[86] Mutations are known in each of these conditions, and direct DNA testing is possible. Each child of an affected person is at 50% risk for inheriting the disease gene and expressing the disease if the individual lives long enough. Age of onset and penetrance characteristics must be taken into consideration. Presymptomatic *APP* mutation testing has been done in a few families on a research basis.[87] DNA tests for *PS-1* mutations (but not APP or *PS-2*) are commercially available. *PS-1* mutations are only likely to be found in patients with early onset AD (<60 years) and a positive family history of early onset dementia. Such testing is complex and includes numerous clinical, psychological, financial, and ethical as well as genetic issues.[86] This testing should be done in the context of experienced professional genetic counseling (see Chapter 22).

## APOLIPOPROTEIN E

The ε4 allele of ApoE has been identified as an important risk factor for AD. The gene for ApoE is on the long arm of chromosome 19 (Fig. 16–2). The ApoE gene has polymorphisms that consist of a single base pair change at codons 112 and 158 that result in three isoforms of the ApoE protein: E2, E3, and E4. Individuals may be heterozygous or homozygous for these alleles. ApoE mediates the binding of lipoproteins to receptors and is involved in lipid transport, and the ε4 allele has been known to be a risk factor for coronary artery disease.[88] An association was found between AD and a polymorphism of the ApoC2 gene, which is adjacent to the ApoE gene on chromosome 19.[89,90] Genetic linkage analysis suggested positive linkage of chromosome 19 markers with late onset FAD.[91] There was then discovered to be a strong association between AD and the ApoE ε4 allele in late onset FAD pedigrees.[92–94] The ε4 allele frequency was 0.52 in affected persons compared with 0.16 in controls. This association of ε4 with late onset AD was rapidly confirmed in many studies, including familial samples,[93,94] AD autopsy cases,[94,97] clinic-based subjects, and community-based cases, including both familial and sporadic AD.[100–106] The ApoE association has also been shown to exist in early onset AD cases with a positive family history (see Table 16–1).[103,104]

The main limitation of association studies is that they do not prove causation. Many aspects of the ApoE–AD association, however, have been extensively investigated and are suggestive of a direct biological role of ApoE in the pathogenesis of AD.

The AD risk associated with ApoE seems to be dose dependent. Compared with the common 3/3 ApoE genotype, odds ratios range from 2.8 to 4.4 for persons with one ε4 allele and from 7.0 to 19.3 for persons with two ε4 alleles (homozygotes).[92,99,100] Each ε4 allele has been shown to lower age of onset by 7 to 9 years in late onset FAD families and by 3 to 7 years in nonfamilial AD. Some studies suggest a different dose effect in males and females.[105,106] In females, one ε4 allele is sufficient to reduce age of onset without further reduction in the presence of a second ε4 allele, whereas in males only 4/4 homozygotes have a younger age of onset. This finding, however, has not been consistent in all studies.[107] ApoE 4/4 homozygotes may also have an accelerated decline in cognitive function.[107a]

A reduced frequency of the ApoE ε2 allele in late onset AD subjects has been observed in some studies.[108–111] This is compatible with the ε2 allele having a protective affect against AD. The 2/2 genotype is rare so most of the evidence for a protective affect comes from persons with the 2/3 genotype. The possible ε2 protective affect has not been found in African Americans or confirmed in all studies.[112–114] Also, the 2/4 genotype seems to impart little or no risk for AD compared with the association with the 3/4 and 4/4 genotypes. Therefore, the relationship between ApoE ε2 and AD remains uncertain.

The ApoE ε4 allele association with AD has been observed in several ethnic groups, including Caucasians, Japanese, and Hispanics. A possible exception are African Americans, but further investigation is required.[113,115] The ε4 allele appears to increase the likelihood of clinical dementia in patients with Down syndrome, especially males.[116]

ApoE interactions have also been evaluated in FAD kindreds with *APP, PS-1,* and *PS-2* mutations. *APP* mutation families are rare, so the data is based on a small number of subjects. In the Swedish mutation *APP670/671* family and in nine pedigrees with *APP717* mutations, the presence of ε4 appears to lower age of onset.[117–121] This does not appear to be the case in the cerebral amyloidosis of the Dutch-type pedigree (*APP693* mutation).[122] In addition, one group has found no association between ApoE 4 and dementia in Down syndrome, whereas another group has reported such an association.[116,123,124] In *PS-1* mutation pedigrees, ApoE genotype has not been found to influence age of onset.[125,126] This

Table 16–1. **Apolipoprotein E (ApoE) Genotyping in Alzheimer's Disease (AD)***

| ApoE | Controls (n = 304) | AD (n = 233) | AD (+ Family History) (n = 85) |
|---|---|---|---|
| 2/2 | 1.3% | 0.0% | 0.0% |
| 2/3 | 12.5 | 3.4 | 3.5 |
| 2/4 | 4.9 | 4.3 | 8.2 |
| 3/3 | 59.9 | 38.2 | 23.5 |
| 3/4 | 20.7 | 41.2 | 45.9 |
| 4/4 | 0.7 | 12.9 | 18.8 |
| 2/– | 18.7 | 7.7 | 11.7 |
| 3/– | 93.1 | 82.8 | 72.9 |
| 4/– | 26.3 | 58.4 | 72.9 |
| 2 (allele freq.) | 9.0 | 3.9 | 5.9 |
| 3 (allele freq.) | 76.5 | 60.5 | 48.2 |
| 4 (allele freq.) | 13.7 | 35.6 | 45.9 |

*Community-based sample aged 48–94 years.
**Source:** Adapted from Jarvik et al.[159]

may be related to the very early onset and aggressive nature of the *PS-1*–related disease, or perhaps it is caused by a pathway that does not involve ApoE. In the VG families with a *PS-2* mutation (N141 I), an ApoE association cannot be excluded but seems unlikely.[72] If ApoE influences disease in *PS-1* families, it appears to be a minor effect. Furthermore, there may be complex interactions between ApoE, AD, cholesterol level, and vascular disease in the overall production of dementia.[127] A biallelic polymorphic site (−491 A allele) in the ApoE promoter region has also shown an association with AD and could be of functional significance.[127a]

## APOLIPOPROTEIN E AND PATHOGENESIS OF ALZHEIMER'S DISEASE

The ApoE isoforms may play a direct biological role in the pathogenesis of AD. There is immunohistochemical evidence that ApoE is present in AD plaques and tangles.[128,129] In AD-affected brains, the amyloid load and plaque density correlate with ε4 dose (homozygotes or heterozygotes), with the highest loads and plaque densities found in 4/4 homozygotes.[130] These histopathological measures do not show high correlation with clinical disease severity.

*In vitro,* ApoE binds to Aβ with high affinity, and in some studies the ApoE4 isoform bound more rapidly and promoted faster Aβ fibril formation than the ApoE3 isoform.[131,132] In another study, ApoE3 bound with greater avidity than ApoE4, leading to the hypothesis of ApoE3 promoting Aβ clearance rather than ApoE4 promoting Aβ deposition.[133] Knock-out of the ApoE gene greatly reduces brain amyloid deposition in transgenic mice overexpressing APP.[134] Whether such interactions occur *in vivo* and whether they are relevant to AD are presently unknown.

A possible independent pathway for ApoE function is interaction with tau, the major protein component of NFT. *In vitro,* ApoE binds to tau, with ApoE3 binding more avidly than ApoE4.[135,136] This could conceivably prevent phosphorylation of tau, a required step in NFT formation. In AD-affected brains, however, ApoE genotype correlates with Aβ load rather than with NFT density.[137] This is more consistent with an ApoE–Aβ interaction than with an

ApoE–tau interaction. Another possible role for ApoE in AD pathogenesis is its known function as a neuronal injury response protein.[138] β amyloid protein is deposited in the brain after severe head injury and ApoE4 may be a risk factor for this deposition.[138a,138b]

## APOLIPOPROTEIN E TESTING

ApoE genotype testing could be of potential value in prediction and diagnosis of AD. Predictive testing is hindered by the fact that only 25% to 40% of subjects with one ε4 allele will develop AD, and those with no ε4 allele are still at risk for AD. Breitner[139] has calculated that 4/4 homozygotes (about 2% of the general population) have approximately a 30% lifetime risk of developing AD. For these reasons, the American College of Medical Genetics/American Society of Human Genetics working group on ApoE and AD has published a consensus statement that the use of ApoE genotyping for predictive testing of AD is not recommended.[140]

The use of ApoE genotyping in the diagnostic evaluation of demented persons is a different issue.[141] Demented individuals who are 4/4 homozygotes may have a 95% or greater risk of having AD, but precise figures require better knowledge of confidence limits for these estimates as well as age and gender influences.[141–143] In addition, ApoE genotype is not completely diagnostic of AD in demented persons. Other causes of dementia are also associated with the ε4 allele (Lewy body dementia, possibly Pick's disease, and perhaps vascular dementia).[144–148] Also, sensitivity of ApoE testing is low in the majority of patients who are not 4/4 homozygotes because at least 35% to 50% of subjects with AD do not have an ApoE ε4 allele. Even in 4/4 homozygotes, in whom dementia is most likely a result of AD, ApoE testing does not preclude the necessity of ruling out treatable causes of dementia such as brain tumor, normal pressure hydrocephalus, metabolic disorders, and vitamin deficiencies.[142]

The American College of Medical Genetics/American Society of Human Genetics working group also did not recommend ApoE genotyping for the diagnosis of AD.[140] An NIA/Alzheimer Association working group,[149] however, suggested that ApoE testing should not be used as a sole diagnostic test for AD, but may have a role as an adjunct to other diagnostic tests in persons with dementia as suggested by Roses.[141] The ApoE 4/4 genotype in a demented person has a high positive predictive value for AD (95% to 99%), but the absence of an ε4 allele has a low negative predictive value (meaning that the person still could have AD).[150] Nevertheless, Mayeux and associates[151] suggest that lack of an ε4 allele in a demented person should encourage further testing for other causes of dementia. Case control [151a] and community based[151b] studies suggest a limited role for ApoE testing in the diagnosis of AD.

Finally, ApoE testing may also become useful in predicting response to therapy or in disease prediction in conjunction with other modalities such as positron emission tomography scans.[152–155] For example, Farlow and coworkers[152] and Poirier and colleagues[153] have preliminary evidence that AD patients with an ε4 allele have a decreased response to tacrine. These fascinating potential clinical applications are presently in the research phase.

## ADDITIONAL GENETIC LOCI

A genomic screen of late onset AD families has suggested that a susceptibility gene for AD may lie on chromosome 12.[156,161] The chromosome 12 gene could be alpha 2-macroglobulin, liproprotein receptor protein, or some other gene in that region.[162–164] This finding requires confirmation, but supports the hypothesis that there are more genes to be found that impact the development of AD. Finally, mutations have been found in the gene coding for tau (microtubule-binding protein) in families with frontotemporal dementia and different types of NFT pathology.[160,165,166] These studies will suggest new strategies for investigating the pathogenesis of AD and begin to address the fascinating issues surrounding the relationship of amyloid plagues to neurofibrillary tangle/tau accumulation.

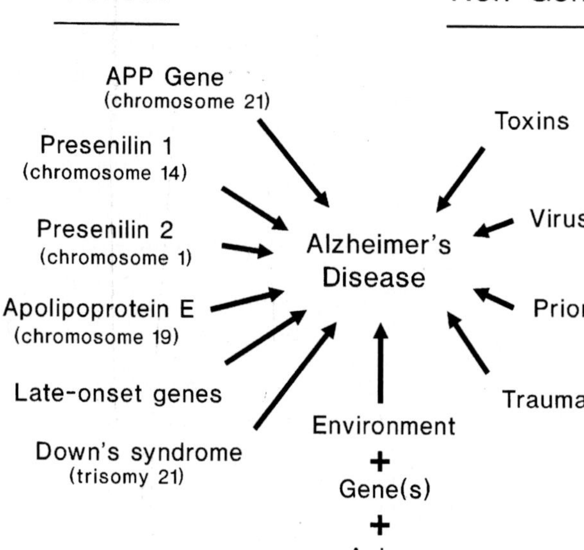


**Figure 16–8.** Schematic diagram illustrating both known and possible causes of Alzheimer's disease. The known genes associated with AD are shown on the left. Possible but presently unproven environmental causes are shown on the right. The bottom of the figure demonstrates that a possible unifying pathogenesis of AD in the general population may be a combination of predisposing genetic factors interacting with environmental influences and the process of aging. (From Bird et al.[157])

## SUMMARY

The essential clinicopathological phenotype of AD is progressive dementia associated with Aβ neuritic plaques, NFT, and cerebral amyloid angiopathy. It is now clear that the genetic background of this AD phenotype is heterogeneous (Fig. 16–8). There are three causative genes in which the presence of a dominantly inherited mutation is sufficient to result in clinical AD. These are the *APP* gene on chromosome 21, the *PS-1* gene on chromosome 14, and the *PS-2* gene on chromosome 1. These are rare causes of AD, but important clues to the pathogenesis of AD. The ApoE gene on chromosome 19 represents an important AD susceptibility factor that is a predisposition for the occurrence of AD and lowers the age of onset.

These genetic factors do not eliminate the importance of possible environmental influences. In fact, the most common cause of AD in the general population may be a complex interaction between genetic predispositions, the aging process, and various environmental insults. Focused investigation of all these factors will lead to a better understanding of the causes of AD and suggest new strategies for treatment and prevention.

## REFERENCES

1. Larson EB, Kukull WA, Katzman RL: Cognitive impairment, dementia and Alzheimer's disease. Annu Rev Public Health 13:431–439, 1992.
2. Hofman A, Rocca WA, Brayne C, et al.: The prevalence of dementia in Europe: A collaborative study of 1980–1990 findings. Int J Epidemiol 20: 736–748, 1991.
3. Hirst C, Yee IML, Sadovnick AD: Familial risk for Alzheimer disease from a population based series. Genet Epidmiol 11:365–374, 1994.
4. Farrer LA, O'Sullivan DM, Cupples LA, et al.: Assessment of genetic risk for Alzheimer's disease among first degree relatives. Ann Neurol 25:485–493, 1989.
5. Hocking LB, Breitner JCS: Cumulative risk of Alzheimer-like dementia in relatives of autopsy-confirmed cases of Alzheimer's disease. Dementia 6:355–356,1995.
6. Mohs R, Breitner J, Silverman J, et al.: Alzheimer's disease—Morbid risk among first degree relatives approximates 50% by 90 years of age. Arch Gen Psychiatry 44:405–408, 1987.
7. Heston LL, Mastri AR, Anderson E, et al.: Dementia of the Alzheimer type. Arch Gen Psychiatry 38: 1085–1090, 1981.
8. Cook RH, Ward BE, Austin JH: Studies in aging of the brain: IV. Familial Alzhiemer disease: Relation to transmissible dementia, aneuploidy, and microtubular defects. Neurology 29:1402–1412, 1979.
9. Nee LE, Polinsky RJ, Eldridge R, et al.: A family with histologically confirmed Alzheimer's disease. Arch Neurol 40:203–208, 1983.
10. Foncin JF, Salmon D, Supino-Viterbo V, et al.: Demence Presenile D'Alzheimer transmise dans

une famille étundue. Rev Neurol 141:194–202, 1985.

11. Bird TD, Sumi SM, Nemens EJ, et al.: Phenotypic heterogeneity in familial Alzheimer's disease: A study of 24 kindreds. Ann Neurol 24:12–25, 1989.
12. Goudsmit JP, White BJ, Weitkamp LR, et al.: Familial Alzheimer's disease in two kindreds of the same geographic and ethnic origin. J Neurol Sci 49:79–89, 1981.
13. Frommelt P, Schnabel R, Kuhne W, et al.: Familial Alzheimer disease: A large, multigeneration German kindred. Alz Dis Assoc Dis 5(1):36–43, 1991.
14. Martin JHJ, Bruyland M, Cras P, et al.: Early-onset Alzheimer's disease in 2 large Belgian families. Neurology 41:62–68, 1991.
15. Lai F, Williams RS: A prospective study of Alzheimer's disease in Down syndrome. Arch Neurol 46: 489–453, 1989.
16. Mann DMA: Association between Alzheimer's disease and Down syndrome: Neuropathological observations. In Berg JM, Karlinsky J, Holland AJ (eds): Alzheimer Disease, Down Syndrome, and Their Relationship. Oxford University Press, Oxford, 193, pp71–92.
17. Bird TD: Clinical genetics of familial Alzheimer's disease. In Terry RD, et al.: (eds): Alzheimer Disease. Raven Press, New York, 1994, pp67–74.
18. Lemaire HG, Salbaum JM, Multhaup G, et al.: The preA4 695 precursor protein of Alzheimer's disease A4 amyloid is encoded by 16 exons. Nucleic Acids Res 1989; 17:517–522.
19. Tanzi RE, Gusella JF, Watkins PC, et al.: Amyloid-B protein gene: cDNA, mRNA distribution, and genetic linkage near the Alzheimer locus. Science 235:880–884, 1987.
20. Tanzi RE, McClatchey AI, Lamperti ED, et al.: Protease inhibitor domain encoded by an amyloid precursor protein mRNA associated with Alzheimer's disease. Nature 311:528–530, 1988.
21. Levy E, Carman MD, Fernandez-Madrid IJ, et al.: Mutation of the Alzheimers' disease amyloid gene in hereditary cerebral hemorrhage, Dutch type. Science 248:1124–1126, 1990.
22. Goate AM, Chartier-Harlene CM, Mullan M, et al.: Segregation of a missense mutation in the amyloid precursor protein gene with familial Alzheimer's disease. Nature 353:844–846, 1991.
23. Naruse S, Igarashi S, Aoki K, et al.: Mis-sense mutation Val Ile in exon 17 of amyloid precursos protein gene in Japanese familial Alzheimer's disease. Lancet 337:978–979, 1991.
24. Yoshioka Y, Miki T, Katsuya T, et al.: The 717 Val Ile substitution in amyloid precursor protine is associated with familial Alzheimer's disease regardless of ethnic groups. Biochem Biphys Res Commun 178:1141–1146, 1991.
25. Karlinsky H, Vaula G, Haines JL, et al.: Molecular and prospective phenotypic characterization of a pedigree with familial Alzheimer's disease and a missense mutation in codon 717 of the β-amyloid precursor protein gene. Neurology 42:1445–1453, 1992.
26. Fidani L, Rooke K, Chartier-Harlin M, et al.: Screening for mutations in the open reading frame and promoter of the beta-amyloid precursor protein gene in familial Alzheimer's disease: Identification of a further family with APP Val 717 Ile. Hum Mol Genet 1:165–168, 1992.
27. Sorbi S, Nacmias B, Forleo P, et al.: APP717 and Alzheimer's disease in Italy. Nat Genet 4:10, 1993.
28. Murrell J, Farlow M, Ghetti B, Benson MD: A mutation in the amyloid precursor protein associated with presenile dementia. Science 254:94–99, 1991.
29. Chartier-Harlin CM, Crawford F, Houlden H, et al.: Early-onset Alzheimer's disease caused by a mutation in codon717 of the beta-amyloid precursor protein gene. Nature 353;844–846, 1991.
30. Mullan M, Crawford F, Axelman K, et al.: A pathogenic mutation for probable Alzheimer's disease in the APP gene at the N-terminus of beta-amyloid. Nat Genet 1:345–347, 1992.

30a. Eckman CB, Meta ND, Crook R, et al.: A new pathogenic mutation in the APP gene 716V increases the relative proportion of A beta 42(43). Hum Mol Genet 6:2087–2089, 1997.

31. St. George-Hyslop PH, Haines JL. Farrar LA, et al.: Genetic linkage studies suggest that Alzheimer's disease is not a single homogeneous disorder. Nature 347:194–197, 1990.
32. Schellenberg GD, Bird TD, Wijsman EM, et al.: Absence of linkage of chromosome 21q21 markers to familial Alzheimer's disease. Science 241:1507–1510, 1988.

32a. Leverenz JB, Raskind MA: Early amyloid deposition in the medial temporal lobe of young Down syndrome patients: A regional quantitative analysis. Exp. Neurol. 150:296–304, 1998.

33. Evenhuis HM: The natural history of dementia in Down's syndrome. Arch Neurol 47:263–276, 1990.
34. Massimo F, Colola M, Piattoni F, et al.: Prevalence of dementia in adult patients with trisomy 21. Am J Med Genet (Suppl) 7:306–308, 1990.
35. Games D, Adams D, Alessandrini R, et al.: Alzheimer-type neuropathology in transgenic mice overexpressing V717F beta-amyloid precursor protein. Nature 373:523–527, 1995.
36. Hsiao KK, Borchelt DR, Olson K, et al.: Age-related CNS disorder and early death in transgenic FVB/N mice overexpressing Alzheimer amyloid precursor proteins. Neuron 15:1203–1218, 1995.
37. Sisodia SS, Koo EH, Beyruther K, et al.: Evidence that β amyloid protein in Alzheimer's disease is not derived by normal processing. Science 248:492–495, 1990.
38. Haass C, Scholssmacher MG, Hung AY, et al.: Amyloid beta peptide is produced by cultutred cells during normal metabolism. Nature 359:322–325, 1992.
39. Shoji M, Golde TE, Ghiso J, et al.: Production of the Alzheimer amyloid protein by normal proteolytic processing. Science 258:126–129, 1992.
40. Citron M, Vego-Pelfrey C, Teplow DB, et al.: Excessive production of amyloid beta protein by peripheral cells of symptomatic and presymptomatic patients carrying the Swedish familial Alzheimer's disease mutation. Proc Natl Acad Sci USA 91: 11993–11997, 1994.
41. Suzuki N, Cheung TT, Cai XD, et al.: An increased percentage of long amyloid beta protein secreted by familial amyloid beta protein precursor (APP717) mutants. Science 264:1336–1340, 1994.

42. Tamaoka A, Odaka A, Ishibashi Y, et al.: APP 717 missense mutation affects the ratio of amyloid beta protein species in familial Alzheimer's disease brain. J Biol Chem 269:32721–32724, 1994.
43. Jarrett JT, Lansbury PT Jr: Seeding "one dimensional crystallization" of amyloid: A pathogenic mechanism in Alzheimer disease and scrapie? Cell 73:1055–1058, 1993.
44. Schellenberg GD, Bird TD, Wijsman EM, et al.: Genetic linkage evidence for a familial Alzheimer's disease locus on chromosome 14. Science 258:668–671, 1992.
45. St. George-Hyslop P, Haines J, Rogaev E, et al.: Genetic evidence for a novel familial Alzheimer's disease locus on chromosome 14. Nat Genet 2:330–334, 1992.
46. Van Broeckhoven C, Backhovens H, Cruts M, et al.: Mapping of a gene predisposing to early-onset Alzheimer's disease to chromosome 14q24.3. Nat Genet 2:335–339, 1992.
47. Mullan M, Houlden H, Windelspecht M, et al.: A locus for familial early-onset Alzheimer's disease maps to the long arm of chromosome 14, proximal to the alpha1-antichymotrypsin gene. Nat Genet 2: 340–342, 1992.
48. Sherrington R, Rogaev EI, Liang Y, et al. Cloning of a gene bearing missense mutations in early-onset familial Alzheimer's disease. Nature 375:754–760, 1995.
49. Boteva K, Vitek M, Mitsuda H: Mutation analysis of presenilin 1 gene in Alzheimer's disease. Lancet 347:130–131, 1996.
50. Perez-Tur J, Froelich S, Prihar G, et al.: A mutation in Alzheimer's disease destroying a splice accceptor site in the presenilin-1 gene. NeuroReport 7;297–301, 1995.
51. Chapman J, Asherov A, Wang N, et al.: Familial Alzheimer's disease associated with S182 codon 286 mutation. Lancet 346:1040, 1996.
52. Campion D, Flaman J-M, Brice A: Mutations of the presenilin I gene in families with early-onset Alzheimer's disease. Hum Mol Genet 4:2373–2377, 1995.
53. Cruts M, Backhovens H, Wabg S-H: Molecular genetic analysis of familial early-onset Alzheimer's disease linked to chromosome 14q24.3. Hum Mol Genet 4:2363–2371, 1995.
54. Gomez-Isla T, Wasco W, Pettingell PD, et al.: A novel mutation in the chromosome 14 familial Alzheimer's disease gene. Neurology 46♣49, 1996.
55. Cervenakova L, Brown P, Kenney K: Identification of AD3 gene point mutations in three early-onset Alzheimer's disease families. Neurology 46:A249, 1995.
56. Sorbi S, Nacmias B, Forleo P, et al.: Missense mutation of S182 in Italian families with early-onset Alzheimer's disease. Lancet 346:439–440, 1996.
57. Tanahashi H, Mitsunaga Y, Takahashi K, et al.: Missense mutation of S182 gene in Japanese familial Alzheimer's disease. Lancet 346:440, 1995.
58. Wasco W, Pettingel WP, Jondro PD, et al.: Familial Alzheimer's disease chromosome 14 mutations. Nat Med 1:848, 1995.
59. Cruts M, VanBrockhoven C: Presenilin mutations in Alzheimer's disease. Hum Mutat 11:183–190, 1998.
60. Lampe TH, Bird TD, Nochlin D, et al.: Phenotype of chromosome 14-linked familial Alzheimer's disease in a large kindred. Ann Neurol 36:368–378, 1994.
61. Lopera F, Ardilla A, Martínez A, et al.: Clinical features of early onset Alzheimer disease in a large kindred with an E208A presenilin-1 mutation. JAMA 277:793–799, 1997.
62. Mann DMA, Iwatsubo T, Cairns NJ, et al.: Amyloid β protein (Aβ) deposition in chromosome 14-linked Alzheimer's disease: Predominance of $A\beta_{42(43)}$. Ann Neurol 40:149–156, 1996.
63. Crook R, Verkkoniemi A, Perez-Tur J, et al.: A variant of Alzheimer's disease with spastic paraparesis and unusual plaques due to deletion of exon 9 of presenilin 1. Nat Med 4:452–455, 1998.
64. Bird TD, Lampe TH, Nemens EJ, et al.: Familial Alzheimer's disease in American descendants of the Volga Germans: Probable genetic founder effect. Ann Neurol 23:25–31, 1988.
65. Bird TD, Nemens EM, Nochlin D, et al.: Familial Alzheimer's disease in Germans from Russia: A model of genetic heterogeneity in Alzheimer's disease. In Boller F, et al. (eds): Heterogeneity of Alzheimer's Disease. Springer-Verlag, Berlin, 1992, pp120–129.
66. Levy-Lahad E, Wijsman EM, Nemens E, et al.: A familial Alzheimer's disease locus on chromosome 1. Science 269:970–973, 1995.
67. Levy-Lahad E, Wasco W, Poorkaj P, et al.: A candidate gene for the chromosome 1 familial Alzheimer's disease locus. Science 269:973–977, 1995.
68. Rogaev EI, Sherrington R, Rogaeva E, et al.: Familial Alzheimer's disease in kindreds with missense mutations in a gene on chromosome 1 related to the Alzheimer's disease type 3 gene. Nature 376:775–778, 1995.
69. Levy-Lahad E, Poorkaj P, Wang K, et al.: Genomic structure and expression of STM2, the chromosome 1 familial Alzheimer's disease gene. Genomics 34:198–204, 1996.
70. Doan A, Thinakaran G, Borchelt DR, et al.: Protein topology of presenilin 1. Neuron 17:1023–1030, 1996.
71. Cruts M, van Dujin CM, Backhovens H, et al.: Estimation of the genetic contribution of presenlin-1 and -2 mutations in a population-based study of presenile Alzheimer disease. Hum Mol Genet 7:43–51, 1998.
71a. Beyer KI, Lao JI, Fernandez-Novoa L, et al.: Identification of a novel mutation (V148I) in the TM2 domain of the presenilin 2 gene in a patient with late onset AD. Neurobiol. Aging 19:45 (360), 1998.
72. Bird TD, Levy-Lahad E, Poorkaj P, et al.: Wide range in age-of-onset for chromosome 1 related familial Alzheimer's disease. Ann Neurol 40:932–936, 1996.
73. Sherrington R, Froelich S, Sorbi S, et al.: Alzheimer's disease associated with mutations in presenilin 2 is rare and variably penetrant. Hum Mol Genet 5:985–988, 1996.
74. Nochlin D, Bird TD, Nemens EJ, et al.: Amyloid angiopathy in a Volga German family with Alzheimer's disease and a presenilin-2 mutation ($N^{141}I$). Ann Neurol 43:131–135, 1998.
75. Schellenberg G, Payami H, Wijsman E, et al.: Chro-

mosome 14 and late onset familial Alzheimer's disease. Am J Hum Genet 53:619–628, 1993.
76. Wragg M, Hutton M, Talbot C, and the Alzheimer's Disease Collaborative Group: Genetic association between intronic polymorphism in the presenilin-1 gene and late-onset Alzheimer's disease. Lancet 347:509–512, 1996.
76a. Tysoe C, Whittaker J, Cairus NJ, et al.: Presenilin-1 intron 8 polymorphism is not associated with autopsy confirmed late-onset AD. Neuroscience Letters 222:68–69, 1997.
77. Kovacs DM, Fausett HJ, Page KJ, et al.: Alzheimer-associated presenilins 1 and 2: Neuronal expression in the brain and localization to intracellular membranes in mammalian cells. Nat Med 2:224–229, 1996.
78. Levitan D, Greenwald I: Facilitation of lin-12–mediated signaling by sel-12, a *Caenorhabditis elegans* S182 Alzheimer's disease gene. Nature 377:351–354, 1995.
79. L'Hernault SW, Arduengo PM: Mutation of a putative sperm membrane protein in *Caenorhabditis elegans* prevents sperm differentiation but not its associated meiotic divisions. J Cell Biol 119:55–68, 1995.
80. Shen J, Bronson RT, Chen DF, et al.: Skeletal and CNS defects in presenilin-1–deficient mice. Cell 89: 629–639, 1997.
81. deStrooper B, Saftig P, Craessaerts K, et al.: Deficiency of presenilin 1 inhibits the normal cleavage of amyloid precursor protein. Nature 391:387–390, 1998.
81a. Wolfe MS, Xia W, Ostaszewski BL, et al.: Two transmembrane aspartates in presenilin-1 required for presenilin endo proteolysis and gamma secretase activity. Nature 398: 513–517, 1999.
81b. De Strooper B, Annaert W, Cupers P, et al.: A presenilin-1 dependent gamma secretase-like protease mediates release of Notch intracellular domain. Nature 398:518–522, 1999.
82. Borchelt DR, Ratovitski T, van Lare J, et al.: Accelerated amyloid deposition in the brains of transgenic mice coexpressing mutant presenilin 1 and amyloid precursor proteins. Neuron 19:939–945, 1997.
83. Scheuner D, et al.: Fibroblasts from carriers of familial AD linked to chromosome 14 show increased A β production. Soc Neurosci Abstr 21: 1500, 1995.
84. Scheuner D, Eckman C, Jensen M, et al.: Secreted amyloid B protein similar to that in the senile plaques of Alzheimer's disease is increased *in vivo* by the presenilin 1 and 2 and APP mutations linked to familial Alzheimer's disease. Nat Med 2: 864–870, 1996.
85. Vito P, Lacana E, D'Adamio L: Interfering with apoptosis: $Ca^{+2}$ binding protein ALG-2 and Alzheimer's disease gene ALG-3. Science 271:521–525, 1996.
86. Bird TD, Bennett RL: Why do DNA testing? Practical and ethical implications of new neurogenetic tests. Ann Neurol 38:141–146, 1995.
87. Lannfelt L, Axelman K, Lilius L, Basun H: Genetic counseling in a Swedish Alzheimer family with amyloid precursor protein mutation. Am J Hum Genet 56:332–335, 1995.
88. Mahley RW, Innerarity TL: Apolipoprotein E. Biochim Biophys Acta 737:197–222, 1983.
89. Schellenberg GD, Deeb SS, Boehnke M, et al.: Association of an apolipoprotein CII allele with familial dementia of the Alzheimer type. J Neurogenet 4:97–108, 1987.
90. Schellenberg GD, Boehnke M, Wijsman EM, et al.: Genetic association and linkage analysis of the apolipoprotein CII locus and familial Alzheimer's disease. Ann Neurol 31:223–227, 1992.
91. Pericak-Vance MA, Bebout JL, Gaskell PC, Yamaoka LH, et al.: Linkage studies in familial Alzheimer's disease: Evidence for chromosome 19 linkage. Am J Hum Genet 41:1034–1050, 1991.
92. Stritmatter WJ, Saunders AM, Schmechel D, et al.: Apolipoprotein E. High avidity binding to beta amyloid and increased frequency of type 4 allele in late onset Alzheimer's disease. Proc Natl Acad Sci USA 90:1977–1981, 1993.
93. Corder EH, Saunders AM, Stritmatter WJ, et al.: Gene dose of the ApolipoproteinE type-4 allele and the risk of Alzheimer's disease in late-onset families. Science 261:921–923, 1993.
94. Saunders AM, Stritmatter WJ Schmechel D, et al.: Association of the apolipoprotein E allele ε4 with late-onset familial and sporadic Alzheimer's disease. Neurology 43:1467–1472, 1993.
95. Yu CE, Payami H, Olson JM, et al.: The apolipoprotein E/CI/CII gene cluster and late-onset Alzheimer's disease. Am J Hum Genet 54:631–642, 1994.
96. Payami H, Kaye J, Heston LL, et al.: Apolipoprotein E genotype and Alzheimer's disease. Lancet 342:738, 1993.
97. Rebeck GW, Reiter JS, Strickland DK: Apolipoprotein E in sporadic Alzheimer's disease: Allelic variations and receptor interactions. Neuron 11: 575–580, 1993.
98. Brousseau T, Legrain S, Berr C, et al.: Confirmation of the e4 allele of the apolipoprotein E gene as a risk factor for late-onset Alzheimer's disease. Neurology 44:342–344, 1994.
99. Poirier J, Davignon J, Bouthillier D, et al.: Apolipoprotein E polymorphisms and Alzheimer's disease. Lancet 342:697–699, 1993.
100. Mayeux R, Stern Y, Ottman R, et al.: The Apolipoprotein e4 allele in patients with Alzheimer's disease. Ann Neurol 34:752–754, 1993.
101. Tsai MS, Tsangalos EG, Petersen RC: Apolipoprotein E: Risk factor for Alzheimer's disease. Am J Hum Genet 54:643–649, 1994.
102. Kuusisto J, Koivisto K, Kervinen K, et al.: Association of Apolipoprotein E phenotypes with with late-onset Alzheimer's disease: Population based study. BMJ 309:636–638, 1994.
103. Van Duijn CM, de Kniff P, Cruts M, et al.: Apolipoprotein e4 allele in a population based study of early-onset Alzheimer's disease. Nat Genet 7:74–78, 1994.
104. Perez-Tur J, Campion D, Martinez M, et al.: Evidence for Apolipoprotein e4 association in early-onset Alzheimer's patients with late-onset relatives. Am J Med Genet 60:550–553, 1995.
105. Payami H, Montee KR Kaye JA, et al.: Alzheimer's disease, Apolipoprotein E e4 and gender. JAMA 271:1316–1317, 1994.

106. Farrer LA, Cupples LA, van Duijn CM: Apolipoprotein E genotype in patients with Alzheimer's disease: Implications for the risk of dementia among relatives. Ann Neurol 38:797–808, 1995.
107. Lucotte G, Aouzirate A, Gerard N, et al.: Allele doses of Apolipoprotein E type e4 in spradic late-onset Alzheimer's disease. Am J Med Genet 60: 566–569, 1995.
107a. Craft S, Teri L, Edland SD, et al.: Accelerated decline in apo E homozygotes with Alzheimer's disease. Neurology 51:149–153, 1998.
108. Corder EH, Saunders AM, Risch NJ: Protective effect of apolipoprotein E type 2 allele for late onset Alzheimer disease. Nat Genet 7:180–184, 1994.
109. Chartier-Harlin MC, Parfitt M, Legrain S, et al.: Apolipoprotein E e4 allele is a major risk factor for sporadic early and late-onset form of Alzheimer's disease: Analysis of the 19q13.2 chromosomal region. Hum Mol Genet 3:568–574, 1993.
110. West HL, Rebeck W Hyman BT. Frequency of the Apoliporotein E e2 allele is diminished in sporadic Alzheimer's disease. Neurosci Lett 175:46–48, 1994.
111. Talbot C, Lendon C, Craddock N, et al.: Protection against Alzheimer's disease with ApoE e2. Lancet 343:1432–1433, 1994.
112. Maestre G, Ottman R, Stern Y, et al.: Apolipoprotein E and Alzheimer's disease: Ethnic variation in genotypic risks. Ann Neurol 37:254–259. 1995.
113. Tang MX, Maestre G, Tsai W-Y, et al.: Relative risk of Alzheimer's disease and age-at-onset distributions, based on ApoE genotpes among elderly African Americans, Caucasians and Hispanics in New York City. Am J Hum Genet 58:574–584, 1996.
114. van Duijn CM, de Knijff P, Wehnert A, et al.: The Apolipoprotein E e2 allele is associated with an increased risk of early onset Alzheimer's disease and a reduced survival. Ann Neurol 37:605–610, 1995.
115. Hendrie HC, Hall KS, Hui S, et al.: Apolipoprotein E genotypes and Alzheimer's disease in a community study of elderly African Americans. Ann Neurol 37:118–120, 1995.
116. Schupf N, Kapell D, Nightingale B, et al.: Earlier onset of Alzheimer's disease in men with Down syndrome. Neurology 50:991–994, 1998.
117. St. George-Hyslop P, McLachlan DC, et al.: Alzheimer's disease and possible gene interaction. Science 263:537, 1994.
118. Alzheimer's disease Collaborative Group: Apolipoprotein E genotype and Alzheimer's disease. Lancet 342:738–739, 1993.
119. Nacmias B, Latorraca S, Piersanti P, et al.: ApoE genotype and familial Alzheimer's disease: A possible influence on age-of-onset in APP Val 717 Ile mutated families. Neurosci Lett 183:1–3, 1995.
120. Sorbi S, Nacmias B, Forleo P, et al.: Epistatic effect of APP717 mutation and Apolipoprotein E genotype in familial Alzheimer's disease. Ann Neurol 38:124–127, 1995.
121. Brooks WS, Martins RN, De Voecht J, et al.: A mutation in codon 717 of the amyloid precursor gene in an Australian family with Alzheimer's disease. Neurosci Lett 199:183–186, 1995.
122. Haan J, Van Broeckhoven C, van Duijn CM, et al.: The Apolipoprotein E e4 allele does not influence the clinical expression of the amyloid precursor protein gene codon 693 and 692 mutation. Ann Neurol 36:434–437, 1994.
123. van Gool WA, Evenhuis HM, van Duijn CM, for the Dutch Study Group on Down's Syndrome and Aging: A case–control study of Apolipoprotein E genotypes in Alzheimer's disease associated with Down's syndrome. Ann Neurol 38:225–230, 1995.
124. Schupf N, Kappel D, Zigman W, et al.: Dementia and decline in adaptive competence is associated with ApoE ε4 in Down's syndrome. Neurology 46 (Supplement):A419(559,005), 1996.
125. Van Broeckhoven C, Backhovens H, Cruts M, et al.: ApoE genotype does not modulate age of onset in families with chromosome 14 encoded Alzheimer's disease. Neurosci Lett 169:179–180, 1994.
126. Levy-Lahad E, Lahad A, Wijsman EM, et al.: Apolipoprotein E genotypes and early-onset familial Alzheimer's disease. Ann Neurol 38:679–680, 1995.
127. Jarvik GP, Wijsman EM, Kukul WA, et al.: Interactions of apolipoprotein E genotype, total cholesterol level, age and sex in prediction of Alzheimer's disease: A case–control study. Neurology 45:1092–1096, 1995.
127a. Bullido MJ, Artiga MJ, Recuero M, et al.: A polymorphism in the regulatory region of ApoE associated with risk for Alzheimer's disease. Nat Genet 18:69–71, 1998.
128. Namba Y, Tomonaga M, Kawasaki H, et al.: Apolipoprotein E immunoreactivity in cerebral amyloid deposits and neurofibrillary tangles in Alzheimer's disease and kuru plaque amyloid in Creutzfeldt-Jacob disease. Brain Res 641:163–166, 1991.
129. Wisniewski T, Frangione B: Apolipoprotein E: A pathological chaperone protein in patients with cerebral and systemic amyloid. Neurosci Lett 135: 235–238, 1992.
130. Schmechel DE, Saunders AM, Strimatter WJ, et al.: Increased amyloid beta-peptide deposition in cerebral cortex as a consequence of ApoE genotype in late-onset Alzheimer's disease. Proc Natl Acad Sci USA 90:9649–9653, 1993.
131. Strittmatter WJ, Saunders AM, Schmechel D, et al.: Binding of human Apolipoprotein E to β A4 peptide: Isoform specific effects and implications for late-onset Alzheimer's disease. Proc Natl Acad Sci Acad USA 90:8098–8102, 1993.
132. Sana DA, Weisgraber KH, Russell SJ, et al.: Apolipoprotein E associates with β amyloid peptide of Alzheimer's disease to form novel monofibrils. Isoform ApoE4 associates more efficiently than ApoE3. JCI 94:860–869, 1994.
133. LaDu MJ, Falduto MT, Manelli AM, et al.: Isoform specific binding of Apolipoprotein E to β β-amyloid. J Biol Chem 269:23403–23406, 1994.
134. Bales KR, Verina T, Dodel RC, et al.: Lack of apolipoprotein E dramatically reduces amyloid β-peptide deposition. Nat Genet 17:263–264, 1997.
135. Roses AD: Apolipoprotein E affects the rate of Alzheimer disease expression: β-Amyloid burden is a secondary consequence dependent on APOE

genotype and duration of disease. J Neuropath Exp Neurol 53:429–437, 1994.
136. Strittmatter WJ, Saunders AM, Goedert M, et al.: Isoform-specific interactions of apolipoprotein E with microtubule associated protein tau: Implications for Alzheimer's disease. Proc Natl Acad Sci USA 91:11183–11186, 1994.
137. Gomez-Isla T, West HL, Rebeck GW, et al.: Clinical and pathological correlates of Apolipoprotein E e4 in Alzheimer's disease. Ann Neurol 39:62–70, 1996.
138. Poirier J: Apolipoprotein E in animal models of CNS injury and Alzheimer's disease. Trends Neurosci 17:525–530, 1994.
138a. Roberts GW, Gentleman SM, Lynch A, et al.: β amyloid protein deposition in the brain after severe head injury: Implications for the pathogenesis of AD. J Neurol Neurosurg Psych, 57:419–425, 1994.
138b. O'Meara ES, Kukull WA, Sheppard L, et al.: Head injury and risk of Alzheimer's disease by apolipoprotein E genotype. Am J Epidem 146: 373–384, 1997.
139. Breitner JCS: ApoE genotying and Alzhiemer's disease. Lancet 347:1184, 1996.
140. American College of Medical Genetics/American Society of Human Genetics Working Group on ApoE and Alzheimer Disease: Statement on use of Apolipoprotein E testing for Alzheimer's disease. JAMA 274:1627–1629, 1995.
141. Roses AD: Apolipoprotein E genotyping in the differential diagnosis, not prediction, of Alzheimer's disease. Ann Neurol 38:6–14, 1995.
142. Bird TD: Apolipoprotein E genotyping in the diagnosis of Alzheimer's disease: A cautionary view. Ann Neurol 38:317–318, 1995.
143. Welsh-Bohmer KA, Gearing M, Saunders AM, et al.: Apolipoprotein E genotypes in a neuropathological series from the consortium to establish a registry for Alzheimer's disease. Ann Neurol 42: 319–325, 1997.
144. Galasko D, Saitoh T, Xia Y, et al.: The Apolipoprotein allele e4 is over-represented in patients with Lewy body variant of Alzheimer's disease. Neurology 44:950–951, 1994.
145. Schneider JA, Gearing M, Robbins RS, et al.: Apolipoprotein E genotyping in diverse neurodegenrative disorders. Ann Neurol 38:131–135, 1995.
146. Frisoni GB, Bianchetti A, Govoni S: Association of Apolipoprotein E e4 with vascular dementia. JAMA 271:1317, 1994.
147. Isoe K, Urakami K, Sato K, et al.: Apolipoprotein E in patients with dementia of the Alzheimer type and vascular dementia. Acta Neurol Scand 93: 133–137, 1996.
148. Noguchi S, Murakami K, Nobuhiro Y: Apolipoprotein E genotype and Alzheimer's disease. Lancet 324:737, 1993.
149. National Institute on Aging/Alzheimer's Association Working Group: Apolipoprotein E genotyping in Alzhiemer's disease. Lancet 347:1091–1095, 1996.
150. Saunders AM, Hulette C, Welsh-Bohmer KA, et al.: Specificity, sensitivity, and predictive value of apolipoprotein-E genotyping for sporadic Alzheimer's disease. Lancet 348:90–93, 1996.
151. Mayeux R, Saunders AM, Shea S, Mirra S, et al.: Utility of the apolipoprotein E genotype in the diagnosis of Alzheimer's disease. N Engl J Med 338:506–511, 1998.
151a. Kukull WA, Schellenberg GD, Bowen JD, et al.: Apo E in Alzheimer disease risk and case detection: A case control study. J Clin Epidem, 49: 1143–1148, 1996.
151b. Tsuang D, Larson EB, Bowen JD, et al.: Apo E genotyping in the diagnosis of Alzheimer's disease in a community based case series. Arch Neurol, 1999, in press.
152. Farlow MR, Lahiri D, Hui S, et al.: Apolipoprotein E genotype predicts response to tacrine in Alzheimer's disease. Neurology 46:A217, 1996.
153. Poirier J, Delissle MC, Quirion R, et al.: Apolipoprotein E4 allele as a predictor of cholinergic deficits and treatment outcome in Alzheimer disease. Proc Natl Acad Sci USA 92:12260–12264, 1995.
154. Amouyel P, Neuman E, Dilleman F, et al.: Characterization of Apolipoprotein E genotypes in a European multicenter trial on Alzheimer's disease with the S-12024-2 (memory enhancer). Neurology 46:A218, 1996.
155. Reiman EM, Caselli RJ, Yun LS, et al.: Preclinical evidence of Alzheimer's disease in persons homozygous for the e4 allele for Apolipoprotein E. N Engl J Med 334:759–762, 1996.
156. Paricak-Vance MA, Bass MP, Yamaoka LH, et al.: Complete genomic screen in late-onset familial Alzheimer disease: Evidence for a new locus on chromosome 12. JAMA 278:1237–1241, 1997.
157. Bird TD, Lampe TH, Wijsman EM, Schellenberg GD: Familial Alzheimer's disease: Genetic studies. In MF Folstein (ed): Neurobiology of Primary Dementia. American Psychiatric Press, Washington, DC, 1998, pp27–42.
158. Levy-Lahad E, Bird TD: Genetic factors in Alzheimer's disease: A review of recent advances. Ann Neurol 40:829–840, 1996.
159. Jarvik GP, Larson EB, Goddard K, et al.: Influences of apolipoprotein E genotype in the transmission of Alzheimer's disease in a community-based sample. Am J Hum Genet 58:1191–200, 1996.
160. Poorkaj P, Bird TD, Wijsman E, et al.: Tau is a candidate for chromosome 17 linked frontotemporal dementia. Ann Neurol 43:815–825, 1998.
161. Wu WS, Holmans P, Wavrant-DeVrieze F, et al.: Genetic studies on chromosome 12 in late-onset Alzheimer disease. JAMA 280:619–622, 1998.
162. Blacker D, Wilcox MA, Laird NM, et al.: Alpha-2 macroglobulin is genetically associated with Alzheimer disease. Nat Genet 19:357–360, 1998.
163. Rogaeva EA, Premkumar S, Grubber J, et al.: An macroglobulin insertion-deletion polymorphism in Alzheimer disease. Nat Genet 22:19–21, 1999.
164. Blacker D, Crystal AS, Wilcox MA, et al.: Reply. Nat Genet 22:21–22, 1999.
165. Hutton M, Lendon CL, Rizzu P, et al.: Association of missense and 5-splice-site mutations in tau with the inherited dementia FTDP-17. Nature 393: 702–705, 1998.
166. Spillantini MG, Murrell JR, Goedert M, et al.: Mutation in the tau gene in familial multiple system tauopathy with presenile dementia. Proc Nat Acad Sci USA 95:7737–7741, 1998.

Chapter 17

# INHERITED EPILEPSIES

Jeffrey R. Buchhalter, MD, PHD



The title of this chapter was chosen to highlight the distinction between the terms *genetic* and *inherited.* Although these terms are frequently used interchangeably, they are not strictly synonymous. *Inherited* refers to variations in the individual genotype that are passed on through generations in the germline (sperm and ova). These variations can predispose an individual to disease in a simple (mendelian) fashion or have a more complex relation to expression of the phenotype. The term *genetic* includes not only variations in the germline but also spontaneous mutations in the somatic line. Thus, an individual could have a mutation in a gene that results in the production of insufficient inhibitory neurotransmitter (e.g., gamma-aminobutyric acid) in neurons leading to neuronal hyperexcitability and epilepsy. The pathophysiology of the epilepsy would be *genetic,* but not inherited. This chapter focuses on those epilepsies for which an inherited predisposition exits.

This topic is approached first with a consideration of the frequencies of the inherited epilepsies to estimate the magnitude of the problem. These epilepsy syndromes are then described with the International Classification of the Epilepsies and Epileptic Syndromes[1] as the organizing principle. More extensive reviews of this topic are available elsewhere.[2,3]

## TERMINOLOGY, CLASSIFICATIONS, AND EPIDEMIOLOGY

Precise diagnosis of individuals with a specific epilepsy type is crucial for elucidating genetic mechanisms. This is due to the necessity of identifying *affected* family members in pedigrees on which linkage analysis is performed. Criteria that are too broad or too narrow can result in a failure to associate a DNA marker with a disease trait. Thus, it is useful to briefly review relevant definitions and classification schemes.

A *seizure* is the motor, sensory, autonomic, or cognitive manifestation of an abnormal, hypersynchronous discharge of neurons. By definition, *epilepsy* refers to recurrent (two or more) unprovoked seizures. An *epilepsy syndrome* is the constellation of seizure type(s), associated electroencephalogram (EEG), developmental history, family history, and response to medication. Classification by seizure type does not provide the prognostic information embedded within epilepsy syndrome identification. Table 17–1 presents the International League Against Epilepsy (ILAE) classification of seizures[4] and epilepsies.[1] It is apparent that both schemes use the mode of seizure onset (starting in one brain location being *partial,* focal, localization-related and starting in both hemispheres simultaneously being *generalized*) as the distinction between two

Table 17–1. **ILAE Classifications of Seizures and Epilepsy Syndromes—Modified**

| Seizures | Epilepsy Syndromes |
|---|---|
| Partial (focal, local) | Localization-related (partial, focal) |
| Simple | Idiopathic |
| Complex | Symptomatic |
| Secondarily generalized tonic-clonic | |
| Generalized | Generalized |
| Tonic | Idiopathic |
| Clonic | Cryptogenic or symptomatic |
| Tonic-clonic | Symptomatic |
| Atonic | |
| Myoclonic | |
| Absence | |
| Unilateral | Undetermined focal or generalized |
| Unclassified | Special syndromes |

ILAE = International League Against Epilepsy.

of the major sub-groups. In recent studies describing seizure etiologies (but not classification), the term *idiopathic* is used to connote the absence of a central nervous system (CNS) injury that is a known precipitant of seizures (i.e., a *symptomatic* seizure).[5] The ILAE classification of the epilepsies, however, uses *idiopathic* to denote epilepsies that have a "presumed genetic etiology" and *cryptogenic* to describe epilepsies of unknown, but presumed symptomatic etiologies.[1] Within this context, the concept of *benign idiopathic* (partial and generalized) epilepsy has arisen. These syndromes are characterized by age-related onset, normal development and cognitive function, normal neurologic examination, and normal brain imaging. A normal interictal EEG and cessation of seizures by the adult years have also been suggested as criteria.

Tables 17–2 and 17–3 list those studies that have used the 1989 ILAE classification of the epilepsies, providing some insight into the frequency of inherited (idiopathic) epilepsies. Of note, the studies by Loiseau and colleagues,[6] Manford and coworkers,[7] and Oka and associates[8] are population based and thus of the greatest epidemiological significance by reducing the biases present in a specialty clinic or referral population. The frequency figures provided by Oka and associates,[8] Ohtsuka and coworkers,[9] and Shah and coworkers[10] have to be interpreted with the knowledge that the upper cut-off age for inclusion was 9 years, 5 years, and 14 years, respectively. Thus, the inherited idiopathic epilepsies that can present beyond these ages are under-represented in these cohorts. The idiopathic epilepsies account for a relatively small proportion of the localization-related epilepsies (mean, 2%; range, 0% to 11%) and a slightly greater fraction of the generalized epilepsies (mean, 16%; range, 3% to 36%). The contribution of the idiopathic epilepsies is even lower when just the population-based studies alone are considered: localization-related, mean, 1%, and generalized, mean, 13%.

Given the relatively low percentages noted above, why are the inherited epilepsies commonly considered to account for approximately 50% of all epilepsies in childhood and for 20% in adults? The reasons for this discrepancy are likely to be at least twofold. First, several of the inherited (idiopathic) epilepsy syndromes identified in the ILAE classification are, in fact, relatively rare (see later). It is likely that a significant number of individuals in whom an inherited predisposition is present do not fit into one of the defined idiopathic syndromes. In addition, much of the epidemiological data is based on clinical descriptions without the benefit of brain imaging and electrophys-

Table 17–2. **Studies Based on the ILAE Classification of the Epilepsies**

| Study* | Senior Author | Year | Country | Age Range | Sample |
|---|---|---|---|---|---|
| 1 | Sander[51] | 1989 | Columbia | NR | Epilepsy clinic |
| 2 | Loiseau[6] | 1990 | France | >2 months | Neuro-pop |
| 3a | Marseille Consensus Group[52] | 1991 | France | All | Private practice |
| 3b | Marseille Consensus Group[52] | 1991 | France | All | Univ-adult neuro |
| 4 | Manford[7] | 1992 | England | >1 month | Population |
| 5 | Shah[10] | 1992 | India | 1 month to 14 years | Out-peds hosp |
| 6 | Ohtsuka[9] | 1993 | Japan | <6 years | Out Univ Neuro |
| 7 | Oka[8] | 1995 | Japan | <10 years | Population |

*As used in Table 17–3.
NR = not recorded; Neuro-pop = data from neurologists and electroencephalographers in a district; Univ-adult neuro = adult neurology clinic in a university hospital; Population = population-based sample; Out Univ Neuro = outpatient clinic in a university child neurology department; Out peds-hosp = outpatient pediatric clinic at a pediatric hospital.

iological data. This could result in "misclassification" by not including a patient with a structural cerebral lesion in the symptomatic group or not including a patient with a characteristic spike-wave pattern in the idiopathic group. Nonetheless, a rough estimate of the portion of individuals with potentially genetically based seizures can be found in several population-based studies.

Several of these studies of the incidence and prevalence of *seizures* have indicated that idiopathic (defined as unknown etiology, but not necessarily genetic) seizures account for 55% to 89% of seizure etiologies.[5,11–14] In a 1993 incidence study of seizures in Rochester, Minnesota, the authors state that most of the cases reported as *idiopathic* would be classified as *cryptogenic* in the 1989 ILAE Classification of the Epilepsies.[12] The idea that cases considered to be cryptogenic could have an inherited/genetic etiology is suggested in two recent studies involving almost 2000 individuals with epilepsy.[15,16] In this cohort (derived from self-referrals to epilepsy-related agencies), no localization-related and "very few"

Table 17–3. **Frequency of Epilepsy Syndromes***

| Type of Syndrome | Study† | | | | | | | |
|---|---|---|---|---|---|---|---|---|
| | 1 | 2 | 3a | 3b | 4 | 5 | 6 | 7 |
| Localization-related | | | | | | | | |
| *Idiopathic* | *2* | *2* | *11* | *1* | *1* | *2* | *0* | *0.2* |
| Symptomatic | 68 | 19 | 13 | 28 | 12 | 24 | 14 | 21 |
| Cryptogenic | 0 | 0 | 18 | 17 | 18 | 27 | 8 | 35 |
| Generalized | | | | | | | | |
| *Idiopathic* | *15* | *8* | *36* | *17* | *7* | *15* | *3* | *26* |
| Cryptogenic or symptomatic | 6 | 2 | 4 | 2 | 0 | 4 | 11 | 7 |
| Symptomatic | <1 | 0 | 3 | 2 | 1 | 7 | 8 | 11 |

*As listed in column one, Table 17–2.
†The frequency of each epilepsy type is presented as the percentage of classifiable individuals in each study. The idiopathic epilepsies, which by definition are presumed to have an inherited etiology, are highlighted with italics. The classification categories of "Undetermined focal or generalized" and "special syndromes" are excluded.

generalized idiopathic syndromes were identified. Thus, the "idiopathic/cryptogenic" category was formed. Relatives of these probands exhibited a significantly greater risk of developing epilepsy than family members of probands with symptomatic epilepsy. In addition, the risk of developing epilepsy disappeared by age 35 years. These two important papers strongly suggest that *(1)* the numeric importance of the inherited epilepsies is probably as high as indicated in the studies of seizure incidence and prevalence cited earlier and *(2)* the current classification system for the epilepsies may have a fundamental weakness with regard to assignment of an inherited etiology.

## INHERITED EPILEPSY SYNDROMES

Several of the major inherited epilepsy syndromes are described in this section. Brief clinical summaries are followed by discussions of what is known about their inheritance patterns and genome localizations. Common syndromes and those that illustrate particularly interesting points about the genetic bases of the inherited epilepsies are emphasized.

### Localization-Related, Idiopathic Epilepsy Syndromes

Several syndromes have been added to this group of epilepsies since 1989, when the ILAE classification was formulated (Table 17–4). Two new syndromes have a chromosomal localization, one a gene product, and another may represent a common inherited syndrome in adults.

#### BENIGN EPILEPSY OF CHILDHOOD WITH CENTROTEMPORAL SPIKES

Benign epilepsy of childhood with centrotemporal spikes (BECTS) is the most commonly recognized idiopathic partial epilepsy syndrome of childhood. The syndrome has gone by several names, including benign epilepsy of childhood with rolandic spikes, sylvian seizures, and lingual epilepsy. The epileptogenic region is located in the inferior rolandic cortex that gives rise to motor and sensory symptoms involving the mouth, tongue, and pharynx. Characteristic events begin with the child's inability to speak despite retention of consciousness. This may be accompanied by a tingling sensation limited to half of the tongue or involving the hypopharynx and cheek. Most of the seizures occur during sleep, but approximately 20% are diurnal. Secondary generalization to a tonic-clonic seizure may occur so rapidly that the initial partial symptoms may not be appreciated. The interictal EEG reveals characteristic di-phasic spikes and sharp waves localized to central and temporal brain regions, although more anterior and posterior locations can be involved. The discharges alternate between hemispheres and usually increase during sleep.

Prognosis is excellent, as greater than 95% of children will stop having seizures by 20 years of age. There is currently an active debate as to the need for anticonvulsant treatment and if so, which medication. The correct syndromic diagnosis allows the clinician to assure the family that the disorder will remit and not be associated with cognitive impairment. Therefore, anticonvulsant therapy, if pursued, should always be monotherapy with no toleration of toxicity.

From the early reports of "temporal-central focal epilepsy," a genetic component was suspected.[17] Although these studies included some individuals with psychomotor seizures, the majority of the cases were clearly BECTS. The frequency of affected family members varied widely, depending on the study and the nature of the relationship (i.e., parents, siblings, offspring). The mode of inheritance of the EEG trait has been considered to be autosomal dominant. This transmission pattern was found in a recent large study in which approximately 30% of siblings and offspring demonstrated a focal EEG abnormality.[18] The penetrance was *age related*, with the peak occurring between 5 and 15 years of age. Only 12% of individuals with the EEG trait, however, had a seizure. This is a very important point for identification of affected individuals (i.e., studying family members of probands who are younger or older than the optimal age of penetrance

Table 17–4. **Localization-Related, Idiopathic (Inherited) Epilepsy Syndromes**

| Syndrome | Transmission | Chromosome | Gene Product |
|---|---|---|---|
| Benign epilepsy of childhood with centrotemporal spikes* | AD | ? | ? |
| Childhood epilepsy with occipital paroxysms* | FH | ? | ? |
| Reading epilepsy* | FH | ? | ? |
| Autosomal dominant nocturnal frontal lobe epilepsy | AD | 20q | α4-NAChR† |
| Partial epilepsy with auditory features | AD | 10q | ? |
| Rolandic epilepsy and speech dyspraxia | AD | ? | ? |
| Familial temporal lobe epilepsy | AD | ? | ? |

*Included in the 1989 International League Against Epilepsy classification of the epilepsies.
†α-NAChR = alpha-4-nictocotinic acetylcholine receptor.
AD = autosomal dominant; FH = family history reported; ? = unknown.

may fail to detect individuals who carry the trait but are asymptomatic). When a population defined by seizures and centrotemporal abnormalities was studied, 68% had family members with seizures, and transmission occurred in an autosomal dominant fashion.[19] A more recent analysis of family members of BECTS probands found that 40% had seizures, but none were of BECTS phenotype (i.e., febrile and generalized seizures).[20] Thus, it appears that a *susceptibility* to seize is inherited, but the specific manifestations can vary.

## CHILDHOOD EPILEPSY WITH OCCIPITAL PAROXYSMS

Childhood epilepsy with occipital paroxysms (CEOP) is also referred to as benign epilepsy with occipital spike waves. This syndrome illustrates the importance of precise clinical definition for genetic studies. As originally described in the ILAE Classification of Epilepsies and Epileptic Syndromes,[1] CEOP is characterized by visual phenomena (amaurosis, scintillations, hallucinations) followed by generalized or hemiclonic seizures. When the patient regains consciousness, a significant pounding headache frequently occurs. The average age of onset is 7 years. The ictal EEG reveals a unilateral spike-wave discharge, whereas the interictal EEG may be completely normal or contain bi-hemispheric spike waves with the eyes closed. Eye opening (i.e., visual fixation), however, can completely eliminate the spike-wave bursts. The seizures remit in approximately 90% of individuals by age 20 years. In the original series of patients, almost 50% had an otherwise unspecified family history of epilepsy,[21] although this was reduced to 37% when patients with evidence of brain injury were included. Insufficient data was provided to suggest a mode of transmission.

Several other age-related occipital lobe syndromes have been recently reported. One is characterized by seizures occurring during sleep, with tonic eye deviation and vomiting.[22] No family history is present. Another syndrome is characterized by occipital seizures induced by visual stimuli (reflex epilepsy). Three of the ten reported patients had first-degree relatives with epilepsy. None of these relations, however, had occipital lobe epilepsy of any type, but rather febrile, BECTS, and idiopathic generalized epilepsy (one each). Thus, the observation of seizure susceptibility rather than specific seizure type made with families identified by a BECTS proband also holds for CEOP.

## READING EPILEPSY

Although uncommon (less than 100 reported cases), reading epilepsy (RE) is one of the most fascinating reflex epilepsies because seizures are induced solely or predominantly by prolonged reading. This epilepsy syndrome includes ictal jaw jerking, secondarily generalized tonic-clonic seizures, normal development, normal neuroimaging, unilateral or bilateral spike-wave discharges, and good response to valproic acid. The age-related onset is from 10 to 46 years. In the largest and most recently reported series, 20% of patients had a family history of epilepsy. The family of one proband consisted of one offspring with RE, and another child had absence and tonic-clonic seizures.[23] Thus, RE is also an epilepsy syndrome in which an inherited predisposition seems operant, but it may be in the form of a general susceptibility rather than a specific syndrome.

## AUTOSOMAL DOMINANT NOCTURNAL FRONTAL LOBE EPILEPSY

Autosomal dominant nocturnal frontal lobe epilepsy (ADNFLE) was defined as a epilepsy syndrome in 1995.[24] The original cohort of patients was considered to have a sleep disorder. The description of five families indicated a wide range of onset (2 months to 52 years), although almost 90% had their first seizure by age 20 years. Motor and cognitive development of all affected individuals was normal. The nocturnal seizures exhibited clonic, tonic, and "hyperkinetic" motor activity. Approximately 80% of the interictal EEGs were normal, with the abnormalities including frontal, central, and temporal epileptiform transients that could be uni- or bi-hemispheric. Like other frontal lobe epilepsies, the ictal recording was relatively nonspecific in that it could reveal bi-hemispheric rhythmic activity, spike wave, or no ictal abnormalities.

Genetic analysis of this syndrome has moved rapidly. An autosomal dominant inheritance pattern with approximately 70% penetrance was determined by segregation analysis in 1994.[25] Within 2 years, exclusion mapping was performed in an affected six-generation family leading to the identification of a candidate gene on chromosome 20q.[26] The identified gene codes for the α-subunit of the α4-nicotinic acetylcholine receptor. Two mutations in this gene have been identified. One is a C to T mutation that affects the M2 domain of the channel,[27] and the other is a GCT triplet insertion.[28] A second locus on chromosome 15q near a region coding for other nictonic acetylcholine receptor subunits has been identified in another family.[29] This recent report, however, excluded the 20q and 15q loci in seven families and seven sporadic cases with the ADNFLE phenotype. Thus it appears that genetic heterogeneity underlies the common phenotype of this disorder. Furthermore, the lack of a demonstrated inherited susceptibility in the sporadic cases complicates genetic counseling for individuals with this phenotype who may have incomplete knowledge of other affected family members.

## PARTIAL EPILEPSY WITH AUDITORY FEATURES

Partial epilepsy with auditory features, reported in 1995, demonstrates the utility of another approach to the genetic analysis of the epilepsies. A genetic–epidemiology project was started in the mid-1980s to ascertain individuals with epilepsy via voluntary organizations. Although the group was biased by factors such as self-referral, age, and seizure and epilepsy types, it provided an opportunity to search for families in which heredity is an important risk factor. Almost 2000 adults were identified, 2% of whom had at least 3 family members with seizures. One family had 17 members with seizures across several generations. As noted in previous chapters in this volume, families of this size are particularly useful for linkage analysis. Among individuals in this family with idiopathic/cryptogenic seizures, a partial epilepsy syndrome was identified in which 91% of individuals had normal cognition. Seizure types included simple partial (auditory, present in approximately 50%), complex partial, and secondarily generalized tonic-clonic (many of which were associated with auditory phenomena).

Linkage analysis was performed with assumptions of autosomal dominant transmission and 71% penetrance. The initial genome screen of affected family members indicated that the disease locus was on the long arm of chromosome 10. When the region of interest was known, additional markers could then be used to narrow down the region to 10 cM. Although the precise gene involved has not yet been identified, this section of chromosome 10 is known to contain genes for adrenergic receptors and genes involved in excitatory amino acid metabolism. One can only speculate that knowledge of the underlying neuropharmacological deficit may lead to more specific anticonvulsant therapy.

### ROLANDIC EPILEPSY AND SPEECH DYSPRAXIA

Recently described in a single family, rolandic epilepsy and speech dyspraxia is characterized by partial motor (face and upper extremity) as well as secondarily generalized tonic-clonic seizures.[30] In the interictal state, expressive and receptive speech difficulties occurred that increase in severity with successive generations. The mode of inheritance is autosomal dominant with virtually 100% penetrance. The increasing severity with each generation suggests the phenomenon of anticipation, which sometimes occurs in neurologic disorders due to expansion of DNA triplet repeats.

### FAMILIAL TEMPORAL LOBE EPILEPSY

When a syndrome (with or without chromosomal localization) is present in a single or a few families, the ability to generalize the findings to a larger population is a concern. Thus, the report of a potentially common and not previously recognized syndrome is of great interest. Familial temporal lobe epilepsy (TLE) was initially noted in an analysis of seizures in twins.[31] The syndrome was then looked for and found in a population of non-twin probands with TLE. Individuals who were ascertained by the standard semiology for this seizure type then identified other family members with seizures.

In contrast to TLE associated with mesial temporal sclerosis, the familial TLE syndrome has onset in the teens to early twenties, is not associated with known precipitants of seizures (febrile seizures, cerebral infection/trauma), presents normal magnetic resonance imaging studies, and is usually well controlled with anticonvulsant medication. An autosomal dominant transmission pattern with age-related penetrance seems likely, although no chromosome location or gene has been identified. This report again illustrates the importance of careful clinical observation and the fact that genetic factors are likely to be even more common than currently appreciated.

## Generalized, Idiopathic Epilepsy Syndromes

Syndromes (Table 17–5) previously referred to as the "primary generalized epilepsies" are now labeled the "generalized, idiopathic epilepsies" in accordance with the

Table 17–5. **Generalized, Idiopathic (Inherited) Epilepsy Syndromes**

| Syndrome* | Transmission | Chromosome | Gene Product | Locus |
|---|---|---|---|---|
| Benign familial neonatal convulsions† | AD | 20q, 8q | K channel | EBN1, EBN2 |
| Benign infantile convulsions | FH | ? | ? | |
| Childhood absence epilepsy† | FH | 8q | ? | |
| Juvenile absence epilepsy† | AD | | ? | |
| Juvenile myoclonic epilepsy† | AD | 6p, 15q | ? | EJM1, ? |
| Generalized tonic-clonic upon awakening† | AD | 6p | ? | EJM1 |
| Generalized tonic-clonic, other | AD | ? | ? | |

*All syndromes described in text except benign infantile convulsions.
†Included in the 1989 International League Against Epilepsy classification of the epilepsies.
AD = autosomal dominant; FH = family history reported; ? = unknown; K = potassium.

ILAE classification system. A range of age dependencies, seizure types, and EEG signatures, with different underlying genetic mechanisms, is found within this large group.

## BENIGN FAMILIAL NEONATAL CONVULSIONS

Although benign familial neonatal convulsions (BFNC) is a relatively uncommon epilepsy syndrome, it illustrates several important points. The initial reports of families with this diagnosis indicated a range of seizure types (generalized and focal), duration of seizures (seconds to minutes), ages of presentation (days to 4 months), and outcome (seizure free/normal cognitive development, febrile and afebrile seizures, learning disabilities). Thus, it seemed plausible that a single gene could have a variety of clinical expressions (phenotypic heterogeneity).

Segregation analysis indicated a likely autosomal dominant mode of inheritance, and linkage analysis strongly supported a locus on chromosome 20q[32] (assuming autosomal dominant inheritance), designated as locus *EBN1*. Subsequent studies of other BFNC pedigrees indicated that families in whom some affected individuals had relatively late onset of epilepsy also mapped to the *EBN1* locus. A large family who did not map to this locus, however, was found to have a phenotype characterized by early onset and freedom from subsequent seizures. This family demonstrated linkage to markers on chromosome 8, which has been referred to as the *EBN2* locus.[33] Recently, mutations in potassium channel genes have been identified with both loci and have been designated as *KCNQ2*[34] (chromosome 20q) and *KCNQ3*[35] (chromosome 8). Thus, this syndrome expands the concepts of genotypic and phenotypic heterogeneity.

These results stimulate hypotheses regarding how different mutations in genes of the same family (e.g., potassium channels) in entirely different locations on the human genome can result in very similar, but not identical clinical presentations. This syndrome also illustrates that the limitations of the current classification scheme (ambiguity of localization-related versus generalized) has no significant impact on our understanding of its genetic basis. It is critical, however, that affected individuals be carefully identified clinically and that the mode of transmission be determined as accurately as possible for linkage analysis to be performed in an informative manner.

## CHILDHOOD ABSENCE EPILEPSY

Childhood absence epilepsy (CAE) is perhaps the most commonly recognized familial epilepsy, usually called *petit mal.* It is also referred to as *typical absence* to distinguish it from the staring (''atypical absence'') associated with the more malignant symptomatic generalized epilepsies. Common features of CAE include onset beginning at age 4 years, many daily staring episodes associated with eyelid fluttering, automatic movements of lips and hands, behavioral arrest, and a 3 Hz spike-wave EEG.

Mendelian transmission is suggested (though not proved) by an apparent autosomal dominant mode of inheritance and high concordance rate (75%) in twins. The risk of a first-degree relative of an affected individual developing seizures is in the range of 8% to 13%.[36,37] The significant methodological issue of identifying family members who should be counted as affected is illustrated by the observation that the EEG trait may be present even though the individual does not have seizures. Among 36 siblings of probands, 72% had spike-wave discharges, whereas only 4% had epilepsy.[38] Furthermore, the timing of obtaining the EEG used for assignment to the affected group may be critical because it is an age-related phenomenon. The possibility of missing affected individuals by performing the EEG too early or too late must be considered.

Although the data is preliminary, it seems likely that the seizure types developed by family members will be of the idiopathic generalized type,[38,39] although the locus on chromosome 6, associated with another common idiopathic generalized epilepsy, juvenile myoclonic epilepsy (see later), has been excluded for this syndrome.[40,41] A report utilizing a large, multigenerational family, however, found linkage of the CAE phenotype and/or a 3 to 4 Hz spike-wave

EEG pattern to chromosome 8q and confirmed this locus in five smaller families.[42] If replicated in other families, this information could be very useful in counseling families as to the risk of developing this or perhaps other idiopathic generalized syndromes in family members of affected individuals.

## JUVENILE ABSENCE EPILEPSY

Juvenile absence epilepsy (JAE) has its onset at 9 to 10 years of age with absences that are similar to those of CAE but with a much lower frequency of occurrence (e.g., several per week).[43] In addition, approximately 80% of children with JAE will have generalized tonic-clonic seizures as a concomitant seizure type within several years of absence onset or as the presenting seizure type. Unlike CAE, the seizures associated with JAE are more difficult to control with medications and usually persist for life. An autosomal dominant inheritance pattern has been postulated, but chromosomal localization has not been achieved.

## JUVENILE MYOCLONIC EPILEPSY

Juvenile myoclonic epilepsy (JME) is the most commonly reported and most intensely studied inherited epilepsy syndrome. Onset is usually in the early teens with several years of myoclonic jerks before the first generalized tonic-clonic seizure brings the individual to medical attention. Absences occur in a small, but significant number of these patients. Cognition is normal. The EEG is characterized by bilateral, synchronous 4 to 6 Hz spike-wave discharges. Despite excellent control with anticonvulsant medication (especially valproic acid), the seizure propensity continues for life at a very variable frequency.

An excellent review of available relevant studies has concluded that the pedigree data is most consistent with a two locus model rather than simple mendelian single-gene transmission.[40] Nonetheless, most studies that utilize linkage analysis assume an autosomal dominant mode with a high degree (>70%) of penetrance. With these assumptions, JME was linked to a locus on the short arm of chromosome 6 by means of HLA markers in 1988.[44] This locus was designated *EJM1.* Although other studies confirmed this localization with DNA markers, it became apparent that not all families mapped to this location.[45] Strong evidence for a locus on chromosome 15q in a region containing a nicotonic acetylcholine receptor gene has raised the possibility that JME may be due to a channelopathy in some pedigrees.[46] Factors important in defining the probands and affected family members in these studies include myoclonic seizures as the predominant seizure type, presence and frequency of absence seizures, and the EEG trait of generalized, 4 to 6 Hz polyspike, and spike-wave discharges.[47–49] Thus, "JME" probably designates a group of phenotypically similar, but genotypically diverse syndromes.

## GENERALIZED TONIC-CLONIC SEIZURES UPON AWAKENING

Generalized tonic-clonic seizures upon awakening is an idiopathic generalized epilepsy syndrome that overlaps with JME with regard to age of onset and seizure occurrence upon awakening from sleep. Generalized tonic-clonic seizures with adolescent onset that occur randomly throughout the sleep-wake cycle is another idiopathic generalized syndrome that is frequently familial. Given the similarity to JME with regard to age of onset and seizure type, it is reasonable to hypothesize that some of these individuals might also map to the *EJM1* locus. A recent study found that only the group with seizures upon awakening shared this locus.[50] The chromosomal localizations of the other, familial generalized tonic-clonic syndromes remains to be determined. This remarkable observation indicates that relatively subtle differences in clinical phenotype may indicate significant genetic heterogeneity.

## COMMENTS

It is apparent from the currently available data that syndromes such as CAE, JAE, JME, and generalized tonic-clonic seizures upon awakening cannot be explained by a simple genetic hypothesis such as a single gene with an age-dependent expression. Even the

Table 17–6. **Progressive Myoclonus Epilepsy Syndromes**

| Syndrome | Transmission | Chromosome | Gene Product | Locus |
|---|---|---|---|---|
| Neuronal ceroid lipofuscinoses | | | | |
| NCL1 (Santavuori) | AR | 1p | ? | *CLN1* |
| NCL2-(Jansky Bielschowsy) (late infantile) | AR | ? | ? | *CLN2* |
| NCL3 (Spielmeyer-Vogt) (juvenile) | AR | 16p | ? | *CLN3* |
| NCL4 (Kufs) (adult) | AR, AD | ? | ? | *CLN4* |
| NCL5 (variant late infantile) | AR | 13q | ? | *CLN5* |
| Unverricht-Lundborg and related syndromes | AR | 21q | Cystatin B | *EPM1* |
| Lafora body | AR | 6q | ? | |
| Northern epilepsy | AR | 8p | ? | *EPMR* |
| Myoclonic epilepsy with ragged red fibers | Maternal | 8344A→G | Cytochrome c oxidase | |
| Sialidosis I | AR | 6p | Neuramini-dase | |

AD = autosomal dominant; AR = autosomal recessive; FH = family history reported; ? = unknown.

role of a gene locus such as *EJM1* is more complex than being present in a subset of families with JME and absent in those with "non-classic" JME, CAE, and JAE. This is illustrated by a recent study[51] of pedigrees ascertained by CAE and JAE probands that included family members with a variety of generalized, idiopathic epilepsies, including JME. No linkage was found with the *EJM1* locus. When a subset of families was selected on the basis of JME as the index syndrome, however, the association with *EJM1* became significant. This interesting data demonstrates the genetic heterogeneity of the generalized, idiopathic epilepsies and shows how a locus may or may not be involved in the expression of a specific phenotype (e.g., JME) within a family.

## Generalized, Cryptogenic, and/or Symptomatic Epilepsy Syndromes

Generalized, cryptogenic, and/or symptomatic epilepsy syndromes include commonly recognized pediatric epilepsies such as West's syndrome (infantile spasms) and Lennox-Gastaut syndrome, which may result from a specific etiology such as tuberous sclerosis or unknown causes. These syndromes are age related in presentation and seizure types. The contribution of inheritance is determined by the specific underlying problem (e.g., meningitis/encephalitis, none; aminoacidopathy, high). A subgroup of the generalized, symptomatic epilepsies includes "specific syndromes" in which seizures are "the presenting or prominent" symptom of the disorder.[1] Several of these (Table 17–6) have been grouped as the "progressive myoclonus epilepsies" due to phenotypic similarities that include myoclonus, seizures, dementia, and ataxia.[52,53] Although relatively uncommon, these entities are described to underscore the genetic diversity (heterogeneity) that can underlie disorders classified by phenotypic and/or neuropathological criteria.

### NEURONAL CEROID LIPOFUSCINOSES

The cytoplasm of neurons in the neuronal ceroid lipofuscinoses (NCLs) contains a material (lipofuscin) that is autofluorescent and appears as yellow granules with hematoxylin–eosin stain under light microscopy. These cytoplasmic inclusions have been described in ultrastructural studies as curvilinear, rectilinear, and fingerprint bodies with several transitional forms. This material can be found in biopsy specimens of brain, skin, conjunctiva, lymphocytes, and rectum. Classification has been based on age of onset (infant to adult), clinical features (especially seizures, myoclonus, visual loss, and dementia) and ultrastructural appearance, with the assumption that all types of NCLs share a common pathophysiology that results in the storage of lipofuscin. Genetic analyses, however, have revealed that several of these disorders are not related on the genomic level. The syndrome names, modes of transmission, chromosome localizations, gene products, and locus designations are provided in Table 17–6.

The multiple types of NCL have recently been described in an excellent textbook regarding metabolic diseases of children.[54] The infantile form (NCL1, Santavuori) begins with visual loss followed by psychomotor deterioration, hypotonia, and death in childhood, with seizures occurring as a late feature. A locus *(CLN1)* on chromosome 1p has been associated with this form. The late infantile type (NCL2, Jansky-Bielschowsy) presents between 2 and 4 years of age, with visual loss and dementia followed by intractable myoclonic and generalized tonic-clonic seizures and ataxia, with death usually occurring before 20 years of age. An autosomal recessive mode of inheritance has been identified, but a chromosomal localization has not been made. A recently reported variant of this type with onset of developmental decline at 4 to 7 years followed by seizures and ataxia has been described in the Finnish population, designated NCL5 and mapped to chromosome 13q.[55] The juvenile form (NCL3, Spielmeyer-Vogt/late onset Batten) presents between 5 and 10 years of age and is characterized by generalized tonic-clonic seizures, myoclonus, blindness, and dementia with the later development of extrapyramidal motor dysfunction.[56] The chromosome locus, *CLN3,* is found on 16p. Finally, the adult type (NCL4, Kufs) is found in two forms, one characterized by seizures, myoclonus, and dementia and the other by disorders of cognition and movement. No chromosomal localization has been made as yet.

## UNVERRICHT-LUNDBORG/ MEDITERRANEAN/BALTIC DISEASES

Until recently, the progressive myoclonus epilepsies of Unverricht-Lundborg, Mediterranean, and Baltic diseases were distinguished more by geographic distribution than by clinical differences. All had onset around adolescence characterized by some combination of seizures, cognitive decline, and ataxia, which progressed at variable rates. The pattern of inheritance is consistently autosomal recessive. Unverricht-Lundborg disease (in the Finnish population) and the Mediterranean and Baltic forms are linked to chromosome 21q (locus *EPM1*). Patients with this phenotype have been reported from multiple other countries, and all have mapped to *EPM1.*

Although rare in most populations, Unverricht-Lundborg disease is present in 1 in 20,000 individuals in the Finland. Given the genetic heterogeneity demonstrated in several of the other syndromes described, the uniformity of the locus underlying this rather broad phenotype is somewhat surprising. In 1996, the *EPM1* locus was identified with the gene coding for cystatin B.[57] Recently, the nature of the mutation was found to be an unstable minisatellite expansion in the gene promotor region.[58] The mechanism by which this ubiquitous protease inhibitor results in the clinical phenotype is unknown.

## LAFORA BODY DISEASE

Lafora body disease, another progressive myoclonus epilepsy, is clinically very similar to the Unverricht-Lundborg–like syndromes described above with the distinguishing features of teenage onset and relatively rapid neurologic deterioration. The defining pathological feature is the presence of cellular inclusions (Lafora bodies) positive for periodic acid–Schiff stain. Failure to map this disorder to the *EPM1* locus led to a genome-wide search in biopsy-confirmed families, and the identification of the EPM2a locus on chromosome 6q occurred in 1995.[59] The EPM2a gene encodes a novel protein tyrosine phosphatase.[59a]

## NORTHERN EPILEPSY SYNDROME

Northern epilepsy syndrome has been described in less than 20 families in northern Finland.[60] It is characterized by onset before age 10 years, generalized tonic-clonic and complex partial seizures, increase in seizure frequency until puberty followed by infrequent seizures as adults, and cognitive deterioration during childhood, progressing to dementia in adults. In contrast to the other progressive myoclonus epilepsy syndromes, in Northern epilepsy syndrome there seems to be a relative slowing of the clinical course during adulthood. Due to the concentration of affected individuals within a few families, it was possible to use linkage analysis techniques to map this disease to a locus on chromosome 8q (locus designation *EPMR*). It should be noted that it was the *clinical* observation that the features of this syndrome were different from the Unverricht-Lundborg–like progressive myoclonus epilepsy (which is much more frequent in the Finnish population) that motivated the search for another chromosomal localization.

### SIALIDOSIS TYPE 1

Sialidosis type 1, which can have associated myoclonic seizures, is traditionally included with the progressive myoclonus epilepsies. It is due to a deficiency of neuraminidase and has been mapped to chromosome 10q.[61]

### MITOCHONDRIAL DISORDERS

Although seizures can be a part of several mitochondrial disorders, the mitochondrial syndrome in which epilepsy is prominent is myoclonic epilepsy with ragged-red fibers (MERRF). MERRF is characterized by a constellation of abnormalities, including weakness (myopathy), myoclonus, ataxia, cognitive abnormalities, and hearing loss presenting in the first two decades of life. Significant clinical heterogeneity within a family with regard to the predominance of one or more symptoms and their severity, however, is common. In the early 1990s it became apparent that the majority of individuals with MERRF have a specific mutation at nucleotide pair 8344 in the mitochondrial genome. It was soon recognized, however, that genetic heterogeneity occurred because some patients with identical symptoms had a different mitochondrial mutation. Furthermore, individuals were found who had the 8344 mutation with different clinical syndromes (i.e., phenotypic heterogeneity).[62,63] Ultimately, it will be necessary to define the pathophysiologies of these disorders to determine how a specific genetic abnormality results in a variety of clinical syndromes.

## GENETIC COUNSELING

Genetic counseling for the epilepsies should take into account the natural history of the disorder, available therapies, and implications for quality of life, in addition to predicting the likelihood of seizure occurrence in a family member.[64] These goals are most readily achieved when a precise epilepsy syndrome can be identified. This may be a syndrome in which epilepsy is the primary manifestation or one in which seizures are part of a multisystem phenotype (e.g., sialidosis type 1). If a mendelian inheritance pattern has been determined, then standard risks (e.g., 50% for autosomal dominant and 25% for autosomal recessive) can be cited for subsequent siblings.

Among the autosomal dominant inherited epilepsies, BFNC comes closest to the expected 50% of siblings affected, verified with pedigree data. Syndromes that have been described in single families, such as ADNFLE and partial epilepsy with auditory features, have been best modeled by an autosomal dominant pattern, but await confirmation in other pedigrees. Other syndromes in which an autosomal dominant mode of inheritance has been postulated show significant variance from that predicted by the autosomal dominant model, for example, CAE (8% to 20%)[36,37] and BECTS (10% to 33%).[18] Risk prediction is complicated in the relatively common syndrome of JME in which autosomal dominant, autosomal recessive, and multilocus models have been suggested.[40] In this situation, meaningful counseling can occur only in the context of a well-defined individual pedigree.

The same complications are present in disorders with proposed autosomal recessive inheritance described above. The "specificity" of counseling is further compromised by the reality that although susceptibility is clearly inherited, the manner in which it will become manifest is not. This is illustrated by the examples provided above (BECTS, CEOP, RE, and generalized idiopathic epilepsies) in which multiple seizure types and epilepsy syndromes can be present within the same family. The ability to predict the likelihood of seizures (independent of type) is even more tenuous for those epilepsies that have a complex inheritance. Unfortunately, these seizure disorders probably represent the majority of inherited epilepsies. Genetic counseling for these families awaits greater understanding of the the genetic–molecular etiologies of seizure susceptibility and expression.

## ANIMAL MODELS

It is apparent from the descriptions of the inherited human epilepsies that a significant amount of phenotypic as well as genotypic heterogeneity exists. The lack of relatively pure "experiments of nature" has made it difficult to elucidate the pathophysiologies and, therefore, mechanism-based treatments of the human epilepsies. Thus, relevant animal models are most useful for elucidating the manner in which genetic variations result in a variety of seizure types. Several examples of these models are briefly described with attention directed to those features that are shared with the human condition. The interested reader is referred elsewhere for more comprehensive reviews.[65–68]

*Papio papio* is a baboon that has myoclonic and tonic-clonic seizures elicited by photic stimulation, thus serving as one of the original models of an inherited reflex epilepsy. Similar to humans, these seizures are effectively prevented with valproic acid. Due to the inherent limitations in breeding, however, more detailed genetic studies have not been possible.

With a faster breeding cycle and comparatively lower costs, rodents have provided the major source of animal investigation. The *genetic epilepsy prone rat (GEPR)* has seizures characterized by behavioral arrest, myoclonus, and tonic-clonic movements in response to auditory stimulation.[65] In addition, the GEPR has spontaneous seizures and a lowered threshold to electrical, chemical, and temperature stimulation. The inferior colliculi have been identified as critical components mediating the auditory response with abnormalities in $\gamma$-aminobutyric acid levels antedating the age-related seizure susceptibility. Phenobarbital, pheytoin, and carbamazepine are effective anticonvulsants. Polygenic and autosomal dominant models of inheritance have been proposed.

The *genetic absence epilepsy rat (GAER)* demonstrates age-related behavioral arrest and staring associated with bi-hemispheric spike-wave discharge on the EEG. The likely pathophysiology of this phenotype involves a calcium current in the lateral thalamic reticular nuclei because blockade of this channel prevents spike-wave discharges.[69,70] Agents effective in human idiopathic generalized epilepsies (valproic acid, ethosuximide, and benzodiazepines) block seizures. The epilepsy phenotype is expressed as an autosomal dominant trait with variable penetrance.

The *epilepsy-like (El)* mouse responds to vestibular stimulation with behavioral arrest, staring, and motor activity seen in the face and the extremities in a manner similar to human complex partial seizures. Metabolic studies have suggested seizure onset in the temporal lobes. Phenytoin and valproate are effective treatments. Extensive breeding studies have provided strong evidence of at least two responsible genetic loci on chromosomes 9 and 2.[71]

Another very productive approach to explore the genetic mechanisms underlying absence epilepsy is to screen bred mice for the absence phenotype associated with a generalized spike-wave pattern on the EEG.[72] Four mouse strains have been identified that meet these criteria. Of great interest, they differ with regard to seizure frequency and duration, associated neurologic features, relevant pharmacological mechanisms, and associated chromosomal aberration. Recently, a mutation in the $\alpha_{1A}$ voltage-sensitive calcium channel gene was demonstrated to be the etiology of absence seizures in the *tottering* strain,[73] whereas a neuronal calcium-channel $\gamma$-subunit mutation underlies a similar phenotype in the *stargazer* mouse.[74] These mice with spontaneously occurring seizures indicate that different ion channel mutations can produce very similar phenotypes that may be used to design specific therapies in the future.

Finally, the ability to target specific genes ("knock-outs") allows study of the multiple steps between a known gene mutation and its clinical manifestations. Such mutations have been produced in mice, which result in seizures as part of a more complex phenotype. These models have been recently reviewed.[75,76] During the last few years, a partial list of targeted gene deletions found to be associated with seizures includes serotonin 2c receptor, synapsins 1 and 2 (synaptic vesicle proteins), Ca/calmodulin protein kinase, and G protein–coupled potassium channel. These demonstrate the multiple potential mechanisms of altering neuronal excitability that can result in seizures. The roles of these mechanisms in any of the human epilepsies are as yet unclear.

## SUMMARY

Although it has long been recognized that genetic factors play a role in a variety of epilepsies, remarkable progress has been made within the last decade. Before this time, a "family history" was acknowledged in some pedigrees, and a suspected mode of inheritance was hypothesized in others. During the last decade, specific syndromes have been linked to different chromosomes, and two human "epilepsy genes" have been identified. It is apparent that significant genetic heterogeneity occurs among families with phenotypically similar epilepsy syndromes. In addition, it appears that it is the susceptibility to have seizures, independent of type or syndrome, that is inherited in some families.

The greatest challenges lie ahead in at least two regards. The genetic/inherited bases of the common epilepsies with complex inheritance patterns remain to be defined. It is likely that multiple genes that control such features as susceptibility, age of expression, degree of penetrance, provoking stimuli, and generalized versus partial mechanisms and possibly gene–environment interactions, will be involved. Finally, definition of the manner in which genetic lesions produce the cascade of events leading the clinical phenotype of seizures should provide a variety of targets to which new therapies can be directed. It is likely that animal models will prove essential to meeting these challenges, as they allow detailed analyses of the cascade of events beginning with alteration of individual and multiple genes, resulting in the cortical hyperexcitability state underlying seizures. Hopefully, understanding this cascade will lead to a new generation of gene-directed, therapeutic interventions and to a greater ability to provide genetic counseling for affected individuals.

## REFERENCES


1. Commission on Classification and Terminology of the International League Against Epilepsy. Proposal for revised classification of epilepsies and epileptic syndromes. Epilepsia 30:389–399, 1989.
2. Dichter MA, Buchhalter JR: The genetic epilepsies. In Rosenberg RN, Prusiner SB, DiMauro S, Barchi RL (eds): The Molecular and Genetic Basis of Neurological Disease. Butterworth-Heinemann, Boston, 1997, pp757–783.
3. Beck-Mannagetta G, Anderson VE, Doose H, Janz D (eds.): Genetics of the Epilepsies. Springer-Verlag, Berlin, 1989.
4. Commission on Classification and Terminology of the International League Against Epilepsy. Proposal for revised clinical and electroencephalographic classification of epileptic seizures. Epilepsia 22:489–501, 1981.
5. Hauser WA, Annegers JF, Kurland LT: Prevalence of epilepsy in Rochester, Minnesota: 1940–1980. Epilepsia 32:429–445, 1991.
6. Loiseau J, Loiseau P, Guyot M, Duche B, Dartigues JF, Aublet B: Survey of seizure disorders in the French Southwest, I: Incidence of epileptic syndromes. Epilepsia 31:391–396, 1990.
7. Manford M, Hart YM, Sander JW, Shorvon SD: The national general practice study of epilepsy—The syndromic classification of the international league against epilepsy applied to epilepsy in a general population. Arch Neurol 49:801–808, 1992.
8. Oka E, Ishida S, Ohtsuka Y, Ohtahara S: Neuroepidemiological study of childhood epilepsy by application of international classification of epilepsies and epileptic syndromes (ILAE, 1989). Epilepsia 36:658–661, 1995.
9. Ohtsuka Y, Ohno S, Ohtahara S: Classification of epilepsies and epileptic syndromes of childhood according to the 1989 ILAE classification. J Epilepsy 6:272–276, 1993.
10. Shah KN, Rajadhyaksha SB, Shah VS, Shah NS, Desai VG: Experience with the International League Against Epilepsy classifications of epileptic seizures (1981) and epilepsies and epileptic syndrome (1989) in epileptic children in a developing country. Epilepsia 33:1072–1077, 1992.

11. Hauser WA, Hesdorffer DC: Epilepsy: Frequency, Causes and Consequences. Demos, New York, 1990.
12. Hauser WA, Annegers JF, Kurland LT: Incidence of epilepsy and unprovoked seizures in Rochester, Minnesota: 1935–1984. Epilepsia 34:453–468, 1993.
13. Cowan LD, Bodensteiner JB, Leviton A, Doherty A: Prevalence of the epilepsies in children and adolescents. Epilepsia 30:94–106, 1989.
14. Haerer AF, Anderson DW, Schoenberg BS: Prevalence and clinical features of epilepsy in a biracial united states population. Epilepsia 27:66–75, 1986.
15. Ottman R, Annegers JF, Risch N, Hauser WA, Susser M: Relations of genetic and environmental factors in the etiology of epilepsy. Ann Neurol 39: 442–449, 1996.
16. Ottman R, Lee JH, Risch N, Hauser WA, Susser M: Clinical indicators of genetic susceptibility to epilepsy. Epilepsia 37:353–361, 1996.
17. Bray PF, Wiser WG: Evidence for a genetic etiology of temporal-central abnormalities in focal epilepsy. N Engl J Med 271:926–933, 1964.
18. Bray PF, Wiser WC, Wood CM, Pusey SB: Hereditary characteristics of familial temporal-central focal epilepsy. Pediatrics 2:207–211, 1965.
19. Heijbel J, Blom S, Rasmuson M: Benign epilepsy of childhood with centrotemporal foci: A genetic study. Epilepsia 16:285–293, 1975.
20. Degen R, Degen HE: Some genetic aspects of rolandic epilepsy: Waking and sleep EEGs in siblings. Epilepsia 31:795–801, 1990.
21. Gastaut H: A new type of epilepsy: Benign partial epilepsy of childhood with occipital spike-waves. Clin Electroencephalogr 13:13–22, 1982.
22. Panayiotopoulos CP: Benign nocturnal childhood occipital epilepsy: A new syndrome with nocturnal seizures, tonic deviation of the eyes, and vomiting. J Child Neurol 4:43–49, 1989.
23. Radhakrishhnan K, Silbert PL, Klass DW: Reading epilepsy: An appraisal of 20 patients diagnosed at the Mayo Clinic, Rochester, Minnesota, between 1949 and 1989, and delineation of the epileptic syndrome. Brain. 118:75–89, 1995.
24. Scheffer IE, Bhatia KP, Lopes-Cendes I, et al.: Autosomal dominant nocturnal frontal lobe epilepsy: A distinctive clinical entity. Brain 118:61–73, 1995.
25. Scheffer IE, Bhatia KP, Lopes-Cendes I, Fish DR, Marsden CD, Andermann F: Autosomal frontal lobe epilepsy misdiagnosed as sleep disorder. Lancet 343:515–517, 1994.
26. Phillips HA, Scheffer IE, Berkovic SF, Hollway GE, Sutherland GR, Mulley JC: Localization of a gene for autosomal dominant nocturnal frontal lobe epilepsy to chromosome 20q13.2. Nat Genet 10:117–118, 1995.
27. Steinlein OK, Mulley JC, Propiing P, et al.: A missense mutation in the neuronal nicotinic acetylcholine receptor α4 subunit is associated with autosomal dominant nocturnal frontal lobe epilepsy. Nat Genet 11:1–5, 1995.
28. Steinlein OK, Magnusson A, Stoodt J, et al.: An insertion mutation of the CHRNA4 gene in a family with autosomal dominant nocturnal frontal lobe epilepsy. Hum Mol Genet 6:943–948, 1997.
29. Phillips HA, Scheffer IE, Crossland KM, et al.: Autosomal Dominant Nocturnal Frontal-Lobe Epilepsy: Genetic Heterogeneity for a Second Locus at 15q24. Am J Hum Genet 63:1108–1116, 1998.
30. Scheffer IE, Jones L, Pozzebon M, Howell RA, Saling MM, Berkovic SF: Autosomal dominant rolandic epilepsy and speech dyspraxia: A new syndrome with anticipation. Ann Neurol 38:633–642, 1995.
31. Berkovic SF, McIntosh A, Howell RA, Mitchell A, Sheffield LJ, Hopper JL: Familial temporal lobe epilepsy: A common disorder identified in twins. Ann Neurol 40:227–235, 1996.
32. Leppert M, Anderson VE, Quattlebaum T, et al.: Benign familial neonatal convulsions linked to genetic markers on chromosome 20. Nature 337: 647–648, 1989.
33. Ryan SG, Wiznitzer M, Hollman C, Torres MC, Szekeresova M, Schneider S: Benign familial neonatal convulsions: Evidence for clinical and genetic heterogeneity. Ann Neurol 29:469–473, 1991.
34. Singh NA, Charlier C, Stauffer D, et al.: A novel potassium channel gene, KCNQ2, is mutated in an inherited epilepsy of newborns. Nat Genet 18:25–29, 1998.
35. Charlier C, Singh NA, Ryan SG, et al.: A pore mutation in a novel KQT-like potassium channel gene in an idiopathic epilepsy. Nat Genet 18:5353–5355, 1998.
36. Doose H, Baier WK: Absences. In Managetta GB (ed): Genetics of the Epilepsies. Springer-Verlag, Berlin, 1989, pp34–42.
37. Metrakos K, Metrakos J: Genetics of convulsive disorders. II. Genetic and electroencephalographic studies in centrencephalic epilepsy. Neurology 11: 474–483, 1961.
38. Degen R, Degen HE, Roth C: Some genetic aspects of idiopathic and symptomatic absence seizures: Waking and sleep EEGs in siblings. Epilepsia 31: 784–794, 1990.
39. Delgado-Escueta AV, Greenberg D, Weissbecker K, et al.: Gene mapping in the idiopathic generalized epilepsies: Juvenile myoclonic epilepsy, childhood absence epilepsy, epilepsy with grand mal seizures, and early childhood myoclonic epilepsy. Epilepsia 31 (suppl 3):S19–S29, 1990.
40. Greenberg D, Durner M, Delgado-Escueta AV: Evidence for multiple gene loci in the expression of the common generalized epilepsies. Neurology 42(suppl 5):56–62, 1992.
41. Serratosa JM, Delgado-Escueta AV, Pascual-Castroviego I, et al.: Childhood absence epilepsy: Exclusion of genetic linkage to chromosome 6p markers. Epilepsia 34(suppl 2):S149, 1993.
42. Fong GCY, Shah PU, Gee MN, et al.: Childhood absence epilepsy with tonic-clonic seizures and electroencephalogram 3–4 Hz spike and multiple-slow wave complexes: Linkage to chromosome 8q24. Am J Hum Genet 63:1117–1129, 1998.
43. Aicardi J: Epilepsy in Children, 2nd ed. Raven Press, New York, 1994.
44. Greenberg DA, Delgado-Escueta AV, Widelitz H, et al.: Juvenile myoclonic epilepsy (JME) may be linked to the BF and HLA loci on human chromosome 6. Am J Med Genet 31:185–192, 1988.
45. Whitehouse WP, Rees M, Curtis D, et al.: Linkage analysis of idiopathic generalized epilepsy (IGE) and marker loci on chromosome 6p in families of

patients with juvenile myoclonic epilepsy: No evidence for an epilepsy locus in the HLA region. Am J Hum Genet 53:652–662, 1993.
46. Elmslie F, Rees M, Williamson MP, et al.: Genetic mapping of a major susceptibility locus for juvenile myoclonic epilepsy on chromosome 15q. Hum Mol Genet 6:1329–1334, 1997.
47. Delgado-Escueta A, Serratosa J, Liu A, et al.: Progress in mapping human epilepsy genes. Epilepsia 35(suppl 1):S29–S40, 1994.
48. Liu AW, Delgado-Escueta AV, Serratosa JM, et al.: Juvenile myoclonic epilepsy locus in chromosome 6p21.2–p11: Linkage to convulsions and electroencephalography trait. Am J Hum Genet 57:368–381, 1995.
49. Serratosa JM, Delgado-Escueta AV, Medina MT, Zhang Q, Iranmanesh R, Sparkes RS: Clinical and genetic analysis of a large pedigree with juvenile myoclonic epilepsy. Ann Neurol 39:187–195, 1996.
50. Greenberg DA, Durner M, Rosenbaum D, Shinnar S: The genetics of idiopathic generalized epilepsies of adolescent onset: Differences between juvenile myoclonic epilepsy and epilepsy with random grand mal and with awakening grand mal. Neurology 45:942–946, 1995.
51. Sander T, Hildmann T, Janz D, et al.: The phenotypic spectrum related to the human epilepsy susceptibility gene "EJM1." Ann Neurol 38:210–217, 1995.
52. Marseille Consensus Group: Classification of progressive myoclonus epilepsies and related disorders. Ann Neurol 28:113–116, 1990.
53. Berkovic SF, Andermann F, Carpenter S, Wolfe LS: Progressive myoclonus epilepsies: Specific causes and diagnosis. N Engl J Med 315:296–305, 1986.
54. Lyon G, Adams RD, Kolodny EH: Neurology of Hereditary Metabolic Diseases of Children, ed 2. McGraw Hill, New York, 1996, pp146–150.
55. Williams R, Vesa J, Jarvela I, et al.: Genetic heterogeneity in neuronal cerid lipofuscinosis (NCL): Evidence that the late-infantile subtype (Jansky-Bielschowsky disease; CLN2) is not an allelic form of the juvenile or infantile sub-types. Am J Hum Genet. 53:931–935, 1993.
56. Mitchison HM, Taschner PE, O'Rawe AM, de Vos N, Phillips HA: Genetic mapping of the Batten disease locus (CLN3) to the interval D16S288-D16S383 by analysis of haplotypes and allelic association. Genomics 22:465–468, 1994.
57. Pennacchio LA, Lehesjoki AE, Stone NE, et al.: Mutations in the gene encoding cystatin B in progressive myoclonus epilepsy (EPM1) [see comments]. Science. 271:1731–1734, 1996.
58. Virtaneva K, D'Amato E, Miao J, et al.: Unstable minisatellite expansion causing recessively inherited myoclonus epilepsy, EPM1. Nat Genet 15:393–396, 1997.
59. Serratosa JM, Delgado-Escueta AV, Posada I: The gene for progressive myoclonus epilepsy of the Lafora type maps to chromosome 6q. Hum Mol Genet 4:1657–1644, 1996.
59a. Minassian BA, Lee JR, Herbrick JA et al.: Mutations in a gene encoding a novel protein tyrosine phosphatase cause progressive myoclonus epilepsy. Nat Genet 20:171–174, 1998.
60. Tahvanainen E, Ranta S, Hirvasniemi A, et al.: The gene for a novel recessively inherited human epilepsy with progressive mental retardation maps to the distal short arm of chromosome 8. Proc Natl Acad Sci USA 91:7267–7270, 1994.
61. Pshezhetsky AV, Richard C, Michaud L, et al.: Cloning, expression and chromosomal mapping of human lysosomal sialidase and characterization of mutations in sialidosis. Nat Genet 15:316–320, 1997.
62. Silvestri G, Ciafaloni E, Santorelli FM, et al.: Clinical features associated wit the A to G transition at nucleotide 8344 of mtDNA ("MERRF mutation"). Neurology 43:1200–1206, 1993.
63. Silvestri G, Moraes CT, Shanske S, Oh SJ, DiMaura S: A new mtDNA mutation in the tRNA(Lys) gene associated with myoclonic epilepsy and ragged-red fibers (MERRF). Am J Hum Genet 51:1213–1217, 1992.
64. Blandfort M, Tsuboi T, Vogel F: Genetic counseling in the epilepsies. I. Genetic risks. Hum Genet 76:303–331, 1987.
65. Jobe P, Mishra P, Ludvig N, Dailey J: Genetic models of the epilepsies. In Schwartzkroin, P (ed). Concepts and Models in Epilepsy Research. Cambridge University Press, Cambridge, 1991 pp.94–140.
66. Buchhalter JR: Animal models of inherited epilepsy. Epilepsia 34(S3):S31–S41, 1993.
67. Engel JJr: Critical evaluation of animal models for localization-related epilepsies. Ital J Neurol Sci 16: 9–16, 1995.
68. Fariello RG: Critical review of the animal models of generalized epilepsies. Ital J Neurol Sci 16:69–72, 1995.
69. Vergnes M, Marescaux C, Depaulis A, Micheletti G, Warter JM: Spontaneous spike and wave discharges in thalamus and cortex in a rat model of genetic petit mal-like seizures. Exp Neurol 96:127–136, 1987.
70. Avanzini G, de Curtis M, Marescaux C, Panzica F, Spreafico R, Vergnes M: Role of the thalamic reticular nucleus in the generation of rhythmic thalamo-cortical activities subserving spike and waves. J Neural Trans Suppl 35:85–95, 1992.
71. Rise M, Frankel W, Coffin J, Seyfried T: Genes for epilepsy mapped in the mouse. Science 253:669–673, 1991.
72. Noebels JL: Single locus mutations in mice expressing generalized spike-wave absence epilepsies. Ital J Neurol Sci 16:623–627, 1995.
73. Fletcher CF, Lutz CM, O'Sullivan TN, et al.: Absence epilepsy in *tottering* mutant mice is associated with calcium channel defects. Cell 87:607–617, 1996.
74. Letts VA, Felix R, Biddlecome GH, et al.: The mouse *stargazer* gene encodes a neuronal $Ca^{2+}$-channel $\gamma$ subunit. Nat Genet 19:340–347, 1998.
75. Noebels JL: Targeting epilepsy genes. Neuron 16: 241–244, 1996.
76. McNamara JO, Puranam RS: Epilepsy genetics: An abundance of riches for biologists. Curr Biol 8: R168–R170, 1998.

Chapter 18

# GENETICS OF PARKINSON'S DISEASE AND OTHER MOVEMENT DISORDERS

Thomas Gasser, MD
Wolfgang H. Oertel, MD



Advances in molecular genetic techniques have lead to a series of exciting discoveries, greatly expanding our knowledge of the molecular basis of genetically determined movement disorders. The chromosomal position of many of the genes responsible for movement disorder syndromes have been determined within the human genome. In many cases, the disease genes themselves and their mutation(s) have been identified. The proteins encoded by these genes and their pathogenic alterations can now be studied, providing new insight into the molecular pathology of their associated diseases. In addition, a new classification based on the nature and the chromosomal location of the genetic defect is now being developed for a number of heterogeneous syndromes. This development is particularly important in the study of movement disorders. Many movement disorder syndromes are etiologically heterogeneous and present overlapping patterns of abnormal movement. Because biological markers are usually not available, it is often difficult to classify a patient based on the clinical picture alone.

The contribution of molecular genetics to diagnosis, classification, and understanding the pathogenesis of movement disorders depends not only on current knowledge of the underlying genetic alterations but also on the degree of etiologic complexity of the disorder. Some diseases are caused by a specific mutation in a single gene. Probably all cases of Huntington's disease, for example, are caused by a trinucleotide repeat expansion in the gene for huntingtin on the short arm of chromosome 4. Other disorders, such as Wilson's disease, are due to a number of different mutations in a single gene, making direct molecular diagnosis and genotype–phenotype correlations more difficult.

Still other disorders, such as the idiopathic torsion dystonias, are genetically heterogeneous. In this case, a mutation in a gene on chromosome 9q34 is responsible for many, but not all, cases of familial generalized torsion dystonia with early onset, and clinical variants of idiopathic dystonias are caused by mutations in other genes. Finally, in complex diseases, such as Parkinson's disease, increasing evidence suggests a genetic contribution to etiology, but the exact nature of this contribution remains unknown. A single-gene defect probably is responsible for such complex disorders in only a small number of families. In most cases, simple mendelian inheritance is unlikely, and the interaction of several genes with each other, or with nongenetic etiologic factors, may be important.

This chapter focuses on recent advances in the molecular genetic analysis of inherited movement disorder syndromes. Some pertinent data on the mapping of genes for hereditary movement disorders is summarized in Table 18–1. Huntington's disease is covered separately in Chapter 13.

## FAMILIAL PARKINSONISM AND IDIOPATHIC PARKINSON'S DISEASE

The first descriptions of the familial occurrence of Parkinson's disease (PD) date back to the nineteenth century. In his classic textbook, Gowers' stated that a hereditary basis may be traced in up to 15% of patients with PD.[1] The first systematic genetic study was carried out by Mjönes. He concluded that PD is a monogenic autosomal dominant disorder with age-related penetrance reaching 60%.[2] This study was later criticized, however, for counting relatives with atypical or minimal symptoms (such as isolated rest and postural tremor) as secondary cases of PD. Subsequent surveys generally failed to demonstrate strong evidence for an increased frequency of PD among relatives of index cases.[3,4] In addition, low concordance rates in twin studies argued against a major genetic contribution to PD.[5–7]

In recent years, however, the role of genetic factors in the etiology of PD has gained increased attention.[8–11] Several epidemiological surveys show a significantly increased risk for PD in relatives of affected individuals, with a risk for first-degree relatives generally in the range of two to three times greater than normal.[12–17] New twin studies (some using $^{18}$F-dopa positron emission tomography [PET] to identify preclinical lesions of the nigrostriatal dopaminergic system) have identified a higher proportion of affected co-twins than previously assumed, providing evidence of an inherited susceptibility to develop PD,[18–20] although the effect of a shared exposure to an environmental toxin cannot be excluded. Finally, it is now well-recognized that parkinsonism may occur as the sole or predominant manifestation of one of several monogenic disorders. It is probable that, like Alzheimer's disease, PD will eventually prove to be etiologically heterogeneous. A small proportion of cases may be caused by highly penetrant mutations in several different genes, but in most cases the interaction of one or more "susceptibility genes" with other (nongenetic) causes are probably necessary to cause the PD phenotype.

### Familial Parkinsonism

Hereditary forms of parkinsonism, more or less closely resembling idiopathic Parkinson's disease, have been described.

#### PARKINSONISM AS A PRESENTATION OF HEREDITARY DISORDERS MORE COMMONLY ASSOCIATED WITH OTHER PHENOTYPES

On rare occasions, parkinsonism may be the consequence of a mutation more commonly associated with other phenotypes. For example, Machado-Joseph disease (MJD), a disorder caused by the expansion

Table 18–1. **Genes Involved in Some Movement Disorder Syndromes**

| Disease | Gene Symbol | Inheritance | Map Position | Gene Product | Mutation | Senior Author |
|---|---|---|---|---|---|---|
| Huntington's disease | *HD* | AD | 4p16.3 | Huntingtin | Trinuc | Huntington's Disease Collaborative Research Group[167] |
| Wilson's disease | *WND* | AR | 13q14.1 | Copper transport protein | pm/del | Huntington's Disease Collaborative Research Group[167] |
| Primary torsion dystonia (early onset generalized) | *DYT1* | AD | 9q34 | TorsinA | GAG-del | Ozelius[88] |
| X-chromosomal dystonia-parkinsonism | *DYT3* | XL | Xq11.2 | Not known | Not known | Graeber[137] |
| Primary torsion dystonia, mixed type | *DYT6* | AD | 8cen | Not known | Not known | Almasy[98] |
| Primary torsion dystonia, adult onset focal | *DYT7* | AD | 18p13 | Not known | Not known | Leube[99] |
| Dopa-responsive dystonia | *DRD* | AD | 14q22.3 | GTP-cyclohydrolase I | pm/ins | Ichinose[53] |
| | *DRD* | AR | 11p15.5 | Tyrosine hydroxylase | pm | Ludecke[113] |
| Paroxysmal dystonia | *FPD1* | AD | 2q | Not known | Not known | Fouad[131] |
| Essential tremor | *ETM* | AD | 2p22–23 | Not known | Not known | Higgins[149] |
| Essential tremor | *FET1* | AD | 3q13 | Not known | Not known | Gulcher[150] |
| Hereditary chin trembling | *GSP* | AD | 9q13–21 | Not known | Not known | Jarman[152] |
| Familial hyperekplexia | *STHE* | AD | 5q | Glycine receptor | pm | Shiang[163] |
| Ponto-pallido-nigral degeneration | *PPND* | AD | 17p21 | MAPTau | pm | Wijker[168] |
| Familial Parkinson's disease | *PARK1* | AD | 4q23 | α-Synuclein | pm | Polymeropoulos[40] |
| Familial Parkinson's disease | *PARK2* | AR | 6q25 | Parkin | pm, del | Kitada[57] |
| Familial Parkinson's disease | *PARK3* | AD | 2p13 | Unknown | Unknown | Gasser[60] |

Abbreviations: AD = autosomal dominant; AR = autosomal recessive; XL = X-linked; pm = point mutations; del = deletions; ins = insertions; trinuc = trinucleotide repeat expansion.

of a triplet repeat sequence in a gene on chromosome 14 that is identical to spinocerebellar ataxia type 3 (SCA3), has been reported to present as levo-dopa-responsive parkinsonism.[21] This is exceptional, however, as most families with inherited parkinsonism, including the one recently described by Sutton and Pulst[21a] do not show an expansion of the MJD repeat.

Another clinical entity that may present with parkinsonism is the disorder initially described as "disinhibition-dementia-ALS-parkinsonism complex" (DDAPC, Wilhelmsen-Lynch disease).[22] This is a neurodegenerative disorder of middle to late adulthood characterized by a predominantly frontal lobe type of dementia and variable signs of motoneuron disease and parkinsonism. The DDAPC disease gene has been mapped to chromosome 17q21–22.[23] The clinical picture of chromosome 17–linked disease was subsequently shown to be rather variable. A recent consensus conference proposed the designation of "frontotemporal dementia and parkinsonism (FTDP).[24] Another rather clinically distinct disorder characterized predominantly by a rapidly progressive akinetic-rigid disorder unresponsive to levo-dopa, called" pontopallido-nigral degeneration (PPND)[25] also maps to this region. Additional neurologic deficits, such as dementia, ocular motility abnormalities, pyramidal tract dysfunction, frontal lobe release signs, perseverative vocalizations, and urinary incontinence, usually help to differentiate this disorder from PD. The course of PPND is exceptionally aggressive, as symptom onset and death consistently occur in the fifth decade. Positron emission tomographic studies with $^{18}$F6-fluoro-levo-dopa showed markedly reduced striatal uptake in PPND patients. Autopsy findings revealed severe neuronal loss with gliosis in the substantia nigra, pontine tegmentum, and globus pallidus, with less involvement of the caudate and the putamen. There were no plaques, tangles, Lewy bodies, or amyloid bodies. In several of these families, which are clinically characterized by a variable degree of dementia, behavioral disturbances, and dementia, mutations in the coding region or in splice sites of the gene for the microtubule-associated protein tau (MAPTau) have been identified.[26]

Finally, dopa-responsive dystonia (DRD) usually presents with leg-onset dystonia in childhood (see later). In some cases, however, the first sign of the disease may be parkinsonism during adult life.[27]

In most cases, the clinical and neuropathologic features of MJD, DDAPC, FTDP, PPND, and DRD are clearly distinct from those of idiopathic PD. These examples show that parkinsonism can be caused by the mutation of a single gene. It is unlikely, however, that mutations in any of these genes play a major role in more typical cases of sporadic or familial PD.

## FAMILIAL PARKINSONISM RESEMBLING IDIOPATHIC PARKINSON'S DISEASE

Families with inherited conditions that are autosomal dominant have been described in whom parkinsonism is the sole or predominant clinical abnormality. In some of these pedigrees, affected individuals exhibit at least some features either clinically [28–30] or neuropathologically [31], that are considered to be atypical for "classic" Lewy body PD. Age at onset may be considerably younger than in typical PD,[28] and in some families additional neurologic signs, such as pyramidal tract dysfunction,[29] dementia, or amyotrophy (family A described by Wszolek and coworkers[32]), are observed in addition to parkinsonism. Therefore, these syndromes could possibly be more precisely called *familial parkinsonism plus syndromes* (PPS).[10] But in other cases, such as the families described by Golbe and coworkers,[33,34] families C and D reported by Wszolek and associates, [32,35] and the family recently described by Markopoulou and associates,[36] the clinical and pathological features more closely resemble true PD.

The relationship of these familial parkinsonian syndromes to sporadic idiopathic PD is unclear. The age at onset and the clinical picture in sporadic, autopsy-proven idiopathic Lewy body PD may be extremely variable.[37] It is therefore conceivable that other, less penetrant mutations in the genes involved in familial parkinsonism are also responsible for apparently sporadic cases of typical PD. Another, more likely possibility is that different genetic or nongenetic factors disturb a common cellular pathway. This eventually leads to the selective degeneration of nigral neurons, which is characteristic of idiopathic PD. The identification of (rare) genetic causes might then help to define this sequence of events.[9]

### FAMILIAL PARKINSON'S DISEASE LINKED TO CHROMOSOME 4q (PARK1)

The mapping of a gene locus[39] in the family described by Golbe and coworkers[38] (to the long arm of chromosome 4 [PARK1]) was an important step in identifying the genetic cause of familial PD. This large family with autosomal dominant inheritance (Fig. 18–1) includes affected people who appear to have typical idiopathic PD both clinically and pathologically except for a relatively early age at onset (46 ± 13 years) and rapid course.

In this family and in three Greek families with inherited parkinsonism, a mutation in the gene for α-synuclein has now been shown to cosegregate with the disease.[40] The α-synuclein gene encodes a protein found in presynaptic nerve terminals and has been identified as a component of the amyloid plaque in Alzheimer's disease.[41] The protein is widely expressed in the brain. Sequence analysis revealed a single base pair change that leads to the substitution of alanine by threonine at position 53 of the protein.[40]

A causative role of α-synuclein mutations in the disease process has been supported by the description of a second, independent mutation (Ala39Pro) in a German family[42] and by the remarkable observation that antibodies to α-synuclein strongly stain the structures that are considered to be the pathological hallmark of PD, the Lewy bodies[43] in familial and sporadic PD. It has therefore been hypothesized that the aggregation of α-synuclein is a crucial step in the pathogenesis of PD. This hypothesis is supported by the observation that α-synuclein aggregates *in vitro*[44] and that the introduction of mutations in the recombinantly expressed protein promotes aggregation.[45]

No evidence for linkage to the PARK1 region (on chromosome 4q) has been found in several other multigenerational families with dominantly inherited parkinsonism[46] and in a cohort of affected pedigree pairs.[47] In addition, the Ala53Thr mutation was not found in 230 European cases of PD with familial clustering, as ascertained by the European Consortium on Genetic Susceptibility in PD[48] and in an independent American sample.[49] Likewise, no mutation was found when the entire sequence of the α-synuclein gene was analyzed in the index patients of 27 multigenerational families with PD.[50] Mutations in this gene appear to be a very rare cause of familial PD.

## Chromosome 6–Linked Autosomal Recessive Juvenile Parkinsonism

Young onset PD has been arbitrarily defined as PD beginning before the age of 40 years, whereas the term *juvenile PD* has been used when onset is before the age of 20.[51] It is now clear that, at least for nosologic purposes, this is not a useful distinction because cases with typical and atypical clinical features and pathology occur in both age groups. The incidence of familial cases appears to be higher in younger patients with parkinsonism, but there are also cases with a sporadic disease with early onset. In some of the familial young-onset cases (onset in the 30s and 40s), pathologically typical Lewy body disease is inherited as a dominant trait (as in the PARK1 families linked to the α-synuclein locus, described above earlier), whereas others (with an onset generally in the 20s and 30s, but sometimes higher) have a recessively inherited form of parkinsonism.

In the latter group, which has been recognized predominantly in Japan,[52] there is a selective and severe degeneration of dopaminergic neurons of the substantia nigra, but no Lewy bodies can be found, indicating that this disorder may be due to a different pathological process. This form has been called *autosomal recessive juvenile parkinsonism* (AR-JP [PARK2]). Clinically, patients suffer from levo-dopa-responsive parkinsonism and show early and severe levo-dopa-induced dyskinesias and motor fluctuations. This is rather characteristic of most patients with early onset PD, but in striking contrast to another dopa-responsive disorder of

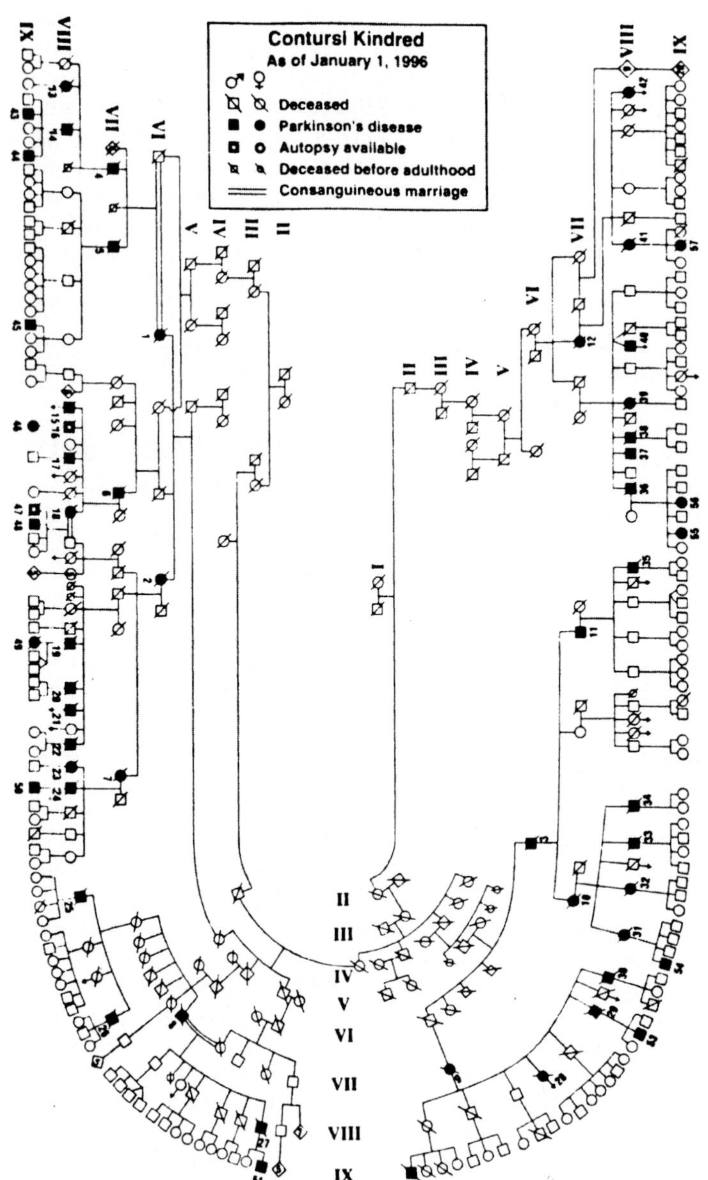


**Figure 18–1.** Pedigree of a large family (the "Contursi kindred") with inherited parkinsonism that is autosomal dominant. In this family, the disease gene has been identified as α-synuclein, which maps to chromosome 4q21–23. (Reproduced with permission from Polymeropoulos et al.[39])

young onset, dominantly inherited DRD, which is caused by mutations in the gene for GTP-cyclohydrolase I on chromosome 14q.[53] In the latter disease, there is excellent and sustained improvement with levo-dopa therapy and no associated motor complications.[54] Other somewhat "atypical" features that have been described in the Japanese population include increased tendon reflexes in the lower extremities.[55]

The genetic locus for AR-JP has been mapped to chromosome 6 in the Japanese population,[56] and mutations have been identified in a large gene in that region with homologies to ubiquitin, which has been called *Parkin*,[57] a novel gene of unknown function. The full range of the clinical spectrum associated with this genetic form of parkinsonism remains to be defined. The (moderate) homology of parts of the Parkin gene to ubiquitin may indicate a role of the proteasomal degradation pathway in the cascade of events leading to nigral degeneration, as has also been suggested by the finding that ubiquitinated α-synuclein is a component of the Lewy body in sporadic and familial PD.[43] That this form of inherited parkinsonism lacks the "neuropathological hallmark" of PD, the Lewy body, in the presence of marked and selective degeneration of nigral neurons raises the interesting question whether this neuropathological feature should be thought of as an essential marker for PD. Of course, nigral degeneration caused by mutations in the Parkin gene could be due to a pathological process different from that leading to typical Lewy body PD. Alternatively, however, this finding could mean that the Lewy body is just a marker for one (arguably the most prevalent) form of PD.

It is already clear that AR-JP is not restricted to the Japanese. A surprisingly high numer of mutations in the Parkin gene have been identified in European cases with young onset parkinsonism.[58,59]

## FAMILIAL PARKINSON'S DISEASE LINKED TO CHROMOSOME 2

Gasser and colleagues[60] described another genetic locus locus in familial parkinsonism (PARK3) on 2p13 with clinical features closely resembling those of sporadic PD including a similar mean age of onset (59 years in these families). The maximum multipoint lod score for all six families in their study was 3.96, considering affected members only. Based on the observation of a common haplotype in two of the linked families originating from Northern Germany and Southern Denmark, respectively, a founder effect appears likely. Analysis of unaffected pedigree members suggested a reduced penetrance of the disease allele (40%). This might indicate that the PARK3 gene may play a role not only in clearly dominant families but also in parkinsonian patients without a clear family history.

## GENETIC FACTORS IN APPARENTLY SPORADIC PARKINSON'S DISEASE

In most instances there is no clear family history of parkinsonism in patients with idiopathic PD. As mentioned earlier, however, the risk to first-degree relatives is about two to three times higher than that of carefully chosen controls.[12–14,16,61] The relative risk is similar in siblings and in offspring, suggesting the presence of a dominant mutation. In contrast to the familial parkinsonian syndromes described in the large families mentioned earlier, Maraganore and coworkers[62] found no difference from sporadic cases when they analyzed the clinical features of 20 British probands with a positive family history of PD (usually two to three affected individuals per family). Segregation analysis was compatible with autosomal dominant inheritence of a single gene with reduced penetrance.[62] It is therefore possible that the cause of the disease in these cases with familial clustering may be directly related to that of sporadic PD. It is generally assumed that in these cases genetic susceptibility interacts with other (environmental?) causes.

## ASSOCIATION STUDIES

A possible clue to the interaction of genetic and environmental factors in the etiology of PD may be the discovery that individuals carrying a particular mutation in the gene for debrisoquine 4-hydroxylase, an enzyme involved in the detoxification of a number of endogenous or exogenous compounds, may be more prone to develop PD. The gene has been termed *CYP2D6*. The so-called B allele of this gene, which is associated with a decreased metabolic activity of the encoded protein, was found to be more prevalent in patients with PD than in healthy controls.[63]

Although confirmed in several independent studies,[64–67] the data is not entirely conclusive. Smith and associates[63] found a higher proportion of homozygotes for the B allele in patients with PD. Armstrong and coworkers[64] observed a higher proportion of heterozygotes with the wild-type *CYP2D6B* genotype, whereas in the study of Kurth and Kurth[68] both homozygotes and heterozygotes are overrepresented among PD patients. Other studies, however, have failed to confirm the initial observation,[69,70] or an association was found only in a particular subgroup (Table 18–2).[65,66,71,72] The B allele is the most prevalent polymorphism

Table 18–2. **Studies on CYP2D6 Association**

| First Author | No. of Patients | No. of Controls | Major Findings |
|---|---|---|---|
| Smith[63] | 229 | 720 | Homozygotes for "poor-metabolizer" alleles (A + B) more prevalent among PD patients |
| Armstrong[64] | 53 | 72 | Heterozygotes for B allele more prevalent among PD patients |
| Kurth and Kurth[68] | 50 | 121 | Heterozygotes and homozygotes for B allele more prevalent among PD patients |
| Planté-Bordeneuve[65] | 48 | 88 | B allele more prevalent among familial PD patients only if compared with controls over 60 years of age |
| Agundez[66] | 123 | 150 | B allele more prevalent among young onset patients only |
| Gasser[69] | 170 | 275 | No difference in allele frequencies between different subgroups (sporadic and familial PD, healthy relatives, community controls) |
| Lucotte[67] | 47 | 47 | "Poor-metabolizer" alleles more prevalent among PD patients (particularly with older onset) |
| Diederich[72] | 80 | 108 | No difference in frequencies of A and B alleles |

associated with the "low-metabolizer" phenotype at least in the Caucasian population, but other mutations may also play a role.[73] The issue is still unclear, and certainly it is far too early to use this information for advising a particular individual about his or her risk to develop PD. Several large multicenter studies are currently underway to identify additional susceptibility loci for PD using the affected sib-pair method.

## DYSTONIAS

Dystonia is defined clinically as a syndrome of sustained involuntary muscle contractions that frequently cause twisting, repetitive movements, or abnormal postures.[74] *Dystonia* therefore is not a disease but a term that describes a type of abnormal movement that may occur as a symptom of a large variety of neurologic disorders. In some cases, dystonia is the consequence of a known structural or metabolic cerebral alteration (i.e., secondary dystonias, many of which have a genetic cause, such as Niemann-Pick disease type C, $GM_2$-gangliosidosis, and many others). More frequently, dystonia in one of its variants (primary or idiopathic torsion dystonia [TD]) may also be the sole manifestation of a disorder with no distinct underlying pathology. Only this group is considered here.

### Primary Torsion Dystonia

Primary torsion dystonia itself is a clinically and genetically heterogeneous group of disorders. Several variants can be distinguished from the "classic" form of primary TD on the basis of additional clinical or pharmacological features, such as dopa-responsive dystonia, myoclonic dystonia (also called "hereditary dystonia with lightning jerks responsive to alcohol" and probably identical to hereditary essential myoclonus) or the paroxysmal dystonias.[75] It is becoming increasingly clear, however, that "classic" primary TD is itself genetically heterogeneous, with different genetic entities presenting with an overlapping range of phenotypes.

The early descriptions of TD date back to the beginning of the twentieth century. The term *dystonia musculorum deformans* was introduced by Oppenheim,[76] who described two siblings of Jewish ancestry presenting during childhood with dystonia in the legs, progressing to generalized dystonia. Many of the early reports of inherited primary TD described the disease among Jewish individuals, and it was suggested that primary TD was more common in Jews.[77] This was confirmed by the first careful genetic study published by Zeman and Dyken[78] in 1967. They estimated a gene frequency of 1/38,000 in the Jewish population, which is approximately five times that in non-Jewish Caucasians (1/200,000), and concluded that the disease was inherited as an autosomal dominant trait with incomplete penetrance. This is now well established in both Jewish and non-Jewish families.[79–82]

## PHENOTYPE OF PRIMARY TORSION DYSTONIA

On a clinical level, it has proved useful to classify primary TD according to either the age at onset of the disease (childhood, adolescence, or adult life) or the physical distribution of symptoms (generalized, segmental, multifocal, and focal dystonia).[74] Childhood onset dystonia tends to present with symptoms in the legs and has a high tendency to progress to the generalized form, whereas adult onset dystonia tends to present with dystonic symptoms in the upper extremity (writer's cramp), neck (spasmodic torticollis), or face (blepharospasm, Meige's syndrome) and usually remains restricted to one or a few parts of the body.

## PRIMARY TORSION DYSTONIA LINKED TO CHROMOSOME 9q34 *(DYT1)*

In 1989, Ozelius and coworkers[83] established linkage between DNA markers on the long arm of chromosome 9 (9q34) and TD in a large non-Jewish family with early onset generalized dystonia. Subsequently, linkage to the same region of chromosome 9 was also demonstrated in 12 Ashkenazi Jewish kindreds.[71] The location of the dystonia gene *(DYT1)* was narrowed down further by the demonstration of a *linkage disequilibrium* between an extended haplotype (a particular combination of alleles at tightly linked loci) around *DYT1* and the disease gene in Ashkenazi Jewish patients with primary TD.[85] Furthermore, this association supports the idea that most, if not all, cases of early onset TD in the Ashkenazi Jewish population are caused by a single mutation. This "founder effect" can also explain the observed high frequency of the disease among Jews. The analysis of the associated marker haplotype (*marking* the mutation-bearing chromosome in this population) together with the known migration patterns of Ashkenazi Jews in Europe led Risch and associates[86] to conclude that the mutation arose in a founder individual living approximately 350 years ago in Lithuania or Byelorussia.[86]

The spectrum of clinical manifestations associated with this particular haplotype has been defined by Bressman and colleagues,[87] who found that the majority of 90 haplotype carriers had dystonia commencing during the first or second decade of life that initially affected a limb (leg and arm equally) and progressed to segmental, multifocal, or generalized dystonia. A minority, however, had initial involvement of neck muscles or of the larynx. No carrier of the founder haplotype presented with other cranial dystonias (jaw, tongue, upper face). Conversely, in almost 80% of Ashkenazi Jewish patients with dystonia who did not carry the founder haplotype, muscles of the face, neck, or larynx were affected at onset. The first symptoms usually appeared after the age of 30 years.

## THE *DYT1* MUTATION

The mutation causing early onset generalized dystonia has recently been identified as the deletion of a single GAG triplet in a novel gene coding for an ATP-binding protein termed *torsinA*. This mutation has been identified in Ashkenazi Jewish patients carrying the founder haplotype as well as in non-Jewish individuals from families with linkage to chromosome 9.[88] Based on haplotype data, it is likely that the *DYT1* mutation has arisen independently in different ethnic populations. No other mutation in the torsinA gene has thus far been detected in dystonia patients. It has therefore been speculated that other mutations in this gene cause a different syndrome, have no phenotype, or are incompatible with life.

## MOLECULAR DIAGNOSIS

Molecular diagnosis by mutational analysis is now easily possible in Jewish and non-Jewish patients with early onset primary TD. It still must be kept in mind, however, that the probability of an individual harboring this mutation to develop symptoms is only 30% and that the severity of the disease cannot be predicted.

It is also clear that the disease is genetically heterogeneous, as several families unlinked to chromosome 9q34 have also been found.[89–91] Therefore, a familial form of primary TD cannot be excluded by a failure to demonstrate a mutation in the torsinA gene.

## Adult Onset Idiopathic Focal and Segmental Dystonia

Overall, adult onset focal and segmental dystonias, such as torticollis, blepharospasm, Meige's syndrome, and writer's cramp, are much more prevalent, at least in non-Jewish European and North American populations, than generalized dystonia.[92] Most of these patients are not aware of a family history of the disease.[93] Several lines of evidence, however, support the view that these dystonias may also be, at least in part, an inherited condition.

Most importantly, although only few patients with focal dystonia volunteer a family history of the disease, a careful study during which as many first-degree relatives as possible were actually examined showed that as many as 25% of patients had affected relatives,[94] most of whom were unaware of the diagnosis of dystonia. Segregation analysis was compatible with autosomal dominant inheritance with reduced penetrance. Also, several families are on record with autosomal dominantly inherited dystonia of adult onset, with a predominantly or purely focal distribution.[95–97]

The GAG deletion in the torsinA gene, however, appears to play no major role in the etiology of late onset focal or segmental dystonias, as Ozelius and coworkers[88] detected no mutation in more than 200 individuals with these forms of dystonia.

## Adult Onset Dystonia Linked to Chromosome 8q

A locus for a form familial dystonia with a predominantly craniocervical phenotype has been mapped to chromosome 8.[98] It has been termed DYT6. Thus far, only two Mennnonite families have been found to be linked to this locus.

## Adult Onset Focal Dystonia Linked to Chromosome 18p

Recently, Leube and coworkers[99] mapped a disease gene to the short arm of chromosome 18 in a German family with adult onset dystonia and a purely focal distribution. It has been termed DYT7.

### PHENOTYPE OF CHROMOSOME 18-LINKED FOCAL DYSTONIA

Age of onset was between 28 and 70 years (mean, 58 years), and the prominent manifestation was torticollis (in six of seven definitely affected people). Spasmodic dysphonia was exhibited in one individual. Postural hand tremor was also found in some affected individuals.

### MAPPING OF THE *DYT7* GENE

Using a haplotype of four closely linked microsatellite markers, Leube and coworkers[99] found evidence of linkage to distal chromosome 18p with a maximum pairwise lod score of 3.17. Analysis of 15 sporadic patients with torticollis from the same geographic region showed that all patients shared portions of a putative founder haplotype identified in family K. The shared haplotype defines a critical region of about 6 cM between D18S1105 and D18S54 for *DYT7*. Allelic association was statistically significant for marker locus D18S1098 and for a haplotype of two marker loci (D18S1098/D18S481), suggesting that the disease in a large proportion of apparently sporadic patients may be due to the same founder mutation.[100] These intriguing findings need to be replicated in independent populations.

At present, the proportion of cases associated with mutations in either of these recently mapped genes (as well as the proportion of genetic cases in general) in adult onset focal dystonia is unknown.

## CLINICAL VARIANTS OF PRIMARY TORSION DYSTONIA

Several variants of inherited primary TD are recognized based on characteristic clinical or pharmacological features. In several cases, the causative genes have now been mapped or cloned.[60]

### Dopa-Responsive Dystonia

The term *dopa-responsive dystonia* (DRD) refers to a distinct subgroup of inherited dystonia with several interesting clinical characteristics.

#### PHENOTYPE OF DOPA-RESPONSIVE DYSTONIA

The usual onset of dystonia is during childhood and nearly always involves the legs, progressing to other body parts in most patients. Some patients exhibit features of parkinsonism (such as bradykinesia and postural instability) later in the course of the disease. Typically, symptoms worsen markedly during the course of the day and improve following sleep.[27] Dramatic and sustained improvement is observed on low doses of levo-dopa.[54,102] Dyskinesias and other complications of levo-dopa therapy do not develop. In some cases, the disease may develop in adult life only.[103] This disease was first described in Japan,[104] but it is now clear that it occurs with probably equal frequency in other parts of the world, with an estimated prevalence of about 0.5 per million.[103] Dopa-responsive dystonia accounts probably for about 5% to 10% of all childhood onset dystonias.

Autosomal dominant inheritance has been reported in the majority of DRD patients. The penetrance of definite dystonia was estimated to be 31%, with girls being more frequently affected than boys. When isolated rigidity was included as a minor disease manifestation, penetrance was close to 100%.[27]

In a single autopsied case of DRD, cell counts and tyrosine hydroxylase (TH) immunoreactivity in the substantia nigra were normal, but dopamine was significantly reduced in the striatum.[105] Therefore, an inherited defect affecting the enzymatic activity of TH has been postulated.

#### THE DRD GENE

The gene for DRD has been mapped by linkage analysis to chromosome 14.[106,107] Ichinose and colleagues[53] and later other groups[108,109] identified point mutations and small insertions in the gene for GTP-cyclohydrolase I (GTP-CH I) in patients with DRD. A variety of different mutations have been identified: missense mutations in conserved regions of the gene, nonsense mutations resulting in a stop codon within the open reading frame, and insertions leading to a frameshift. Furukawa and colleagues found a G to A transition at the splice acceptor site for intron 1, leading to exon 2 skipping and frameshift.[108]

GTP-CH I catalizes the first step in the *de novo* formation of tetrahydrobiopterin, an essential cofactor of TH that in turn is the rate-limiting enzyme of dopamine biosynthesis. Mutations in its structural gene found in patients with DRD are associated with a reduction of enzyme activity of TH in PHA-activated mononuclear blood cells to less than 50% of controls.[110] Reduced levels of CSF neopterin and total biopterin in patients with DRD reflect this enzyme deficiency.[111] The cofactor deficiency may in turn lead to a critical reduction of dopamine biosythesis without degeneration of dopaminergic neurons and eventually to the clinical manifestations of dystonia and parkinsonism.

#### MOLECULAR DIAGNOSIS OF DOPA-RESPONSIVE DYSTONIA

Molecular diagnosis of DRD is complicated by the fact that no frequent common mutation has been found, so that sequencing of all six exons of the structural gene for GTP-CH I is necessary to confirm the diagnosis. In addition, in some patients mutations are located in the nontranslated regions of the gene and probably result in aberrant splicing of the mRNA.[108]

Juvenile onset levodopa-sensitive parkinsonism (which is defined as parkinsonism with onset before 40 years of age) resembles

DRD in that it often presents with dystonic symptoms (most frequently gait disturbance due to foot dystonia), but it differs from typical DRD in the need for increasing doses of levodopa and the appearance of treatment-associated complications such as motor response fluctuations and dopa-induced dyskinesias.[111] Thus far, mutations in the GTP-CH I gene have not been identified in patients with juvenile onset parkinsonism with dystonia, so that this disorder is probably not allelic to DRD.[112]

#### DOPA-RESPONSIVE DYSTONIA CAUSED BY MUTATIONS IN THE GENE FOR TYROSINE HYDROXYLASE

A rare recessive variant of DRD may be caused by a mutation in the gene for TH.[113] Two brothers with DRD have been identified who are homozygous for a missense mutation in the TH gene. When expressed in *Escherichia coli,* the mutant enzyme represents a kinetic variant form with a reduced affinity for L-tyrosine and a residual enzyme activity of 15%.[114]

## Myoclonus-Dystonia Syndrome

Brief, shock-like movements have long been recognized to be a part of the spectrum of abnormal movements observed in idiopathic TD.[115] Over the years, however, a number of families have been described with a condition dominated by myoclonic jerks commencing during the first two decades of life, with little progression, accompanied in some, but not all, cases by more sustained involuntary movements that fit the description of dystonia. These families have been described variously under the titles of "hereditary essential myoclonus," "hereditary myoclonic dystonia," or even "benign hereditary chorea."

Quinn and Marsden[116] described patients from six families with myoclonus-dystonia syndrome, reviewed the subject, and discussed the confusing terminology. Based on the published clinical and electrophysiological descriptions, they thought that at least some of the families published under different headings probably represent a single clinical and genetic entity for which they used the term *hereditary dystonia with lightning jerks responsive to alcohol.*[117] Until the nosologic boundaries of the diseases characterized by the occurrence of myoclonus and dystonia have been clarified with molecular genetic studies, it may be better to use the more neutral term *myoclonus-dystonia syndrome.*[118]

### PHENOTYPE

Age at onset is usually in the first and second decade, and typically the disease runs a relatively benign course and is essentially nonprogressive over many years.[119] Remissions have been described in affected members of some families.[116]

Symptoms include proximal, action-induced bilateral myoclonic jerks, usually involving the arms and axial muscles more than the legs and gait. Stimulus sensitivity to loud, sudden noise has frequently been described. In some cases, myoclonus could be provoked by tactile stimuli.[120] Relatively mild dystonic symptoms, such as torticollis or writer's cramp, in addition to myoclonus are common. Rarely, dystonia may be the only manifestation of the disease.[116,120] Relief of myoclonus by alcohol in many but not all affected people seems to be a relatively characteristic feature of the disease.[117] Improvement has also been reported with anticholinergics[121] and with clonazepam.[120,122,123]

All of the published families who fit this category[119,120,124,125] exhibited autosomal dominant inheritance with variable expressivity and high, but incomplete penetrance.[116,122] Males and females are equally affected in most families. However, in a family we recently studied, males were affected (n = 10) more than females (n = 1), suggesting nearly complete penetrance in males and lower penetrance in females.[119]

### LINKAGE ANALYSES

Genetic linkage analyses have been reported in several families with myoclonus-dystonia syndrome. Current evidence suggests that the disorder is genetically distinct from primary torsion dystonia linked to chromosome 9q34, as the entire candidate region of the *DYT1* gene in a Swedish and a German family with myoclonic dystonia has been excluded.[119,126] Other chromosomal regions bearing genes that encode receptor subunits for inhibitory neurotransmitters such as GABA and glycine have been excluded in one family.[119] A genomic screen in two large families has excluded major parts of the genome,[127] but definite proof of linkage to an autosomal locus is still lacking.

## Paroxysmal Dystonia/Paroxysmal Choreoathetosis

*Paroxysmal dyskinesias* are a clinically heterogeneous group of disorders. Phenotypically, a variety of hyperkinetic involuntary movements, ranging from dystonic posturing to athetoid and choreic movements, may be observed during attacks. Attacks differ widely in duration and intensity and are provoked by different stimuli.

### PHENOTYPE

In *paroxysmal kinesigenic dystonia*, attacks are short (seconds to minutes), precipitated by abrupt voluntary movement, and usually respond to anticonvulsants. Involuntary movements may be mild and almost unnoticeable to the observer. It is frequently described as a sporadic disorder, but occasionally familial occurrence has been noted, and both autosomal dominant[128] and autosomal recessive[129] patterns of inheritance have been proposed. In contrast, *paroxysmal nonkinesigenic dystonia*, which was first described by Mount and Reback,[130] is most frequently inherited as an autosomal dominant trait. In this form, the attacks are longer lasting (minutes to hours) and may occur up to several times per day. They are often provoked by ingestion of caffeine, chocolate, or alcohol and to a lesser extent, by exercise, fatigue, and emotional stress. The attacks may respond to azetazolamide or low doses of benzodiazepines. Between attacks, affected people are neurologically normal.

### FAMILIAL PAROXYSMAL DYSKINESIA LINKED TO CHROMOSOME 2q

Recently, a gene locus for familial (nonkinesigenic, benzodiazepine-sensitive) paroxysmal dyskinesia *(FPD1)* was located on chromosome 2q by two independent groups of investigators.[131,132] The nature of the disorder suggests that the causative gene may encode an ion channel, as other episodic disturbances of motility, such as episodic ataxia[133] and the periodic paralyses and myotonias,[134,135] have been shown to be caused by mutations in potassium, sodium, and chloride channels.

### PAROXYSMAL CHOREOATHETOSIS WITH SPASTICITY LINKED TO CHROMOSOME 1p

In a single family with a more complex phenotype, including paroxysmal choreoathetosis accompanied by imbalance, dysarthria, and paresthesias, as well as in some patients a persistent spastic paraplegia, Auburger and colleagues[136] reported linkage to the short arm of chromosome 1. This chromosomal region contains a cluster of potassium channel genes. It is not unlikely that the disease may be caused by a mutation in one of these genes. Until the question of possible genetic heterogeneity is settled, molecular diagnosis is restricted to the few families in whom the gene locus has been mapped.

## X-Linked Dystonia-Parkinsonism Syndrome (LUBAG, DYT3)

An X-linked syndrome of focal dystonia of the face, neck, trunk, or limbs, progressing within a few years to a generalized form, has been described in natives of the Philippine island of Panay. Onset is usually in early to middle adult life. As the disease progresses, parkinsonism, which usually does not respond to levodopa, occurs. Parkinsonian features may also be the presenting symptom. The disease has been mapped to a small pericentromeric region of the X chromosome.[137] Neuropathologically, neuronal loss and astrocytosis was seen in the caudate and putamen.[138] This disease may be exclusive to the Ilongo ethnic group in the Philippines. Most, if not all, patients with this condition share a common ancestor, who had a mutation on chromosome Xq12–13.1.

## ESSENTIAL TREMOR

Essential tremor (ET) is a frequent disorder characterized by postural tremor predominantly involving the upper limbs but sometimes also the head, legs, jaw, and tongue. Essential tremor is one of the most common movement disorders, with prevalence estimates ranging from 1% to 2% of individuals over 65 years of age.[139] The pathogenesis of ET is unknown. In PET studies, a bilateral increase in metabolic activity in deep cerebellar structures has been found, even when the individual is at rest and there is no visible tremor.

It is frequently stated in the literature that about 50% of patients with ET have relatives affected with tremor, and this claim certainly is supported by clinical experience. In different studies, however, the estimates range from 17% to 100%, and the published investigations are hampered by methodological problems: Criteria for the diagnosis of ET are often not specified precisely, and no control group (e.g., relatives of the spouses of the index patients) have been investigated. Therefore, the frequency of ET in relatives of patients with this disorder is still unknown.[139]

Age-dependent penetrance has been reported. Larsson and Sjögren[140] suggested that penetrance was not complete until the age of 70 years. Some,[141,142] but not all,[143] studies noted that patients with a positive family history for ET had an earlier age of onset, supporting the existence of two separate types of ET. It is also possible, however, that the greater availability of antecedents of young onset patients could produce a bias in favor of a positive family history.

Although ET is frequent, only a few large multicase families have been reported in the recent literature.[144–146] Autosomal dominant inheritance has been assumed in most instances. No formal segregation analysis, however, has been performed in the families of an unselected population with ET. The selection of families with multiple affected members may lead to a faulty specification of the genetic model, and autosomal recessive or complex inheritance may still be a possibility. Anticipation (successively younger age at onset in subsequent generations) has been described in at least one family. This raises the question of the possible contribution of an expanded trinucleotide repeat sequence as a cause of ET. Anticipation has been refuted by other authors, however, and all neurologic disorders caused by expanded trinucleotide repeats that have been identified thus far have degenerative features, which have not been found in autopsies of patients with ET.[147]

An interesting question concerns the relationship between essential (postural) tremor and other movement disorders. Associations have been described for PD and dystonia.[141] Recent PET studies suggest that in a minority of cases pure ET may be associated with a decreased striatal $^{18}$F-dopa uptake. One of these patients later developed akinesia and rigidity, so that the authors concluded that isolated postural tremor may be an early and mild manifestation of PD.[148] Patients with familial ET, however, had normal nigrostriatal function. This finding argues against an association of familial tremor with PD.

Recently, two gene loci were mapped in ET. In one large family of Eastern European descent with clear autosomal dominant inheritance, the disease was mapped to the short arm of chromosome 2.[149] In another study, a disease gene was mapped to chromosome 3q13 in a set of 13 Icelandic families.[150] The relevance of these respective loci to the ET population in general remains to be determined.

Hereditary chin trembling ("geniospasm") has been classified as a variant of ET. Clinical features of this benign disorder, however are distinct enough to justify its nosologic classification as a distinct entity.[151] The gene for this disorder has very recently been mapped to the long arm of chromosome 9.[152]

## WILSON'S DISEASE

Wilson's disease (WD) is an autosomal recessive disorder caused by abnormal depo-

Table 18–3. **Presenting Symptoms in 31 Patients with Wilson's Disease**

| Symptom | Proportion of Patients (%) |
|---|---|
| Dysarthria | 97 |
| Dystonia | 65 |
| Dysdiadochokinesia | 58 |
| Rigidity | 52 |
| Gait disorder | 42 |
| Hypomimia | 39 |
| Tremor | 32 |
| Oculomotor dysfunction | 32 |
| Hyperreflexia | 29 |
| Bradykinesia | 23 |
| Motor impersistence | 19 |
| Frontal lobe dysfunction | 19 |
| Paresis | 16 |
| Athetosis | 10 |
| Pyramidal tract dysfunction | 10 |
| Sensory dysfunction | 3 |

**Source:** Modified from Starosta-Rubinstein et al.[169]

sition of copper in different organs, particularly in the liver and the brain. In approximately one-third of patients, signs of central nervous system dysfunction predominate, leading to variable combinations of dysarthria, tremor, dystonia, parkinsonism, and ataxia.[153]

## Phenotype

About one-third of patients with WD present with hepatic, neurologic, or psychiatric abnormalities, respectively. Neurologic dysfunction appears during childhood, adolescence, or early adulthood (usually between ages 4 and about 25 years), but late manifestations (up to 60 years) have been described. Symptoms are extremely variable, but extrapyramidal dysfunction usually predominates the clinical picture. Typically, bradykinesia and rigidity, a coarse tremor of the extremities of the action or postural type (sometimes referred to as *flapping tremor*), dysarthria, dysphagia, or a generalized or focal dystonic syndrome can be seen. The frequencies of neurologic signs and symptoms in a series of 31 patients described by Brewer and Yuzbasiyan and Gurkan[153] are summarized in Table 18–3.

## The Wilson's Disease Gene (*ATP7B*)

After genetic linkage studies located the gene on chromosome 13, several groups identified a gene, coding for a protein involved in active transmembrane copper transport (a P-type ATPase called ATP7B), which maps to this chromosomal region.[154,155] Identification of the *ATP7B* gene was greatly facilitated by the cloning of the gene responsible for another disorder of copper metabolism: Menke's ("kinky hair") disease. Menke's disease is an X-linked, recessive disorder characterized by neurologic and connective tissue manifestations due to a defective intracellular copper transport mechanism.

A portion of the Menke gene was used as a probe to identify a homologous gene in the critical WD region, which then turned out to harbor mutations in patients with WD. A large number of different mutations have been identified in patients with WD along the entire open reading frame of this gene (Table 18–4). Depending on the exact nature of the mutation, its functional effect on the encoded protein may vary, probably contributing to the wide clinical variability of the disease. Nonsense mutations, causing the premature termination of the translation, are more frequently associated with childhood onset hepatic disease, whereas missense mutations, causing the exchange of amino acids in a normal-length gene product, seem to predispose to later onset neurologic symptomatology. This correlation is relatively loose.[156]

## Molecular Diagnosis

In principle, molecular diagnosis with direct gene sequencing to search for mutations is now possible in sporadic and familial cases. The large number of different mutations that may cause WD, however, complicates molecular testing. In addition,

Table 18–4. **Mutations in the Gene for *ATP7B****

| Mutation | Domain | Exon | Predicted Effect | Ethnic Groups | No. | Percent Frequency (N. Euro.) |
|---|---|---|---|---|---|---|
| **Insertion/Deletion** | | | | | | |
| 846delC | Cu3 | 2 | Frameshift | Iranian, Greek | 2 | — |
| 1747delAT | Cu6 | 5 | Frameshift | British | 1 | 1 |
| 1748insT | Cu6 | 5 | Frameshift | Indian | 1 | — |
| 2161delA† | Tm3 | 8 | Frameshift | Italian | 1 | — |
| 2302insC† | Tm4 | 8 | Frameshift | Italian, British | 3 | 2 |
| 3088delAC | Ph | 14 | Frameshift | British | 1 | — |
| 3149delC | ATP loop | 14 | Frameshift | Indian | 2 | — |
| 3403delC‡ | ATP loop | 15 | Frameshift | Ukrainian | 1 | 1 |
| 3629del4 | ATP pocket | 17 | Frameshift | Swedish | 1 | 1 |
| 3651del6 | ATP pocket | 17 | Disrupts ATP binding | British | 1 | 1 |
| 4094delTG | After Tm7 | 20 | Frameshift | British | 1 | 1 |
| **Nonsense** | | | | | | |
| Leu937ter† | Tm5 | 12 | Truncates protein | Saudi, Greek | 3 | — |
| Arg1320ter | ATP–Tm7 | 19 | Truncates protein | British | 1 | 1 |
| **Splice site** | | | | | | |
| 1711−1G→C | Cu6 | 5 | Skips exon 5 | Indian | 2 | — |
| 2576+1G→C | Td | 10 | Includes intron 10 | British | 1 | 1 |
| 3559+1G→A | ATP pocket | 16 | Includes intron 16 | British | 1 | 1 |
| **Missense** | | | | | | |
| Arg779Leu† | Tm4 | 8 | Disrupts Tm4 | Chinese | 3 | — |
| Gly944Ser† | Tm5 | 12 | Disrupts Tm5 | Bangladeshi | 2 | — |
| His1070Gln‡ | Loop motif (SEHPL) | 14 | Disrupts ATP binding | Eastern European, German, French, British | 19 | 28 |
| Gly1102Arg | ATP loop | 15 | Disrupts ATP binding | Indian | 2 | |
| Ile1103Thr | ATP loop | 15 | Disrupts ATP binding | Indian | 2 | — |
| Gly1267Lys | ATP hinge | 18 | Disrupts ATP hinge | French, British | 7 | 10 |
| Asn1271Ser‡ | ATP hinge | 18 | Disrupts ATP hinge | Italian | 1 | — |

*Numbering of base pairs and amino acids begins at the published ATG initiation codon. Domains are as described. Number of chromosomes on which each mutation was found is given. Frequency of the mutation in the northern European population is given. The frequencies in other populations were not determined due to small sample size.

†Mutations presenting in exons that undergo alternative splicing.

‡Mutations described.

many patients may have a different mutation in each of their *ATP7B* genes ("compound heterozygotes"). The search for individual mutations in this large gene (>4.1 kb of coding sequence spread out in 22 exons along more than 80 kb of genomic DNA) may be extremely costly and time consuming, so that indirect genetic testing with closely linked polymorphic DNA markers is still an option for presymptomatic or prenatal testing in families with one already affected child.[157]

Nevertheless, depending on the population studied, a few predominant mutations may be found on a relatively large proportion of disease chromosomes, as shown by haplotype analysis.[156] This figure may be as high as 85% in more isolated populations, such as in Sardinians The identification of one of these known haplotypes, which is usually associated with a particular mutation, may guide molecular diagnosis in many cases, as the associated mutation can then be directly confirmed by sequencing or by restriction analysis.[158]

## RESTLESS LEGS SYNDROME

Restless legs syndrome (RLS) is a frequent and probably underdiagnosed cause of insomnia. It is a heterogeneous syndrome, which is hereditary in approximately half of all cases. Recently, efforts have been undertaken to more clearly define the clinical features of RLS. As minimal criteria for diagnosis, the RLS Study Group proposed the following four features: *(1)* desire to move the extremities, often associated with paresthesias/dysesthesias; *(2)* motor restlessness; *(3)* worsening of symptoms at rest with at least temporary relief by activity; and *(4)* worsening of symptoms in the evening or night. Other features commonly seen in RLS include sleep disturbance, periodic limb movements in sleep and similar involuntary movements while awake, a normal neurologic examination in the idiopathic form, a tendency for the symptoms to be worse in middle to older age.

Restless legs syndrome is idiopathic in most patients, but it may be the presenting feature of iron deficiency. It is also common in uremia, pregnancy, diabetes mellitus, rheumatoid arthritis, and polyneuropathy. For patients with severe symptoms, levodopa, bromocriptine mesylate, opioids, carbamazepine, clonazepam, and clonidine hydrochloride have proved to be effective.[159] In 25% to 50% of cases, a family history suggestive of an autosomal dominant mode of inheritance is found.[160] Clinical variability within families is thought to be high.[161]

Because there is no biological marker for RLS and mild feelings of restlessness may be extremely common in the general population, the assignment of affection status in any given case in a family study is often in doubt. In addition, the number of nongenetic phenocopies is likely to be high, and the genetic parameters such as prevalence and penetrance are unknown. This considerably complicates genetic linkage studies, which have been undertaken to localize the genetic defect.

## STARTLE DISORDERS

Familial startle disease (also known as *hyperekplexia* and *congenital "stiff man* or *"stiff person" syndrome*) is an autosomal dominant disorder characterized by an exaggerated startle reaction to sudden, unexpected auditory or tactile stimuli; affected neonates also have severe and occasionally fatal hypertonia. Patients with symptoms frequently respond to clonazepam treatment. Linkage analysis has provided evidence for tight linkage between the disease locus and polymorphic genetic markers on chromosome 5q33–q35.[162] Several genes encoding neurotransmitter receptor components have been physically mapped to the subtelomeric region of chromosome 5q and are thus candidates for the startle disease gene.

Based on this combined genomic screen/candidate gene approach, Shiang and coworkers[163] identified two point mutations in the gene encoding the $\alpha_1$-subunit of the glycine receptor *(GLRA1)* in patients from four different families. The mutations occurred in the same base pair of exon 6 and resulted in the substitution of an uncharged amino acid (leucine or glutamine) for Arg271 in the mature protein.[163] Subsequently, a third mutation in two other families with clinically typical autosomal dominant hyperekplexia has been identified.[164] One patient with seemingly sporadic hyperekplexia was identified who was homozygous for a novel mutation in *GLRA1.* This patient was the result of a consanguinous mating, supporting the idea that autosomal recessive as well as dominant forms of hyperekplexia may be caused by mutations in *GLRA1.*[165] Interestingly, a patient homozygous for a *GLRA*1$^{null}$ mutation has been identified who also showed clinical symptoms of hyperekplexia, but proprioceptive and exteroceptive inhibition of muscle activity previously correlated to glycinergic mechanisms were not affected.

In addition to the "major" form of hyperekplexia, which was described earlier, a "minor" form has been recognized in which patients show an abnormal startle response but lack associated stiffness. No mutations in the *GLRA*1 gene have been identified in the minor form.[166] Also, in several sporadic and in clinically atypical cases, no alteration was found in the *GLRA1* gene.[164]

## SUMMARY

Recent advances in molecular genetics have greatly expanded our knowledge of the genetic basis of movement disorders. Direct molecular diagnosis by mutational analysis is now possible for several diseases, such as Huntington's chorea, primary generalized torsion dystonia, and WD. In addition, a genetic classification of heterogeneous movement disorder syndromes, such as the primary torsion dystonias and ET, is being developed.

In PD, several genes for monogenically inherited forms have been mapped or cloned. The identification of these genes and their mutations provides insight into the degenerative process affecting nigral dopaminergic neurons and will eventually lead to novel therapeutic strategies.

## REFERENCES


1. Gowers WR. Diseases of the Nervous System. Philadelphia, P. Blakiston, Son & Co, 1888, p.996.
2. Mjönes H: Paralysis agitans. A clinical genetic study. Acta Psychiatr Neurol Scand 54:1–195, 1949.
3. Martin WE, Young WI, Anderson VE: Parkinson's disease. A genetic study. Brain 96:495–506, 1973.
4. Martilla RJ, Rinne UK: Arteriosclerosis, heredity and some previous infections in the etiology of Parkinson's disease. Clin Neurol Neurosurg 79:46–56, 1976.
5. Marsden CD: Parkinson's disease in twins. J Neurol Neurosurg Psychiatry 50:105–106, 1986.
6. Duvoisin RC, Eldridge R, Williams A, et al: Twin study of Parkinson disease. Neurology 31:77–80, 1981.
7. Ward CD, Duvoisin RC, Ince SE, et al: Parkinson's disease in twins. Adv Neurol 40:341–344, 1984.
8. Golbe LI: The genetics of Parkinson's disease. Rev Neurosci 4:1–16, 1993.
9. Duvoisin RC, Golbe LI: Kindreds of dominantly inherited Parkinson's disease: Keys to the riddle. Ann Neurol 38:355–356, 1995.
10. Denson MA, Wszolek ZK: Familial parkinsonism: Our experience and a review of the literature. Parkinsonism Rel Disord 1:35–46, 1995.
11. Gasser T: Genetics of Parkinson's disease. Clin Genet 54:259–265, 1998.
12. Vieregge P, Heberlein I: Increased risk of Parkinson's disease in relatives of patients. Ann Neurol 37:685–685, 1995.
13. Payami H, Larsen K, Bernard S, et al: Increased risk of Parkinson's disease in parents and siblings of patients. Ann Neurol 36:659–661, 1994.
14. Lazzarini AM, Myers RH, Zimmerman TR, Jr, et al: A clinical genetic study of Parkinson's disease: Evidence for dominant transmission. Neurology 44: 499–506, 1994.
15. Bennett P, Bonifati V, Bonuccelli U, et al: Direct genetic evidence for involvement of tau in progressive supranuclear palsy. European Study Group on Atypical Parkinsonism Consortium. Neurology 51: 982–985, 1998.
16. Bonifati V, Fabrizio E, Vanacore N, et al: Familial Parkinson's disease: A clinical genetic analysis. Can J Neurol Sci 22:272–279, 1995.
17. Marder K, Tang MX, Mejia H, et al: Risk of Parkinson's disease among first-degree relatives: A community-based study. Neurology 47:155–160, 1996.
18. Burn DJ, Mark MH, Playford ED, et al: Parkinson's disease in twins studied with 18F-dopa and positron emission tomography. Neurology 42:1894–1900, 1992.
19. Vieregge P, Schiffke KA, Friedrich HJ, et al: Parkinson's disease in twins. Neurology 42:1453–1461, 1992.
20. Piccini P, Morrish PK, Turjanski N, et al: Dopaminergic function in familial Parkinson's disease: A clinical and 18F-dopa positron emission tomography study. Ann Neurol 41:222–229, 1997.
21. Tuite PJ, Rogaeva EA, St George Hyslop PH, et al: Dopa-responsive parkinsonism phenotype of Machado-Joseph disease: Confirmation of 14q CAG expansion. Ann Neurol 38:684–687, 1995.

21a. Sutton JP, Pulst SM: Atypical parkinsonism in a family of Portuguese ancestry: Absence of CAG repeat expansion in the MJD1 gene. Neurology 48: 1285–1290, 1997.

22. Lynch T, Sano M, Marder KS, et al: Clinical characteristics of a family with chromosome 17–linked disinhibition-dementia-parkinsonism-amyotrophy complex. Neurology 44:1878–1884, 1994.
23. Wilhelmsen KC, Lynch T, Pavlou E, et al: Localization of disinhibition-dementia-parkinsonism-amyotrophy complex to 17q21–22. Am J Hum Genet 55:1159–1165, 1994.
24. Foster NL, Wilhelmsen K, Sima AA, et al: Frontotemporal dementia and parkinsonism linked to chromosome 17: A consensus conference. Conference Participants. Ann Neurol 41:706–715, 1997.
25. Wszolek ZK, Pfeiffer RF, Bhatt MH, et al: Rapidly progressive autosomal dominant parkinsonism and dementia with pallido-ponto-nigral degeneration. Ann Neurol 32:312–320, 1992.
26. Hutton M, Lendon CL, Rizzu P, et al: Association of missense and 5'-splice-site mutations in tau with the inherited dementia FTDP-17. Nature 393:702–705, 1998.
27. Nygaard TG, Trugman JM, de Yebenes JG, et al: Dopa-responsive dystonia: The spectrum of clinical

manifestations in a large North American family. Neurology 40:66–69, 1990.
28. Waters CH, Miller CA: Autosomal dominant Lewy body parkinsonism in a four-generation family. Ann Neurol 35:59–64, 1994.
29. Nisipeanu P, Kuritzky A, Korczyn AD: Familial levodopa-responsive parkinsonian-pyramidal syndrome. Mov Disord 9:673–675, 1994.
30. Takahashi H, Ohama E, Suzuki S, et al: Familial juvenile parkinsonism: Clinical and pathologic study in a family. Neurology 44:437–441, 1994.
31. Dwork AJ, Balmaceda C, Fazzini EA, et al: Dominantly inherited, early-onset parkinsonism: Neuropathology of a new form. Neurology 43:69–74, 1993.
32. Wszolek ZK, Cordes M, Calne DB, et al: Hereditary Parkinson disease: Report of 3 families with dominant autosomal inheritance. Nervenarzt 64:331–335, 1993.
33. Golbe LI, Di Iorio G, Bonavita V, et al: A large kindred with autosomal dominant Parkinson's disease. Ann Neurol 27:276–282, 1990.
34. Golbe LI, Lazzarini AM, Schwarz KO, et al: Autosomal dominant parkinsonism with benign course and typical Lewy-body pathology. Neurology 43: 2222–2227, 1993.
35. Wszolek ZK, Pfeiffer B, Fulgham JR, et al: Western Nebraska family (family D) with autosomal dominant parkinsonism. Neurology 45:502–505, 1995.
36. Markopoulou K, Wszolek ZK, Pfeiffer RF: A Greek-American kindred with autosomal dominant, levodopa-responsive parkinsonism and anticipation. Ann Neurol 38:373–378, 1995.
37. Sage JI, Miller DC, Golbe LI, et al: Clinically atypical expression of pathologically typical Lewy-body parkinsonism. Clin Neuropharmacol 13:36–47, 1990.
38. Golbe LI, Di Iorio G, Sanges G, Lazzarini A, LaSala S, Bonavita V, Duvoisin R. Clinical genetic analysis of Parkinson's disease in the Contursi kindred. Ann Neurol 40: 767–775. 1996.
39. Polymeropoulos MH, Higgins JJ, Golbe LI, et al: Mapping of a gene for Parkinson's disease to chromosome 4q21–23. Science 274:1197–1199, 1996.
40. Polymeropoulos MH, Lavedan C, Leroy E, et al: Mutation in the α-synuclein gene identified in families with Parkinson's disease. Science 276:2045–2047, 1997.
41. Ueda K, Fukushima H, Masliah E, et al: Molecular cloning of cDNA encoding an unrecognized component of amyloid in Alzheimer disease. Proc Natl Acad Sci USA 90:11282–11286, 1993.
42. Krüger R, Kuhn W, Müller T, et al: Ala39Pro mutation in the gene encoding α-synuclein in Parkinson's disease. Nat Genet 18:106–108, 1998.
43. Spillantini MG, Schmidt ML, Lee VM, et al: Alpha-synuclein in Lewy bodies. Nature 388:839–840, 1997.
44. Hashimoto M, Hsu LJ, Sisk A, et al: Human recombinant NACP/alpha-synuclein is aggregated and fibrillated *in vitro*: Relevance for Lewy body disease. Brain Res 799:301–306, 1998.
45. El-Agnaf OM, Jakes R, Curran MD, et al: Effects of the mutations Ala30 to Pro and Ala53 to Thr on the physical and morphological properties of alpha-synuclein protein implicated in Parkinson's disease. FEBS Lett 440:67–70, 1998.
46. Gasser T, Müller-Myhsok B, Wszolek Z, et al: Genetic complexity and Parkinson's disease. Science 277:388–389, 1997.
47. Scott WK, Stajich, JM, Yamaoka L-H, et al: Genetic complexity in Parkinson's disease. Science 277: 387–388, 1997.
48. Vaughan JR, Durr A, Gasser T, et al: The a-synuclein Ala53Thr mutation is not a common cause of familial Parkinson's disease: A study of 230 European cases. Ann Neurol 44:270–273, 1998.
49. Chan P, Tanner CM, Jiang X, et al: Failure to find the alpha-synuclein gene missense mutation (G209A) in 100 patients with younger onset Parkinson's disease. Neurology 50:513–514, 1998.
50. Vaughan JR, Farrer M, Wszolek EK, et al: Sequencing of the alpha-synuclein gene in a large series of families with familial Parkinson's disease fails to reveal any further mutations. Hum Mol Genet 7:751–753, 1998.
51. Golbe LI: Young-onset Parkinson's disease: A clinical review. Neurology 41:168–173, 1991.
52. Ishikawa A, Tsuji S: Clinical analysis of 17 patients in 12 Japanese families with autosomal-recessive type juvenile parkinsonism. Neurology 47:160–166, 1996.
53. Ichinose H, Ohye T, Segawa M, et al: GTP cyclohydrolase I gene in hereditary progressive dystonia with marked diurnal fluctuation. Neurosci Lett 196:5–8, 1995.
54. Nygaard TG, Marsden CD, Fahn S: Dopa-responsive dystonia: Long-term treatment response and prognosis. Neurology 41:174–181, 1991.
55. Ishikawa A, Takahashi H: Clinical and neuropathological aspects of autosomal recessive juvenile parkinsonism. J Neurol 245:4–9, 1998.
56. Matsumine H, Saito M, Shimoda-Matsubayashi S, et al: Localization of a gene for an autosomal recessive form of juvenile parkinsonism to chromosome 6q25.2–27. Am J Hum Genet 60:588–596, 1997.
57. Kitada T, Asakawa S, Hattori N, et al: Mutations in the parkin gene cause autosomal recessive juvenile parkinsonism. Nature 392:605–608, 1998.
58. Lucking CB, Abbas N, Durr A, et al: Homozygous deletions in parkin gene in European and North African families with autosomal recessive juvenile parkinsonism. The European Consortium on Genetic Susceptibility in Parkinson's Disease and the French Parkinson's Disease Genetics Study Group [letter]. Lancet 352:1355–1356, 1998.
59. Abbas N, Lücking CB, Ricard S, et al: A wide variety of mutations in the parkin gene are responsible for autosomal recessive parkinsonism in Europe. Hum Mol Genet 8:567–574, 1999.
60. Gasser T, Müller-Myhsok B, Wszolek ZK, et al: A susceptibility locus for Parkinson's disease maps to chromosome 2p13. Nat Genet 18:262–265, 1998.
61. De Michele G, Filla A, Marconi R, et al: A genetic study of Parkinson's disease. J Neural Transm Suppl 45:21–25, 1995.
62. Maraganore DM, Harding AE, Marsden CD: A clinical and genetic study of familial Parkinson's disease. Mov Disord 6:205–211, 1991.
63. Smith CA, Gough AC, Leigh PN, et al: Debrisoquine hydroxylase gene polymorphism and suscep-

tibility to Parkinson's disease. Lancet 339:1375–1377, 1992.
64. Armstrong M, Daly AK, Cholerton S, et al: Mutant debrisoquine hydroxylation genes in Parkinson's disease. Lancet 339:1017–1018, 1992.
65. Planté-Bordeneuve V, Davis MB, Maraganore DM, et al: Debrisoquine hydroxylase gene polymorphism in familial Parkinson's disease. J Neurol Neurosurg Psychiatry 57:911–913, 1994.
66. Agundez JA, Jimenez Jimenez FJ, Luengo A, et al: Association between the oxidative polymorphism and early onset of Parkinson's disease. Clin Pharmacol Ther 57:291–298, 1995.
67. Lucotte G, Turpin JC, Gerard N, et al: Mutations frequencies of the cytochrome Cyp2D6 gene in Parkinson disease patients and in families. Am J Med Genet 67:361–365, 1996.
68. Kurth MC, Kurth JH: Variant cytochrome P450 CYP2D6 allelic frequencies in Parkinson's disease. Am J Med Genet 48:166–168, 1993.
69. Gasser T, Müller-Myhsok B, Supala A, et al: The CYP2D6B-allele is not over-represented in a population of German patients with idiopathic Parkinson's disease. J Neurol Neurosurg Psychiatry 61: 518–520, 1996.
70. Sandy MS, Armstrong M, Tanner CM, et al: CYP2D6 allelic frequencies in young-onset Parkinson's disease. Neurology 47:225–230, 1996.
71. Akhmedova SN, Pushnova EA, Yakimovsky AF, et al: Frequency of a specific cytochrome P4502D6B (CYP2D6B) mutant allele in clinically differentiated groups of patients with Parkinson disease. Biochem Mol Med 54:88–90, 1995.
72. Diederich N, Hilger C, Goetz CG, Keipes M, Hentges F, Vieregge P, Metz M: Genetic variability of the CYP2D6 gene is not a risk factor for sporadic Parkinson's disease. Ann Neurol 40:463–465, 1996.
73. Iwahashi K, Miyatake R, Tsuneoka Y, et al: A novel cytochrome P-450IID6 (CYPIID6) mutant gene associated with multiple system atrophy [letter]. J Neurol Neurosurg Psychiatry 58:263–264, 1995.
74. Fahn S, Bressman SB, Marsden CD: Classification of dystonia. Adv Neurol 78:1–10, 1998.
75. Fahn S: Clinical variants of idiopathic torsion dystonia. J Neurol Neurosurg Psychiatry Suppl:96–100, 1989.
76. Oppenheim H: Über eine eigenartige Krampfkrankheit des kindlichen und jugendlichen Alters (Dysbasia lordotica progressiva, Dystonia musculorum deformans). Neurol Centralblatt 30:1090–1107, 1911.
77. Zador J: Le spasme de torsion: parallèle des tableaux clinicques entre la race juive et les autres races. Rev Neurol 66:365–389, 1936.
78. Zeman W, Dyken P: Dystonia musculorum deformans: Clinical, genetic, and pathoanatomical studies. Psychiatr Neurol Neurochir 10:77–121, 1967.
79. Zilber N, Korczyn AD, Kahana E, et al: Inheritance of idiopathic torsion dystonia among Jews. J Med Genet 21:13–20, 1984.
80. Bressman SB, de Leon D, Brin MF, et al: Idiopathic dystonia among Ashkenazi Jews: Evidence for autosomal dominant inheritance. Ann Neurol 26: 612–620, 1989.
81. Pauls DL, Korczyn AD: Complex segregation analysis of dystonia pedigrees suggests autosomal dominant inheritance. Neurology 40:1107–1110, 1990.
82. Kramer PL, Heiman GA, Gasser T, et al: The DYT1 gene on 9q34 is responsible for most cases of early limb-onset idiopathic torsion dystonia in non-Jews. Am J Hum Genet 55:468–475, 1994.
83. Ozelius L, Kramer PL, Moskowitz CB, et al: Human gene for torsion dystonia located on chromosome 9q32–q34. Neuron 2:1427–1434, 1989.
84. Kramer PL, de Leon D, Ozelius L, et al: Dystonia gene in Ashkenazi Jewish population is located on chromosome 9q32–34. Ann Neurol 27:114–120, 1991.
85. Ozelius LJ, Kramer PL, de Leon D, et al: Strong allelic association between the torsion dystonia gene (DYT1) and loci on chromosome 9q34 in Ashkenazi Jews torsion dystonia genes in two populations confined to a small region on chromosome 9q32–34. Am J Hum Genet 49:366–371, 1991.
86. Risch N, deLeon D, Fahn S, et al: ITD in Ashkenazi Jews—Genetic drift or selection? [letter]. Nat Genet 11:13–15, 1995.
87. Bressman SB, de Leon D, Kramer PL, et al: Dystonia in Ashkenazi Jews: Clinical characterization of a founder mutation. Ann Neurol 36:771–777, 1994.
88. Ozelius L, Hewett JW, Page CE, et al: The early-onset torsion dystonia gene (Dyt1) encodes an ATP-binding protein. Nat Genet 17:40–48, 1997.
89. Bressman SB, Hunt AL, Heiman GA, et al: Exclusion of the DYT1 locus in a non-Jewish family with early-onset dystonia. Mov Disord 9:626–632, 1994.
90. Warner TT, Fletcher NA, Davis MB, et al: Linkage analysis in British and French families with idiopathic torsion dystonia. Brain 116:739–744, 1993.
91. Ahmad F, Davis MB, Waddy HM, et al: Evidence for locus heterogeneity in autosomal dominant torsion dystonia. Genomics 15:9–12, 1993.
92. Nutt JG, Muenter MD, Aronson A, et al: Epidemiology of focal and generalized dystonia in Rochester, Minnesota. Mov Disord 3:188–194, 1988.
93. Chan J, Brin MF, Fahn S: Idiopathic cervical dystonia: Clinical characteristics. Mov Disord 6:119–126, 1991.
94. Waddy HM, Fletcher NA, Harding AE, et al: A genetic study of idiopathic focal dystonias. Ann Neurol 29:320–324, 1991.
95. Forsgren L, Holmgren G, Almay BG, et al: Autosomal dominant torsion dystonia in a Swedish family. Adv Neurol 50:83–92, 1988.
96. Uitti RJ, Maraganore DM: Adult onset familial cervical dystonia: Report of a family including monozygotic twins. Mov Disord 8:489–494, 1993.
97. Leube B, Kessler KR, Goecke T, et al: Frequency of familial inheritance among 488 index patients with idiopathic focal dystonia and clinical variability in a large family. Mov Disord 12:1000–1006, 1997.
98. Almasy L, Bressman SB, Raymond D, et al: Idiopathic torsion dystonia linked to chromosome 8 in two Mennonite families. Ann Neurol 42:670–673, 1997.
99. Leube B, Rudnicki D, Ratzlaff T, et al: Idiopathic torsion dystonia: Assignment of a gene to chromosome 18p in a German family with adult onset,

autosomal dominant inheritance and purely focal distribution. Hum Mol Genet 5:1673–1677, 1996.

100. Leube B, Hendgen T, Kessler KR, et al: Evidence for DYT7 being a common cause of cervical dystonia (torticollis) in Central Europe. Am J Med Genet 74:529–532, 1997.
101. Gasser T: Idiopathic, myoclonic and dopa-responsive dystonia. Curr Opin Neurol 10:357–362, 1997.
102. Segawa M, Nomura Y, Kase M: Hereditary progressive dystonia with marked diurnal fluctuation: Clinicopathophysiological identification in reference to juvenile Parkinson's disease. Adv Neurol 45:227–34:227–234, 1987.
103. Nygaard T: Dopa-responsive dystonia. In Tsui JKC, Calne DB (eds): Handbook of Dystonia. New York, Marcel Dekker, 1995, pp213–226.
104. Segawa M, Hosaka A, Miyagwa F, et al: Hereditary progressive dystonia with marked diurnal variation. Adv Neurol 14:251–233, 1976.
105. Rajput AH, Gibb WR, Zhong XH, et al: Dopa-responsive dystonia: Pathological and biochemical observations in a case [see comments]. Ann Neurol 35:396–402, 1994.
106. Nygaard TG, Wilhelmsen KC, Risch NJ, et al: Linkage mapping of dopa-responsive dystonia (DRD) to chromosome 14q. Nat Genet 5:386–391, 1993.
107. Tanaka H, Endo K, Tsuji S, et al: The gene for hereditary progressive dystonia with marked diurnal fluctuation maps to chromosome 14q. Ann Neurol 37:405–408, 1995.
108. Furukawa Y, Shimadzu M, Rajput AH, et al: GTP-cyclohydrolase I gene mutations in hereditary progressive and dopa-responsive dystonia. Ann Neurol 39:609–617, 1996.
109. Bandmann O, Nygaard T, Surtees R, et al: Dopa-responsive dystonia in British patients: New mutations of the GTP-cyclohydrolase I gene and evidence for genetic heterogeneity. Hum Mol Genet 5:403–406, 1996.
110. Ichinose H, Ohye T, Takahashi E, et al: Hereditary progressive dystonia with marked diurnal fluctuation caused by mutations in the GTP cyclohydrolase I gene. Nat Genet 8:236–242, 1994.
111. Furukawa Y, Mizuno Y, Narabayashi H: Early-onset parkinsonism with dystonia. Clinical and biochemical differences from hereditary progressive dystonia or DOPA-responsive dystonia. Adv Neurol 69:327–337, 1996.
112. Bandmann O, Daniel S, Marsden CD, et al: The GTP cyclohydrolase I gene in atypical parkinsonian patients: A clinico-genetic study. J Neurol Sci 141:27–32, 1996.
113. Ludecke B, Dworniczak B, Bartholome K: A point mutation in the tyrosine hydroxylase gene associated with Segawa's syndrome. Hum Genet 95: 123–125, 1995.
114. Knappskog PM, Flatmark T, Mallet J, et al: Recessively inherited L-DOPA–responsive dystonia caused by a point mutation (Q381K) in the tyrosine hydroxylase gene. Hum Mol Genet 4:1209–1212, 1995.
115. Fahn S: The varied clinical expressions of dystonia. Neurol Clin 2:541–553, 1984.
116. Quinn NP, Marsden CD: Dominantly inherited myoclonic dystonia with dramatic response to alcohol. Neurology 34:236–237, 1984.
117. Quinn NP, Rothwell JC, Thompson PD, et al: Hereditary myoclonic dystonia, hereditary torsion dystonia and hereditary essential myoclonus: An area of confusion. Adv Neurol 50:391–401, 1988.
118. Gasser T: Inherited myoclonus-dystonia syndrome. Adv Neurol 78:325–334, 1998.
119. Gasser T, Bereznai B, Müller B, et al: Linkage studies in alcohol-responsive myoclonic dystonia. Mov Disord 12:363–370, 1996.
120. Kurlan R, Behr J, Medved L, et al: Myoclonus and dystonia: A family study. Adv Neurol 50:385–389, 1988.
121. Duvoisin RC: Essential myoclonus: Response to anticholinergic therapy. Clin Neuropharmacol 7: 141–147, 1984.
122. Kyllerman M, Forsgren L, Sanner G, et al: Alcohol-responsive myoclonic dystonia in a large family: Dominant inheritance and phenotypic variation. Mov Discord 5:270–279, 1990.
123. Lundemo G, Persson HE: Hereditary essential myoclonus. Acta Neurol Scand 72: 176–179, 1985.
124. Mahloudji M, Pikielny RT: Hereditary essential myoclonus. Brain 90:669–674, 1967.
125. Fahn S, Sjaastad O: Hereditary essential myoclonus in a large Norwegian family. Mov Disord 6:237–247, 1991.
126. Wahlstrom J, Ozelius L, Kramer P, et al: The gene for familial dystonia with myoclonic jerks responsive to alcohol is not located on the distal end of 9q. Clin Genet 45:88–92, 1994.
127. Wilhelmsen KC, Nygaard T, Weeks DE, et al: Progress in genetic localization of the gene for hereditary essential myoclonus. Mov Disord 9: 132–132, 1994.
128. Keretz A: Paroxysmal kinesigenic choreoathetosis. Neurology 17:680–690, 1967.
129. Goodenough DJ, Fariello RG, Annis BL, et al: Familial and acquired paroxysmal dyskinesias. A proposed classification with delineation of clinical features. Arch Neurol 35:827–831, 1978.
130. Mount LA, Reback S: Familial paroxysmal chreoathetosis: Preliminary report on a hitherto undescribed clinical syndrome. Arch Neurol Psychiatry 44:841–847, 1940.
131. Fouad GT, Servidei S, Simon D, et al: A gene for familial paroxysmal dyskinesia (FDP1) maps to chromosome 2q. Am J Hum Genet 59:135–139, 1996.
132. Fink Jk, Rainier S, Wilkowski J, et al: Paroxysmal dystonic choreoathetosis: Tight linkage to chromosome 2q. Am J Hum Genet 59:140–145, 1996.
133. Browne DL, Gancher ST, Nutt JG, et al: Episodic ataxia/myokymia syndrome is associated with point mutations in the human potassium channel gene, KCNA1. Nat Genet 8:136–140, 1994.
134. Fontaine B, Khurana TS, Hoffman EP, et al: Hyperkalemic periodic paralysis and the adult muscle sodium channel alpha-subunit gene. Science 250:1000–1002, 1990.
135. Koch MC, Steinmeyer K, Lorenz C, et al: The skeletal muscle chloride channel in dominant and recessive human myotonia. Science 257:797–800, 1992.

136. Auburger G, Ratzlaff T, Lunkes A, et al: A gene for autosomal dominant paroxysmal choreoathetosis/spasticity (CSE) maps to the vicinity of a potassium channel gene cluster onchromosome 1p, probably within 2 cM between D1S443 and D1S197. Genomics 31:90–94, 1996.
137. Graeber MB, Muller U: The X-linked dystonia-parkinsonism syndrome (XDP): Clinical and molecular genetic analysis. Brain Pathol 2:287–295, 1992.
138. Waters CH, Takahashi H, Wilhelmsen KC, et al: Phenotypic expression of X-linked dystonia-parkinsonism (lubag) in two women. Neurology 43:1555–1558, 1993.
139. Louis ED, Ottman R: How familial is familial tremor? The genetic epidemiology of essential tremor. Neurology 46:1200–1202, 1996.
140. Larsson T, Sjögren T: Essential tremor: A clinical and genetic population study. Acta Psychiatr Neurol Scand 36:1–176, 1960.
141. Koller WC, Busenbark K, Miner K: The relationship of essential tremor to other movement disorders: Report on 678 patients. Essential Tremor Study Group. Ann Neurol 35:717–723, 1994.
142. Rautakorpi I, Marttila RJ, Rinne UK: Epidemiology of essential tremor. In Findley LJ, Capildeo R (eds): Movement Disorders: Tremor. London and Basingstoke, Macmillan, 1984, pp211–218.
143. Lou JS, Jankovic J: Essential tremor: Clinical correlates in 350 patients. Neurology 41:234–238, 1991.
144. Bain PG, Findley LJ, Thompson PD, et al: A study of hereditary essential tremor. Brain 117:805–824, 1994.
145. Critchley W: Observations on essential (heredofamilial) tremor. Brain 72:113–119, 1949.
146. Critchley E: Clinical manifestations of essential tremor. J Neurol Neurosurg Psychiatry 35:365–372, 1972.
147. Rajput AH, Rozdilsky B, Ang L, et al: Clinicopathologic observations in essential tremor: Report of six cases. Neurology 41:1422–1424, 1991.
148. Brooks DJ, Playford ED, Ibanez V, et al: Isolated tremor and disruption of the nigrostriatal dopaminergic system: An 18F-dopa PET study. Neurology 42:1554–1560, 1992.
149. Higgins JJ, Pho LT, Nee LE: A gene (ETM) for essential tremor maps to chromosome 2p22–p25. Mov Discord 12:859–864, 1997.
150. Gulcher JR, Jonsson P, Kong A, et al: Mapping of a familial essential tremor gene, FET1, to chromosome 3q13. Nat Genet 17:84–87, 1997.
151. Danek A: Geniospasm: Hereditary chin trembling. Mov Disord 8:335–338, 1993.
152. Jarman PR, Wood NW, Davis MT, et al: Hereditary geniospasm: Linkage to chromosome 9q13–q21 and evidence for genetic heterogeneity. Am J Hum Genet 61:928–933, 1997.
153. Brewer GJ, Yuzbasiyan Gurkan V: Wilson disease. Medicine (Baltimore) 71:139–164, 1992.
154. Petrukhin K, Lutsenko S, Chernov I, et al: Characterization of the Wilson disease gene encoding a P-type copper transporting ATPase: Genomic organization, alternative splicing, and structure/function predictions. Hum Mol Genet 3:1647–1656, 1994.
155. Tanzi RE, Petrukhin K, Chernov I, et al: The Wilson disease gene is a copper transporting ATPase with homology to the Menkes disease gene. Nat Genet 5:344–350, 1993.
156. Thomas GR, Roberts EA, Walshe JM, et al: Haplotypes and mutations in Wilson disease. Am J Hum Genet 56:1315–1319, 1995.
157. Vidaud D, Assouline B, Lecoz P, et al: Misdiagnosis revealed by genetic linkage analysis in a family with Wilson disease. Neurology 46:1485–1486, 1996.
158. Figus A, Angius A, Loudianos G, et al: Molecular pathology and haplotype analysis of Wilson disease in Mediterranean populations. Am J Hum Genet 57:1318–1324, 1995.
159. O'Keeffe ST: Restless legs syndrome. A review. Arch Intern Med 156:243–248, 1996.
160. Godbout R, Montplaiser J, Poirier G: Epidemiologic data in familial restless legs syndrome. Sleep Res 16:228–228, 1987.
161. Walters AS, Picchietti D, Hening W, et al: Variable expressivity in familial restless legs syndrome. Arch Neurol 47:1219–1220, 1990.
162. Ryan SG, Sherman SL, Terry JC, et al: Startle disease, or hyperekplexia: Response to clonazepam and assignment of the gene (STHE) to chromosome 5q by linkage analysis. Ann Neurol 31:663–668, 1992.
163. Shiang R, Ryan SG, Zhu YZ, et al: Mutations in the alpha 1 subunit of the inhibitory glycine receptor cause the dominant neurologic disorder, hyperekplexia. Nat Genet 5:351–358, 1993.
164. Shiang R, Ryan SG, Zhu YZ, et al: Mutational analysis of familial and sporadic hyperekplexia. Ann Neurol 38:85–91, 1995.
165. Rees MI, Andrew M, Jawad S, et al: Evidence for recessive as well as dominant forms of startle disease (hyperekplexia) caused by mutations in the alpha 1 subunit of the inhibitory glycine receptor. Hum Mol Genet 3:2175–2179, 1994.
166. Tijssen MA, Shiang R, van Deutekom J, et al: Molecular genetic reevaluation of the Dutch hyperekplexia family. Arch Neurol 52:578–582, 1995.
167. Huntington's Disease Collaborative Research Group: A novel gene containing a trinucleotide repeat that is expanded and unstable on Huntington's disease chromosomes. Cell 72:971–983, 1993.
168. Wijker M, Wszolek ZK, Wolters EC, et al: Localization of the gene for rapidly progressive autosomal dominant parkinsonism and dementia with pallido-ponto-nigral degeneration to chromosome 17q21. Hum Mol Genet 5:151–154, 1996.
169. Starosta-Rubinstein S, Young AB, Kluin K, et al. Clinical assessment of 31 patients with Wilson's disease. Correlation with structural changes on magnetic resonance imaging. Arch Neurol 44: 365–373, 1987.

# Chapter 19

# MULTIPLE SCLEROSIS AND OTHER DEMYELINATING DISEASES

A. Dessa Sadovnick, PhD
D. Dyment, MSc



This chapter focuses on demyelinating diseases of the central nervous system (CNS) (diseases in which normal functional myelin sheaths are broken down) for which genetic factors play important roles in the etiology. (These diseases are referred to as "inherited" diseases, although it is recognized that nongenetic factors may also be important). The most common of these diseases is multiple sclerosis (MS), which occurs in approximately 0.1% of Caucasians of northern and central European ancestry. A few inherited demyelinating diseases that are less common than MS are discussed briefly. These include Krabbe's disease (globoid cell leukodystrophy), metachromatic leukodystrophy, Leber's hereditary optic neuropathy, and X-linked adrenoleukodystrophy. The reader is referred to Scriver and coworkers[1] for a wider overview of inherited demyelinating diseases. Inherited myelin diseases of the peripheral nervous system (PNS), such as Charcot-Marie-Tooth disease, or dysmyelinating diseases (i.e., diseases associated with failure to initially form normal functional myelin) are not discussed in this chapter.

Myelin is the lipid-rich insulator that surrounds axons in the CNS and PNS. Oligodendrocytes are cells that produce and maintain the myelin sheath, which increases axonal impulse conduction by "saltatory conduction." Depolarization of the axon membrane occurs between myelin segments in the "nodes of Ranvier," the unmyelinated axonal segments. It must still be resolved whether the initial attack in MS is on the myelin, the oligodendrocyte, or both. At present, data supports the hypothesis that the primary attack is on the myelin sheath, with oligodendrocyte death being the secondary event. Conduction velocity is diminished in unmyelinated fibers compared with myelinated ones (for further discussion, see Morell and coworkers[2]).

Central nervous system myelin protein is largely made up of proteolipid protein (PLP) and myelin basic protein (MBP). Relatively minor myelin proteins include MAG (myelin-associated glycoprotein) and MOG (myelin/oligodendrocyte glycoprotein). As is discussed, MBP is one of several candidate genes that have been proposed for MS.

## MULTIPLE SCLEROSIS

Multiple sclerosis is a putative autoimmune disease, but the actual mechanism(s) leading to inflammatory demyelination in the CNS and the subsequent signs and symptoms must yet be determined.[3] In fact, there is little correlation between regions of demyelination and the clinical signs and symptoms of MS.

The terms *multiple* and *disseminated* describe the basic spatial and temporal characteristics of the CNS lesions found in MS. Typically, there are many (multiple) focal demyelinating lesions (plaques) throughout the white and gray matter. The primary lesions are not scars, as implied by the term *sclerosis,* but are probably inflammatory. The most common areas for MS plaques to occur are the optic nerves, spinal cord, and cerebral hemispheres. Over time, initially isolated plaques may coalesce and become confluent.

As MS plaques age and develop, the degree of inflammation decreases and gliosis begins. Despite early beliefs that the axon is preserved in MS, it is now recognized that as gliosis continues, axonal degeneration can take place.[4] Remyelination, once thought to be irreversible, may be possible in MS.[4]

Most MS patients have a monosymptomatic onset (one symptom, frequently motor or sensory), but polysymptomatic onset is not uncommon. The spectrum of symptoms representing the onset of MS is wide and can include sensory symptoms (numbness, tingling), visual disturbances (optic neuritis, diplopia), spasticity, weakness, fatigue, ataxia and intention tremor, and bowel and/or bladder disturbances.

The clinical course of MS can be very variable, ranging from a fulminating disorder that can be fatal within months to an asymptomatic condition only recognized at autopsy. The typical clinical course is initially characterized by relapses and remissions but becomes progressive over time. Other relatively common clinical courses include "benign," "long-term relapsing-remitting," and "primary chronic progressive." Although MS is not usually a fatal disease, disability and decreased quality of life are common.

Innumerable epidemiological studies have been conducted on MS. The nonrandom geographic distribution as illustrated by the "north–south" gradient in the northern hemisphere,[5] migration,[6] the identification of "resistant" populations,[7] and different MS rates within similar latitudes[8,9] have been known for decades. The decisive conclusions about the geography and prevalence of MS from the available epidemiological data are as follows: *(1)* a north–south gradient exists in the northern hemisphere; *(2)* major differences in prevalence occur in the absence of latitude differences; *(3)* individuals from the same ethnic derivation have either similar prevalence rates or very different prevalence rates in widely separated geographical areas, and *(4)* specific resistant isolates are shown to exist regardless of latitude. This information leads to the almost inescapable conclusion that the epidemiology of MS on a population basis cannot be explained by any single known environmental or genetic factor in isolation but rather results from a heterogeneous distribution (and probably interaction) of both genetic and environmental factors.[10–12] (For more detailed reviews, Sadovnick and colleagues.[12,13]) The role of any transmissible agent in MS now appears unlikely (Table 19–1).

Although the increased familial aggregation of MS has been well established for many years, the explanation for this observation has remained unclear. Familial aggregation can be explained in several ways, including *(1)* the increased genetic sharing among biological relatives (i.e., nature); *(2)* common shared nongenetic factors (i.e., nurture); or *(3)* a combination of nature and nurture. Results of two recent studies[14,15] described below now clearly show that the excess of MS among relatives (i.e., familial aggregation) is explained by nature (i.e., the increased genetic sharing among relatives) rather than nurture or a combination of nature and nurture.

## Data From Adoption Studies

Adoption studies provide an important method to discriminate between nature and nurture in the etiology of both normal variation and disease. The only known adoption study for MS was conducted by Ebers and associates[14] as part of the Canadian Collaborative Project on Genetic Susceptibility to MS (CCPGSMS).[16] With data from the

Table 19–1. **Evidence Against a Transmissible Etiology in Multiple Sclerosis**

Low concordance rate in monozygotic twins[55,56]

Low rate of MS among spouses (i.e., conjugal MS)[85]

Groups resistant to MS in "high-risk areas," e.g., Amerindians (North America)[86]; Asians, e.g., Chinese, Japanese (North America)[87]; Lapps (Scandinavia)[88]

Birth order position data[89,90]

Age of onset among siblings concordant for MS[91]

Nonbiological (adopted) first-degree relatives have a risk for MS similar to that for the general population rather than for biological relatives[14]

Half-siblings have a risk for MS that is consistent with their decreased genetic sharing compared with full siblings[15]

Half-sibling risks do not vary according to whether the half-siblings have lived together[15]

See Sadovnick et al.[12] for detailed discussions about this evidence.

CCPGSMS, it was possible to compare MS rates in biological and nonbiological first-degree relatives of MS patients (index cases). The term *nonbiological first-degree relative* refers to an adopted parent, sibling, or child of the MS index case who does not share any genetic material with the index case.

Specifically, the study[14] looked at *(1)* adopted MS index cases and their adopting parents, adoptive siblings, and adopted children; and *(2)* nonadopted index cases and their adopted siblings and adopted children. The hypothesis being tested was that the familial aggregation (excess of MS among relatives) is genetic (nature). The study found only one case of MS among 1201 nonbiological first-degree relatives studied. This finding was significantly lower than that predicted for biological relatives ($P = 2.5 \times 10^{-10}$), but not different from the expected 1.2 affected individuals based on the general population prevalence of 0.1%.

This adoption data can therefore be interpreted as support for the hypothesis. Nevertheless, MS literature has been plagued by studies that could not be replicated. For this reason, it was important to test this hypothesis with another approach. The CCPGSMS database[16] provided a unique opportunity to conduct a half-sibling study[15] in MS.

## Data From Half-Sibling Studies

Half-siblings have only one parent in common and therefore share 25% rather than 50% of their genetic material. Half-siblings are also of special interest because they may or may not be raised together within a common family environment. For example, in some families such as when there is an acrimonious break-up, half-siblings may only spend time together on rare occasions, if ever. In other situations, such as the death of parent when the child is very young and subsequent remarriage of the surviving parent, half-siblings can be raised together in the family environment. Half-siblings therefore allow the testing of the effects of both reduced genetic sharing and different environmental sharing on the familial aggregation of MS. In addition, maternal half-siblings (common mother) allow an assessment of the effect of common uterine environment and maternal inheritance on the familial aggregation of MS.

The results of the half-sibling study[15] are summarized in Table 19–2. The age-adjusted risk for *half-siblings* (1.32%; SD = 0.31) was statistically lower than for *full siblings* of the same MS index cases (3.46%; SD = 0.54), G = 12.69, $p < 0.001$. The age-adjusted risk for *half-siblings who lived together* was 1.17% (SD = 0.41), which was not statistically different from that for *half-siblings who did not live together* (1.47%; SD = 0.46), G = 0.25, $0.50 < p < 0.75$. The age-adjusted risk for *maternal* half-siblings of MS index cases was 1.42% (SD = 0.42), not statistically different from that for *paternal* half-siblings (1.19%; SD = 0.45), G = 0.14, $0.90 < p < 0.95$.

The results of the half-sibling study pro-

Table 19–2. **Half-Siblings Studies in Multiple Sclerosis**

| Relationship to Index Case | No. | No. With MS | Age-Adjusted Risk% (S.D.) |
|---|---|---|---|
| *Full Siblings versus Half-Siblings* | | | |
| Full Siblings | 1395 | 39 | 3.46% (0.55) |
| Half-siblings | 1839 | 18 | 1.32% (0.31) |
| | G = 12.69, $p < 0.001$ | | |
| *Half-Siblings Raised Together versus Half-Siblings Raised Apart* | | | |
| Half-siblings who lived together | 897 | 6 | 1.17% (0.41) |
| Half-siblings who never lived together | 942 | 10 | 1.47% (0.46) |
| | G = 0.25; $0.50 < p < 0.75$ | | |
| *Maternal versus Paternal Half-Siblings* | | | |
| Maternal half-siblings | 1033 | 11 | 1.42% (0.42) |
| Paternal half-siblings | 806 | 7 | 1.19% (0.45) |
| | G = 0.14, $0.90 < p < 0.95$ | | |

**Source:** Sadovnick et al.[15]

vide strong evidence that shared nongenetic factors (environment or "nurture") do not account for the familial aggregation of MS, thereby supporting the results of the adoption study. The data also shows that maternal factors (e.g., intrauterine and/or perinatal factors such as breast-feeding, genomic imprinting, mitochondrial inheritance) have no demonstrable effect on the familial aggregation of MS.

## The Search for Candidate Genes

To plan linkage studies of a complex disease such as MS, it is important to have some understanding of the likelihood of finding linkage under the constraints imposed by the nature of the problem.[12] The likelihood of finding linkage depends on *(1)* the number of loci involved in MS susceptibility, *(2)* the magnitude of their individual effects, *(3)* the population frequencies of high-risk alleles, *(4)* the relationship of genotypes at multiple loci to risk (encompassing concepts of genetic heterogeneity and/or epistasis where genes at different loci may or may not interact in producing risk), *(5)* the density (map distance) of the di (tri, tetra) nucleotide repeat map (and other restriction fragment length polymorphisms), and *(6)* the polymorphism content of the markers involved (for further discussion, see Sadovnick and coworkers[12]).

Despite nearly three decades of searching for candidate genes in MS, the only unambiguous association remains the class II major histocompatibility complex (MHC), located on chromosome 6.[17] Nevertheless, existing data strongly indicates that additional loci that influence both susceptibility and outcome will be identified.

The following is a brief review of some of the suggested candidate loci for MS. These candidates (and others) have been put forward largely because of their role in either the immune process[18] or myelin formation.[2] This is not meant to be a comprehensive list of either all suggested candidate genes or all studies per candidate.

### HUMAN LEUKOCYTE ANTIGEN

Human leukocyte antigen (HLA) molecules play a key role in the immune system's response against foreign antigens. They regulate the development and maturation of the T-cell repertoire within the thymus and are also involved in the activation of the cell-mediated immune response of the periphery. The mature T cell will initiate (or not initiate) an immune response depending on the class of HLA (i.e., class I or class II) and whether the presented antigen is a foreign antigen (or a self-antigen). As the normal immune response depends on HLA, the genes of the HLA locus have been proposed as candidate genes for MS susceptibility.

Early studies demonstrated an association between MS and HLA antigens.[17,19] In contrast to association studies, the results of linkage studies have been contradictory.[20–22] The genome-wide screen conducted in the United States[23] confirmed a role for HLA in MS pathogenesis. This finding was supported by a smaller study in Finland[24] and to a lesser extent by Canadian and United Kingdom genome-wide screens.[25,26]

The contribution of HLA to the risk of developing MS is believed to be modest at best. A rough estimate of this contribution of HLA to MS, based on 336 published[20–22,27–29] affected sibling pairs, based on the methods of Risch,[30] concluded that "other determinants" contribute more to the relative risk of MS than does HLA.

## $TCR_\alpha$ AND $TCR_\beta$ CHAIN POLYMORPHISMS

The T-cell receptor (TCR) has an important role in immunity (for a more detailed discussion of immunity with respect to MS, see Ebers[18]). Briefly, the T-cell receptor, a transmembrane glycoprotein on T lymphocytes, recognizes the HLA complex and binds to it. The T-cell receptor is made up of two pairs of polypeptide chains: $TCR_{ga}$ (chromosome 14q) and $TCR_\beta$ (chromosome 7q).

Association, classic linkage, and affected sibling pair (ASP) linkage studies have been done for both $TCR_\alpha$ and $TCR_\beta$ with conflicting results (Table 19–3). Taken together, the data suggests that $TCR_\alpha$ chain polymorphisms do not contribute to MS susceptibility and $TCR_\beta$ chain polymorphisms contribute relatively little to MS susceptibility, and the contribution is likely dependent on the presence of other loci.

Table 19–3: **Selected Studies of $TCR_\alpha$ and $TCR_\beta$ in Multiple Sclerosis**

| Association | Classic Linkage | Linkage Affected Sibling Pair |
|---|---|---|
| *$TCR_\alpha$ (chromosome 14q)* | | |
| Oksenberg[92]† | Lynch† | Hashimoto[94]† |
| Hillert[93]† | | |
| Hashimoto[94]† | | |
| *$TCR_\beta$ (chromosome 7q)* | | |
| Beall[96]* | Lynch[103]† | Seboun[104]† |
| Charmley[97]* | | |
| Fugger[98]† | | |
| Hillert[99]† | | |
| Martinez-Naves[100]* | | |
| Beall[101]* | | |
| Wei[102]* | | |

*Significant results, $p < 0.05$.
†Nonsignificant results, $p \geq 0.05$.

## MYELIN BASIC PROTEIN

Myelin basic protein is a major component of the myelin sheath and has been proposed as a candidate gene in MS. It has been suggested that an autoimmune reaction against MBP may occur in MS patients.[31]

Association, classic linkage, and ASP linkage studies have been done for MBP with conflicting results (Table 19–4). Taken together, the data suggests that, at least for non-Finnish populations, MBP does not contribute to MS susceptibility.

Table 19–4. **Selected Studies of Myelin Basic Protein (Chromosome 18q) in Multiple Sclerosis**

| Association | Classic Linkage | Linkage Affected Sibling Pair |
|---|---|---|
| Boylan[105]* | Tienari[106]* | Wood[108]† |
| Tienari[106]* | Rose[110]† | Eoli[109]† |
| Graham[107]† | Eoli[109]† | |
| Wood[108]† | | |
| Eoli[109]† | | |

*Significant results, $p < 0.05$.
†Nonsignificant results, $p \geq 0.05$.

## IMMUNOGLOBULIN HEAVY CHAIN

Immunoglobulins, found on B cells, are secreted as antibodies. They recognize and

Table 19–5. **Selected Studies of Immunoglobulins in Multiple Sclerosis**

| Association | Determinant |
|---|---|
| Propert[111*] | Gm1, Gm1, 2 |
| Sandberg-Wollheim[112*] | Gm1, 2, 21 |
| Sesboue[113†] | Gm1, Gm2, Gm3 |
| Salier[114†] | Gm1, Gm2, Gm3 |
| Francis[115†] | Gm1 (1, 2, 3, 17) |
| Francis[115†] | Gm3 (5, 10, 11, 13, 14, 21) |
| Gaiser[116*] | Constant region |
| Walter[117*] | Variable region |
| Hillert[118†] | Constant region |
| Yu[119†] | Constant region |
| *Linkage Affected Sibling Pair Study* | |
| Yu[119†] | Variable region |

*Significant results, $p < 0.05$.
†Nonsignificant results, $p \geq 0.05$.

bind to foreign antigens, thus triggering the immune response.

An immunoglobulin is made up of two chains, a heavy chain and a light chain. The heavy chain has two parts: *(1)* the constant region, which defines the specific function of the antibody; and *(2)* the variable region, which binds to the antigen.

Different constant regions are *isotypes*. Polymorphisms within an isotype are *allotypes*. The following observations suggest that immunoglobulins are involved in MS: Immunoglobulin G (an isotype) is restricted to the cerebrospinal fluid (CSF) of MS patients,[32] and autoantibodies may be involved in the destruction of myelin.[33]

Taken together, results of association and ASP linkage studies for the immunoglobulins (Table 19–5) suggest that constant region polymorphisms do not contribute to MS susceptibility. Variable region polymorphisms need further confirmation from independent samples before any conclusions can be made.

### TUMOR NECROSIS FACTOR

Tumor necrosis factor-α (TNF-α) has been put forward as a possible candidate gene based on observations of the role of TNF-α at the CNS lesions of MS patients[34] and the levels of TNF in their CSF and sera.[35,36] This remains speculative.[37,38]

### GENOME SCREENS

With advances in the techniques of molecular genetics, it is now possible to conduct total genome screens with microsatellite markers. In August 1996, the initial results of genome screens in multiplex families from Canada,[25] the United States,[23] and the United Kingdom[26] were simultaneously published in *Nature Genetics*. The Canadian group[25] was able to exclude 88% of the genome, and the United Kingdom group[23] was able to exclude 93% of the genome, given the methodological limitations described in the papers.

Table 19–6 lists several regions of interest identified by the three groups.[23,25,26] Taken together, the initial findings are consistent with genetic epidemiological data in that they support the idea of multiple genes, each having a relatively small individual effect that interacts epistatically to determine the total heritable susceptibility.[39]

## Animal Models

For a more detailed review of animal models in MS, see Kastrukoff and Rice.[40] A specific peptide of MBP can induce a chronic relapsing experimental allergic encephalomyelitis (EAE) in certain strains of susceptible mice and rats.[41] This chronic EAE model shows MS-like pathology in the CNS and the lymphocyte infiltrate.[42] Experimental allergic encephalomyelitis differs from MS in that EAE does not occur spontaneously. The animal must be inoculated with the MBP and/or myelin protein mixture or have MBP-restricted T cells adoptively transferred from an affected animal. Several genes are involved in EAE susceptibility, including those in the MHC (e.g., *eae1*) and those outside the MHC (e.g., *eae2, eae3*).[43]

Transgenic mouse models exist for EAE. Goverman and colleagues[44] constructed a strain of mouse that expressed a T-cell receptor specific for MBP. These mice developed EAE if they were inoculated with MBP, Freund's adjuvent, and pertussis toxin. It

Table 19–6. **Some Regions of Interest Identified From Genome Screens in Multiplex Multiple Sclerosis Families**

| Chromosome No. | Marker | Chromosome |
|---|---|---|
| 1 | | 1 cen‡ |
| 2 | 2S119* | |
| 3 | D3S1261* | |
| 5 | D5S406* | |
| | D5S815† | 5q13–23 |
| | | 5 cen‡ |
| 6 | | 6p21(MHC)‡ |
| 7 | D7S554† | 7q21–22 |
| | D7S523† | 7q32–34 |
| | | 7p‡ |
| 10 | D10S212* | |
| 11 | D11S2000* | |
| | D11S922† | 11p15 |
| 12 | PAH† | 12q24 |
| | D12S392† | 12q24-qter |
| | | 12p‡ |
| 17 | | 17q22‡ |
| 19 | D19S219† | 19q13 |
| | APOC2† | 19q13 |
| 22 | | 22q‡ |
| X Chromosome | DXS1068* | |

*Canada.[25]
†United States.[23]
‡United Kingdom.[26]

was also noted that mice housed in nonsterile cages developed EAE spontaneously, suggesting a relationship between sanitation and EAE, as has also been suggested for MS.[13]

Lafaille and associates[45] developed a transgenic mouse deficient in Rag1, which is responsible for the expression of rearranged TCR gene products. In these mice, only the TCR transgene expressed its rearranged TCR gene product, but all the mice (100%) developed spontaneous EAE. In contrast, only 14% of the TCR transgenic mice that were also Rag1+ developed spontaneous EAE. These results suggest that the MBP-specific CD4+ T cells are sufficient to develop EAE and that there may be other populations of T cells (present in the Rag1+ mice) that provide a protective effect.

Another animal model often used in MS research is the Theilers murine encephalitis virus–induced demyelinating disease model (TMEV). There are similarities with EAE as TMEV resembles MS in terms of pathology and immunology and occurs in EAE-susceptible strains of rodents.[46] The TMEV model differs from EAE in that a virus (picornvirus) rather than a protein mixture is needed to induce TMEV. Nevertheless, it is important to remember that no virus has been consistently identified in MS patients.[47] A recent study[48] identified four markers within a 20 cM region of chromosome 14 in TMEV. These findings may be interpreted to support the possibility that two loci in this region are involved in controlling demyelination.

## Genetic Counseling

As genetic factors are recognized to have important roles in both the overall etiology and the familial aggregation of MS, neurologists, family physicians, and genetic counselors are increasingly being asked about family risks for MS. Although data is available for more distant relatives (e.g., second and third degree) of individuals with MS, genetic counseling information is most accurate and is in fact most often requested for children and siblings of persons with MS.

Lifetime risks for children and siblings, controlling for the amount of genetic sharing, are given in Table 19–7. Depending on the amount of genetic sharing, the relative risk for these individuals compared with the general population can range from 1× (adopted siblings and children who share no genetic material with the MS patient) to 190× (monozygotic co-twins who share 100% of their genetic material with the MS patient).

When counseling biological full siblings of MS patients, one can refine the risks from those given in Table 19–7 provided that information is available on the age of MS onset in the affected family member and whether or not one parent has MS[49] (Table 19–8). Research is underway as part of the CCPGSMS[16] to determine the effects of covariates on risks for other categories of

Table 19–7. **Comparison of Age-Adjusted Lifetime Risks by Percentage of Genetic Sharing With the Individual Having Multiple Sclerosis (MS)**

| Relationship to the Individual With MS | Approximate Risk (%) | Relative Risk to General Population | % Genetic Sharing with the Affected Individual |
|---|---|---|---|
| General Population | 0.2 | 1 | 0 |
| First-degree relative | 3–5 | 15–25 | 50 |
| Dizygotic twin | 3–5 | 15–25 | 50 |
| Monozygotic twin | 38 | 190 | 100 |
| "Adopted" first-degree relative | 0.2 | 1 | 0 |
| Half-siblings | 1.3 | 6.5 | 25 |

**Source:** Sadovnick et al.[12]

relatives such as children of MS patients. At present, genetic counseling for MS must be based on empiric data rather than theoretical models. It is now recognized that the familial aggregation of MS results from the genetic sharing among biological relatives. For more discussion on this topic, see Sadovnick and associates.[49a]

## Predictive Testing

At this time, it is not possible to identify an asymptomatic individual who has a very high likelihood to develop symptomatic MS. Results of MRI scans and cerebrospinal fluid analyses, even for asymptomatic monozygotic co-twins of MS patients, remain ambiguous with respect to "prediction." At present, there is no known cure, long-term effective treatment, or prevention for MS. Subclinical MS is known to occur in individuals who never develop symptoms over a long lifespan.[50] Ongoing research on the ramifications of being able to predict which asymptomatic individuals have a high risk to develop a common, complex disorder, such as MS or Alzheimer's disease, is underway.[51]

## Conclusions

Results from ongoing research, much of which has used the classic genetic epide-

Table 19–8. **Observed Multiple Sclerosis (MS) Lifetime Risks for Siblings of MS Patients, Controlling for Covariates of Age of MS Onset and Parental MS Status**

| | Brothers | | Sisters | |
|---|---|---|---|---|
| Age of MS Onset in Proband (Years) | One Parent With MS Risk (SE) (%) | No parent With MS Risk (SE) (%) | One Parent With MS Risk (SE) (%) | No Parent With MS Risk (SE) (%) |
| <20 | — | 2.71 (2.06) | 50.00 (25.00) | 7.74 (2.79) |
| 21–30 | 12.73 (9.58) | 1.22 (0.50) | 15.29 (10.30) | 3.51 (0.70) |
| 31–40 | — | 1.65 (0.58) | 7.26 ( 4.98) | 2.53 (0.63) |
| >40 | — | 0.53 (0.37) | — | 1.45 (0.59) |

SE = standard error.

*This data does not apply to conjugal MS (both parents affected).

**Source:** Adapted from Sadovnick et al.[49]

miological approach, have led to the following conclusions with respect to the role of genetic factors in the etiology of MS:

1. Genetic and nongenetic factors are involved in the etiology of MS on a population basis.
2. The familial aggregation of MS (excess of MS among biological relatives) appears to be genetic.
3. Maternal factors do not seem to influence the risk for siblings to develop MS.
4. MS appears to be oligogenic (having more than one locus).

Taken together,[14,49,52–56] comparative data on age-corrected rates of MS among relatives of index cases according to the amount of genetic sharing (see Table 19–3) supports an oligogenic or polygenic disease model. To date, the number of loci, mode of inheritance, and mechanism of inheritance remain largely unknown.[12] Despite ongoing research and genome screens,[23–26] no candidate genes have yet been definitively identified.

The data (e.g., from twin and half-sibling studies) presented in this chapter, in addition to showing the importance of genetic factors in the etiology of MS, also implies major environmental factor(s) that operate broadly at the population level conferring different MS risks on susceptible individuals depending on where they live rather than on more family-specific environmental factors. There are relatively few broad factors that would act at the level of the population to differentiate "at-risk" groups. Indeed, climate (or its indirect consequences), diet, or these two factors together seem to be the most attractive possibilities. Our interpretation of the available data, including those on migrants, is that MS susceptibility is determined at an early age. Accordingly, it may well be that the timing of putative environmental factors occurs early (and perhaps *very* early) in the life of a person who develops MS. Research is presently in progress as part of the CCPGSMS[16] that hopefully will allow the dissection of early life experience for MS patients with a view to identifying infrequent events that are either over-represented (i.e., predisposing) or under-represented (i.e., protective) among the MS population compared with a control population.[16]

## INHERITED DEMYELINATING DISEASES OTHER THAN MULTIPLE SCLEROSIS

The discussion in this section focuses on some of the more common and better understood inherited diseases associated with demyelination, namely, Krabbe's disease, metachromatic leukodystrophy, Leber's hereditary optic neuropathy, and X-linked adrenoleukodystrophy.

### Krabbe's Disease (Globoid Cell Leukodystrophy)

Krabbe's disease (globoid cell leukodystrophy [GLD]) is an autosomal recessive lysosomal disorder. Affected individuals rarely survive the second year of life, although atypical (late onset) forms of the disease have been recognized. Early symptoms are often nonspecific and include irritability or hypersensitivity to external stimuli. As the disease progresses, severe psychomotor deterioration is observed. Pathologically, the disease is characterized by multinucleated globoid cells in the white matter (macrophages of mesodermal origin containing undigested galactocerebroside). The defect has been identified as a deficiency of galactocerebroside β-galactosidase (galactocerebrosidase), the lysosomal enzyme that degrades galactocerebroside, a major component of myelin, to galactose and ceramide. It is the accumulation of psychosine (galactosylsphingosine) that becomes highly cytotoxic and is responsible for the destruction of myelin cells and the resultant demyelination.

Clinically, there appear to be four forms of Krabbe's disease based on the age of onset, with the most common being infantile (onset age 3–6 months; average duration less than 1 year). Late infantile (onset age 6–36 months; average duration 1–3 years), juvenile (onset age 3–10 years; average duration 5 years), and adult (onset age 10–35 years; average duration 2–5 years) forms of Krabbe's disease also exist. All four are characterized by a deficiency of galactocerebrosidase,[57,58] although the expression of late onset GLD can be variable.[59,60]

The disease locus for GLD has been

mapped to chromosome 14.[61] Recently, Rafi and coworkers[57] identified a large deletion in the GALC gene beginning within intron 10 together with a polymorphic C–T transition at position 502 that changes the codon arginine to cysteine. The majority (but not all) of individuals identified to date with this deletion plus the C–T transition are of northern European ancestry.[57]

Although prenatal diagnosis is possible for at-risk couples, identification of carriers is not always unequivocal. "Pseudodeficiency," that is, low GALC activity in unaffected individuals, is also recognized.[62]

The *twitcher* mouse[63] is the murine model used for studying GLC. As in humans, GLD in the mouse is inherited as an autosomal recessive disorder. The gene has been mapped to chromosome 12. Study of the *twitcher* mouse has increased our understanding of demyelination and human GLD. For example, it was determined that GLD is caused by the excess galactosylceramide resulting from the enzyme deficiency. Very recently, research on the *twitcher* mouse raised the possibility of retroviral-mediated gene therapy for the treatment of Krabbe's disease.[64] (See Suzuki[65] and Suzuki and Taniike[66] for reviews of the murine model for GLD.)

## Metachromatic Leukodystrophy

Metachromatic leukodystrophy (MLD) is characterized by loss of myelin sheaths, reduction of interfascicular oligodendrocytes, and accumulation of metachromatic granules in the CNS. Although atypical cases of MLD have been described (for discussion, see Scriver and coworkers[1]), common types based on the amount of enzyme activity are *(1)* late infantile MLD, usually beginning during the first or second year of life with no enzyme activity; *(2)* juvenile MLD, usually beginning between the ages of 4 and 12 years; and *(3)* adult onset MLD, with onset typically over the age of 16 years and with some enzyme activity, although this is reduced.

Clinically, infantile MLD shows signs and symptoms that have come to be expected for white matter disease such as spastic diplegia, and most cases show peripheral nerve involvement.[67] Juvenile MLD is usually characterized by mental regression and/or behavioral changes.[67]

The age of clinical onset for adult onset MLD ranges from 16 to 63 years.[67,68] Adult onset MLD usually presents with dementia and/or psychiatric disturbance. Adult onset MLD should be considered in the differential diagnosis of early onset dementia, particularly when a family history of dementia is present among siblings and/or *(1)* the parental mating was either consanguineous or *(2) one or both* of the parents are either older than the age of clinical onset in their children or *(3) one or both* of the parents died after the age of onset in their children. Sadovnick and associates[69] presented two case reports to emphasize this fact. Amaducci and associates[70] have even suggested that the initial case report of Alzheimer's disease[71] may have in fact been adult onset MLD. Table 19–9 compares and contrasts two individuals with Alzheimer's disease and MLD, respectively, seen at a specialized dementia clinic. The MLD patient was initially referred with a diagnosis of Alzheimer's disease.

Although the various forms of MLD show autosomal recessive inheritance (25% risk to siblings of affected individuals; unaffected siblings have a 67% chance of being a carrier; males are affected as often as females; parental consanguinity noted on occasion), each form appears to be a distinct genetic entity. Identified arylsulfatate (ARA) mutations are $ARA^I$ or $ARA^O$ and $ARA^A$ or $ARA^R$. These are extremely rare and are allelic with the relatively more common (7.5% to 15% gene frequency) pseudodeficient allele ($ARA^P$). In the recessive state, $ARA^I$/ARA$^I$ is associated with late infantile MLD (no functional gene product) and $ARA^A$/ARA$^A$ is associated with adult MLD (small amounts of residual enzyme activity). Juvenile MLD is associated with the genotype $ARA^I$/ARA$^A$. The pseudodeficient mutation ($ARA^P$) can occur in the heterozygote state with the wild-type allele ($ARA^+$) or with either of the mutant alleles ($ARA^I$ or $ARA^A$). $ARA^+$, ARA$^I$, ARA$^A$, and $ARA^P$ are allelic and have been mapped to chromosome 22q13.[72] (For a more detailed discussion, see Kolodny and Fluharty.[73])

Pseudo-arylsulphatase A deficiency

Table 19–9. **Comparison of Clinical Features for Familial Alzheimer's Disease (AD) and Adult Onset Metachromatic Leukodystrophy (MLD)**

| Feature | AD | MLD |
|---|---|---|
| Year of birth | 1940 | 1941 |
| Age of onset | 40 years | 40 years |
| Initial diagnosis, psychiatric | Unipolar depression | Schizophrenia |
| Presenting diagnosis | Pseudodementia | AD |
| Final diagnosis | AD | MLD |
| Selected results from neuropsychological assessments | | |
| New learning capacity | Deficits noted | Relatively preserved; on initial tests deterioration with retesting over time |
| Global cognitive decline | Relatively rapid | Relatively unchanged |
| Aggressiveness/hostility | Progressive | Fluctuating |

**Source:** Adapted from Sadovnick et al.[69]

(pseudodeficiency of arylsulphatase A) has been reported in individuals who otherwise have neither clinical nor preclinical MLD. Identified individuals with pseudo-arylsulphatase A deficiency are generally asymptomatic older relatives of MLD patients who have an arylsulphatase A activity of 5% to 15% of normal. These values are well below the range for MLD carriers and within the range for individuals showing classic MLD.[74]

## Leber's Hereditary Optic Neuropathy

Leber's hereditary optic neuropathy (LHON) was named for the German ophthalmologist Theodor Leber. Congenital optic atrophy and retrobulbar neuritis must be considered in the differential diagnosis. The age of onset varies, but most cases are seen in patients between the ages of 18 and 25 years. Clinically, LHON is characterized by poor vision (less than 6/60, large central visual field defects, and poor color vision.[75] In most cases, both eyes are affected simultaneously. If, however, only one eye is initially affected, the second eye is usually affected within 1 year. The visual loss generally has an insidious onset, although this may progress more rapidly, mimicking retrobulbar neuritis. Although individuals have a dense central scotomata, total blindness rarely occurs. At times, the visual function can stabilize or even improve to a certain degree, but recovery is rare.

LHON is characterized by degeneration of the central part of the optic nerve from papillae to the lateral geniculate bodies, with the papillomacular bundles being especially affected. It is assumed that the axis cylinders and myelin degenerate together.

Maternal transmission is well documented in LHON, with at least 11 mitochondrial (mt) DNA gene mutations having been identified. Up to 70% of LHON cases in Europe and over 90% of Japanese cases result from a guanine to alanine (G to A) transition of mtDNA basepair number 11,778 in the *ND4* gene.[76] The second most common cause of LHON is a G to A transition mutation in the *ND1* gene at mtDNA basepair 3,460.[77,78]

Some features of LHON, such as the male preponderance among affected individuals and the high number of mutant mtDNA in unaffected relatives of patients, cannot be entirely explained by mitochondrial inheritance. It has been suggested that an interacting "X-linked visual loss susceptibility locus" may exist.[75] To date, results of various studies have not been definitive.[79]

## X-Linked Adrenoleukodystrophy

X-linked adrenoleukodystrophy (ALD) is a neurodegenerative disorder with a wide range of phenotypes.[80] The two most common forms are the childhood form and the adult form (Table 19–10). Signs and symptoms of childhood ALD include hyperactivity, emotional liability, weakness, ataxia, impaired vision, and seizures. The child progresses into a vegetative state within 2 to 4 years, and this is followed by an early death. The adult form of ALD is characterized by a slowly progressive paraparesis, dementia, and/or psychosis. Rarer forms include adrenal insufficiency without neurologic involvement, psychotic or dementing illness in adults, and localized cerebral defect. Approximately 5% to 10% of individuals in whom the biochemical defect is identified remain asymptomatic well into adulthood. The clinical phenotype can vary among and within families, but the reason for this is not well understood.

ADL is characterized by demyelination in the CNS, adrenal insufficiency, accumulation of very-long-chain fatty acids, and variable phenotypes within families.[81] Intragenic deletions of the ALD gene and several point mutations[82,83] have been identified. It is estimated that perhaps up to 7% of cases represent new mutations.[81] A recent French study of 44 unrelated X-linked ALD families[84] identified mutations in 37 of 44 ALD patients and confirmed that the de novo mutation frequency was approximately 7% and that ALD mutations are widely distributed over the entire coding region. The majority of families have unique gene mutations.

## SUMMARY

Myelin is the lipid-rich insulator that surrounds axons in the CNS, thus increasing axonal impulse conduction. Demyelination

Table 19–10. **Comparison of Childhood and Adult Adrenoleukodystrophy (ADL)**

| | Childhood ADL | Adult ADL |
|---|---|---|
| Frequency | 60% ADL cases | 21% ADL cases |
| Mean age of onset | 7.2 ± 1.7 years | 29 ± 7 years |
| Impaired adrenal function | 85% | 70% |
| Dementia or psychosis | — | 20–30% |
| Mean age of death | 2.8 ± 2 years | |
| Course | Progresses to a vegetative state in 1.9 ± 2 years | Slowly progressive |
| Signs and symptoms | Hyperactivity<br>Emotional lability<br>Impaired vision<br>Impaired auditory discrimination<br>Weakness<br>Ataxia<br>Seizures | Paraparesis<br>Urinary incontinence or retention<br>Impotence<br>Peripheral neuropathy |

**Source:** Adapted from Buyse.[80]

(breakdown of normal functional myelin sheaths) lessens conduction velocity.

This chapter focused on inherited demyelinating diseases of the CNS, the most common being MS. Multiple sclerosis is representative of a wide range of common (with respect to prevalence), complex (with respect to etiology) disorders increasingly being recognized to have genetic components in their etiologies. It is only within the last decade or so that objective, reproducible findings have not only clearly illustrated the importance of genetic factors in MS but have also better described the type of non-genetic factors believed to be involved.

Other very less common inherited demyelinating diseases discussed are Krabbe's disease (globoid cell leukodystrophy), metachromatic leukodystrophy, Leber's hereditary optic neuropathy, and X-linked adrenoleukodystrophy. It is not uncharacteristic for these disorders to show genetic and phenotypic heterogeneity. Families must therefore be carefully characterized before a definitive diagnosis is made.

## REFERENCES


1. Scriver CR, Beaudet AL, Sly WS, Valle D: The Metabolic and Molecular Bases of Inherited Disease. McGraw Hill, New York, 1995.
2. Morell P, Quarles RH, Norton WT: Myelin formation, structure and biochemistry. In Siegel GJ, Agranoff BW, Albers RW, Molinoff PB (eds): Basic Neurochemistry: Molecular, Cellular, and Medical Aspects, ed 5. Raven Press, New York, 1994, pp117–143.
3. Paty DW, Ebers GC (eds): Multiple Sclerosis. F.A. Davis, Philadephia, 1997.
4. Moore GRW: Neuropathology and pathophysiology of the multiple sclerosis lesion. In Paty DW, Ebers GC (eds): Multiple Sclerosis. F.A. Davis, Philadephia, 1997, pp257–328.
5. Kurtzke JF, Beebe GW, Norman JE: Epidemiology of multiple sclerosis in U.S. veterans. 1. Race, sex and geographic distribution. Neurology 29:1228–1235, 1979.
6. Alter M, Hapern L, Kurland LT, et al: Multiple sclerosis in Israel: Prevalence among migrants and native inhabitants. Arch Neurol 7:253–263, 1962.
7. Detels R, Visscher BR, Haile RW, et al: Multiple sclerosis and age at migration. Am J Epidemiol 108: 386–393, 1978.
8. Dean G, Grimaldi G, Kelly R, et al.: Multiple sclerosis in southern Europe. I. Prevalence in Sicily in 1975. J Epidemiol Comm Health 33:107–110, 1979.
9. Vassallo L, Elian M, Dean G: Multiple sclerosis in southern Europe. II. Prevalence in Malta in 1978. J Epidemiol Comm Health 33:111–113, 1979.
10. Bulman DE, Ebers GC: The geography of multiple sclerosis reflects genetic susceptibility. J Trop Geogr Neurol: 2:66–72, 1992.
11. Ebers GC, Sadovnick AD: The geographical distribution of multiple sclerosis. Neuroepidemiology 12:1–5, 1993.
12. Sadovnick AD, Dyment D, Ebers GC: Genetic epidemiology of multiple sclerosis. Epidemiol Rev 19: 99–106, 1997.
13. Sadovnick AD, Ebers GC: Epidemiology of multiple sclerosis: A critical overview. Can J Neurol Sci 20: 17–29, 1993.
14. Ebers GC, Sadovnick AD, Risch NJ, and the Canadian Collaborative Study Group: Familial aggregation in multiple sclerosis is genetic. Nature 377: 150–151, 1995.
15. Sadovnick AD, Ebers GC, Dyment DA, Risch NJ, and the Canadian Collaborative Study Group: Evidence for genetic basis of multiple sclerosis. Lancet 347:1728–1730, 1996.
16. Sadovnick AD, Risch NJ, Ebers GC, and the Canadian Collaborative Study Group: Canadian Collaborative Project on Genetic Susceptibility to MS, phase 2: Rationale and method. Can J Neurol Sci 25:216–221, 1998.
17. Jersild C, Svejgaard A, Fog T: HLA antigens and multiple sclerosis. Lancet 1:1240–1215, 1972.
18. Ebers GC: Immunology. In Paty DW, Ebers GC (eds): Multiple Sclerosis. F.A. Davis, Philadephia, 1997, pp403–426.
19. Olerup O, Hillert J: HLA class II–associated genetic susceptibility in multiple sclerosis: A critical evaluation. Tissue Antigens 38:1–15, 1991.
20. Tienari P, Wikstrom J, Koskimies S, et al.: Reappraisal of HLA in multiple sclerosis: Close linkage in multiplex families. Eur J Hum Genet 1:257–268, 1993.
21. Ebers G, Paty D, Stiller C, et al.: HLA-typing in multiple sclerosis sibling pairs. Lancet 1:88–90, 1982.
22. Kellar-Wood H, Wood N, Holmans P, et al.: Multiple sclerosis and the HLA-D region: Linkage and association studies. J Neuroimmunol 58:183–190, 1994.
23. The Multiple Sclerosis Genetics Group: Complete genomic screen for multiple sclerosis underscores a role for the major histocompatibility complex. Nat Genet 13:469–471, 1996.
24. Kuokkanen S, Sundvall M, Terwilliger JD, et al.: A putative vulnerability locus to multiple sclerosis maps to 5p14–p12 in a region syntetic to the murine locus *Eae2.* Nat Genet 13:477–480, 1996.
25. Ebers GC, Kukay K, Bulman DE, et al.: A full genome search in multiple sclerosis. Nat Genet 13: 472–476, 1996.
26. Sawcer S, Jones HB, Feakes R, et al.: A genome screen in multiple sclerosis reveals susceptibility on chromosome 6p21 and 17q22. Nat Genetics 13: 464–468, 1996.
27. Compston A, Howard S: HLA typing in multiple sclerosis. Lancet 1:661, 1982.
28. Stewart G, McLeod J, Basten A, Bashir H: HLA family studies and multiple sclerosis: A common

gene, dominantly expressed. Hum Immunol 3:13–29, 1981.

29. Goverts A, Gony J, Martin-Mondiere C, et al.: HLA and multiple sclerosis: Population and family studies. Tissue Antigens 25:187–199, 1985.
30. Risch N: Assessing the role of HLA linked and unlinked determinants of disease. Am J Hum Genet 40:1–14, 1987.
31. Olsson T, Sun J, Hillert J, Hojeberg B, Ekre HP: Increased numbers of T cells recognizing multiple myelin basic protein epitopes in multiple sclerosis. Eur J Immunol 22:1083–1087, 1992.
32. Link H, Tibling G: Principles of albumin and IgG analysis in neurological diseases. II. Evaluation of IgG synthesis within CNS of MS patients. Scand J Clin Lab Invest 37:397–401, 1971.
33. Ollson T, Baig S, Hojeberg B, Link H: Antimyelin basic protein and antimyelin antibody-producing cells in multiple sclerosis. Ann Neurol 20:20–25, 1990.
34. Selmaj K, Raine CS, Cannella B, Brosnan CF: Identification of lymphotoxin and tumor necrosis factor in multiple sclerosis lesions. J Clin Invest 87:949–954, 1991.
35. Sharief MK, Hentges R: Association between tumor necrosis factor-alpha and disease progression in patients with multiple sclerosis. N Engl J Med 326: 272–273, 1992.
36. Sharief MK, Thompson EJ: *In vivo* relationship of tumor necrosis factor alpha to blood–brain barrier damage in patients with active multiple sclerosis. J Neuroimmunol 38:27–33, 1992.
37. Fugger L, Morling N, Sandberg-Wolheim M, Ryder LP, Svejaard A: Tumor necrosis factor alpha gene polymorphism in multiple sclerosis and optic neuritis. J Neuroimmunol 27:85–88, 1990.
38. Weinshenker BG, Liu Q, Schaid DJ, Summer S: Polymorphism of the promotor region of the tumor necrosis factor alpha gene and the outcome of multiple sclerosis. J Neuroimmunol s1:77, 1995.
39. Bell JI, Lathrop GM: Multiple loci for multiple sclerosis. Nat Genet 13:377–378, 1996.
40. Kastrukoff LF, Rice GPA: Virology. In Paty DW, Ebers GC (eds): Multiple Sclerosis. F.A. Davis, Philadephia, 1997, pp370–402.
41. Jansson L, Olsson T, Hojeberg B, Holmdahl R: Chronic experimental autoimmune encephalomyelitis induced by the 89–101 myelin basic protein peptide in B10R111 (H-2r) mice. Eur J Immunol 21: 693–699, 1991.
42. Owens T, Sriram S: The immunology of multiple sclerosis and its animal model experimental allergic encephalomyelitis. Neurol Clin 13:51–73, 1995.
43. Sundvall M, Jirholt J, Yang H, Jansson L, Engstrom A, Pettersson U, Holmdahl R: Identification of murine loci associated with susceptibility to chronic experimental allergic encephalomyelitis. Nat Genet 10:313–317, 1995.
44. Goverman J, Woods A, Larson L, Weiner L, Hood L, Zaller D: Transgenic mice that express a myelin basic protein–specific T cell receptor develp spontaneous autoimmunity. Cell 72:551–560, 1993.
45. Lafaille J, Nagashima K, Katsuki M, Tongegawa S: High incidence of spontaneous autoimmune encephalomyelitis in immunodeficient anti-myelin basic protein T cell receptor transgenic mice. Cell 78:399–408, 1994.
46. Tienari PJ, Tertwilliger JD, Ott J, Palo J, Peltonen L: Two-locus linkage analysis in multiple sclerosis (MS). Genomics 19:320–325, 1994.
47. Souberbielle B, Szawlowski P, Russell W: Is there a case for a virus aetiology in mutliple sclerosis? Scot Med J 40:55–62, 1995.
48. Bureau J-F, Drescher KM, Pease LR, et al.: Chromsosome 14 contains determinants that regulate susceptibility to Theiler's virus-induced demyelination in the mouse. Genetics 1998 148:1941–1949.
49. Sadovnick AD, Yee IML, Ebers GC, Risch NJ: The effect of age onset and parental disease status on sib risks for multiple sclerosis. Neurology 50:719–723, 1998.
49a. Sadovnick AD, Dircks A, Ebers GC: Genetic counselling in multiple sclerosis: Risks to Sibs and children of affected individuals. Clinical Genetics, in press, 1999.
50. Gilbert JJ, Sadler M: Unsuspected multiple sclerosis. Arch Neurol 40:533–536, 1983.
51. Post SG, Whitehouse PJ, Binstock RH, et al.: Consensus statement: The clinical introduction of genetic testing for Alzheimer disease. *JAMA* 277:832–840, 1997.
52. Sadovnick AD, Baird PA, Ward RH: Multiple sclerosis: Updated risks for relatives. Am J Med Genet 29:533–541, 1988.
53. Carton H, Vlietinck R, Debruyne J, de Keyser JD, D'Hooghe M-B, Loos R, Medaer R, Truyen L, Yee IML, Sadovnick AD: Risks of multiple sclerosis in relatives of patients in Flanders, Belgium. J Neurol Neurosurg Psychiatry 62:329–333, 1997.
54. Robertson NM, Fraser M, Deans J, Clayton D, Walker N, Comptston DAS: Age-adjusted recurrence risks for relatives of patients with multiple sclerosis. Brain 119:449–455, 1996.
55. Sadovnick AD, Armstrong H, Rice GPA, et al.: A population-based study of multiple sclerosis in twins: Update. Ann Neurol 33:281–285, 1993.
56. Mumford CJ, Wood NW, Kellar-Wood H, Thorpe JW, Miller DH, Compston DAS: The British Isles survey of multiple sclerosis in twins. Neurology 44: 11–15, 1994.
57. Rafi MA, Luzi P, Chen YQ, Wenger DA: A large deletion together with a point mutation in the GALC gene is a common mutant allele in patients with infantile Krabbe disease. Hum Mol Genet 4: 1285–1289, 1995.
58. Suzuki K, Suzuki Y, Suzuki K: Galactosylceramide lipidosis: Globoid-cell leukodystrophy (Krabbe disease). In Scriver CR, Beaudet AL, Sly WS, Valle D (eds): The Metabolic and Molecular Bases of Inherited Disease. McGraw-Hill, New York, 1995, pp2671–2692.
59. Arvidsson J, Hagberg B, Mansson J-E, Svennerholm L: Late onset globoid cell leukodystrophy (Krabbe's disease): Swedish case with 15 years of follow-up. Acta Paediatr 84:218–221, 1995.
60. Lyon G, Hagberg B, Evrard PH, Allaire C, Pavone L, Vanier M: Symptomatology of late onset Krabbe's leukodystrophy: The European experience. Dev Neurosci 13:240–244, 1991.
61. Zlotogora J, Chakraborty S, Knowlton RG, Wenger DA: Krabbe disease locus mapped to chromosome

14 by genetic linkage. Am J Hum Genet 47:37–44, 1990.
62. Wenger DA, Riccardi VM: Possible misdiagnosis of Krabbe disease. J Pediatr 88:76–79, 1976.
63. Duchen LW, Eicher EM, Jacobs JM, Scaravilli F, Teixeira F: Hereditary leucodystrophy in the mouse. The new mutant twitcher. Brain 103:695–710, 1980.
64. Sosa MAG, De Gasperi R, Undevia S, et al.: Correction of the galactocerebrosidase deficiency in globoid cell leukodystrophy–cultured cells by SL3-3 retroviral-mediated gene transfer. Biochem Biophys Res Commun 218:766–771, 1996.
65. Suzuki K: A genetic demyelinating disease globoid cell leukodystrophy: Studies with animal models. J Neuropathol Exp Neurol 53:359–363, 1994.
66. Suzuki K, Taniike M: Murine model of genetic demyelinating disease: The twitcher mouse. Microsc Res Tech 32:204–214, 1995.
67. Aicardi J: The inherited leukodystrophies: A clinical overview. J Inherit Metab Dis 16:733–743, 1993.
68. Baumann N, Masson M, Carreau V, Lefevre M, Herschkowitz N, Turpin JC: Adult forms of metachromatic leukodystrophy: Clinical and biochemical approach. Dev Neurosci 13:211–215, 1991.
69. Sadovnick AD, Tuokko H, Applegarth DA, Toone JR, Hadjistavropoulos T, Beattie BL: The differential diagnosis of adult onset metachromatic leukodystrophy and early onset familial Alzheimer's disease in an Alzheimer's clinic population. Neurol Sci 20:312–318, 1993.
70. Amaducci L, Sorbi S, Piacentini S, Bick KL: The first Alzheimer disease case: A metachromatic leukodystrophy? Dev Neurosci 13:186–187, 1991.
71. Alzheimer A: Uber eine eigenartige Erkkrankung der Hirnrinde. Allgemeine Z Psychiatrie Psychish-Gerlichtliche Med 64:146–148, 1907.
72. Phelan MC, Thomas GR, Saul RA, et al: Cytogenetic, biochemical and molecular analyses of a 22q13 deletion. Am J Med Genet 43:872–876, 1992.
73. Kolodny EH, Fluharty AL: Metachromatic leukodystrophy and multiple sulphatase deficiency: Sulfatide lipidosis. In Scriver CR, Beaudet AL, Sly WS, Valle D (eds): The Metabolic and Molecular Bases of Inherited Disease. McGraw-Hill, New York, 1995, pp2693–2739.
74. Kappler J, Leinekugel P, Conzelmann E, et al.: Genotype–phenotype relationship in various degrees of aryl sulfatase A deficiency. Hum Genet 86: 463–470, 1991.
75. Harding AE, Sweeney MG, Govan GG, Riordan-Eva P: Pedigree analysis in Leber hereditary optic neuropathy families with a pathogenic mitochondrial DNA mutation. Am J Hum Genet 57:77–86, 1995.
76. Wallace DC, Singh G, Lott MT, et al.: Mitochondrial DNA mutation associated with Leber's hereditary optic neuropathy. Science 242:1427–1430, 1988.
77. Howell N, Bindoff LA, McCullough DA, et al.: Leber hereditary optic neuropathy: Identification of the same mitochondrial ND1 mutation in six pedigrees. Am J Hum Genet 49:939–950, 1991.
78. Huoponen K, Vilkki J, Aula P, Nikoskelainen EK, Savontaus ML: A new mtDNA mutation associated with Leber hereditary optic neuropathy. Am J Hum Genet 48:1147–1153, 1991.
79. Chalmers RM, Davis MB, Sweeney MG, Wood NW, Harding AE: Evidence against an X-linked visual loss susceptibility locus in Leber hereditary optic neuropathy. Am J Hum Genet 59:103–108, 1996.
80. Buyse ML (ed): Adrenoleukodystrophy, X-linked. In Birth Defects Encyclopedia. Blackwell Scientific, Cambridge, MA, 1990, pp61–62.
81. Moser HW, Smith KD, Moser AB: X-linked adrenoleukodystrophy. In Scriver CR, Beaudet AL, Sly WS, Valle D (eds): The Metabolic and Molecular Bases of Inherited Disease. McGraw-Hill, New York, pp2325–2349, 1995.
82. Cartier N, Sarde C-O, Douar A-M, Mosser J, Mandel J-L, Aubourg P: Abnormal messenger RNA expression and a missense mutation in patients with X-linked adrenoleukodystrophy. Hum Mol Genet 2:1949–1951, 1993.
83. Yasutake T, Yamada T, Furuya H, Shinnon N, Goto I, Kobayashi T: Molecular analysis of X-linked adrenoleukodystrophy patients. J Neurol Sci 131:58–64, 1995.
84. Feigenbaum V, Lombard-Platet G, Guidoux S, Sarde C-O, Mandel J-L, Aubourg P: Mutational and protein analysis of patients and heterozygous women with X-linked adrenoleukodystrophy. Am J Hum Genet 58:1135–1144, 1996.
85. Robertson NP, O'Riordan JI, Chataway J, Kingsley DPE, Miller DH, Clayton D, Compston DAS: Offspring recurrence rates and clinical characteristics of conjugal multiple sclerosis. Lancet 349:1587–1590, 1997.
86. Hader WJ, Feasby TE, Noseworthy JH, Rice GPA, Ebers GC: Multiple sclerosis in Canadian Native people. Neurology 35: (suppl 1):300, 1985.
87. Detels R, Visscher BR, Malmgren RM, Coulson AH, Lucia MV, Dudley JP: Evidence for lower susceptibility to multiple sclerosis in Japanese Americans. Am J Epidemiol 105:303–310, 1977.
88. Gronning M, Mellgren SI: Multiple sclerosis in the two northernmost counties of Norway. Acta Neurol Scand 72:321–327, 1985.
89. Gaudet JPC, Hashimoto L, Sadovnick AD, Ebers GC: A study of birth order and multiple sclerosis in multiplex families. Neuroepidemiology 14:188–192, 1995.
90. Gaudet JPC, Hashimoto L, Sadovnick AD, Ebers GC: Is multiple sclerosis caused by late childhood infection: A case–control study of birth order in sporadic cases of multiple sclerosis. Acta Neurol Scand 91:19–21, 1995.
91. Bulman DE, Sadovnick AD, Cripps J, Ebers GC: Age of onset in siblings concordant for multiple sclerosis. Brain 114:937–950, 1991.
92. Oksenberg JR, Sherritt M, Begovich AB, Erlich HA, Bernard CC, Cavalli-Sforza LL, Steinman L: T-cell receptor V alpha and C alpha alleles associated with multiple sclerosis and myasthenia gravis. Proc Natl Acad Sci USA 86:988–992, 1989.
93. Hillert J, Chummao L, Olerup O: T cell receptor alpha chain germline gene polymorphisms in multiple sclerosis. Neurology 42:80–84, 1992.
94. Hashimoto LL, Mak TW, Ebers GC: T-cell alpha chain polymorphisms in multiple sclerosis. J Neuroimmunol 40:41–48, 1992.
95. Lynch SG, Rose JW, Petajan JH, Stauffer D, Kamerath C, Leppert M: Discordance of T-cell recep-

tor alpha-chain gene in familial multiple sclerosis. Neurology 42:839–844, 1992.
96. Beall SS, Concannon P, Charmley P, McFarland HF, Gatti RA, Hood LE, McFarlin DE, Biddison WE: The germline repertoire of T cell receptor beta chain genes in patients with chronic progressive multiple sclerosis. J Immunol 21:59–66, 1989.
97. Charmley P, Beall SS, Concannon P, Hood L, Gatti RA: Further localization of a multiple sclerosis susceptibility gene on chromosome 7q using a new T cell receptor beta chain polymorphism. J Neuroimmunol 32:231–240, 1991.
98. Fugger LM, Sandberg-Wollheim M, Morling N, Ryder LP, Svejgaard A: The germline repertoire of T-cell receptor beta chain genes in patients with relapsing/remitting multiple sclerosis or optic neuritis. Immunogenetics 31:278–280, 1990.
99. Hillert J, Leng C, Olerup O: No association with germ line T cell receptor B-chain gene alleles or haplotypes in Swedish patients with multiple sclerosis. J Neuroimmunol 31:141–147, 1991.
100. Martinez-Naves E, Victoria-Gutierrez M, Uria DF, Lopez-Larrea C: The germline repertoire of T cell B chain genes in multiple sclerosis patients from Spain. Neuroimmunology 47:9–14, 1993.
101. Beall S, Biddison W, McFarlin D, McFarland H, Hood L: Susceptibility for multiple sclerosis is determined, in part, by inheritance of a 175 Kb region of the TCR Vb chain locus and the HLA class II genes. J Neuroimmunol 45: 53–60, 1993.
102. Wei S, Charmley P, Birchfield R, Concannon P: Human T cell receptor Vb gene polymorphism and multiple sclerosis. Am J Hum Genet 56: 963–969, 1995.
103. Lynch SG, Rose JW, Petajan JH, Stauffer D, Kamerath C, Leppert M: Discordance of T-cell receptor beta-chain gene in familial multiple sclerosis. Ann Neurol 30:402–410, 1991.
104. Seboun E, Robinson MA, Doolittle TH, Ciulla TA, Kindt TJ, Hauser SL: A susceptibility locus for multiple sclerosis is linked to the T cell receptor beta chain complex. Cell 57:1095–1100, 1989.
105. Boylan KB, Takahashi N, Paty DW, Sadovnick AD, Diamond M, Hood LE, Prusiner SB: DNA length polymorphism 5' to the myelin basic protein gene is associated with multiple sclerosis. Ann Neurol 27:291–297, 1990.
106. Tienari PJ, Wikstrom J, Sajantila A, Palo J, Peltonen L: Genetic susceptibility to multiple sclerosis is linked to the myelin basic protein gene. Lancet 2:987–991, 1992.
107. Graham CA, Kirk CW, Nevin NC, Droogan AG, Hawkins SA, McMillan SA, McNeill TA: Lack of association between myelin basic protein gene microsatellite and multiple sclerosis. Lancet 2:1596, 1993.
108. Wood NW, Homans P, Roberston N, Compston DAS: No linkage or association between multiple sclerosis and the myelin basic protein gene in affected sib pairs. J Neurol Neurosurg Psychiatry 57: 1191–1199, 1994.
109. Eoli M, Pandolfo M, Milanese C, Gasparini P, Salmaggi A, Zeviani M: The myelin basic protein gene is not a major susceptibility locus for multiple sclerosis in Italian patients. J Neurol 241:615–619, 1994.
110. Rose J, Gerken S, Lynch S, Pisani P, Varvil T, Otterud B, Leppert M: Genetic susceptibility in familial multiple sclerosis not linked to the myelin basic protein gene. Lancet 2:1179–1181, 1993.
111. Propert DW, Bernard CCA, Simons MJ: Gm allotypes and multiple sclerosis. J Immunogenet 9: 359–361, 1982.
112. Sandberg-Wollheim M, Baird LG, Schanfield M, Knoppers M, Youker K, Tachovsky T: Association of CSF IgG concentration and immunoglobulin allotype in multiple sclerosis and optic neuritis. Clin Immunol Immunopathol 31:212–221, 1984.
113. Sesboue R, Davea M, Degos JD, Martin-Mondiere C, Goust JM, Schuller E, Rivat-Peran L, Coquerel A, Dujardin M, Salier JP: IgG (Gm) allotypes and multiple sclerosis in a French population: Phenotype distribution and quantitative abnormalities in CSF with respect to sex, disease severity and presence of intrathecal antibodies. Clin Immunol Immunopathol 37:143–153, 1985.
114. Salier JP, Sesboue R, Martin-Mondiere C, Daveau M, Cesaro, P. Cavalier B, Coquerel A, Legrand L, Goust JM, Degos JD: Combined susceptibility of Gm and HLA phenotypes upon MS susceptibility and severity. J Clin Invest 78:533–538, 1986.
115. Francis DA, Brazier DM, Batchelor JR, McDonald WI, Downie AW, Hern JEC: Gm allotypes in multiple sclerosis influence susceptibility in HLA-DQw1–positive patients from the North-East of Scotland. Immunol Immunopathol 41:409–416, 1986.
116. Gaisner CN, Johnson MJ, DeLange G, Rassenti L, Cavalli-Sforza LL, Steinman L: Susceptibility to multiple sclerosis associated with immunoglobulin gamma 3 restriction fragment length polymorphism. Clin Invest 79:309–313, 1987.
117. Walter MW, Gibson WT, Ebers GC, Cox DW: Susceptibility to multiple sclerosis is associated with the proximal immunoglobulin heavy chain variable region. J Clin Invest 87:1266–1273, 1991.
118. Hillert J: Immunoglobulin gamma constant gene region polymorphisms in multiple sclerosis. J Neuroimmunol 43:9–14, 1993.
119. Yu JS, Pandey JP, Massacesi L, Lincoln R, Usuku K, Seboun E, Hauser S: Segregation of immunoglobulin heavy chain constant region genes in MS sibling pairs. J Neuroimmunol 42:113–116, 1993.

Chapter 20

# THE GENETICS OF MIGRAINE

Robert W. Baloh, M. D.



Despite the long-standing clinical impression that migraine is inherited, some skeptics still question the role of genetic factors in the cause of migraine. A recent letter to the editor of the *British Medical Journal*[1] entitled "Migraine runs in families . . . but is it inherited?" illustrates this controversy. In a response to an article showing increased family aggregation with migraine,[2] W. E. Waters concluded that the jury is still out on the importance of hereditary and environmental factors in the production of migraine.

## OVERVIEW

With a prevalence as high as 15% to 20% in the general population,[3] migraine could affect multiple members of the same family without necessarily being inherited. Furthermore, common environmental factors could lead to increased family aggregation. The final confirmation requires identification of the gene(s).

Before the specific evidence that migraine is inherited is reviewed, it is useful to consider whether migraine is a disease or a variety of diseases, some of which are inherited, some of which are not. The situation is analogous to asking whether epilepsy is inherited. Some seizure syndromes are inherited and genetic factors are important for most types of epilepsy, but anyone can have a seizure with adequate provocation. Similarly, several inherited syndromes are associated with migraine headaches, and genetic factors are important in determining the threshold for a migraine headache, but structural lesions such as vascular malformations and vasculopathies can probably trigger migraine headaches in anyone.

As is discussed later, hemiplegic migraine is clearly inherited in an autosomal dominant fashion, and locus heterogeneity has already been established for this syndrome. There is also good evidence that migraine with visual aura is inherited as an autosomal dominant trait with decreased penetrance. These syndromes are defined based on the presence of either hemiplegic episodes or episodes of visual aura that accompany migraine headaches. Within such families, however, other members may have only migraine headaches, indicating that there is also phenotypic heterogeneity with migraine. Discussions as to whether migraine with aura (MA) is a different disease than migraine without aura (MO) may miss the point. Probably both syndromes can be caused by the same gene and both can be

Table 20–1. **Inherited Neurologic Syndromes Associated with Migraine Headaches***

| Syndrome | Abnormal Gene | Chromosome Locus |
|---|---|---|
| Hemiplegic migraine | *CACNA1A* | 19p |
| Familial episodic ataxia | *CACNA1A* | 19p |
| Cerebral autosomal dominant arteriopathy with subcortical infarcts and leukoencephalopathy (CADASIL) | *Notch3* | 19p |
| Familial migraine, episodic vertigo, and essential tremor | Unknown | Unknown (not 19p) |
| Mitochondrial encephalopathy, lactic acidosis, and strokes (MELAS) | *tRNA* | Mitochondrial DNA |

*See text for references and discussion.

caused by different genes. Not surprisingly, because headache is the least specific symptom of the different migraine syndromes, the genetic basis for MO has been most difficult to obtain. Table 20–1 lists some inherited neurologic syndromes that are associated with migraine headaches.

## FAMILY AGGREGATION

Numerous studies over the years have documented familial aggregation of migraine, and some neurologists have suggested that a positive family history should be part of the diagnostic criteria.[4] Most studies have not separated patients with MA from those with MO, which may confuse interpretation. In nearly all studies, the incidence of a positive family history in patients with migraine headaches was significantly greater than that in controls. The incidence of a positive family history varied from approximately 40% to 90% compared with approximately 5% to 20% in controls.[4–9] The percentage of positive family histories tended to be greater in those studies in which family members were individually interviewed than in studies that relied on questionnaires or on the recall of the proband.

In probably the most complete study of familial aggregation of migraine, Russell and Olesen[9] identified a sample of 3000 men and 1000 women aged 40 years from the Danish Central Person Registry. From this population, they identified 137 probands with MA and they selected an equivalent number of probands with MO for comparison. Probands who had never had migraine were selected as a random sample of controls. The proband supplied information about his or her spouse and first-degree relatives; these individuals were interviewed by telephone. The interviewers were blinded regarding the relatives' status. The operational diagnostic criteria of the International Headache Society (IHS)[10] were used. Compared with the general population, the first-degree relatives of probands with MO had 1.9 times the risk of MO and 1.4 times the risk of MA. The first-degree relatives of probands with MA had nearly 4 times the risk of MA and no increased risk of MO. The first-degree relatives of probands who had never had migraine had no increased risk of migraine either with or without aura. They concluded that MO was caused by a combination of genetic and environmental factors, whereas MA is determined largely by genetic factors.

## TWIN STUDIES

Studies of monozygotic and dizygotic twins with migraine suffer from the same limitations as the studies of familial aggregation.[9] Most were completed before the introduction of the standard IHS criteria for the diagnosis of migraine, and most used questionnaires rather than direct interviews to determine the presence or absence of migraine. For example, Harvald and Hauge[11] found that 12 of 24 monozygotic twins were concordant for migraine, whereas only 6 of 60 dizygotic twins were concordant for migraine. The diagnosis of migraine was based on a questionnaire that simply asked whether the twins had migraine. The authors selected all twins born in Denmark during the years 1870 to 1910 and each set of twins was traced to their place of residence or to their deaths. When a pair of twins had been traced, a questionnaire was sent to each of the twins or, in the case of death, to the nearest living relative.

More recently, Ulrich and colleagues[12] used the population based new Danish Twin Register to identify 2,026 monozygotic twins and 3,334 same-sex dizygotic twins born from 1953 to 1960 to study the genetic influences on the cause of MA. They used a validated questionnaire to initially screen for migraine, obtaining an 87% response rate in both the monozygotic and dizygotic twins. All twin pairs with at least one twin with possible MA were then interviewed by an experienced physician using IHS criteria. Of the 211 twin pairs identified with MA, 77 were monozygotic pairs (33 male and 44 female pairs) and 134 were dizygotic pairs (58 male and 76 female pairs). The concordance rate for MA was 26 of 77 for the monozygotic pairs (34%) and 16 of 134 for the dizygotic pairs (12%) ($p$ = 0.003). These findings emphasize the importance of genetic factors in MA, but also suggest that environmental factors are important since the concordance rate was less than 100% in the monozygotic pairs.

Possibly the most convincing evidence for a genetic cause for MA comes from the report of two monozygotic twin pairs reared apart so that they had no contact with their biological parents or siblings during childhood.[13] The biological mothers and several siblings had migraine. Each pair of twins developed MA at approximately the same age (10 and 12 years, and 15 and 16 years, respectively).

## PREVALENCES IN DIFFERENT RACIAL GROUPS

The prevalence of migraine in African and Asian populations is lower than in European and North American populations.[14–17] These differences among racial groups are probably due to genetic rather than to cultural or environmental factors because they persist in the United States.[18] Stewart and coworkers[18] randomly selected and interviewed (by telephone) 12,328 individuals 18 to 65 years of age living in Baltimore County, Maryland. The IHS criteria were used for the diagnosis of migraine. Migraine prevalence was significantly higher in Caucasians than in African or Asian Americans (Table 20–2). African Americans

Table 20–2. **Migraine Prevalence by Gender and Race in Baltimore County, Maryland**

| | **Women** | | | **Men** | | |
|---|---|---|---|---|---|---|
| | **Number*** | **Crude Prevalence** | **Adjusted Prevalence†** | **Number** | **Crude Prevalence** | **Adjusted Prevalence** |
| Caucasian | 1069 | 20.4 | 1.00 | 318 | 8.6 | 1.00 |
| African American | 285 | 16.2 | 0.73§ | 66 | 7.2 | 0.76‡ |
| Asian American | 7 | 9.2 | 0.49‡ | 3 | 4.8 | 0.60 |
| Other | 18 | 19.6 | 0.88 | 9 | 11.4 | 1.39 |

*Number of subjects who met IHS criteria for migraine.
†Prevalence ratio adjusted for age, race, and education.
‡$p$ value $<$ 0.05 difference compared with Caucasians.
§$p$ value $<$ 0.01 difference compared with Caucasians.
**Source:** Stewart et al.[18]

reported a higher level of headache pain but were less likely to report nausea and vomiting with their attacks than were Caucasians. The African Americans were less disabled by their attacks than Caucasians were. Asian Americans and Caucasians did not have significant differences in associated features.

## MODE OF INHERITANCE

Although genetic factors have generally been accepted in the pathogenesis of migraine, the mode of inheritance remains controversial. As noted earlier, numerous families with familial hemiplegic migraine with an autosomal dominant pattern of inheritance have been reported.[19–23] In addition, families with cluster headache,[24] migraine headaches and episodic vertigo,[25] and migraine headaches with periodic ataxia[26] have also been reported to show an autosomal dominant pattern of inheritance.

The issue is less clear with the more common syndromes of MA and MO. An autosomal dominant pattern with reduced penetrance has been suggested for both of these disorders, but the penetrance of the gene would have to be very low in most studies to support an autosomal dominant inheritance. For example, in a recent study of migraine patients from two Mexican populations,[8] one urban and one rural, among 381 siblings of index cases only 31 were found to be affected. As with most of these studies, a questionnaire was used to determine the affected status, so that underreporting was probable. Another problem with a simple autosomal dominant inheritance is the female to male preponderance with migraine of 2–3 to 1.[3] Hormonal changes in women are well known triggers for migraine symptoms, however, and hormonal factors could account for increased penetrance in women.

### Segregation Analysis

Classic segregation analysis has been performed in three recent studies. Devoto and associates[27] performed segregation analysis in 128 families with migraine (they did not distinguish between MA and MO). Their results were not compatible with either an autosomal dominant or an autosomal recessive inheritance, but rather suggested a polygenic inheritance. Mochi and coworkers[28] concluded that an autosomal recessive model best fit their data for both MA and MO. Russell and coworkers[29] performed complex segregation analysis on the families of 126 probands with MO and 127 probands with MA and concluded that both of these disorders have multifactorial inheritance. There was a significantly better fit to a multifactorial model than to a sporadic model.

It should be noted that classic segregation analysis cannot detect whether one phenotype is caused by different genotypes and does not analyze for reduced penetrance. Clearly this type of analysis does not exclude the possibility that some families have a simple mendelian pattern of inheritance while others do not. Because migraine is almost certainly not a single disease, by grouping families together one could easily miss individual families with a clear autosomal dominant pattern of inheritance.

### Are Migraine with Aura and Migraine without Aura Different Genetic Diseases?

As noted earlier, there is still debate about whether MA and MO are distinct syndromes, different manifestations of the same disorder, or part of a continuum. Patients have both types of attacks (with or without aura), and not infrequently both types of migraine run in the same family. Furthermore, the headache pain phases of both types of migraine are almost identical, and the same treatments are usually effective for both types of migraine. On the other hand, certain epidemiological characteristics, overall familial aggregation, and varying pathophysiological findings suggest that these two types of migraine are separate entities.[30]

One way to address the issue of genetic heterogeneity with migraine is to study a single, large, well-documented family for the mode of inheritance. The advantages and difficulties of such a study are illustrated by the family pedigree shown in Figure 20–1.[25] The goal of documenting such families is to perform linkage analysis to ultimately identify the mutated gene. The pattern of inheritance in this family with migraine, episodic vertigo, and essential tremor is consistent with an autosomal dominant trait. All affected members had the onset of symptoms before age 25 years. Of the 15 subjects who met the IHS criteria for migraine headaches, 6 also had classic visual aura, 8 had recurrent episodes of vertigo, and 9 had essential tremor. The vertigo spells in affected members lasted seconds to hours and nearly always occurred separately from the visual aura or headaches. Essential tremor typically began in adolescence or early adulthood. All symptoms, including headache, visual aura, vertigo, and essential tremor, responded to treatment with acetazolamide.

Within this pedigree, some members with MA gave rise to offspring with MO (Example, II-4 and III-10) and some members with MO had offspring with MA (Example, I-2 and II-8). At least within this family, it seems that the same gene can result in migraine either with or without aura. It is unlikely that the association between migraine and essential tremor in this family was a chance occurrence because only members with migraine had essential tremor, and both types of symptoms responded to acetazolamide. It is unclear how the same gene could result in such varied symptoms as migraine headaches, episodic vertigo, and essential tremor, although a basic neuronal defect such as an ion channel disorder could be the explanation (see later).

## INHERITED SYNDROMES WITH MIGRAINE HEADACHES

### Familial Hemiplegic Migraine

#### PHENOTYPE

Familial hemiplegic migraine (FHM) is an autosomal dominant disease characterized by headache attacks preceded by, or accompanied by, episodes of hemiplegia, sometime lasting days.[10] Unlike those of MO and MA, the prevalence rate for FHM is the same in men and women. Within reported families with FHM, some affected members have interictal nystagmus, ataxia, and essential tremor.[19–22] Episodes of hemiplegia and MA may alternate within individuals and co-occur within families. Based on this observation, Russell and Olesen[9] concluded that the pathophysiologies and etiology of FHM and uncomplicated migraine are probably the same.

Haan and associates[31] questioned whether FHM was a hereditary form of basilar migraine. They studied aura symptoms in 83 patients from 6 unrelated families with FHM and found that 55 of the patients

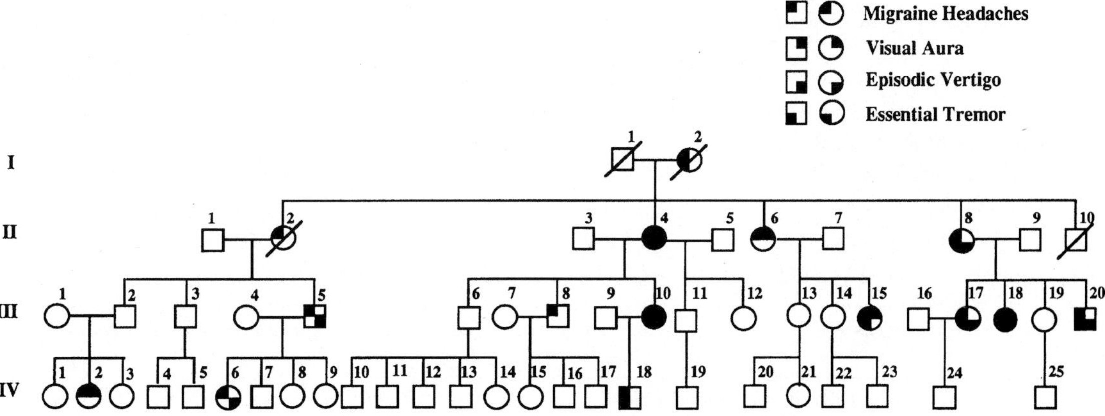


**Figure 20–1.** Pedigree of a family with migraine headaches, episodic vertigo, and essential tremor.[20] See text for details.

reported symptoms that met the IHS criteria for basilar migraine.[10] Consistent with this interpretation, angiography performed during an FHM attack in a single patient showed spasm of the basilar artery.

### GENOTYPE

The genetic defect in four families with hemiplegic migraine (two of which also had cerebellar ataxia) was linked to markers on chromosome 19p.[22] The genetic abnormality in 4 other families with hemiplegic migraine, however, was not linked to 19p; that is, there is genetic heterogeneity with FHM.[23] Terwindt and coworkers[32] compared clinical characteristics in three families with FHM linked to chromosome 19p with those of two families not linked to 19p and found only minor differences (Table 20–3). Patients from linked families had more frequent episodes of unconsciousness, and attacks were more often triggered by mild head trauma. This suggested a genetically determined lower threshold for external triggering of migraine attacks in the variety linked to 19p. Recently, FHM families linked to 19p were found to have different missense mutations in conserved functional domains of the gene coding for an $\alpha_1$-subunit *(CACNA1A)* of a voltage-gated calcium channel (Figure 20–2).[33,34] A second FHM locus has been found on chromosome 1q and other families with FHM are not linked to 19p or 1q.[35,36]

## Familial Episodic Ataxia

### PHENOTYPE

Familial episodic ataxia (EA) is a dominantly inherited neurologic disorder characterized by bouts of ataxia, usually with mild interictal neurologic findings. At least two distinct forms have been identified: families with brief episodes of ataxia (seconds to minutes) and interictal myokymia (EA-1) and families with longer episodes of ataxia (hours to days) and interictal nystagmus (EA-2).[37] Both syndromes typically respond to treatment with acetazolamide. EA-2 has been associated with migraine headaches (MO occurs in about 50% of patients),[38] and there is overlap in the clinical features of EA-2 and FHM.[38,39] Both EA-2 and FHM are associated with typical symptoms of basilar migraine, and both can have interictal nystagmus and progressive cerebellar ataxia.

Table 20–3. **Comparison of Clinical Characteristics in Familial Hemiplegic Migraine Linked and Not Linked to Chromosome 19**

| | Linked Families | Nonlinked Families |
|---|---|---|
| No. of patients (M, male; F, female) | 46 (16M/30F) | 20 (10M/10F) |
| Age at onset (years) | Mean 9.3 (range 2–30) | Mean 11.7 (range 4–19) |
| Frequency attacks (per year) | Mean 8.7 (range <1–48) | Mean 8.1 (range <1–52) |
| Duration of total attack | Hours to days (weeks) | Hours to days |
| Duration of paresis | Minutes to hours (weeks) | Minutes to hours |
| Basilar migraine symptoms* | Present | Present |
| No. with unconsciousness | 18 (39%) | 3 (15%)† |
| No. with attacks after minor head trauma | 32 (70%) | 8 (40%)† |
| Associated features | Cerebellar ataxia (one family) | Infantile convulsions (one family) |

*Bilateral paresis or paresthesia, bilateral visual symptoms, dysarthria, vertigo, tinnitus, loss of balance when walking, drop attacks, crossed or switching symptoms.

†Significant difference ($p < 0.05$) between linked families and nonlinked families.

**Source:** Terwindt et al.[32]

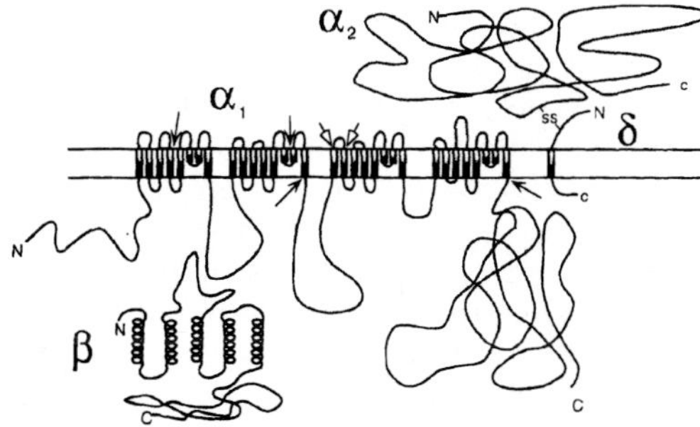


**Figure 20–2.** Subunits of a typical brain voltage-gated calcium channel (Adapted from Perez-Reyes and Schneider,[73] with permission). The location of mutations in the $\alpha_1$-subunit that cause familial hemiplegic migraine (FHM) and episodic ataxia type-2 (EA-2) are marked.[33] Closed arrows indicate FHM; open arrows indicate EA-2.

### GENOTYPE

Episodic ataxia type 1 is due to mutations in a $K^+$ channel *(KCNA1)* gene on chromosome 12p.[40] This was the first inherited neurologic disorder shown to result from mutations in a brain ion channel gene. Recently, patients with EA-2 were found to have mutations in the same voltage-gated $Ca^{2+}$ channel gene on chromosome 19p that is defective in FHM (Fig. 20–2)[33,41,42]. Unlike like the missense mutations in *CACNA1A* found with FHM, however, most of the mutations with EA-2 disrupt the reading frame and are predicted to yield a truncated $\alpha_1$-subunit. This presumably leads to a decrease in the density of $Ca^{2+}$ channels normally heavily expressed in the cerebellum,[38] possibly explaining the episodic and progressive ataxia seen with EA-2. How missense mutations in the same gene can lead to FHM and EA-2 is unclear, although the location of the mutation is a key factor.[42] Although most heavily expressed in the cerebellum, *CANCA1A* is also expressed in the brain stem and spinal cord.[43]

## Cadasil

### PHENOTYPE

Cerebral autosomal dominant arteriopathy with subcortical infarcts and leukoencephalopathy (CADASIL) is a progressive neurologic disorder characterized by subcortical infarcts and progressive neuropsychiatric symptoms and signs.[44] It is associated with a characteristic granular eosinophilic and osmiophilic deposit in the smooth muscle layer of small arteries.[45] Families with CADASIL can have migraine headaches and basilar migraine-like attacks; in some families, migraine is an early and prominent feature.[46] A characteristic finding with CADASIL is subcortical $T_2$-intense lesions on magnetic resonance imaging, a finding sometimes seen in patients with migraine.[47]

### GENOTYPE

Although linked to the same general region on chromosome 19p as FHM and EA-2,[48] CADASIL is due to missense mutations in another nearby gene, *Notch3*.[49] In *Drosophila,* this gene codes for a glycosylated transmembrane receptor that is involved in cell-fate specification during development.[50] Its function in humans and how mutations lead to development of CADASIL and migraine headaches are unknown.

## Melas

### PHENOTYPE

The syndrome of mitochondrial encephalopathy, lactic acidosis, and stroke (MELAS) is one of several diseases affecting mitochondrial function that have diverse clinical manifestations including migraine-like headaches. Initial descriptions of MELAS mentioned severe headaches associated with vomiting and abdominal pain,[51] but later reports[52,53] emphasized that the neurologic events were often preceded by prolonged migraine-like headaches, sometimes occurring in clusters lasting days. Montogna and colleagues[53] suggested that the frequent occurrence of MO and MA with MELAS might be explained on the basis of mitochondrial abnormalities in the smooth muscle of cerebral blood vessels.

### GENOTYPE

Mitochondrial DNA disorders such as MELAS exhibit a characteristic maternal transmission that should be easily identified when examining a pedigree.[51–53] MELAS is associated with an A to G transition mutation at nucleotide pair 3243 in the dihydrouridine loop of the mitochondrial tRNA Leu(UUR) gene.[54] Mosewich and coworkers[55] recently reported a large family with the 3243 point mutation; several members had migraine headaches, but only one exhibited a stroke-like episode. These investigators suggested that the severity of clinical features may depend on the percentage of mutated mitochondrial DNA and its tissue distribution.

## LINKAGE STUDIES IN FAMILIES WITH MIGRAINE WITH AND WITHOUT AURA

Despite the high prevalence of uncomplicated migraine, there have been relatively few linkage studies in large, well-documented families. The assignment of the FHM locus to chromosome 19p provided a promising genetic locus to consider for MO and MA. Hovatta and associates.[56] excluded the 19p locus for the disease gene in four Finnish families with uncomplicated migraine. Three of the families had some members with MA and others with MO, while the fourth family had only members with MO. Each of the families was relatively small, however, and the individual lod scores, although negative, were not conclusive.

The total lod scores for the four families for $\theta = 0.00$ ranged between $-2$ and $-2.5$ for the four most informative markers. The family with migraine headaches, episodic vertigo, and essential tremor shown in Figure 20–1 also was not linked to chromosome 19p. Lod scores for informative markers in the critical area on 19p were all less than $-4$ for $\theta = 0.01$.[25]

May and coworkers[57] tested for the involvement of the chromosomal 19p region in 28 unrelated families with both MA and MO by following the transmission of a single highly informative marker on 19p (D19S394). Sib-pair analysis showed that affected siblings shared the same marker allele more frequently than expected by chance. The overall lod score of marker D19S394 was 1.38 for $\theta = 0.00$, but a major contribution to this total lod score came from one family that had a maximum lod score of 1.29. Most of the families were uninformative with this marker. Although more families need to be studied, it seems apparent that the 19p locus is not associated with most families with uncomplicated migraine. Furthermore, Kim and colleagues[58] screened CACNA1A for mutations in 9 families with migraine and episodic vertigo and no mutations were found.

Thus far there have been no reports of standard linkage analysis with modern microsatellite markers that span the entire human genome in well-documented families with uncomplicated migraine. A few early studies focused on the HLA system on chromosome 6,[59–61] and a more recent study by Pardo and associates[62] investigated 11 genetic markers scattered over the human genome in 112 unrelated patients with migraine (50 with aura and 62 without aura). The only significant associations were found between the patients with migraine and the group-specific component GC on chromosome 4q and esterase D on chromosome 13q. Although neither of these genes is likely involved in the pathogenesis of migraine, other nearby genes, such as β-thromboglobulin (BTG) and platelet factor 4 on chromosome 4q, and the $5HT_{2A}$ receptor gene on chromosome 13q, are candidate genes for migraine. Subsequent studies, however, have ruled out linkage with the $5HT_{2A}$ locus on chromosome 13q (see later). Peroutka and colleagues[63] found an increased frequency of the dopamine $D_2$ receptor allele, DRD2 NcoIC in patients with MA compared to controls suggesting that the DRD2 receptor may play a role in the pathophysiology of MA.

## CANDIDATE GENES

Before the candidate genes for MO and MA are considered, it is useful to briefly consider the pathophysiology of migraine as it is currently understood. Probably the most characteristic of migraine symptoms is the classic visual aura. It typically begins with a small scintillating scotoma that gradually enlarges over 20 to 30 minutes. There is convincing evidence that the visual aura is secondary to a spreading wave of cortical depression beginning at the occipital pole, which gradually spreads across the cortex before stopping at the central sulcus.[64,65] Although decreased cerebral perfusion is associated with the spreading wave of depression, it is probably a secondary phenomenon rather than a primary process. The spreading wave of cortical depression is associated with a marked accumulation of extracellular potassium that must be cleared before neural activity can return to normal. Although the exact mechanism for the spreading wave of depression is not known, most agree that the initial event is a local build-up of potassium in the extracellular space.[65]

Nearby synaptic terminals then depolarize in response to the high extracellular potassium, and both excitatory and inhibitory neurotransmitters are released. This release in turn leads to the opening of subsynaptic channels, resulting in further ionic exchange between the intracellular and extracellular fluids. During the spreading wave of depression, neurons are completely silent for approximately 1 minute, and they then slowly recover their predepression level of firing. The rate of movement of the spreading wave of depression across the visual cortex nicely correlates with the rate of enlargement of the scintillating scotoma observed by the patient. Recently a spreading wave of cortical depression was observed using positron emission tomography (PET) in a patient during a typical MO.[66]

Consistent with a basic neuronal defect, patients with migraine have cortical abnormalities not only during their attacks but also in the interictal period. Paroxysmal slowing on interictal electro encephalography (EEG) is commonly seen in migraine, and the clinical association of migraine and epilepsy is well-documented.[67] Interestingly, identical paroxysmal slowing on EEG is seen in patients with EA-2.[26] Magnetic resonance spectroscopy shows decreased interictal energy metabolism in the cortex of patients with migraine with or without aura.[68,69] Single-photon emission computed tomography (SPECT) and other techniques for measuring cerebral blood flow have shown areas of regional hypoperfusion, not only during migraine attacks but also in the interictal phase.[70] These changes were found in migraine without visual aura, with visual aura, and with episodes of hemiplegia. Acetazolamide reversed these interictal areas of hypoperfusion in all three classes of migraine patients.[63]

Moskowitz[71,72] proposed a mechanism to explain how the spreading wave of depression and associated increase in extracellular potassium could lead to a typical migraine headache. He introduced the concept of the trigeminal vascular system in the pathogenesis of vascular headaches. Trigeminal nerve fibers surrounding pial arteries on the ventral surface of the brain are depolarized by the high potassium concentration. This in turn leads to the release of neurotransmitters such as substance P and calcitonin gene–related peptide by both orthodromic and antidromic conduction. The result is an increase in vascular permeability, dilation of cerebral vessels, and a local inflammatory response further activating pain-provoking fibers of the trigeminal vascular system. Thus the headache of migraine could be a secondary phenomenon, the end result of a local increase in extracellular potassium concentration.

## Ion Channels

One way to explain the heterogeneity of migraine syndromes is to postulate a group of defects in genes that code for a family of proteins with similar properties and functions. A family of ion channels is appealing because many of the migraine syndromes share the clinical features of the known inherited ion channel disorders (Table 20–4).[25] With the finding of an abnormal voltage-gated $Ca^{2+}$ channel gene in FHM and EA-2, mutations in other $Ca^{2+}$ channel genes are prime candidates for other migraine syndromes, including MO and MA. These channels are remarkably diverse in their conductance and gating mechanisms, and most neurons express several subtypes that are characterized by different functional and pharmacologic properties (Fig. 20–2).[73]

A defective $Ca^{2+}$ channel could explain

Table 20–4. **Clinical Features of Known Inherited Ion Channel Disorders**

| |
|---|
| Autosomal dominant inheritance |
| Reduced penetrance |
| Periodic symptoms determined by where abnormal channels are expressed |
| Episodes triggered by stress |
| May or may not have interictal findings |
| Response to acetazolamide |

the local build-up of extracellular potassium that initiates the spreading wave of depression in migraine. As $Ca^{2+}$ enters neurons, potassium exits. Many of the well-known triggers for migraine symptoms, including stress and menstruation, could result from hormonal influences on the defective calcium channels. Finally, prophylactic drugs such as β-blockers, calcium channel blockers, acetazolamide, and tricyclic amines might work by stabilizing the abnormal calcium channels. Acetazolamide presumably works in EA-2 by stabilizing calcium channels through changes in cerebellar pH.[74]

## Serotonin

Several different types of evidence implicate alterations in the metabolism of serotonin (5HT) in the pathogenesis of migraine.[75,76] For example, platelets release serotonin, and urinary excretion of 5-hydroxyidoleacetic acid (5HIAA), a breakdown product of 5HT, is increased during an attack. Migraine headaches can be precipitated by reserpine, which releases serotonin from body stores. Stabilization of serotonin neurotransmission by altering the activity of serotonergic neurons may be a common mechanism of action of several drugs effective in treating migraine. These drugs alter serotonin's effective bioavailability by different means, including receptor agonism and antagonism, prolongation of biological half-life, inhibition of release, and activation of cyclic adenosine monophosphate (cAMP). Serotonin receptors are present both in intracranial blood vessels and within nerve terminals throughout the central nervous system.[77]

Fozard and Kalkman[78] proposed a role for serotonin in producing migraine headaches based on stimulation of a specific receptor subtype ($5HT_{2C}$) present on endothelial cells lining the cerebral vasculature. The $5HT_{2C}$ receptor (originally called $5HT_{1C}$) has close sequence homology to a $5HT_2$ receptor of the rat fundus ($5HT_{2B}$).[77] These receptors couple with G proteins, which activate phospholipase C. The human $5HT_{2C}$ receptor gene is located on chromosome Xq.[79] Stimulation of the $5HT_{2C}$ receptor leads to the local release of nitrous oxide and the initiation of a sterile inflammatory response. The theory of Fozard and Kalkman[78] is based on two key observations:

1. An experimental drug, m-chlorophenylpiperazine (mCPP), triggers migraine headaches in selected subjects at doses that yield peak plasma concentrations at which the only relevant action of mCPP is agonism of the $5HT_{2C}$ receptors.
2. Several pharmacological agents with a high affinity for the $5HT_{2C}$ receptors protect against migraine when given prophylactically.

They proposed that activation of $5HT_{2C}$ receptors by mCPP or endogenous serotonin derived from perivascular neurons arising from nuclei in the brain stem would induce nitrous oxide release, activation of sensory neurons, and initiation of the sterile inflammatory response typical of migraine. Thus this model is consistent with the trigeminal neurovascular model of Moskowitz and colleagues.

Buchwalder and colleagues.[79] found no evidence of linkage for the chromosomal regions overlapping the $5HT_{2A}$ (13q14–q22) and $5HT_{2C}$ (Xq22–25) receptors in families with migraine. Furthermore, they analyzed the coding region of the $5HT_{2A}$ and $5HT_{2C}$ receptor genes in migraine patients and unaffected controls, using polymerase chain reaction and direct sequencing, and did not find any mutations in either receptor in the patients with migraine. Nyholt and associates[80] also ruled out linkage to the $5HT_{2A}$ locus of chromosome 13q in 3 families with uncomplicated migraine. Other 5HT genes, including those coding for other receptors, 5HT transporters, and 5HT metabolizers, remain candidate genes for migraine.

## SUMMARY

Migraine is not a disease but a syndrome that undoubtedly has multiple causes. Several migraine syndromes have a clear autosomal dominant pattern of inheritance, and recently an abnormal calcium channel gene was identified in families with FHM and EA-2. Familial aggregation and twin studies in families with other more common migraine syndromes (migraine with and without visual aura) show that genetic factors are important in most cases, although the mode of inheritance is not always clear.

Classic segregation analysis performed on such families suggests a multifactorial inheritance. This type of analysis does not exclude the likelihood that some families have a simple mendelian pattern of inheritance, whereas others do not. The first critical step in identifying a "migraine gene" is to carefully document more families with a clear mendelian pattern of inheritance. One can then consider potential candidate genes, such as those associated with ion channels and serotonin metabolism. Defects in the group of genes coding for different voltage-gated calcium channel subunits is a good working hypothesis to explain the diversity of migraine syndromes. Because most of these genes have been cloned and sequenced[73] and their locations in the human genome are known,[81] it is a straightforward hypothesis to test.

## REFERENCES

1. Waters WE: Migraine runs in families–but is it inherited? Letter to the Editor. BMJ 311:1227, 1995.
2. Russell MB, Olesen J: Increased familial risk and evidence of genetic factor in migraine. BMJ 311: 541–544, 1995.
3. Russell MB, Rasmussen BK, Thorvaldsen P, Olesen J: Prevalence and sex-ratios of the subtypes of migraine. A population based epidemiologic survey of four thousand 40 year old males and females. Int J Epidemiol 24:612–618, 1995.
4. Refsum S: Genetic aspects of migraine. In Vinken PP, Bruyn G (eds): Handbook of Clinical Neurology, Vol 5. North Holland Publishing, Amsterdam, 1975, pp258–261.
5. Allan W: The inheritance of migraine. Arch Intern Med 13:590–599, 1930.
6. Goodell H, Lewontin R, Wolff HG: Familial occurrence of migraine headache. A study of heredity. Arch Neurol Psychiatry 72:325–334, 1954.
7. Dalsgaard-Nielsen T, Ulrich T: Prevalence and heredity of migraine and migrainoid headaches among 461 Danish doctors. Headache 4:168–172, 1973.
8. Vilatela MEA, Pedroza FG, Ziegler DK, Mendez AG: Familial migraine in a Mexican population. Neuroepidemiology 11:46–49, 1992.
9. Russell MB, Olesen J: The genetics of migraine without aura and migraine with aura. Cephalalgia 13:245–248, 1993.
10. Headache Classification Committee of the International Headache Society: Classification and diagnostic criteria for headache disorders, cranial neuralgias and facial pain. Cephalalgia 8:1–97, 1988.
11. Harvald B, Hauge M: A catamnestic investigation of Danish twins. A preliminary report. Br Med Bull 3:150–158, 1956.
12. Ulrich, V, Gervil M, Kyvik KO, Olesen J, Russell MB: Evidence of a genetic factor in migraine with aura: A population-based Danish Twin Study. Ann Neurol 45:242–246, 1999.
13. Juel-Nielsen N: Individual and environmental. A psychiatric investigation of monozygotic twins reared apart. Acta Psychiatr Scand 40 (suppl 183): 1–292, 1964.
14. Osuntokun BO, Schoenberg BS, Nottidge VA, et al.: Migraine headache in a rural community in Nigeria: Results of a pilot study. Neuroepidemiology 1:31–19, 1982.
15. Levy LM: An epidemiological study of headache in an urban population in Zimbabwe. Headache 23: 2–9, 1983.
16. Zhao F, Tsay JY, Cheng XM, et al.: Epidemiology of migraine: A survey of 21 provinces of the People's Republic of China, 1985. Headache 28:558–656, 1988.
17. Tokio S, Hisanori K, Toshiya N, Kazuro T: Prevalence of migraine in western Japan [Abstract]. Cephalalgia 13 (suppl 13):10, 1993.
18. Stewart WF, Lipton RB, Liberman J: Variation in migraine prevalence by race. Neurology 47:52–59, 1996.
19. Ohta M, Shukuro A, Kuriowa Y: Familial occurrence of migraine with a hemiplegic syndrome and cerebellar infarctions. Neurology 17:813–817, 1967.
20. Zifkin B, Andermann E, Andermann F, Kirkham T: An autosomal dominant syndrome of hemiplegic migraine, nystagmus and tremor. Ann Neurol 8:329–332, 1980.
21. Bisgård C, Jensen TS, Dupont E, Hertz JM: Familial hemiplegic migraine associated with cerebellar ataxia. A distinct inherited disease entity? Acta Neurol Scand 85 (suppl 138):29, 1992.
22. Joutel A, Bousser M-G, Biousse V, et al.: A gene for familial hemiplegic migraine maps to chromosome 19. Nat Genet 5:40–45, 1993.
23. Joutel A, Ducros A, Vahedi K, et al.: Genetic heterogeneity of familial hemiplegic migraine. Am J Hum Genet 55:1166–1172, 1994.

24. Russell MB, Andersson PG, Thomsen LL: Familial occurrence of cluster headache. J Neurol Neurosurg Psychiatry 58:341–343, 1995.
25. Baloh RW, Foster CA, Yue Q, Nelson SF: Familial migraine with vertigo and essential tremor. Neurology 46:458–460, 1996.
26. Zasorin NL, Baloh RW, Myers LB: Acetazolamide-responsive episodic ataxia syndrome. Neurology 33:1212–1214, 1993.
27. Devoto M, Lozita A, Staffa G, et al.: Segregation analysis of migraine in 128 families. Cephalalgia 6: 101–105, 1986.
28. Mochi M, Sangiorgi S, Cortelli P, et al.: Testing models for genetic determination in migraine. Cephalalgia 13:389–394, 1993.
29. Russell MB, Iselius L, Olesen J: Inheritance of migraine investigated by complex segregation analysis. Hum Genet 96:726–630, 1995.
30. Rassmussen BK: Migraine with aura and MO are two different entities. Cephalalgia 15:183–186, 1995.
31. Haan J, Terwindt GM, Ophoff RA, et al.: Is familial hemiplegic migraine a form of basilar migraine? Cephalalgia 15:477–481, 1995.
32. Terwindt GM, Ophoff RA, Haan J, Frants RR, Ferrari MD: Familial hemiplegic migraine: A clinical comparison of families linked and unlinked to chromosome 19p. Cephalalgia 16:153–155, 1996.
33. Ophoff RA, Terwindt GM, Vergouwe MN, et al.: Familial hemiplegic migraine and episodic ataxia type-2 are caused by mutations in the $Ca^{2+}$ channel gene *CACNL1A4*. Cell 87:543–553, 1996.
34. Ducros A, Denier C, Joutel A, et al.: Recurrence of the T666M calcium channel CACNAIA gene mutation in familial hemiplegic migraine with progressive ataxia. Am J Hum Genet 64:89–98, 1999.
35. Ducros A, Joutel A, Vahedik, et al.: Mapping of a second locus for familial hemiplegic migraine to 1q21–q23 and evidence of further heterogeneity. Ann Neurol 42:885–890, 1997.
36. Gardner K, Hoffman EP: Current Status of genetic discoveries in migraine: Familial hemiplegic migraine with progressive cerebellar ataxia. Am J Hum Genet 64:89–98, 1999.
37. Kramer PL, Yue Q, Gancher ST, et al.: A locus for the nystagmus-associated form of episodic ataxia maps to an 11-cM region on chromosome 19p. Am J Hum Genet 57: 182–185, 1995.
38. Baloh RW, Yue Q, Furman JM, Nelson SF: Familial epsiodic ataxia: Clinical heterogeneity in four families linked to chromosome 19p. Ann Neurol 41:8–16, 1997.
39. Elliott MA, Peroutka SJ, Welch S, May EF: Familial hemiplegic migraine, nystagmus, and cerebellar atrophy. Ann Neurol 39:100–106, 1996.
40. Browne DL, Gancher ST, Nutt JG, et al.: Episodic ataxia/myokymia syndrome is associated with point mutation in the human potassium channel gene KCNA1. Nat Genet 8:136–140, 1994.
41. Yue Q, Jen JC, Thwe MM, Nelson S, Baloh RW: De novo mutation in CACNA1A caused acetazolamide-responsive episodic ataxia. Am J Med Genet 77: 298–301, 1998.
42. Yue Q, Jen JC, Nelson S, Baloh RW: Progressive ataxia due to a missense mutation in a calcium channel gene. Am J Hum Genet 61:1078–1087, 1997.
43. Mori Y, Friedrich T, Kim M-S, et al.: Primary structure and functional expression from a complementary DNA of a brain calcium channel. Nature 350: 398–402, 1991.
44. Tournier-Lasserve E, Joutel A, Melki J, et al.: Cerebral autosomal dominant arteriopathy with subcortical infarcts and leukoencephalopathy (CADASIL) maps on chromosome 19q12. Nat Genet 3:256–259, 1993.
45. Ruchoux M-M, Guerouaou D, Vandenhaute B, et al.: Systemic vascular smooth muscle cell impairment in cerebral autosomal dominant arteriopathy with subcortical infarcts and leukoencephalopathy. Acta Neuropathol 89:500–512, 1995.
46. Vérin M, Rolland Y, Landgraf F, et al.: New phenotype of the cerebral autosomal dominant arteriopathy mapped to chromosome 19: Migraine is a prominent clinical feature. J Neurol Neurosurg Psychiatry 59:579–585, 1995.
47. Chabriat H, Tournier-Lasserve E, Vahedi K, et al.: Autosomal dominant migraine with MRI white-matter abnormalities mapping to the CADASIL locus. Neurology 45: 1086–1091, 1995.
48. Ducros A, Nagy T, Alamowitch S, et al.: Cerebral autosomal dominant arteriopathy with subcortical infarcts and leukoencephalopathy, genetic homogeneity, and mapping of the locus within a 2-cM interval. Am J Hum Genet 458: 171–181, 1996.
49. Joutel A, Corpechot C, Ducros A, et al.: *Notch3* mutations in CADASIL, a hereditary adult-onset condition causing stroke and dementia. Nature 383: 707–710, 1996.
50. Gridley T: Notch, stroke and dementia. Nature 383: 673, 1996.
51. Pavlakis SG, Phillips PC, Di Mauro S, De Vivo DC, Rowland LP: Mitochondrial myopathy, encephalopathy, lactic acidosis, and stroke-like episodes: A distinctive clinical syndrome. Ann Neurol 16: 4881–488, 1984.
52. Dvorkin GS, Andermann F, Carpenter S, et al.: Classical migraine, intractable epilepsy and multiple strokes: A syndrome related to mitochondrial encephalopathy. In Andermann F, Lugaresi E (eds): Migraine and Epilepsy. Butterworths, Boston, 1987, pp203–232.
53. Montagna P, Gallassi R, Medori R, et al.: MELAS syndrome: Characteristic migrainous and epileptic features and maternal transmission. Neurology 38: 751–754, 1988.
54. Goto Y, Nonaka I, Horal S: A mutation in the tRNA Leu(UUR) gene associated with the MELAS subgroup of mitochondrial encephalomyopathies. Nature 348: 651–653, 1990.
55. Mosewich RK, Donat RJ, DiMaurio S, et al.: The syndrome of mitochondrial encephalopathy, lactic acidosis, and strokelike episodes presenting without stroke. Arch Neurol 50: 275–278, 1993.
56. Hovatta I, Kallela M, Färkkilä M, Peltonen L: Familial migraine: Exclusion of the susceptibility gene from the reported locus of familial hemiplegic migraine on 19p. Genomics 23: 707–709, 1994.
57. May A, Ophoff RA, Terwindt GM, et al.: Familial hemiplegic migraine locus on 19p13 is involved in

the common forms of migraine with and without aura. Hum Genet 96: 604–608, 1995.

58. Kim J-S, Yue Q, Jen JC, Nelson SF, Baloh RW: Familial migraine with vertigo: no mutations found in CACNA1A. Am J Med Genet 79: 148–151, 1998.
59. Kudrow L: HLA antigens in cluster headache and classical migraine. Headache 18: 167–168, 1978.
60. O'Neill BP, Kapur JJ, Good AE: HLA antigens in migraine. Headache 19: 71–31, 1979.
61. Giacovazzo M, Valeri M, Piazza A, et al.: Elevated frequency of HLA-shared haplotypes in migraine families. Headache 27: 575–577, 1987.
62. Pardo J, Carracedo A, Muñoz I, et al.: Genetic markers: Association study in migraine. Cephalalgia 15: 200–204, 1995.
63. Peroutka SJ, Wilhoit T, Jones K: Clinical susceptability to migraine with aura is modified by dopamine D2 receptor (DRD2) NcoI alleles, Neurology 49: 201–206, 1997.
64. Leao AAP: Spreading depression of activity in cerebral cortex. J Neurophysiol 7: 359–390, 1944.
65. Lauritzen M: Pathophysiology of migraine aura. Brain 117: 119–210, 1994.
66. Woods RP, Iacoboni MI, Mazziotta JC: Bilateral spreading cerebral hypoperfusion during spontaneous migraine headache. N Engl J Med 331: 1689–1692, 1994.
67. Lipton RB, Ottman R, Ehrenberg BL, Hauser WA: Comorbidity of migraine: The connection between migraine and epilepsy. Neurology 44 (suppl 7): S28–S32, 1994.
68. Welch KMA, Levine SR, D'Andrea G, Schultz LR, Helpern JA: Preliminary observations on brain energy metabolism in migraine studied by *in vivo* phosphorous 31p NMR spectroscopy. Neurology 39: 538–541, 1989.
69. Montagna P, Cortelli P, Barbiroli B: Magnetic resonance spectroscopy studies in migraine. Cephalalgia 14: 184–193, 1994.
70. Schlake H-P, Bottger IG, Grotemeyer K-H, et al.: The influence of acetazolamide on cerebral low-flow regions in migraine—An interictal 99mmTc-HMPAO SPECT study. Cephalalgia 12: 284–288, 1992.
71. Moskowitz MA: The neurobiology of vascular head pain. Ann Neurol 16: 157–168, 1984.
72. Moskowitz MA: Basic mechanisms in vascular headache. Neurol Clin 8: 801–815, 1990.
73. Perez-Reyes E, Schneider T: Calcium channels: Structure, function, and classification. Drug Dev Res 33: 295–318, 1994.
74. Bain PG, O'Brien MD, Keevil SF, Porter DA: Familial periodic cerebellar ataxia: A probable of cerebellar intracellular pH homeostasis. Ann Neurol 31: 147–154, 1992.
75. Ferrari MD, Saxena PR: On serotonin and migraine: A clinical and pharmacological review. Cephalalgia 13: 151–165, 1993.
76. Humphrey PPA: 5-Hydroxytryptamine and the pathophysiology of migraine. J Neurol 238: S38–S44, 1991.
77. Humphrey PPA, Hartig PR, Hoyer D: A proposed new nomenclature for 5-HT receptors. Trends Pharmacol Sci 14: 233–236, 1993.
78. Fozard JR, Kalkman HO: 5-Hydroxytryptamine (5-HT) and the initiation of migraine: New perspectives. Naunyn Schmiedebergs Arch Pharmacol 350: 225–229, 1994.
79. Buchwalder A, Welch SK, Peroutka SJ: Exclusion of the 5-$HT_{2A}$ and 5-$HT_{2C}$ receptor genes as candidate genes for migraine. Headache 36: 254–258, 1996.
80. Nyholt DR, Curtain RP, Gaffney PT, et al.: Migraine association and linkage analyses of the 5-hydroxytryptamine ($5HT_{2A}$) receptor gene. Cephalalgia 16: 463–467, 1996.
81. Diriong S, Lory P, Williams ME, et al.: Chromosomal localization of the human genes for $\alpha_{1A}$, $\alpha_{1B}$, and $\alpha_{1E}$ voltage-dependent $Ca^{2+}$ channel subunits. Genomics 30: 605–609, 1995.

# Chapter 21

# GENETICS OF CEREBROVASCULAR DISEASE

Jeffrey L. Saver, MD
Titi Tamburi, MD



Stroke is the third leading cause of death and the leading cause of adult disability in the developed world. Reflecting the complete pathogenesis of cerebrovascular disease, over 110 heritable disorders, 175 genetic loci, and 2050 unique mutations predisposing to stroke are known. Systematic investigation of genetic causes of cerebrovascular disease is essential to the management of pediatric stroke, stroke in the young adult, familial stroke, and "cryptogenic" stroke. In this chapter, a diverse array of genetic determinants of cerebrovascular disease are reviewed and classified; those of greatest clinical or genetic import are examined in depth.

Stroke is quintessentially a complex genetic disorder. Both environmental and genetic factors contribute to cerebrovascular disease, and the genetic effects are often polygenic—related to multiple interacting genes.[1] Many of the major risk factors for stroke, such as hypertension, diabetes mellitus, atherosclerosis, and obesity, are themselves synthetic, polygenic traits that further interact in the production of cerebrovascular disease. As a result, assessing the total burden of genetic disposition to stroke in most individuals is exceedingly problematic. In addition to polygenic influences, the cerebral vasculature is vulnerable to numerous single-gene disorders, in which an isolated gene defect exerts a predominating clinical effect, inherited in strict mendelian fashion. Though individually rare or uncommon, together these disorders account for a substantial portion of stroke cases and elucidate critical components of the biology of the cerebral vessels. Because they provide unique insights into vascular biology and in aggregate contribute to stroke in many patients, diseases due to single-gene defects are a major focus here. In particular, disorders in which cerebrovascular manifestations are a leading or frequent feature will be emphasized, with briefer reviews of conditions in which stroke is a minor or inconstant manifestation.

## GENERAL HERITABLE TENDENCY TO STROKE

The general tendency toward familial aggregation of stroke, without considering stroke subtype or mechanism (or firmly separating environmental from genetic influence), was first well-characterized, by studies of the Framingham population cohort.[2] Offspring of a parent with a stroke or transient ischemic attack (TIA) had a 1.90 crude relative risk and a 1.56 multivariate-adjusted relative risk of a cerebrovascular event. Individuals with siblings who suffered stroke or TIA were 1.5 times as likely to experience a cerebrovascular event as those without a sibling history and 1.2 times as likely when multivariate adjustments, including blood pressure, were made. Convergent findings from the British Regional Heart Study demonstrated that a history of parental death from stroke increased personal risk of stroke 1.4-fold among prospectively followed middle-aged men.[3] Similarly, the Family Heart Study found that paternal history of stroke increased the odds ratio for stroke in offspring to 2.0 and maternal history of stroke increased the odds ratio to 1.4.[3a]

Twin studies also provide strong evidence of heritable influences on stroke. Among 15,948 male twin pairs in the National Academy of Sciences–National Research Council Twin Registry, the stroke concordance rate for monozygotic pairs was 17.7% versus 3.6% for dizygotic pairs, a 4.3-fold increase in relative risk.[4] This increased risk for monozygotic pairs declined with aging of the cohort,[5] consistent with a growing influence of nongenetic factors related to aging and environment on strokes in later life.

Table 21–1. **Selected Genetic Causes of Accelerated Cervicocephalic Atherosclerosis**

| |
|---|
| Dyslipoproteinemias |
|   Low-density lipoprotein (LDL) |
|     Familial hyupercholesterolemia (LDL receptor gene defects) |
|     Apolipoprotein B gene defects |
|     Familial combined hyperlipidemia |
|   Apolipoprotein E (ApoE) |
|     Familial dysbetalipoproteinemia (ApoE2 homozygosity) |
|     Apolipoprotein E2 heterozygosity |
|   Lipoprotein(a) (Lp[a]) |
|     Lp(a) polymorphism |
|   High-density lipoprotein |
|     Familial dyslipidemia |
|     Familial hypoalphalipoproteinemia |
|     Apoliprotein A-I deficiency |
|     Tangier disease |
|     Paraoxonase polymophism |
| Cerebrotendinous xanthomatosis |
| Homocyst(e)ine metabolism |
|   Homocystinuria/homocyt(e)inemia |
|     Cystathione β-synthetase deficiency |
|     Methylene tetrahydrofolate deficiency |
| Premature aging syndromes |
|   Progeria (Hutchinson-Gilford syndrome) |
|   Werner's syndrome |

## CEREBRAL INFARCTION

### Accelerated Atherosclerosis

Major risk factors for cerebrovascular atherosclerosis—hypertension, diabetes mellitus, dyslipidemia, and obesity—are in large measure genetically determined. Furthermore, epidemiological investigations suggest strong additional genetic influences on cerebrovascular atherogenesis beyond that mediated by these risk factors. In one study, heritability of classic risk factors such as hypertension and diabetes explained only 10% to 25% of phenotypic variation in carotid artery intimal–medial thickness variation, but additional genetic influences, not mediated through standard risk factors, accounted for 66% to 75% of variation.[6] Selected monogenic causes of accelerated cervicocephalic atherosclerosis are listed in Table 21–1.

#### HYPERTENSION

After age, hypertension is the most powerful risk factor for stroke in the Western world, increasing the risk of both cerebral infarction and cerebral hemorrhage 5- to 7-fold. Genetic factors account for 20% to 60% of observed variances in blood pressure.[7a] Although numerous renal, endocrine, and neurologic disorders may secondarily produce hypertension, essential hypertension of unknown etiology accounts for more than 90% of cases. Individuals with essential hypertension are twice as likely to have a hypertensive parent than are normotensives. Blood pressure correlations between monozygotic twins (0.55 to 0.7) are more than twofold greater than those between dizygotic twins. More than 40 monogenic causes of hypertension are known.[7b] The most common single-gene disorder leading to hypertension is autosomal dominant polycystic kidney disease, which produces hypertension in 75% of cases.

A deletion polymorphism in the gene encoding the angiotensin I–converting enzyme (ACE) is an independent risk factor for myocardial infarction and has been linked to cerebral infarction. An important regulator of blood pressure and salt and water metabolism, ACE catalyzes the conversion of angiotensin I to angiotensin II, a potent vasopressor, and inactivates bradykinin, a vasodilator. The human ACE gene on chromosome 17 contains 26 exons.[8] A deletion/insertion (D/I) polymorphism in intron 16 is strongly associated with variation in circulating ACE levels. Combined segregation and linkage analysis suggests that this polymorphism is a marker in strong linkage disequilibrium with a major ACE gene variant that accounts for 44% of the variability in plasma ACE level. Small case–control studies provide conflicting evidence for an association of ACE gene polymorphism and cerebrovascular disease, with some associating the *DD* genotype with intima–media thickening of the common carotid arteries, parental history of stroke, and lacunar infarction.[9] Meta-analyses of these studies suggest that the D allele, acting recessively, is a modest, independent risk factor for ischemic stroke.[9a,9b] Conversely, absence of the D allele may increase the risk of intracranial saccular aneurysm.[9c] Although ACE genetic variation affects blood pressure in rodents, a strong effect on blood pressure in humans has not yet been demonstrated. Alternative mechanisms that may mediate the adverse effects of elevated serum ACE levels include modulation of local vascular tone, induction of vascular smooth muscle proliferation, and reduction of fibrinolysis by increasing plasma levels of plasminogen activator inhibitor-1.[10]

## DIABETES MELLITUS

Diabetes mellitus is an independent risk factor for cerebral infarction, conferring a relative risk of 1.5 to 3.0. Diabetes increases the risk of both large vessel and lacunar infarction by accelerating cervicocerebral atherosclerosis and cerebral microangiopathy. Hyperglycemia is a feature of more than 60 rare genetic syndromes, indicating that mutations at many genetic loci can disrupt glucose homeostasis. Genetic factors play a modest role in type 1 insulin-dependent diabetes, which, a widely held view suggests, is the outcome of a genetic predisposition and a viral or other environmental insult producing T cell–mediated destruction of pancreatic islet cells.[11] Genetic factors appear to play a very strong role in type 2, noninsulin-dependent diabetes.[10,11] Up to 60% of cases of maturity onset diabetes of the young are due to mutations in the glucokinase gene. Insulin gene, insulin receptor gene, and mitochondrial DNA mutations are rare causes of type 2 diabetes, with more than 40 insulin receptor mutations known. All single-gene disorders characterized to date, however, account for only a small portion of type 2 diabetes.

## DYSLIPOPROTEINEMIAS

In general, two types of genetic influence on lipids and atherosclerosis may be distinguished: rare mutations that powerfully raise choleresterol levels irrespective of environmental exposures and more common genetic polymorphisms that modestly affect cholesterol metabolism in interaction with diet, tobacco, exercise, and other environmental factors.[12] Information on stroke risk in the uncommon, potent familial dysplipidemia syndromes is surprisingly sparse, likely in part because early cardiac death often supervenes before cerebrovascular disease can manifest. In contrast, epidemiological studies have linked several genetic polymorphisms to cerebrovascular atherosclerosis.

Family and twin studies demonstrate that half the population variance in low-density lipoprotein (LDL) cholesterol levels is genetic. Known mutations in the LDL receptor, Apolipoprotein B (ApoB), and Apolipoprotein E (ApoE) account for 7% of the variance, with the preponderance due to as yet unidentified genetic factors.[10] Familial hypercholesterolemia (type IIa hyperlipoproteinemia) is an autosomal dominant disorder due to a defective LDL receptor gene on chromosome 19q13.[13,14] The 45 kb gene contains 18 exons and 17 introns and codes for an 866 amino acid polypeptide. Homozygotes exhibit total cholesterol levels of 650 to 1000, sixfold elevations in LDL cholesterol, and fatal myocardial infarction generally by age 30 years. A distinctive planar cutaneous xanthoma develops in childhood. Heterozygotes account for up to 5% of cases of adult myocardial infarction, and 75% develop nodular xanthomas of the Achilles or other tendons. The estimated prevalence of heterozygosity in the general population is 1:500. Early stroke and accelerated cervicocerebral atherosclerosis has been observed anecdotally.[15] More than 150 different LDL receptor mutations have been described. Some patients with phenotypic familial hypercholesterolemia have mutations in the ApoB gene on chromosome 2p24, disrupting LDL binding to the LDL receptor.

Familial combined hyperlipidemia (type IIb hyperlipoproteinemia) is the most common genetic hypercholesterolemia, characterized by elevations of both LDL cholesterol and very-low-density lipoprotein (VLDL) triglyceride, and is present in about 10% of myocardial infarction patients under age 60 years. Information on cerebrovascular manifestations is scanty. The precise genetic defect is not known.

Familial dysbetalipoproteinemia (type III hyperlipoproteinemia) is characterized by elevated total cholesterol, elevated triglycerides, reduced LDL cholesterol, and plasma accumulation of chylomicron and VLDL remnants.[13,14] In addition to an increased susceptibility to severe premature coronary artery disease and peripheral vascular disease, instances of early cerebral infarction have been frequently documented.[16] Pathognomonic yellow–orange discolorations of palm and finger creases (xanthoma striata palmaris) may occur. Disruption of ApoE on the surface of chylomicron and intermediate-density lipoprotein (IDL) particles, preventing their hepatic clearance, underlies this disorder and is most frequently the result of homozygosity for the ApoE2 phenotype.[17]

ApoE is encoded by a gene cluster on chromosome 19q13 that also encodes apolipoproteins CI and CII. The human ApoE gene is 3.7 kb in length, contain four exons and three introns, and codes for an ApoE polypeptide that includes an 18 amino acid signal peptide and a 299 amino acid mature protein. Three ApoE alleles are common in the general population: E2 (8% of Caucasians), E3 (77%), and E4 (15%). The ApoE2 allele encodes a protein with a cysteine for arginine substitution at residue 158 in the ApoE sequence that exhibits only 1% to 2% of normal receptor binding activity. Approximately 1 in 50 of E2/2 individuals cannot compensate for impaired ApoE function and develop fasting lipid elevations and accelerated atherosclerosis. These individuals likely have additional IDL cholesterol metabolism impairments in addition to the E2/2 genotype, related to such factors as aging, obesity, glucose intolerance, exogenous estrogen, or heterozygosity for another genetic defect.

Genetic variation in ApoE accounts for 3% to 5% of variance in serum LDL cholesterol levels. Compared with individuals with the most common E3/3 genotype, those with E3/4 have LDL cholesterol levels 5 to 20 mg/dL higher, and those with E3/2 have LDL cholesterol levels 10 to 20 mg/dL lower. Heterozygosity for E4 has been linked to cerebrovascular disease, increasing the odds of ischemic stroke and vascular dementia.[18,18a]

Lipoprotein (a) (Lp[a]) is a lipoprotein particle quite similar to LDL except that it has one molecule of Apolipoprotein(a) (Apo[a]) attached. The wide variations in serum levels of Lp(a) observed in the general population, from less than 0.1 to more than 200 mg/dL, are almost completely genetically determined. Lp(a) is an independent risk factor for premature coronary artery disease. In addition, a robust body of case–control studies demonstrates an association of Lp(a) with carotid atherosclerosis and with ischemic stroke in Caucasian,

Chinese, and Japanese populations.[19] Apo(a) contains multiple repeats of a protein domain resembling the kringle 4 domain of plasminogen and one copy of a domain similar to the kringle 5 domain of plasminogen. The Apo(a) gene lies near the plasminogen gene on chromosome 6. More than 100 Apo(a) gene alleles in the population have been posited.[20] Apo(a) and plasminogen are members of the plasminogen gene superfamily. Evolutionarily, these genes likely arose by duplication of an ancestor gene. Several are regulatory proteases in the coagulation or fibrinolytic pathways, and all have a serine protease domain and a sequence of kringles.

Disorders affecting high-density lipoprotein (HDL) include familial dyslipidemia (observed in 15% of patients with premature heart disease), familial hypoalpalipoproteinemia (observed in 4% of patients with premature heart disease), the uncommon Apolipoprotein A-I (ApoA-I) deficiency states, and Tangier disease. Precise information on stroke incidence in these conditions is lacking except for Tangier disease. Tangier disease is a rare, autosomal codominant form of HDL deficiency characterized by extremely low levels of HDL cholesterol and ApoA-I. Homozygotes accumulate massive quantities of cholesterol esters in macrophages throughout the body, including tonsils, lymph nodes, liver, spleen, intestinal mucosa, and Schwann cells. Leading clinical features are orange tonsils, hepatosplenomegaly, and peripheral neuropathy. In addition, a tendency to early cardiac and cerebral vascular disease is noted. The precise genetic defect in Tangier disease has not been identified. Paraoxonase is a protein tightly associated with HDL that reduces the accumulation of lipid oxidation products on LDL. The paraoxonase gene is located at chromosome 7q21–22. Polymorphisms at positions S4 and 191 in paroxonase have been associated with coronary heart disease, and the Leu-Met54 polymorphism was associated with carotid atherosclerosis in an Austrian population.[20a]

## HOMOCYSTINURIA

Homocystinuria is a rare, autosomal recessive disorder characterized by severe increases in blood and urine of homocyteine, homocystine, and methionine. Homocysteine is a sulfur-containing amino acid produced by the demethylation of methionine. Affected homozygous individuals develop mental retardation, usually mild, dislocation of the lenses, and often a tall, thin, marfanoid habitus. Thromboembolism affecting the heart, brain, and veins is common and is the presenting feature in 15% of cases. In a survey of over 600 patients with inherited homocystinuria, more than half suffered a vascular event before age 30 years, and ischemic stroke accounted for 60% of the recorded arterial events.[21] Homocyst(e)inemia may promote infarction through several potential mechanisms that have been identified in vitro, including *(1)* accelerating atherogenesis, by inducing vascular smooth muscle proliferation, oxidizing LDL, and increasing incorporation of Lp(a) into fibrin; *(2)* disrupting endothelial function, by impairing production of endothelium-derived relaxing factor and tissue factor activity; and *(3)* producing a hypercoagulable state, by altering clotting proteins including protein C, thrombomodulin, antithrombin III, fibrinogen, and factor VIIc. Treatment with methionine dietary restriction and folate and pyridoxine vitamin supplementation reduces the incidence of thromboembolism by age 15 years by more than 50% and the incidence of fatal outcome by age 30 years by 80%. Homocystinuria results from inherited deficiency of cystathionine β-synthetase (which catabolizes homocysteine to cysteine) or of enzymes involved in the methylation of vitamin B6 and B12 (which serve as cofactors for the remethylation of homocysteine to methionine). The most common genetic defect is cystathionine β-synthetase deficiency, with a prevalence about 1: 332,000.[22] More than 17 mutations in this gene have been identified.[23]

Recognition of the vascular manifestations of homocystinuria led to the hypothesis that more moderate elevations in plasma total homocysteine constitute an independent risk factor for coronary, peripheral, and cerebral vascular disease in the general population. Numerous epidemiological studies now support this contention, including several cross-sectional and case–control studies linking serum homocyst(e)ine with carotid intimal-medial wall thickening and cerebral infarction.[24] Moderate hyperhomocyst(e)inemia may result from acquired nutritional deficiencies of folate, pyridoxine, or cobalamin or from one of several genetic defects.[25] Heterozygosity for the enzymatic defect that most commonly causes severe homocystinuria, cystathione β-synthetase deficiency, is a cause of moderate hyperhomocyst(e)inemia, but is present in only 0.3% of the population. A far more common genetic mechanism for moderate hyperhomocyst(e)inemia is a homozygous defect of methylenetetrahydrofolate reductase, an enzyme involved in the remethylation of homocysteine to form methionine. In addition to rare, severe mutations, methylenetetrahydrofolate reductase is subject to a frequent, mild mutation that produces a thermolabile form of the enzyme with an alanine to valine missense substitution.[26] Thermolabile methylenetetrahydrofolate reductase is present in 5% of the general population and accounts for more than 60% of subjects with moderate hyperhomocyst(e)inemia. The mutation has been associated with ischemic stroke.[26a,26b]

### CEREBROTENDINOUS XANTHOMATOSIS

Cerebrotendinous xanthomatosis is a lipid storage disease with multiorgan involvement and autosomal recessive transmission. Clinical onset is generally during the second decade of life, with cognitive deterioration, pyramidal and cerebellar dysfunction, peripheral neuropathy, juvenile cataracts, recurrent bone fractures, and tendon xanthomas. Premature atherosclerosis is a common feature, with symptomatic cardiac disease in 10% of cases, although symptomatic cerebrovascular disease is apparently rare.[27] Cerebrotendinous xanthomatosis is caused by mutations in the gene encoding sterol 27 hydroxylase, a bile acid biosynthetic enzyme that also plays a role in eliminating excess cholesterol from human macrophages.[28]

### SYNDROMES OF PREMATURE AGING

Accelerated atherosclerosis is seen in inherited syndromes of premature aging. Progeria (Hutchinson-Gilford syndrome) is a rare disorder in which children exhibit growth retardation, characteristic facies, balding, loss of eyebrows, decreased subcutaneous fat, and restricted joint mobility. Severe, accelerated atherosclerosis is a leading feature. The median age of death is 12 years, and more than 80% of deaths are due to myocardial infarction or congestive heart failure. Several cases of cerebral infarction due to atherosclerosis of the internal carotid or vertebral arteries have been described, occurring between ages 4 and 12.[29] Cell cultures from progeria patients exhibit defective DNA repair. The underlying genetic defect producing progeria remains unknown. Both autosomal dominant and autosomal recessive modes of inheritance have been proposed.

Werner's syndrome is a rare, autosomal recessive disorder characterized by early onset of cataracts, premature graying of hair, generalized hair loss, hypogonadism, scleroderma-like loss of skin elasticity, osteoporosis, short stature, neoplasia, and atherosclerosis and arteriosclerosis. The cellular basis of Werner's syndrome is faulty DNA replication and repair. The gene responsible for Werner's syndrome is the *WRN* gene on chromosome 8, which encodes a polypeptide member of the RecQ subfamily of DExH-box–containing helicases.[30] RecQ helicases unwind DNA duplexes to permit protein access to DNA strands and are central to maintenance of genomic stability. At least six Werner's syndrome–causing mutations of *WRN* have been described.

## Nonatherosclerotic Arteriopathies

The heritable nonatherosclerotic vasculopathies may be classified by the type of blood vessel affected and the evident pathological process (Table 21–2).[31]

### CADASIL

Cerebral autosomal dominant arteriopathy with subcortical infarcts and leukoencephalopathy (CADASIL) is an autosomal dominant arterial disease of the brain. Though recognized only in 1977, the dis-

Table 21–2. **Selected Inherited Nonatheroslcerotic Vasculopathies**

Aorta and large arteries
- Marfan syndrome
- Supravalvular aortic stenosis

Medium arteries
- Moyamoya
- Ehlers-Danlos syndrome type IV
- Pseudoxanthoma elasticum
- Polycystic kidney disease
- Fabry's disease
- Osteogenesis imperfecta
- Down syndrome
- William's syndrome
- Ito's hypomelanosis
- Neurofibromatosis
- Menke's disease
- Kohlmeier-Degos disease
- Fanconi's anemia

Small arteries
- CADASIL
- Cerebral amyloid angiopathy
  - Familial Alzheimer's disease
  - Down syndrome
  - HCHWA–Dutch type
  - HCHWA-Icelandic type
  - HCHWA-Flemish type
- Familial cavernous angiomas
- Klippel-Trenauney-Weber syndrome
- HERNS

Capillaries and venules
- Hereditary hemorrhagic telangectasia
- Sturge-Weber syndrome

Vascular neoplasia
- von Hippel-Lindau disease

CADASIL = cerebral autosomal dominant arteriopathy with subcortical infarcts and leukoencephalopathy; HCHWA = hereditary cerebral hemorrhage with amyloidosis; HERNS = hereditary endotheliopathy with retinopathy, nephropathy, and stroke.

ease appears to be fairly common, with well over 120 families now described. The prototypical course is attacks of migraine with aura beginning in the third decade of life, onset of recurrent ischemic stroke 10 years later, dementia 20 years after onset, and early death in the sixth decade, though clinical expression is quite variable.[32] Migraine with aura occurs in about one-fifth of patients. Ischemic subcortical events, either transient or permanent, appear in four-fifths. Dementia of subcortical type supervenes in 80% before death. Bipolar or monopolar mood disturbance occurs in one-fifth.

Neuroimaging studies disclose multiple small subcortical infarcts in basal ganglia and cerebral white matter and patchy or diffuse leukoaraiosis. Magnetic resonance changes often precede clinical symptoms, and the neuroimaging penetrance of CADASIL is virtually complete between ages 30 and 40 years. Pathological studies demonstrate a nonatherosclerotic, nonamyloid angiopathy mainly involving small cerebral arteries, with marked thickening of the arterial wall, eosinophilic deposits in the media, and reduplication of the internal elastic lamella.[33]

CADASIL is caused by mutations in the human *Notch3* gene at a locus on chromosome 19q12.[34] The *Notch3* gene is 5.6 kb in length with 34 exons. Products of the *Notch* gene family had previously been shown to be essential for proper embryonic development in insects, nematodes, and mammals, but actions in adult vasculature had not been identified. Proteins in the Notch family are transmembrane receptors whose extracellular domains contain many tandem repeats of an epidermal growth factor (EGF) motif, and intracellular domains contain six copies of the Cdc10/ankyrin motif. In 50 unrelated CADASIL families, 23 different missense mutations in the *Notch3* gene were identified.[34a] The mutations tend to cluster in exons 3 and 4, which encode the first five EGF repeats.

## MOYAMOYA

Moyamoya is an uncommon, chronic, occlusive intracranial vasculopathy characterized by progressive obliteration of the arteries about the circle of Willis. Stenoses typically initially involve the intracranial internal carotid arteries bilaterally and progress to encompass the middle and posterior cerebral arteries. An abnormal, dense network of small collateral channels develops at the base of the brain. Clinically, moyamoya has two modes of presentation, one in childhood generally during the first decade of life and the other in young adulthood with a peak onset during the third decade.

Children generally present with recurrent

cerebral ischemia, both TIAs and completed infarctions, sometimes provoked by valsalva or hyperventilation. Seizures are present in 5% to 10%. Cerebral hemorrhage occurs in only 5%. Adults typically present with hemorrhage, most commonly ganglionic, thalamic, or intraventricular. Fragile, abnormal collateral vessels are the presumed source of bleeding. Cerebral ischemia appears in 25%. Intracranial aneurysms are often associated with moyamoya, particularly in the posterior circulation, and may produce subarachnoid hemorrhage.

Pathologic studies of moyamoya show noninflammatory fibrocellular intimal and medial thinning of basal cerebral arteries and enhanced angiogenesis. The incidence of moyamoya is much higher in Japanese than in Western populations.

The cause of most cases of moyamoya is unknown. A genetic contribution is strongly suggested by familial clustering, with familial occurrences accounting for 6% to 9% of all cases. The incidence of moyamoya is 3% among siblings of a proband with the disease and 2.4% among offspring of an affected parent.[35] More than 14 pairs of monozygotic twins concordant for moyamoya have been reported.[35] An association of human leukocyte antigen B51 with moyamoya also supports a genetic etiology. Atypical moyamoya vascular changes are also known to occur with higher than expected frequency in several diseases that have a genetic basis, including Down syndrome, Williams' syndrome, Turner's syndrome, Ito's hypomelanosis, neurofibromatosis, tuberous sclerosis, pseudoxanthoma elasticum, retinitis pigmentosa, polycystic kidney disease, glycogen storage disease type 1, Fanconi's anemia, thalassemia, and sickle cell anemia.

## FIBROMUSCULAR DYSPLASIA

Fibromuscular Dysplasia (FMD) is an uncommon, systemic vasculopathy characterized by nonatherosclerotic abnormalities of smooth muscle and fibrous and elastic tissue in small- and medium-sized arteries. Cervical, renal, visceral, iliac, femoral, axillary, subclavian, and internal mammary arteries and the aorta may be affected. Cervicocephalic vessels are implicated in one-fourth of cases, the most frequent site after renal arteries. Cervicocephalic FMD most often presents as an incidental finding at angiography of irregularly spaced concentric narrowings, alternating with mural dilations, yielding a "string of pearls" appearance. The lumen caliber is usually reduced only mildly. Symptomatic presentations including TIAs or cerebral infarction, pulsatile tinnitus, Raeder's syndrome, dissection, saccular or giant aneurysms, and carotid-cavernous fistulas. Fibromuscular dysplasia accounts for 15% of internal carotid artery dissections, and saccular aneurysms have been reported in 20% to 50% of FMD patients. Pathological studies in FMD demonstrate smooth muscle hyperplasia, elastic fiber destruction, fibrous tissue proliferation, and arterial wall disorganization.

The etiology of FMD is unknown. A strong female predominance is noted, with women accounting for 85% of cerebrovascular FMD. Though a preponderance of cases appear sporadic, genetic factors are suggested by several reports of familial FMD and FMD in monozygotic twins.[36] Autosomal dominant inheritance with reduced penetrance in males has been suggested. Occurrence of FMD in patients with Ehlers-Danlos syndrome and Turner's syndrome has been noted.

## CERVICOCEPHALIC DISSECTIONS

Cervicocephalic dissections transpire when blood extrudes into the wall of an artery supplying the brain, producing an intramural hematoma.[37] When subintimal, the intramural hemorrhage bulges inward, narrowing the vessel lumen. When subadventitial, the intramural hematoma pushes outward, producing an arterial dilation (dissecting aneurysm). Exposure of flowing blood to thromboplastin and other highly thrombogenic tissue molecules in the vessel wall often precipitates vigorous local thrombus formation and distal embolization. Dissections account for 10% to 25% of ischemic strokes in young adults and probably 1% to 2% of all cerebral infarctions. The typical clinical presentation is of neck pain or headache, sometimes precipitated by minor trauma or intense physical activity, followed in a few hours or days by one or more episodes of cerebral ischemia.

Although most spontaneous dissections occur in healthy subjects, underlying arteriopathies account for a substantial proportion of patients. Fibromuscular dysplasia is present in 15% of cases and is especially frequent in patients with simultaneous, spontaneous dissection of multiple cervicocephalic arteries. Cervicocephalic dissections have been associated with several heritable connective tissue disorders, including Marfan's syndrome, Ehlers-Danlos syndrome types IV and VI, polycystic kidney disease, and osteogenesis imperfecta. An association has also been noted with autosomal dominant $\alpha_1$-antitrypsin deficiency.

Familial occurrence of cervicocephalic arterial dissections has been observed on at least five occasions.[38] In one case–control study, 18.2% of patients with carotid artery dissection had a family history of cervical artery dissection or cerebral aneurysm versus only 2.6% of controls.[38] Three of eight families in a Mayo Clinic series exhibited clustering of cervicocephalic arterial dissection, aortic dissection, and congenitally bicuspid aortic valves, and two of eight exhibited a syndrome of arterial dissection and multiple lentigines, suggesting an underlying developmental abnormality of the neural crest.[39]

## MARFAN SYNDROME

Marfan syndrome is an autosomal dominant, highly pleiotropic disorder of connective tissue. Skeletal, ocular, and cardiovascular abnormalities that are leading features include tall stature, long limbs and arachnodactyly, prognathism, high-arched palate, kyphoscoliosis, pectus excavatum or carinatum, joint hyperextensibility, myopia, ectopia lentis, aortic and mitral valve insufficiency, aortic root dilation, and aortic dissection. The most common neurovascular manifestation, developing in 10% to 20% of cases, is extension of aortic dissection into the common carotid and innominate arteries, producing cerebral ischemia, or into spinal artery ostia, producing spinal ischemia.[40] Isolated cervical internal carotid and vertebral artery dissections have also been described. Tortuosity and ectasia of cervical arteries is a common angiographic finding. Intracranial aneuryms have been frequently associated with Marfan syndrome. Most often noted are giant aneurysms arising from the cavernous carotid artery and presenting with mass effect, although subarachnoid hemorrhage from saccular aneurysms is also encountered.[40]

Mutations in the gene for fibrillin-1 *(FBN1)* are the cause of both familial and sporadic Marfan syndrome. Sporadic cases, due to new mutations in the paternal germline, account for 15% to 35% of cases and are associated with increasing paternal age. Fibrillin, a large glycoprotein, is one of the major components of microfibrils that provide structural support in multiple elastin-containing tissues, including the media of the aorta and other arteries. The fibrillin-1 gene lies in chromosome band 15q21.1. The gene contains 65 exons and covers 110 kb of genomic DNA. More than 125 mutations have been identified, including missense mutations clustering in EGF-like and TGF$\beta$-binding protein-like motifs, and stop codon and splice site mutations distributed over the entire gene.[41,41a]

## EHLERS-DANLOS SYNDROME

Ehlers-Danlos Syndrome (EDS) is a heterogenous collection of connective tissue disorders characterized by joint laxity, bruisability, fragile and hyperextensible skin, and dystrophic scarring. Eleven major types of EDS are presently recognized based on clinical, genetic, and biochemical criteria. Neurovascular complications are a leading feature of type IV EDS. Isolated reports also link types I and VI to cerebral aneurysms or cervicocephalic artery dissection. Common nonvascular clinical manifestations of autosomal dominant type IV EDS are translucent, fragile skin with normal extensibility, easy bruising, joint hypermobility, uterine and bowel rupture, pneumothorax, and a characteristic facies.

Vascular complications of EDS type IV include spontaneous rupture, dissection, or aneurysm formation of large- and medium-sized arteries throughout the body and friable, varicose veins. Average lifespan is 35 years, and arterial complications are the cause of death in a preponderance of cases. Leading neurovascular complications are carotid-cavernous fistula, intracranial aneurysm, and dissection.[40] Spontaneous carotid-cavernous fistula is probably the most common complication, typically arising in the third or fourth decade, from rupture of a cavernous-carotid artery aneurysm or less often from transmural dissection of the cavernous-carotid artery. Intracranial saccular aneurysms are also a common complication of EDS type IV and may present with subarachnoid hemorrhage. The most common aneurysm site is the cavernous-carotid artery, where they may present with ocular motor nerve palsies. Spontaneous dissections of the cervical carotid and vertebral arteries have been reported occasionally in type IV EDS. An additional commonly encountered angiographic finding is ectasia and tortuosity of cervical arteries, without overt aneurysm or dissection. Pathological examination of affected vessels in EDS type IV demonstrates disarrangement of collagen fibers and intimal fragmentation.

The molecular basis of EDS type IV is an abnormality in type III collagen, a major element of the extracellular matrix of distensible tissues, including blood vessels, skin, and hollow viscera. Type III procollagen consists of three pro-$\alpha_1$-chains, encoded by the *COL3A1* gene mapped to chromosome 2q24.3. More than 33 mutations in the *COL3A1* gene, producing qualitative or quantitative defects in type III collagen, have been recognized in patients with EDS type IV.[42]

## OSTEOGENESIS IMPERFECTA

Osteogenesis imperfecta (OI) is a group of generalized connective tissue disorders typified by bone fragility, bluish sclerae, short stature, and dentinogenesis imperfecta. Osteogenesis imperfecta is divided into four major types on the basis of clinical and genetic features. Cerebrovascular manifestations of OI have been reported infrequently, including multivessel cervicocephalic dissections and carotid-cavernous fistula.[40,43] Platybasia is common in OI and may mechanically compromise blood flow through the vertebral artery to produce posterior circulation ischemia. Abnormalities in type I collagen are the underlying molecular defect in OI. Type I procollagen is comprised of two pro-$\alpha_1$ (I) chains encoded by the *COL1A1* gene on chromosome 17 and one pro-$\alpha_2$ (I) chain encoded by the *COL1A2* gene on chromosome 7. Osteogenesis imperfecta type I is almost invariably associated with mutations in the *COL1A1* gene, while in OI types II to IV mutations in either *COL1A1* or *COL1A2* may be identified.

## POLYCYSTIC KIDNEY DISEASE

Polycystic kidney disease is characterized by multiple, bilateral renal cysts and occurs in autosomal dominant and autosomal recessive forms. Cerebrovascular complications have been described only in autosomal dominant polycystic kidney disease (ADPKD). In ADPKD, cysts may appear in many parts of the body in addition to the kidneys, including liver, spleen, pancreas, pineal gland, and subarachnoid space. Inguinal hernias, diverticulosis of the colon, and colonic rupture occur relatively commonly. Cardiovascular complications include mitral valve prolapse, aortic dissection, aortic root enlargement, aortic aneurysm, and coarctation of the aorta.

The most common neurovascular complication is saccular intracranial aneurysm.[40,44] Screening of asymptomatic ADPKD patients with magnetic resonance angiography reveals aneurysms in about 10%, and intracranial aneurysms are found in one-fourth of ADPKD patients at autopsy. ADPKD accounts for 2% to 8% of cases in series of intracranial aneurysms. An individual with ADPKD is more likely to be harboring an aneurysm if there is a family history of intracranial aneurysms and possibly if extensive polycystic liver disease is present. A male predominance among ADPKD patients with intracranial aneurysms is noted, and aneurysm rupture occurs at an earlier age than with sporadic cerebral aneurysms. Less common cerebrovascular complications include persistent fetal carotid-basilar anastomoses, moyamoya syndrome, arteriovenous malformations, cervicocephalic arterial dissection, and intracranial vascular ectasia. In patients with poorly controlled hypertension from renal impairment in ADPKD, intracerebral hemorrhage may occur. Intracranial aneurysms, however, appear primarily to result from an underlying connective tissue defect, not hypertensive disease.

ADPKD is one of the most common of all genetic diseases, with a prevalence of 1 in 400 to 1000. Approximately 85% to 90% of cases are due to defects in the *PKD1* gene on chromosome 16p13.3. *PKD1* is 52 kb in length and contains 46 exons.[45] It encodes a 4302/3 amino acid protein, designated polycystin. Its amino acid sequence suggests an integral membrane protein with many extracellular domains involved in cell–cell or cell–matrix interactions. Stop, frameshifting, and deletion mutations predominate among the first dozen *PKD1* mutations described. In families without *PKD1* abnormalities, a second gene for ADPKD has been identified, on chromosome 4, *PKD2,* that encodes a 968 amino acid protein with homologies to polycystin and to voltage-activated calcium channels.[46] The PKD1 locus is responsible for approximately 85% and the PKD2 locus for approximately 15% of cases of ADPKD.[46a]

## PSEUDOXANTHOMA ELASTICUM

Pseudoxanthoma elasticum (PXE) is a heterogenous group of disorders of elastic fibers in the skin, eyes, and arteries. General clinical manifestations include yellow, xanthoma-like papular, and reticulated skin lesions, retinal angioid streaks, lower extremity claudication, abdominal angina, and early onset hypertension. Early myocardial infarction is uncommon. The most frequent neurovascular manifestation is cerebral infarction due to premature carotid and vertebral artery stenosis or occlusion.[40] Both extracranial and intracranial vessels may be affected, with cerebral ischemia usually presenting in the fifth decade or later.

Pseudoxanthoma elasticum has been linked to intracranial aneurysms in several reports, with a predilection for the cavernous segment of the internal carotid artery. Occasional cases have been reported of congenital carotid hypoplasia with formation of rete mirabile, a dense network of anastomotic vessels between the intracranial internal carotid artery and the external carotid artery or the extracranial internal carotid artery. Cervical vertebral artery dissection in PXE has been noted at least once Pseudoxanthoma elasticum additionally may produce tortuosity and ectasia of cervical arteries without frank aneurysm formation.

The prevalence of PXE is around 1 per 100,000, and PXE is genetically heterogenous, with two autosomal dominant and two autosomal recessive types recognized. Vascular abnormalities appear to be more common in one of the autosomal dominant varieties. The basic genetic defect in PEX is unknown. Linkage mapping of both autosomal dominant and autosomal recessive varieties implicated a gene at chromosome 16p13.1.[46b]

## FABRY'S DISEASE

Fabry's disease, or angiokeratoma corporis diffusum, is a rare X-linked disorder of glycosphingolipid metabolism. Deficient activity of α-galactosidase A, a lysosomal hydrolase, leads to accumulation of glycosphingolipids in many visceral tissues, especially in lysosomes of the vascular endothelium. In classically affected hemizygous males, the major disease manifestations include angiokeratoma, acroparesthesias, and vascular disease of the heart, kidney, and brain, with early demise in adulthood. In a review of all 53 cases of cerebrovascular complications of Fabry's disease reported through 1996, Mitsias and Levine[47] found the average age of onset of cerebrovascular symptoms to be 34 years for hemizygous males (four-fifths of cases) and 40 years for heterozygous females (one-fifth of cases).

The predominant clinical and radiographic finding was dolichoectasia of the vertebrobasilar artery, attributed to vascular smooth muscle injury from glycosphingolipid deposition. Stenosis and occlusion of small penetrating intracranial arteries was also observed. Vertebrobasilar infarcts were common, reflecting stretching and distortion of stenotic vertebrobasilar branch vessels. Nonischemic, compressive complications of dolichoectatic intracranial arteries included hydrocephalus, optic atrophy, trigeminal neuralgia, and cranial nerve palsies. Multiple small, deep cerebral infarcts, large anterior circulation infarcts, and cerebral hemorrhage were additional modes of presentation.

The human α-galactosidase A gene is localized at Xq22. The 14 kb sequence contains seven exons and 12 intronic Alu repetitive elements. More than 25 varieties of molecular lesion producing classic Fabry's disease have been identified, including partial gene rearrangements, RNA processing defects, nonsense mutations, and missense mutations.[48] Atypical variants of Fabry's disease with reduced, but not absent, enzyme activity have been described that produce relatively isolated middle to late life hypertrophic cardiomyopathy. Prenatal diagnosis by assay of enzyme activity in amniocytes and chorionic villi is available.

## HEREDITARY HEMORRHAGIC TELANGIECTASIA

Hereditary hemorrhagic telangiectasia (HHT), or Rendu-Osler-Weber disease, is an autosomal dominant vascular dysplasia characterized by telangiectasias of the skin, mucous membranes, and viscera. The most common clinical manifestation is recurrent systemic hemorrhage, including melena, genital bleeding, and, especially, epistaxis. The most common neurovascular complications are due to pulmonary arteriovenous malformations, present in 15% to 25% of patients. Paradoxical embolization of clots, air, or septic material through pulmonary arteriovenous malformations produces TIAs or cerebral infarctions. Additional causes of cerebral ischemia in select patients are high-output cardiac failure due to hepatic or other visceral arteriovenous fistulas and polycythemia due to chronic pulmonary shunting. Central nervous system vascular malformations also occur with substantial frequency. In a review of 215 patients with neurologic complications of HHT, 25% had cerebral vascular malformations including cavernous angiomas and telangiectasias, 8% had spinal vascular malformations, and 3% had cerebral aneurysms.[49] Hereditary hemorrhagic telangiectasia occurs in 1 to 2 per 100,000, with a penetrance of 97% by age 40 years, and it is genetically heterogenous, with at least three causative genetic loci identified. The *ORW1* gene at chromosome 9q3 encodes endoglin and the *ORW2* gene on chromosome 12 encodes activin receptor–like kinase[50,51] Both protein products are members of the transforming growth factor-beta receptor family and are strongly expressed on endothelial cell surtaces.[51a] A third HHT gene is located on chromosome 3p22.

## DOWN SYNDROME

Ischemic stroke episodes are uncommon complications in Down syndrome, related to congenital heart disease, infections, and occasionally moyamoya vascular changes.[52] Cerebral hemorrhage occurs frequently in patients over age 40 years from cerebral amyloid angiopathy, a component of the accelerated Alzheimer-like brain changes universal in Down syndrome by the sixth decade.[53]

## NEUROFIBROMATOSIS

The genetics and leading neurologic manifestations of neurofibromatosis are reviewed in Chapter 9. Cerebrovascular complications occur in neurofibromatosis type 1 and include, in roughly descending order of frequency, stenosis or occlusion of the intracranial circulation, often with a moyamoya collateral pattern; extracranial carotid or vertebral aneurysms; cervical vessel arteriovenous fistulas; and intracranial saccular aneurysms.[40]

## STURGE-WEBER SYNDROME

Sturge-Weber syndrome is a neurocutaneous disease in which an angiomatous malformation involves the face, the choroid of the eye, and the leptomeninges. Cardinal features are a port-wine stain in the area of the trigeminal nerve and ipsilateral leptomeningeal angiomatosis. Characteristic neurologic manifestations are seizures, hemiparesis, mental retardation, cerebral hemiatrophy, and hemicalcification. Cerebrovascular complications are uncommon, but include recurrent venous occlusion with infarction in brain regions adjacent to leptomeningeal angiomas, recurrent arterial thrombotic episodes, arteriovenous malformations, and venous and dural sinus abnormalities.[54] Sturge-Weber syndrome is most often sporadic, but a few familial cases have been reported, without a defined dominant or recessive pattern of inheritance.

### OTHERS

Hereditary endotheliopathy with retinopathy, nephropathy, and stroke (HERNS) is a recently described autosomal dominant syndrome characterized by migraine, mood disorders, dementia, retinopathy, nephropathy, and multiple subcortical white matter strokes.[54a] Ultrastructural studies suggest systemic basement membrane abnormalities and generalized vascular endothelial dysfunction with disruption of the integrity of capillaries and arterioles.

Hereditary cerebroretinal vasculopathy is an earlier described, autosomal dominant disorder with similar clinical features, except for absence of nephropathy, and may or may not represent the same disorder.[54b]

Menke's disease (kinky-hair disease) is an X-linked recessive disorder of copper metabolism. In addition to other neurologic manifestations, there is a tendency to tortuosity and occlusion of cerebral and systemic arteries.

Bonnayan-Zonana syndrome is a rare, autosomal dominant condition with macrocephaly, lipomas, and hemangiomas of skin, viscera, and brain. Arteriovenous malformations and cerebral hemorrhage have been rarely reported.[55]

Kohlmeier-Degos disease (malignant atrophic papulosis) is a rare small- and medium-sized vessel proliferative–occlusive vasculopathy, producing skin, gastrointestinal, and cerebral infarcts. Familial clustering has been observed and an autosomal dominant mode of inheritance proposed.[56]

## Cardiac Disorders Producing Stroke

Mitral valve prolapse (MVP) is a putative risk factor for embolic stroke, though not fully substantiated by well-controlled, population-based studies.[57] Mitral valve prolapse is present in 5% to 10% of the population. For most cases of MVP as an isolated defect, both autosomal dominant and polygenic modes of inheritance have been suggested.[58] The rare condition of X-linked myxomatous valvular dystrophy has been mapped to chromosome Xq28.[58a] It may also appear as a component of other hereditable disorders, including EDS, Marfan syndrome, OI, Pseudoxanthromoelasticum Duchenne's and Becker's muscular dystrophies, von Willebrand's disease, and fragile-X syndrome.

A variety of cardiac conduction and rhythm disorders that may produce embolic stroke have a monogenetic basis (Table 21–3).[59] From 2% to 6% of sick sinus syndrome patients evidence an autosomal dominant

Table 21–3. **Selected Genetic Causes of Cardioembolic Stroke**

Cardiac valvulopathies
- Mitral valve prolapse
- X-linked myxomatous valvular dystrophy

Ventricular and atrial septal defects
- Holt-Oram syndrome
- Autosomal dominant atrioventricular septal defect
- Conotruncal anomaly face syndrome
- Down syndrome

Cardiomyopathies
- Autosomal dominant hypertrophic obstructive cardiomyopathy
- Autosomal dominant familial dilated cardiomyopathy
- Hereditary systemic amyloidoses
- Dystrophinopathies
  - Duchenne's muscular dystrophy
  - Becker's muscular dystrophy
  - X-linked dilated cardiomyopathy
- Emery-Dreifuss muscular dystrophy
- Limb-girdle muscular dystrophy
- Myotonic dystrophy
- Friedreich's ataxia
- Kearns-Sayre syndrome

Cardiac conduction and rhythm disorders
- Autosomal dominant sick sinus syndrome
- Familial atrioventricular node dysfunction
- Autosomal dominant atrial fibrillation

Intracardiac tumors
- Familial atrial myxoma
- Carney complex
- Tuberous sclerosis

inheritance pattern.[60] Rare syndromes of familial atrioventricular node dysfunction, producing atrioventricular block and sinus arrhythmias (including atrial fibrillation), have been described.[61] An autosomal dominant form of atrial fibrillation has been mapped to chromosome 10q22–24.[61a]

A number of mendelian disorders produce congenital ventricular and atrial septal defects that can cause cerebral infarction through paradoxical emboli, associated cardiac arrhythmias, and chronic polycythemia. These include Holt-Oram syndrome,[62,63] autosomal dominant atrioventicular septal defect,[64,64a] conotruncal anomaly face syndrome,[65] and Down syndrome.[66]

Many cardiomyopathies are inherited as single-gene disorders and can produce embolic stroke from mural thrombi adhering to abnormal myocardium or from associated arrhythmias. Hypertrophic obstructive cardiomyopathy, when isolated, is often inherited as an autosomal dominant disorder[41a,167] and may appear in larger genetic syndromes including glycogen storage diseases, Friedriech's ataxia, mitochondrial myopathies, and Turner's syndrome. The incidence of stroke is 0.6% yearly, higher if atrial fibrillation supervenes. The most common form of inherited dilated cardiomyopathy is autosomal dominant familial dilated cardiomyopathy, with disease-causing loci mapped to sites in chromosomes 1, 9 and 10.[67a] Several inherited neuromuscular disorders may be complicated by dilated cardiomyopathy and cardiac rhythm disturbances, leading to stroke, congestive heart failure, and sudden cardiac death.[68,68a] These disorders include Duchenne's and Becker's muscular dystrophies,[69,68a] Emery-Dreifuss muscular dystrophy,[68a,70] myotonic dystrophy,[68a] limb-girdle muscular dystrophy,[68a] Friedriech's ataxia, and Kearns-Sayre syndrome.[68a,71] X-linked dilated cardiomyopathy in some pedigrees has been shown to be an isolated cardiac phenotype of defects in the Duchenne's muscular dystrophy gene encoding dystrophin.[68a]

Intracardiac tumors are a rare cause of cerebral infarction. Left atrial myxomas, or right atrial myxomas with associated septal defects, can produce stroke by tumor or thrombus embolization. Although most atrial myxomas are sporadic, both autosomal dominant and autosomal recessive forms have been described.[72] Carney complex is the association of cardiac myxomas with lentiginosis, and in autosomal dominant form is often due to a mutation at chromosome 17q2.[72a] Cardiac rhabdomyomas develop in up to two-thirds of patients with tuberous sclerosis and may produce embolic cerebral infarction, albeit rarely.[73] Intracranial cerebral aneurysms have also been reported in tuberous sclerosis (see Chapter 9).

## Migraine

Migraine is an independent risk factor for stroke, especially in young women.[74] Familial clustering of migraine is well-known. Migraine is further discussed in Chapter 20.

## Vasculitis

Genetic predispositions likely contribute to autoimmune dysmodulation in most vasculitides. Many vasculitic syndromes affecting the cervicocephalic vasculature have been reported to exhibit familial clustering or other evidence of genetic factors. For example, Takayasu's arteritis has a strong predilection to appear in young Oriental women and is associated with HLA antigens Bw52 and Dw12. There are more than 20 reported cases of familial occurrence, including three concordant monozygotic twins.[75] In giant cell (temporal) arteritis, familial clustering has been reported, with siblings of patients having a tenfold increased incidence of disease over controls.[76] Additional cerebral vasculitides for which there is evidence of familial clustering or genetic factors include Wegener's granulomatosis, polyarteritis nodosa, systemic lupus erythematosus, X-linked lymphoproliferative syndrome, ulcerative colitis, and Crohn's disease.

## Hypercoagulable States

Although most of the hypercoagulable states are associated with an increased incidence of venous thrombosis, arterial throm-

Table 21–4. **Selected Genetic Causes of Hypercoagulable State and Cerbral Venous or Arterial Stroke**

Coagulation disorders
- Antithrombin III deficiency
- Protein C deficiency
- Protein S deficiency
- Resistance to activated protein C
- Prothrombin gene mutation
- Heparin cofactor II deficiency

Disorders of fibrinolysis
- Dysfibrinogenemia
- Fibrinogen polymorphism
- Plasminogen deficiency
- Plasminogen activator deficiency
- Factor XII (prekallikrein) deficiency
- Platelet Defects
  - GPIIIa polymorphism
  - Platelet-activating factor acetylhydrolase deficiency

Hemoglobinopathies
- Sickle cell anemia
- Sickle-C disease
- β-Thalassemia

Chronic myeloproliferative disorders
- Polycythemia vera
- Essential thrombocythemia

bosis has been observed as well. Genetic causes of hypercoagulable states are listed in Table 21–4.

## COAGULATION INHIBITION DEFECTS

Antithrombin III (AT-III) is a glycoprotein that acts as a natural anticoagulant by inhibiting thrombin and clotting factors IXa, Xa, Xia, and XIIa. Antithombin III deficiency may be acquired, as in liver disease or nephrotic syndrome, or inherited in an autosomal dominant fashion and results in venous and less often arterial thrombosis.[77,78] Neurovascular complications are uncommon, but more than 20 cases have been reported. Cerebral venous thrombosis is most frequent, and cerebral arterial thrombosis may also occur.[79] Treatment is with heparin, warfarin, or antithrombin concentrates. Functional and immunologic criteria divide AT-III deficiency into quantitative (type 1) and qualitative (type II) forms. Genetic defects in AT-III are present in 1 per 2000 to 5000 in the general population and account for about 5% of patients presenting with venous thrombosis. The gene coding for AT-III lies on chromosome 1q23–25, contains seven exons, and encodes a 432 amino acid protein that belongs to the serine proteinase inhibitor family.[80] More than 229 frameshift missense nensense and genedetetion mutations in the *AT3* gene have been characterized.[80a]

Protein C is a vitamin K–dependent glycoprotein that exerts a natural anticoagulant effect by forming a protein C/S complex that inactivates factors Va and VIIIa. Inheritance of protein C deficiency is autosomal dominant. Homozygosity may cause life-threatening thrombosis in neonates, purpura fulminans. Heterozygous protein C deficiency is present in 0.1% to 0.5% of the general population, in both quantitative (type I) and qualitative (type II) forms, and is responsible for 2% to 5% of cases of venous thrombosis. Most heterozygotes are symptom free, but, among those belonging to families with a history of symptomatic thrombosis, 50% will experience thrombotic complications.

Recurrent deep vein thrombosis and pulmonary embolism are the most common manifestations. In the cerebral vasculature, cerebral venous thrombosis is the most frequent presentation. Arterial cerebral infarction also occurs. Protein C deficiency accounted for 2% of arterial ischemic strokes among 311 patients across 8 young stroke series.[81] Treatment in symptomatic patients is with heparin or warfarin. Warfarin should be initiated at very low doses in conjunction with heparin to prevent skin and fat necrosis from transient initial prothrombotic effects.

The protein C gene maps to chromosome 2q13–14, spans 11 kb, and comprises of 9 exons.[80] More than 160 *PROC* gene mutations have been described, of which 67% are missense mutations, 7% splice site mutations, 5% nonsense mutations, and 4% frameshift deletions.[82] The large number of unique mutations suggests a high rate of *de novo* mutation in the protein C gene.

Protein S is a vitamin K–dependent glycoprotein that acts as a cofactor for activated protein C in the inactivation of factors

V and VIII.[77,78] Protein S deficiency is transmitted in an autosomal dominant fashion. Homozygotes may develop purpura fulminans shortly after birth. Deep venous thrombosis and pulmonary embolism are the most common general presentations in heterozygotes, and protein S deficiency is found in 5% to 10% of individuals under age 45 years with unexplained venous thrombosis. Protein S deficiency appears to affect the cerebral vasculature more frequently than protein C or AT-III deficiency. Cerebral venous thrombosis is the most frequent result, but arterial cerebral infarction also is seen. Protein S deficiency accounted for 12% of ischemic strokes in young adults in large series.[81] Anticoagulation with heparin or warfarin is recommended for symptomatic patients. To avoid the very rare complication of warfarin skin necrosis, warfarin should be introduced slowly with concomitant heparin. Protein S deficiency is classified into quantitative (type I) and qualitative (type II) forms. The gene for protein S, *PSα,* maps to chromosome 3, spans 80 kb, and encompasses 15 exons. Nearby on chromosome 3 lies a pseudogene, PSβ, that shows 97% homology with PSα coding sequences but no open reading frame.[80] More than 90 disease-causing mutations in the *PSα* gene have been identified, with point mutations predominating.[83]

First described only in 1993, resistance to activated protein C (APC) is a remarkably frequent cause of a prothrombotic state, five to ten times more common in young venous thrombosis patients than protein C, protein S, or AT-III deficiency. Resistance to APC is an important risk factor for cerebral venous thrombosis, present in 14% of 114 consecutive patients in three recent series.[84,84a] In patients with cerebral arterial thrombosis, the incidence is much lower, and findings conflict as to whether APC resistance constitutes a modest independent risk factor for infarction.[84b] In at least 90% of cases of APC resistance, the responsible defect is a single point mutation in the gene for factor V.[85] This mutation alters codon 506, resulting in substitution of arginine by glycine. This mutation has been christened the factor V Leiden gene mutation, reflecting the condition's first recognition in the Leiden population. The Leiden mutation renders factor Va resistant to APC-mediated inactivation. Resistance to APC is highly prevalent in the general population, present in 2% to 5% of individuals, and is inherited as an autosomal dominant trait. Homozygotes have an approximately 80-fold increased risk of thrombosis, and heterozygotes an 8- to 10-fold increased risk. Presumptive treatment with warfarin in stroke patients found to have APC resistance seems judicious, although data from large scale treatment studies is currently lacking.

Prothrombin, or factor II, is a vitamin K-dependent zymogen that is activated by factor Va to form thrombin, a serine protease. Thrombin plays numerous roles in the coagulation system, including platelet activation, activation of factors V, VIII, XI, and XIII, the conversion of fibrinogen to fibrin, and thrombomodulin modulation. The prothrombin gene is located on chromosome 11. A genetic polymorphism in the 3'-untranslated region of the prothrombin gene producing a G→A transition at nucleotide position 20210 is almost as common a cause of venous thrombosis as the factor V Leiden mutation. The G20210A prothrombin gene mutation is a frequent contributor to cerebral venous thrombosis. Among 85 patients with cerebral venous thrombosis in two recent series, the mutation was present in 14%.[85a,85b] Studies suggest that the G20210A prothrombin gene mutation may also be a risk factor for arterial cerebral infarction in young, but not middle-aged, individuals.[85c,85d] The G20210A prothrombin gene mutation appears frequently in Caucasian populations, but is virtually absent in non-Caucasian populations. Evolutionary population studies suggest a founder effect, with a single genetic origin arising from a mutational event 21,000–34,000 years ago.[85e]

Heparin cofactor II (HCII) is a plasma glycoprotein that inactivates thrombin. Heparin cofactor II deficiency is inherited as an autosomal dominant trait and is a rare cause of unexplained venous thrombosis.[77] The HCII gene is located on chromosome 22q11 and contains five exons. Association with cerebral ischemia has been reported rarely.[86]

Most individuals with dysfibrinogenemia, a hereditary disorder of fibrinogen production, are asymptomatic or exhibit a mild to moderate hemorrhagic disorder, reflecting a decreased tendency of abnormal fibrinogen to form fibrin clots. However, 10% to 20% of dysfibrinogenemias are associated with thrombosis due to increased thrombin levels resulting from defective binding of thrombin to fibrin and to resistance of clots composed of abnormal fibrin to tissue plasminogen activator–mediated fibrinolysis. More than 100 different dysfibrinogenemias have been characterized. Most of the scattered reports of stroke are in the setting of cerebral venous thrombosis, but large cerebral arterial thromboses in young individuals have also been noted. Dysfibrinogenemia is inherited in autosomal dominant fashion. Fibrinogen is a dimer of three pairs of peptides, encoded by three separate genes on chromosome 4. Several causative mutations in each gene have been identified.[87]

A large body of epidemiologic evidence links elevations in plasma fibrinogen to ischemic stroke, myocardial infarction, and peripheral vascular disease. Heritable factors account for 30%–50% of the variation in individual plasma fibrinogen level. Particular genetic polymorphisms in the β fibrinogen gene have been implicated in determination of individual plasma fibrinogen level and in thrombotic events. Among these, the G/A-455 polymorphism has been associated with ischemic stroke and the C/T-148 polymorphism with carotid atherosclerosis.[87a,87b]

Plasminogen is a plasma glycoprotein of molecular weight 90,000 that when converted into the serine protease plasmin performs fibrin clot digestion. Congenital plasminogen deficiency accounts for as many as 2% of cases of unexplained deep venous thrombosis in young patients. Hypoplasminogenemia occurs in both absent and dysfunctional forms.[77] Plasminogen deficiency is a rare cause of cerebral ischemia, more often venous thrombosis than arterial. Plasminogen deficiency was present in 0.5% of young arterial thrombosis ischemic stroke patients across five series.[81] The gene coding for plasminogen is localized on chromosome 6q26–27, and transmission is autosomal dominant.

More rarely reported inherited fibrinolytic defects predisposing to thrombosis that can affect the cerebral circulation include plasminogen activator deficiency and factor XII (prekallikrein) deficiency.[77]

The antiphospholipid antibody (aPL) syndrome is a thrombophilic disorder that causes both venous and arterial occlusions.[84] Antiphospholipid antibodies are detectable in 2% of normal individuals, at high titer in 0.2%. In contrast, aPL are found in 35% to 50% of systemic lupus erythematosus patients, approximately 10% of unselected ischemic stroke patients, and 25% to 50% of young stroke patients. One half of patients with the aPL syndrome have the disorder on a primary basis, and one half have secondary disease, appearing in the setting of lupus or lupus-like disease. The pathological hallmark of the aPL syndrome is noninflammatory thrombotic occlusion of small or large vessels, venous, arterial, or both. Unlike most other hypercoagulable states, arterial thrombosis is a major feature of the aPL syndrome, and cerebral infarct is the most common manifestation of arterial thrombosis. Treatment is with high-dose warfarin, with a target International Normalized Ratio of 3.0 to 4.0. The relative contributions of environmental and genetic factors to the aPL syndrome remains ill-defined. Evidence for a genetic predisposition includes familial clustering, especially in the setting of systemic lupus erythematosus, and concordance in monozygotic twins and triplets.[88] Modeling studies in familial aPL syndrome suggest a susceptibility gene is inherited in autosomal dominant fashion.[88a]

Platelet aggregation requires the binding of fibrinogen and von Willebrand factor to a receptor on the platelet surface consisting of two glycoproteins, GPIIb and GPIIIa. A common polymorphism on exon 3 of the GPIIIa results in a proline (P1A2) for leucine (P1A1) substitution in 16%–20% of individuals. The P1A2 polymorphism has been associated with early onset ischemic cerebral infarction and early onset myocardial ischemia in some, but not all, studies.[88b–88e]

Platelet-activating factor (PAF) is a phospholipid that causes platelet and leukocyte activation, vasodilation or vasoconstriction, and endothelial cell-blood cell interaction. Platelet-activating factor is inactivated by the enzyme platelet-activating factor acetylhydrolase. A missense mutation ($Val^{279}$→Phe) has been identified that causes PAF acetylhydrolase deficiency in Japanese populations. A recent case control study found that this mutation is a risk factor for non-cardioembolic cerebral infarction.[88f]

Hemoglobinopathies may lead to either thrombotic or hemorrhagic stroke. Hemoglobin variants that cause sickling of erythrocytes and hyperviscous sludging in microvasculature include HbSS (sickle cell anemia), HbSC (sickle-C disease), and HbSA (sickle cell trait). Sickle cell disease is inherited in an autosomal recessive fashion. Sickle cell disease is due to a point mutation in the beta hemoglobin gene on chromosome 11 and affects 0.3% to 8.0% of the world's black population. Strokes develop in 6% to 9% of patients with sickle cell anemia by age 20 years.[89] Cerebral infarction is most common, especially under age 15 years. Intracerebral and subarachnoid hemorrhage occurs more frequently in adults. In addition to microcirculatory derangements, large vessel occlusive disease is frequent, and a moyamoya-type angiographic pattern is occasionally seen. The anterior cortical arterial border zone is a favored site of infarction. Dural venous thrombosis also occurs. Prophylactic transfusions in patients with evidence of anterior circulation vasculopathy on transcranial Doppler ultrasound can prevent first stroke in children with sickle cell disease.[89a] Neurovascular manifestations occur less frequently in sickle-C disease. Several case reports link sickle cell trait to cerebral infarction, especially in settings of dehydration, severe hypoxia, and heat stress. Controlled epidemiological studies, however, have failed to identify HbSA as a major risk factor for stroke.

β-Thalassemia, a recessive trait, has been associated with cerebrovascular infarction, particularly in association with blood transfusions.[90]

Although most often an acquired disorder, polycythemia vera can occur on a familial basis, associated with mutant hemoglobins, enhanced erythropoietin production, or abnormal 2,3-diphosphoglycerate metabolism. Both autosomal dominant and autosomal recessive patterns have been noted. Stroke is not common in hereditary polycythemia, but has been reported.[72] Essential thrombocythemia may produce spontaneous thrombosis and/or hemorrhage involving arterial and venous circulations. The neurovascular manifestations are mainly ischemic and are likely mediated by qualitative proaggregrant platelet defects and hyperviscosity in small vessels. Though usually a nongenetic disorder, a familial form of thrombocytosis has been described, with cerebral ischemia as one manifestation.[91]

## METABOLIC DISORDERS

Mitochondrial encephalopathy, lactic acidosis, and stroke-like episodes (MELAS) is a mitochondrial disorder that, in addition to the features highlighted in its name, frequently exhibits exercise intolerance, a myopathy with ragged red fibers on modified Gomori's trichrome stain, and seizures. The stroke-like events are acute in onset, often transient, and occasionally associated with a febrile illness.[92] Neuroimaging demonstrates multiple areas of low attenuation on computed tomography (CT) and $T_2$ hyperintensity on magnetic resonance imaging (MRI) that do not correspond to major cerebral vascular territories and often are transient. Lesions favor temporoparietal and occipital cortices and subjacent white matter. Basal ganglia calcification and generalized atrophy are also seen. Cerebral angiography is generally normal or shows focal capillary blush or early venous filling in affected cortical regions. Cerebral blood flow studies have variously found diminished, normal, or increased flow to regions structurally abnormal on CT or MRI.

Pathologic examination demonstrates multiple cortical and subjacent subcortical ischemic regions, spongiform degeneration of cortex, and calcium deposition in capillary walls of globus pallidus. Endothelial and smooth muscle cells of pial arterioles and small arteries exhibit increased numbers of structurally abnormal mitochondria, and capillary lumens are narrowed due to endothelial hypertrophy. Competing theories for the pathogenesis of MELAS propose either a primary neuronal oxidative metabolic derangement or a primary mitochondrial cerebral angiopathy, with defective arteriolar autoregulation and capillary lumen compromise. Cardiomyopathy due to mitochondrial disease may contribute to stroke-like events in some cases. Treatment is with coenzyme Q and possibly idebenone.

The inheritance pattern for MELAS is maternal. At least eight responsible mtDNA point mutations and one microdeletion mutation have been identified to date, five in the transfer RNA for leucine, two in the transfer RNA for valine, and two in subunit III cytochrome oxidase.[93] The genetics of MELAS are further discussed in Chapter 15.

Rarely, stroke-like events have been reported in other mitochondrial diseases, including Leigh's disease and Kearns-Sayre syndrome.[72] Stroke or stroke-like episodes have also been infrequently reported in the autosomal recessive organic acidemias methylmalonic acidemia, proprionic acidemia, and isovaleric acidemia and in autosomal recessive sulfite oxidase deficiency.[72]

## CEREBRAL HEMORRHAGE

### Cerebrovascular Malformations

#### ARTERIOVENOUS MALFORMATIONS

Arteriovenous malformations (AVMs) are generally accepted to represent a disorder of embryogenesis, but evidence for a major genetic contribution is sparse. The incidence of familial clustering is surprisingly low, with only seven families, encompassing 15 affected individuals, reported through 1990.[94] Arteriovenous malformations are occasionally encountered in diverse larger genetic syndromes, including autosomal dominant polycystic kidney disease, HHT, Bannayan-Zonana syndrome, and Sturge-Weber syndrome. These disorders were reviewed earlier.

Spinal arteriovenous malformations are an occasional feature of Klippel-Trenaunay-Weber syndrome (angio-osteohypertrophy syndrome). This syndrome is a rare, congential angiodysplasia characterized by the triad of cutaneous hemangiomas, varicosities, and hemihypertrophy of bones and soft tissues. In addition to multiple spinal AVMs, less common cerebrovascular manifestations include cerebral AVMs, cerebral aneurysm, and carotid aplasia. Most cases Klippel-Trenaunay-Weber syndrome are sporadic, but familial occurrence has been described and multifactorial and paradominant modes of transmission proposed.[95]

#### CAVERNOUS ANGIOMAS

Cerebral cavernous angiomas are clusters of large vessels with a single layer of endothelium and little or no intervening neural parenchyma. Present in approximately 0.4% of all individuals, they account for 5% to 15% of cerebrovascular malformations. Clinical modes of presentation are seizures, hemorrhage, focal neurologic deficits, and headache. Cavernous angiomas occur in two forms: sporadic, generally producing a single, isolated lesion; and autosomal dominant, frequently producing multiple lesions.[96] The inherited form accounts for up to 50% of all cases of cavernous angioma. Familial cavernous angioma is genetically heterogenous, with at least three disease-causing loci. Linkage analysis mapped one familial cerebral cavernous angioma gene to a 15 cM region on chromosome 7q11–22.[97] A founder effect related to this mutation is responsible for the especially high frequency of familial cavernous angiomas in Mexican-American families.[98] In non-Hispanic Caucasian kindreds, additional cavernous angioma loci have been mapped to chromosome 7p13–15 and chromosome 3q25.2–27.[98a]

#### CAPILLARY TELANGIECTASIAS

Capillary telangiectasias are rare causes of cerebral hemorrhage. Autosomal dominant occurrence is a feature of HHT (Rendu-Osler-Weber disease), discussed earlier.

#### VON HIPPEL-LINDAU DISEASE

von Hippel-Lindau disease is an autosomal dominant disorder characterized by central nervous system hemangioblastomas and a variety of visceral tumors.[99] Stroke is a rare complication of von Hippel-Lindau disease. Ischemic stroke may occur secondary to polycythemia and is present in 5% to 20% of patients with cerebral hemangioblastomas. Hemorrhage may appear due to disruption of vessel integrity within a hemangioblastoma or to hypertension from an associated pheochromacytoma. von Hippel-Lindau disease is further discussed in Chapter 9.

### CEREBRAL ANEURYSMS

Several lines of evidence suggest a genetic contribution to cerebral aneurysms. Family occurrence has been documented in over 250 families, and large series indicate that 2% to 20% of cerebral aneurysms are familial. Concordance for cerebral aneuysms in monozygotic twins has been observed. In a segregation analysis of all kindreds reported through 1994, mode of inheritance could not be unequivocally established, although autosomal dominant and autosomal recessive models best fit available data.[100] In a population-based epidemiological study, first-degree relatives of individuals with aneuysmal subarachnoid hemorrhage had a fourfold increased risk of aneurysmal subarachnoid hemorrhage.[101] The incidence of aneurysms among first-degree relatives of index patients with aneurysms is about 9%.[102]

Familial intracranial aneurysms appear to have some characteristics different from those that are sporadic, including a tendency to rupture at a lower age, less frequent occurrence at the anterior cerebral artery complex, greater female predominance, and possibly a tendency to rupture at a smaller size. Within families, intracranial aneuryms often arise within the same arterial distribution and often rupture within the same decade of life. Cost–benefit analyses have yielded conflicting findings regarding the merits of screening for unruptured aneurysms with magnetic resonance angiography in individuals with a family history of cerebral aneuryms.[103a]

Cerebral aneurysms are a feature of several conditions with well-defined genetic origins. They are present in 10% to 25% of patients with polycystic kidney disease and in Ehlers-Danlos syndrome, Marfan syndrome, PXE, and neurofibromatosis, as discussed earlier. A link with $\alpha_1$-antitrypsin deficiency has also been suggested.[40]

Table 21–5. **Selected Genetic Causes of Hemostasis Abnormalities and Hemorrhagic Stroke**

| |
|---|
| Clotting factor deficiencies |
| Factor VIII deficiency (hemophilia A) |
| Factor IX deficiency (hemophilia B) |
| Factor V deficiency |
| Factor VII deficiency |
| Factor X deficiency |
| Factor XI deficiency |
| Factor XIII deficiency |
| Disorders of fibrinolysis |
| Dysfibrinogenemia |
| Afirinogenemia |
| Platelet–fibrinogen interaction defects |
| von Willebrand's disease, types 1–3 |
| Platelet defects |
| Glanzmann's thrombasthenia |
| Bernard-Soulier syndrome |

## Coagulation Disorders

Inherited causes for abnormal hemostasis with the potential for hemorrhagic stroke are listed in Table 21–5.

### HEMOPHILIA

The hemophilias are X-linked bleeding disorders resulting from a deficiency of factor VIII (hemophilia A, classic hemophilia) or factor IX (hemophilia B, Christmas disease). Spontaneous bleeding may occur into joints, muscles, and internal organs. Cerebral hemorrhage occurs in 2% to 8% of patients, most often under the age of 20 years.[104] Hemophilia A, the most common severe coagulopathy in humans, occurs in 1 to 2 per 10,000 births. The gene for factor VIII is located on chromosome Xq28, is 186 kb in length, and contains 26 exons.[105] Although more than 290 unique mutations of the factor VIII gene have been described, almost 50% of severe hemophilia A results from a major X chromosome inversion with one breakpoint situated within intron 22 or the factor VIII gene. The gene for factor IX is situated at Xq27, is 33.5 kb long, and contains 8 exons. More than 673 factor IX gene mutations have been described.

### ADDITIONAL COAGULAPATHIES

Other heritable coagulation disorders that have been associated with cerebral hemorrhage include factor V, VII, X, XI, and XIII deficiencies, afibrinogenemia, dysfibrinogenemia, and von Willebrand's disease.[72,106]

### PLATELET DISORDERS

A variety of uncommon, inherited defects of platelet number and function are associated with recurrent bleeding events, occasionally involving the cerebrum. These disorders include Glanzmann's thrombasthenia, due to an autosomal recessive defect in the GPIIa IIIb platelet fibrinogen receptor; and Bernard-Soulier syndrome, due to defects in the GpIb-IX-V receptor for von Willebrand's factor.[106]

## Cerebral Amyloid Angiopathy

Cerebral amyloid angiopathy (CAA) is characterized by the accumulation of amyloid in the media and adventitia of cortical and leptomeningeal medium and small arteries, arterioles, and veins and is responsible for up to 10% of nontraumatic brain hemorrhage. Cerebral amyloid angiopathy appears in brain aging and as a main pathological feature of Alzheimer's disease (including heritable familial Alzheimer's disease) and Down syndrome. Rare familial forms with distinctive clinical syndromes have been described. Most cases of CAA in the elderly occur sporadically. Some studies suggest a disease-modifying effect of ApoE alleles on sporadic CAA, with the $\varepsilon 4$ allele associated with more frequent and earlier onset lobar hemorrhage.[107,107a] A recent report similarly linked an intronic polymorphism in the presenilin-1 gene (a cause of familial AD) with increased severity of CAA in the elderly.[107b]

### HEREDITARY CEREBRAL HEMORRHAGE WITH AMYLOIDOSIS–DUTCH TYPE

Hereditary cerebral hemorrhage with amyloidosis–Dutch type (HCHWA-D) has been described in several families in two Netherlands coastal fishing villages, with an autosomal dominant inheritance pattern. Symptomatic onset is in the fourth to sixth decades. The most common clinical manifestation is intracerebral hemorrhage, often irregular in shape, situated in the parietal lobe, and exhibiting a tendency to gradual progression.[108] Recurrent hemorrhage is seen in one-third. Ischemic strokes occur in 13%, and leukoaraiosis is common. Cognitive deterioration often precedes strokes. As in sporadic CAA, the main component of vascular amyloid in HCWHA-D is amyloid β protein (Aβ). The genetic basis for HCHWA-D is a mutation in the β amyloid precursor protein gene located on chromosome 21. A G to C codon 693 point mutation causes amino acid substitution at residue 1852 of the β amyloid precursor protein and at corresponding residue 22 of the Aβ protein.[109] This mutations in the β amyloid precursor protein is distinct from those at codons 670/671 and 717 that cause early onset familial Alzheimer's disease. A point mutation at codon 692 has been identified in Flemish families that produces an intermediate syndrome with features of both HCHWA-D and Alzheimer's disease.[110] The incidence of *de novo* appearance of the HCHWA-D mutation in non-Dutch patients appears to be low.[111]

### HEREDITARY CEREBRAL HEMORRHAGE WITH AMYLOIDOSIS–ICELANDIC TYPE

Hereditary cerebral hemorrhage with amyloidosis–Icelandic type (HCWHA) is an autosomal dominant disease characterized by multiple cerebral hemorrhages, dementia, and death before age 50 years. Onset is typically in the third decade. Amyloid is actually deposited in various tissues throughout the body, but clinical symptomatology is primarily cerebral. The vascular amyloid in

HCHWA-I is composed of a fragment of cystatin C, a 120 amino acid serum protein found in all body fluids and tissues. (The term *hereditary cystatin C amyloid angiopathy* has been advanced as an alternative designation for HCHWA-I.) Cystatin C is a member of the cystatin protein superfamily of cysteine-protease inhibitors. The genetic substrate for HCHWA-I is an A for T point mutation at codon 68 in the gene for cystatin C on chromosome 20p11.[112] The same mutation has been identified in nine Icelandic families with 150 affected members, indicating a founder effect. Few *de novo* appearances of the mutation have been described.[113]

### FAMILIAL OCULO-LEPTOMENINGEAL AMYLOIDOSIS

Familial oculo-leptomeningeal amyloidosis is a unique form of extracerebral, leptomeningeal amyloidosis in which vascular amyloid composed of transthyretin appears in vitreous, retina, leptomeninges, and other organs, but not brain parenchymal vessels. A wide spectrum of clinical manifestations in North American and Japanese kindreds includes ischemic strokes, dementia, seizures, peripheral neuropathy, myelopathy, blindness, and deafness. Intracerebral hemorrhage is rare. Mutations in the transthyretin gene on chromosome 18 are responsible.

## DIAGNOSTIC EVALUATION FOR GENETIC ETIOLOGIES OF STROKE

Diagnostic evaluation for genetic etiologies of stroke is tailored to the individual clinical setting. It is not necessary to consider all causes for every patient. History taking should include detailed analysis of the patient's pedigree and consideration of whether the patient belongs to a national or ethnic population with increased incidence of particular candidate disorders. For many entities, physical examination will reveal cutaneous, skeletal, or ocular manifestations of dysmorphogenetic syndromes in which stroke may be a feature (Table 21–6).

Neuroimaging is mandatory for all patients being considered for genetic etiologies of stroke to exclude nonvascular causes of focal deficits and to establish the stroke type—arterial infarct, venous infarct, or cerebral hemorrhage. In arterial ischemic stroke, the differential diagnosis is then narrowed by investigation of the vascular system—cervicocephalic vessels and the heart—to further categorize stroke mechanism. Magnetic resonance angiography, carotid and transcranial ultrasonography, cerebral angiography, and transthoracic and transeophageal echocardiography are all useful modalities. Results of brain and vessel imaging permit assignment of stroke mechanism among the categories of atherosclerotic, nonatherosclerotic arteriopathic, cardioembolic, and hypercoagulable for ischemic strokes. Blood and urine screening for genetic causes of these mechanisms (see Tables 21–1 through 21–5) may then be undertaken.

## GENE THERAPY FOR CEREBROVASCULAR DISEASE: PRELIMINARY PROSPECTS

Advances in molecular vascular biology promise to transform stroke therapy as well as diagnosis. Potential therapeutic genes for major cerebrovascular pathophysiological processes are listed in Table 21–7. Highly efficient methods for genetic modification of the endothelium and other components of the vascular wall have been developed in experimental models, including catheter devices for local delivery of viral vectors to diseased vessel segments.[114,115] Gene transfer of potentially therapeutic vasoactive agents to blood vessels and neuroprotective agents to brain tissues has been accomplished in a variety of animal models of vascular disease.[116,116a,116b] A pilot clinical trial of gene therapy for familial hypercholesterolemia demonstrated prolonged reductions in LDL in three of five patients.[117] Pilot trials of vascular endothelial growth factor gene transfer in humans have shown improved collateral flow and reduced symp-

Table 21–6. **Distinctive Cutaneous, Skeletal, or Ocular Manifestations of Select Heritable Syndromes Causing Stroke**

| Syndrome | Physical Signs |
|---|---|
| Familial dyslipidemias | Xanthoma, xanthalasma |
| Tangier disease | Orange tonsils, hepatosplenomegaly, peripheral neuropathy |
| Homocystinuria | Dislocation of lenses, tall stature, thin body habitus, mental retardation |
| Cerebrotendinous xanthomatosis | Cataracts, xanthomas, bone fractures, cognitive deterioration |
| Progeria | Growth retardation, balding, loss of eyebrows, decreased subcutaneous fat, decreased joint mobility |
| Werner's syndrome | Cataracts, early gray hair, hair loss, hypogonadism, short stature |
| Marfan's syndrome | Tall stature, arachnodactyly, high-arched palate, joint hyperextensibility, ectopic lenses |
| Ehlers-Danlos type IV | Translucent skin, joint hypermobility, characteristic facial appearance |
| Osteogenesis imperfecta | Bluish sclerae, short stature, dentinogenesis imperfecta |
| Pseudoxanthoma elasticum | Pseudoxanthomas, retinal angioid streaks |
| Fabry's disease | Angiokeratoma, hyperhidrosis, corneal opacity |
| Hereditary hemorrhagic telangiectasia | Telangiectasias on skin and mucosal surfaces |
| Down syndrome | Epicanthic folds, simian crease, cryptorchidism, protruded tongue |
| Neurofibromatosis type 1 | Neurofibromas, café-au-lait spots, axillary freckling, Lisch nodules, scoliosis |
| Sturge-Weber syndrome | Facial angioma |
| Holt-Oram syndrome | Triphalangeal or absent thumb, foreshortened arm |
| Duchenne muscular dystrophy | Limb-girdle weakness, calf pseudohypertrophy, scoliosis |
| Myotonic dystrophy | Thin cheeks, inverted V-shaped upper lip, cataracts |
| Klippel-Trenauney-Weber syndrome | Cutaneous hemangiomas, varicosities, hemihypertrophy of bones and soft tissue |
| Hemophilia | Hemarthrosis |

toms in patients with myocardial and limb ischemia.[117a,117b]

## SUMMARY

The complex web of genetically determined physiological processes responsible for optimal function of the blood and cerebral vasculature is vulnerable to diverse pathogenetic mechanisms. More than[110] heritable disorders etiologic for cerebrovascular disease have been catalogued and classified in this chapter. Though individually uncommon, collectively these disorders account for a substantial proportion of strokes, particularly in the pediatric and young adult populations. Recognizing a genetic cause of stroke provides intellectual satisfaction to both patient and physician. More importantly, a genetic diagnosis has critical, practical implications—determining long-term prognosis, guiding selection of effective treatment to prevent recurrence, and allowing presymptomatic identification of family members at risk. The heritable entities reviewed in this chapter should be considered

Table 21–7. **Examples of Candidate Agents for Gene Therapy of Cerebrovascular Disease**

| Process | Gene Product |
|---|---|
| Ischemia | Angiogenic factors<br>Vascular endothelial growth factor<br>Fibroblast growth factor<br>Neuroprotectives<br>Superoxide dismutase<br>Heat shock protein<br>Interleukin-1 receptor antagonist protein<br>Antiaptotics<br>Protein bc 1-2 |
| Atherosclerotic plaque stabilization | Low-density lipoprotein receptor<br>High-density lipoprotein<br>Soluble vascular cell adhesion molecule 1 |
| Vasopasm | Vasodilators<br>Nitric oxide synthase<br>Calcitonin gene–related peptide |
| Restenosis | Dominant-negative growth factor receptors<br>Platelet-derived and fibroblast growth factors, ras<br>Cell replication inhibitors<br>Retinoblastoma, cyclins, p53<br>Growth inhibitors<br>Nitric oxide generators<br>Gene converting drug to toxic metabolite<br>HSV-tk + ganciclovir |
| Thrombosis | Thrombomodulin<br>Tissue plasminogen activator |

in the differential diagnosis of all patients presenting with otherwise cryptogenic stroke, familial stroke, and stroke at an early age.

## REFERENCES


1. Alberts MJ: Genetic aspects of cerebrovascular disease. Stroke 22:276–280, 1991.
2. Kiely DK, Wolf PA, Cupples A, Beiser AS, Myers R: Familial aggregation of stroke: The Framingham study. Stroke 24:1366–1371, 1993.
3. Wannamethee SG, Shaper AG, Ebrahim S: History of parental death from stroke or heart trouble and the risk of stroke in middle-aged men. Stroke 27: 1492–1498, 1996.

3a. Liao D, Myers R, Hunt S, et al.: Familial history of stroke and stroke risk. Stroke 28:1908–1912, 1997.

4. Brass LM, Isaacsohn JL, Merikangas KR, Robinette CD: A study of twins and stroke. Stroke 23:221–223, 1992.
5. Brass LM, Carrano D, Hartigan PM, Concato J, Page WF: Genetic risk for stroke: A follow-up study of the National Academy of Sciences/Veteran Administration twin registry. Neurology 46:A212, 1996.
6. Duggirala R, Villapando CG, O'Leary DH, Stern MP, Blangero J: Genetic basis of variation in carotid artery wall thickness. Stroke 27:833–837, 1996.
7. Kurtz TW: Genetics of essential hypertension. Am J Med 194:77–84, 1993.

7a. Svetkey LP, O'Riordan E, Conlon PJ, Emovon O: Genetics of hypertension. In Alberts MJ (ed): Genetics of Cerebrovascular Disease. Futura Publishing Company, Armonk, New York, 1999, pp.57–80.

7b. Auburger G: New genetic concepts and stroke prevention. Cerebrovasc Dis 8(suppl 5):28–32, 1998.

8. Corvol P, Michaud A, Soubrier F, Williams TA: Re-

cent advances in knowledge of the structure and function of the angiotensin I converting enzyme. J Hypertens 13(suppl 3):3–10, 1995.
9. Markus HS, Barley J, Lunt R, et al.: Angiotensin-converting enzyme gene deletion polymorphism: A new risk factor for stroke but not carotid atheroma. Stroke 26:1329–1333, 1995.
9a. Sharma P: Meta-analysis of the ACE gene in ischaemic stroke. J Neurol Neurosurg Psychiat 64: 227–230, 1998.
9b. Staessen JA, Wang JG, Ginocchio G, et al.: The deletion/insertion polymorphism of the angiotensin converting enzyme gene and cardiovascular-renal risk. J Hypertens 15:1579–1592, 1998.
9c. Takenaka K, Yamakawa H, Sakai H, et al.: Angiotensin I-converting enzyme gene polymorphism in intracranial aneurysm individuals. Neurol Res 20: 607–611, 1998.
10. Breslow JL, Dammerman M: Genetic determinants of myocardial infarction. In Longenecker JB, Kritchevsky D, Drezner MK (eds): Nutrition and Biotechnology in Heart Disease and Cancer. Plenum Press, New York, 1995, pp65–78.
11. Aitman TJ, Todd JA: Molecular genetics of diabetes mellitus. Baillieres Clin Endocrinol Metab 9:631–656, 1995.
12. Humphries SE, Peacock RE, Talmud PJ: The genetic determinants of plasma cholesterol and response to diet. Baillieres Clin Endocrinol Metab 9: 797–823, 1995.
12a. Graffagnino C: Molecular genetics of lipid metabolism. In Alberts MJ (ed): Genetics of Cerebrovascular Disease. Futura Publishing Company, Armonk, New York, 1999, pp81–115
13. Schaefer EJ, Genest JJ, Ordovas JM, Salem DN, Wilson PWF: Familial lipoprotein disorders and premature coronary artery disease. Atherosclerosis 108(suppl):41–54, 1994.
14. Breslow JL: Genetics of lipoprotein disorders. Circulation 87(suppl III):16–21, 1993.
15. Perla C, Sanchez R, Alfaro A, Gilsanz A, Dominguez F: Striatocapsular infarct in a young patients with heterozygous familial hypercholesterolemia and Klinefelter's syndrome. Med Clin 101:746–749, 1993.
16. Brown MS, Goldstein JL, Fredrickson DS: Familial type 3 hyperlipoproteinemia. In Stanbury JB, Wyngaarden JB, Frederickson DS, et al (eds): The Metabolic Basis of Inherited Disease, ed 5. McGraw-Hill, New York, 1983, pp655–671.
17. Knecht TP, Glass CK: The influence of molecular biology on our understanding of lipoprotein metabolism and the pathobiology of atherosclerosis. Adv Genet 32:141–198, 1995.
18. Pedro-Botet J, Serti M, Rubies-Prat J: Apolipoprotein Epolymorphism and ischemil cerebrovascular disease. Stroke 25:521, 1994.
18a. Frisoni GB, Calabresi L, Geroldi C, et al.: Apolipoprotein E espilon4 allele in Alzheimer's disease and vascular dementia. Dementia 5:240–242, 1994.
19. Jurgens G, Taddei-Peters WC, Koltringer P, et al.: Lipoprotein(a) serum concentration and Apolipoprotein(a) phenotype correlate with severity and presence of ischemic cerebrovascular disease. Stroke 26:1841–1848, 1995.
20. Cohen JC, Chiesa G, Hobbs HH: Sequence polymorphisms in the apolipoprotein(a) gene: Evidence for dissociation between apolipoprotein(a) size and plasma lipoprotein(a) levels. J Clin Invest 91:1630–1636, 1993.
20a. Schmidt H, Schmidt R, Niederkorn K, et al.:Paraoxonase PON1 polymorphism Leu-Met54 is associated with carotid atherosclerosis. Stroke 29:2043–2048, 1998.
21. Mudd SH, Skovby F, Levy HL, et al.: The natural history of homocystinuria due to cystathione β-synthetase deficiency. Am J Hum Genet 37:1–31, 1985.
22. Homocyst(e)ine and arterial occlusive diseases. J Intern Med 236:603–617, 1994.
23. Kluijtmans LAJ, Blom HJ, Boers GHJ, Van Oost BA, Trijbels FJM, Van den Heuvel LPWJ: Two novel missense mutations in the cystathione β-synthetase gene in homocystinuric patients. Hum Genet 96: 249–250, 1995.
24. Perry IJ, Refsum H, Morris RW, Ebrahim SB, Ueland PM, Shaper AG: Prospective study of serum total homocysteine concentration and risk of stroke in middle-aged British men. Lancet 346: 1395–1398, 1995.
25. Dudman NPB, Kim MH, Wang J, et al.: Thermolabile methylenetetrahydrofolate reductase causes mild hyperhomocyst(e)inemia in patients with vascular disease. Am J Hum Genet 52:899, 1993.
26. Frosst P, Blom HJ, Milos R, et al.: A candidate genetic risk factor for vascular disease: A common mutation in methylenetetrahydrofolate reductase. Nat Genet 10:111–113, 1995.
26a. Harmon DL, Doyle RM, Meleady R, et al.: Genetic analysis of the thermolabile variant of 5, 10-methylenetetrahydrofolate reductase as a risk factor for ischemic stroke. Arterioscler Thromb Vasc Biol 19:208–211, 1999.
26b. Morita H, Karihara H, Tsubaki S, et al.: Methylenetetrahydrofolate reductase gene polymorphism and ischemic stroke in Japanese. Arterioscler Thromb Vasc Biol 18:208–211, 1998.
27. Kuriyama M, Fujiyama J, Yoshidome H, et al.: Cerebrotendinous xanthomatosis: Clinical and biochemical study of 8 patients and review of the literature. J Neurol Sci 102:225–232, 1991.
28. Meiner V, Meiner Z, Reshef Z, Marais DA, Bjorkhem I, Leitersdorf E: Cerebrotendinous xanthomatosis: Molecular diagnosis enable pre-symptomatic detection of a treatable disease. Neurology 44:288–290, 1994.
29. Smith AS, Wiznitzer M, Karaman BA, Horwitz SJ, Lanzieri CF: MRA detection of vascular occlusion in a child with progeria. AJNR 14:441–443, 1993.
30. Yu CE, Oshima J, Fu YH, et al.: Positional cloning of the Werner's syndrome gene. Science 272:258–262, 1996.
31. Shvolin CL, Scott J: Inherited diseases of the vasculature. Annu Rev Physiol 58:483–507, 1996.
32. Charbriat H, Vahedi K, Iba-Zizen MT, et al.: Clinical spectrum of CADASIL: A study of 7 families. Lancet 346:934–939, 1995.
33. Baudrimont M, Dubas F, Joutel A, Tournier-Lasserve E, Bousser M-G: Autosomal dominant leukoencephalopathy and aubcortical ischemic stroke: A clinicopathologic study. Stroke 24:122–125, 1993.

34. Joutel A, Corpechot C, Ducros A, et al.: *Notch3* mutations in CADASIL, a hereditary adult-onset condition causing stroke and dementia. Nature 383: 707–710, 1996.
34a. Joutel A, Vahedi K, Corpechot C, et al.: Strong clustering and stereotyped nature of *Notch3* mutations in CADASIL patients. Lancet 350:1511–1515, 1997.
35. Houkin K, Tanaka N, Takahashi A, Kamiyama H, Abe H, Kajii N: Familial occurrence of moyamoya disease. Child Nerv Syst 10:421–425, 1994.
36. Ouchi Y, Tagawa H, Yamakado M, et al.: Clinical significance of cerebral aneurysm in renovascular hypertension due to fibromuscular dysplasia: Two cases in siblings. Angiology 40:581–588, 1989.
37. Saver JL, Easton JD: Dissections and trauma of cervicocerebral arteries. In Barnett HJM, Stein BM, Mohr JP, Yatsu FM (eds): Stroke: Pathophysiology, Diagnosis and Management, ed 3. Churchill Livingstone, New York, 1998, pp769–786.
38. Majamaa K, Portimojarvi H, Sotaniemi KA, Myllyla VV: Familial aggregation of cervical artery dissection and cerebral aneurysm. Stroke 25:1704–1705, 1994.
39. Familial aorto-cervicocephalic arterial dissections and congenitally bicuspid aortic valve. Stroke 26: 1935–1940, 1995.
40. Schievink WI, Michels VV, Piepgras DG: Neurovascular manifestations of heritable connective tissue disorders. Stroke 25:889–903, 1994.
41. Nijbroek G, Sood S, McIntosh I, et al.: Fifteen novel *FBN1* mutations causing Marfan syndrome detected by heteroduplex analysis of genomic amplicons. Am J Hum Genet 57:8–21, 1995.
41a. Maron BJ, Moller JH, Seidman CE, et al.: Impact of molecular diagnosis on contemporary diagnostic criteria for genetically transmitted cardiovascular diseases: Hypertrophic cardiomyopathy, long-QT syndrome, and Marfan syndrome. Circulation 98: 1460–1471, 1998.
42. Beighton P: The Ehlers-Danlos syndromes. In Beighton P (ed): McKusick's Heritable Disorders of Connective Tissue, ed 5. CV Mosby, St Louis, 1993, pp189–251.
42a. Schwarze U, Goldstein JA, Byers PH: Splicing defects in the Col3A1 gene: Marked preference for 5' (donor) splice-site mutations in patients with exon-skipping mutations and Ehlers-Danlos syndrome type IV. Am J Human Genetics 61:1276–1286, 1997.
43. Mayer SA, Rubin BS, Starman BJ, Byers PH: Spontaneous multivessel cervical artery dissection in a patient with a substitution of alanine for glycine (G13A) in the $\alpha1$(I) chain of type I collagen. Neurology 47:552–556, 1996.
44. Lozano AM, Leblanc R: Cerebral aneurysms and polycystic kidney disease: A critical review. Can J Neurol Sci 19:222–227, 1992.
45. Harris PC, Ward CJ, Peral B, Hughes J: Polycystic kidney disease, 1: Identification and analysis of the primary defect. J Am Soc Nephrol 6:1125–1133, 1995.
46. Mochizuki T, Wu G, Hayashi T, et al.: *PKD2,* a gene for polycystic kidney disease that encodes an integral membrane protein. Science 272: 1339–1342, 1996.
46a. Calvet JP: Molecular genetics of polycystic kidney disease. J Nephrol 11:24–34, 1998.
46b. Struk B, Neldner KH, Rao VS, St Jean P, Lindpaintner K: Mapping of both autosomal recessive and autosomal dominant variants of pseudoxanthoma elasticum to chromosome 16p13.1. Human Molecul Genet 6:1823–1828, 1997.
47. Mitsias P, Levine SR. Cerebrovascular complications of Fabry's disease. Ann Neurol 40:8–17, 1997.
48. Okumiya T, Ishii S, Kase R, Kamei S, Sakuraba H, Yoshiyuki S: α-Galactosidase gene mutations in Fabry disease: Heterogenous expressions of mutant enzyme proteins. Hum Genet 95:557–561, 1995.
49. Roman G, Fisher M, Perl DP, Poser CM: Neurological manifestations of hereditary hemorrhagic telangiectasia. Ann Neurol 4:130–144, 1978.
50. Haitjema T, Westermann CJ, Overtoom TT, et al.: Hereditary hemorrhagic telangiectasia (Osler-Weber-Rendu disease): New insights in pathogenesis, complications, and treatment. Arch Intern Med 156:714–719, 1996.
51. Johnson DW, Berg JN, Baldwin MA, et al.: Mutations in the activin receptor-like kinase 1 gene in hereditary hemorrhagic telangiectasia type 2. Nat Genet 13:189–195, 1996.
51a. Marchuk DA: Genetic abnormalities in hereditary hemorrhagic telangectasia. Curr Opin Hematol 5: 332–338, 1998.
52. Pearson E, Lenn NJ, Cail WS: Moyamoya and other cuases of stroke in patients with Down syndrome. Pediatr Neurol 1:174–179, 1985.
53. Hyman BT: Down syndrome and Alzheimer disease. Prog Clin Biol Res 379:123–142, 1992.
54. Love BB: Rare genetic disorders predisposing to stroke. In Biller J, Mathews KD, Love BB (eds): Stroke in Children and Young Adults. Butterworth-Heineman, Boston, 1994, pp147–164.
54a. Jen J, Cohen AH, Yue A, et al.: Hereditary endotheliopathy with retinopathy, nephropathy, and stroke (HERNS). Neurology 49:1322–1330, 1997.
54b. Gutmann DH, Fischbeck KH, Sergott RC: Hereditary retinal vasculopathy with cerebral white matter lesions. Am J Med Genet 34:217–220, 1989.
55. Miles JH, Zonana J, MacFarlane JP, et al.: Macrocephaly with hamartomas: Bannayan-Zonana syndrome. Am J Genet 19:225–234, 1984.
56. Blecic S, Bogousslavsky J: Kohlmeier-Degos disease (malignant atrophic papulosis). In Bogousslavsky J, Caplan L (eds): Stroke Syndromes. Cambridge University Press, Cambridge, MA, 1995, pp448–452.
57. Orencia AJ, Petty GW, Khandheria BK, et al.: Risk of stroke with mitral valve prolapse in population-based cohort study. Stroke 26:7–13, 1995.
58. Wilcken DEL: Genes, gender and geometry and the prolapsing mitral valve. Aust NZ J Med 22:556–561, 1992.
58a. Kyndt F, Schott J-J, Trochu J-N, et al.: Mapping of X-linked myxomatous valvular dystrophy to chromsome Xq28. Am J Hum Genet 62:627–632, 1998.
59. Gunteroth WG, Motulsky AG: Inherited primary disorders of cardiac rhythm and conduction. Prog Med Genet 5:381–402, 1983.
60. Lehmann H, Kelin UE: Familial sinus node dysfunction and autosomal dominant inheritance. Br Heart J 40:1314–1316, 1978.

61. Bharati S, Surawicz B, Vidaillet H, Lev M: Familial congenital sinus rhythm anomalies: Clinical and pathological correlations. Pac Clin Electrophysiol 15:1720–1729, 1992.
61a. Brugada R, Tapscott T, Czernuszewicz GZ, et al.: Identification of a genetic locus for familial atrial fibrillation. New Engl J Med 336:905–911, 1997.
62. Basson CT, Cowley GS, Solomon SD, et al.: The clinical and genetic spectrum of the Holt-Oram syndrome (heart-hand syndrome). N Engl J Med 330:885–891, 1994.
63. Li QY, Newbury-Ecob RA, Terrett JA, et al.: Holt-Oram syndrome is caused by mutations in TBX5, a member of the Brachyury (T) gene family. Nat Genet 1997;15:21–29.
64. Wilson L, Curtis A, Korenberg JR, et al.: A large, dominant pedigree of atrioventricular septal defect (ASVD): Exclusion from the Down syndrome critical region on chromosome 21. Am J Hum Genet 53:1262–1268, 1993.
64a. Benson DW, Sharkey A, Fatkin D, et al.: Reduced penetrance, variable expressivity, and genetic heterogeneity of familial atrial septal defects. Circulation 97:2043–2048, 1998.
65. Momma K, Kondo C, Matusoka R, Takao A: Cardiac anomalies associated with a chromosome 22q11 deletion in patients with conotruncal anomaly face syndrome. Am J Cardiol 78:591–594, 1996.
66. Hyett J, Moscoso G, Nicolaides K: Abnormalities of the heart and great arteries in first trimester chromosomally abnormal fetuses. Am J Med Genet 69: 207–216, 1997.
67. Watkins H: Multiple disease genes cause hypertrophic cardiomyopathy. Br Heart J 72(suppl):4–9, 1994.
67a. Mestroni L, Rocco C, Vatta M, et al. Advances in molecular genetics of dilated cardiomyopathy. Cardiol Clin 16:611–621, 1998.
68. Biller J, Ionasecu V, Zellweger H, et al.: Frequency of cerebral infarction in patients with inherited neuromuscular diseases. Stroke 18:805–807, 1987.
68a. Cox GF, Kunkel LM. Dystrophies and heart disease. Curr Opin Cardiol 12:329–343, 1997.
69. Nigro G, Comi L, Politano L, Bain R: The incidence and evolution of cardiomyopathy in Duchenne muscular dystrophy. Int J Cardiol 26:271–277, 1990.
70. Rakovec P, Zidar J, Sinkovec M, Zupan I, Brecelj A: Cardiac involvement in Emery-Dreifuss muscular dystrophy. PACE 18:1721–1724, 1995.
71. Provenzale J, VanLandingham K: Cerebral infarction associated with Kearns-Sayre syndrome-related cardiomyopathy. Neurology 46:826–828, 1996.
72. Natowicz M, Kelley RI: Mendelian etiologies of stroke. Ann Neurol 22:175–192, 1987.
72a. Casey M, Mah C, Merliss AD, et al.: Identification of a novel locus for familial cardiac myxomas and Carney complex. Circulation 98:2560–2566, 1998.
73. Roach ES: Neurocutaneous syndromes. Pediatr Neurol 39:591–620, 1992.
74. Chang CL, Donaghy M, Poulter N: Migraine and stroke in young women: (Ase-control study. Brit Med J 318:13–18, 1999.
75. Numano F: Hereditary factors of Takayasu arteritis. Heart Vessels 7(suppl): 68–72, 1992.
76. Wernick R, Davey M, Bonafede P: Familial giant cell arteritis. Report of an HLA-typed sibling pair and a review of the literature. Clin Exp Rheum 12: 63–66, 1994.
77. Bick RL, Pegram M: Syndromes of hypercoagulability and thrombosis: A review. Semin Thromb Hemost 20:109–132, 1994.
78. Schafer AI: Hypercoagulable states: Molecular genetics to clinical practice. Lancet 344:1739–1742, 1994.
79. Coull BM, Clark WM: Abnormalities of hemostasis in ischemic stroke. Med Clin North Am 77:77–94, 1993.
80. Aiach M, Gandrille S, Emmerich J: A review of mutations causing deficiencies of antithrombin, protein C, and protein S. Thromb Haemost 74:81–89, 1995.
80a. Lane DA, Bayston T, Olds RJ et al.: Antithrombin mutation database: Second (1997) update. Thromb Haemostasis 77:197–211, 1997.
81. Barinagarrementeria F, Cantu-Brito C, De La Pena A, Izaguirre R: Prothrombotic states in young people with idiopathic stroke. Stroke 25:287–290, 1994.
82. Reitsma PH, Bernardi F, Doig RG, et al.: Protein C deficiency: A database of mutations, 1995 update. Thromb Haemost 73:876–889, 1995.
83. Gandrille S, Borgel D, Ireland LT, et al.: Protein S deficiency: A database of mutations. Thromb Haemost 77:1201–1214, 1997.
84. Saver JL: Emerging risk factors for stroke: Patent foramen ovale, aortic arch atherosclerosis, antiphospholipid antibodies, and resistance to activated protein C. J Stroke Cerebrovasc Dis (in press), 1997.
84a. Ludemann P, Nabavi DG, Junker R, et al.: Factor V Leiden mutation is a risk factor for cerebral venous thrombosis: A case-control study of 55 patients. Stroke 29:2507–2510, 1998.
84b. Nabavi DG, Junker R, Wolff E, et al.: Prevalence of Factor V Leiden mutation in young adults with cerebral ischemia: a case-control study on 225 patients. J Neurol 245:653–658, 1998.
85. Dahlback B: New molecular insights into the genetics of thrombophilia. Thromb Haemost 74:139–148, 1995.
85a. Martinelli I, Sacchi E, Landi G, et al.: High risk of cerebral-vein thrombosis in carriers of a prothrombin-gene mutation and in users of oral contraceptives. N Engl J Med 338:1793–1797, 1998.
85b. Reuner KH, Ruf A, Grau A, et al.: Prothrombin gene G20210→A transition is a risk factor for cerebral venous thrombosis. Stroke 29:1764–1769, 1998.
85c. De Stefano V, Chiusolo P, Paciaroni K, et al.: Prothrombin G20210A mutant genotype is a risk factor for cerebrovascular ischemic disease in young patients. Blood 91:3562–3565, 1998.
85d. Ridker PM, Hennekens CH, Miletich JP: G20210A mutation in prothrombin gene and risk of myocardial infarction, stroke, and venous thrombosis in a large cohort of US men. Circulation 99:999–1004, 1999.
85e. Zivelin A, Rosenberg N, Faier S, et al.: A single genetic origin for the common prothrombotic G20210A polymorphism in the prothrombin gene. Blood 92:1119–1124, 1998.

Chapter 22

# GENETIC COUNSELING AND DNA TESTING

Thomas D. Bird, MD
Robin L. Bennett, MD



Genetic counseling is an important aspect of the management of every patient with a neurogenetic disorder. Such counseling may sometimes be relatively brief and uncomplicated. For example, a patient with isolated, well-documented, multiple sclerosis (MS) may inquire about the risk for MS in his or her children. A brief discussion of multifactorial inheritance and reference to an empiric table of risks for MS (indicating that the risk is about 2 to 3%) would be satisfactory.[1] On the other hand, many families with neurogenetic disorders raise complex issues that require detailed and time-consuming counseling by an experienced professional with knowledge of both the disease process and the genetic factors.[2–5]

It is often assumed that genetic counseling refers only to providing families with genetic risk estimates; however, it is really a process that includes aspects of both patient education and clinical practice (Table 22–1) The first step is to establish or confirm the correct diagnosis of the disease occurring in a given family. Giving detailed counseling for an incorrect diagnosis is obviously an error that the counselor must avoid. Even this initial step can be complex and time consuming, because diagnostic accuracy can often be confusing or problematic. We have seen hereditary ataxias mistaken for Huntington's disease (HD), leukodystrophies for MS, myotonic dystrophy for amyotrophic lateral sclerosis (ALS), and porphyria for lead poisoning.

Once the correct diagnosis has been established, genetic counseling then becomes an educational process related to providing information about both the genetic and clinical aspects of the disease. Family members are informed about their individual risks for inheriting the disease gene. The recurrence risks for the major patterns of inheritance are discussed in Chapter 1. Different family members may have different genetic risks based on the disease's pattern of inheritance, their gender, and their genetic relationship to affected persons. Autosomal dominant inheritance is usually straightforward, but autosomal recessive and X-linked inheritance patterns can be confusing and often require repetition and explanation from

Table 22–1. **Genetic Counseling: Process of and Areas to Consider**

Diagnosis
Education regarding
- Estimation of disease recurrence risks in other family members
- Variable expression
- Penetrance
- Natural history and prognosis

Need for further testing
- Of other family members
- DNA tests
- Other tests

Further genetic options
- Prenatal testing
- Adoption
- Artificial insemination

Referal to consultants
Support group information
Long-term follow-up

different perspectives. Diagrams and drawings of the various inheritance patterns often help. Demonstration of the inheritance possibilities step by step with the actual family pedigree or a hypothetical family pedigree can be most instructive. A detailed description of the construction and interpretation of medical family pedigrees is available.[5a]

*Variable expression* refers to the different clinical characteristics that may occur with the inheritance of a single disease gene. For example, tuberous sclerosis may cause mental retardation, seizures, skin changes, all of these, or any combination. The various possibilities need to be explained. The likelihood of each clinical possibility should be mentioned, as well as the influence of factors such as gender, age, diet, and drugs. It is often helpful to describe a severe clinical scenario, a mild scenario, and a typical or average scenario.

*Penetrance* refers to the proportion of gene carriers who express any clinical signs of a disease. Some disorders have a well-recognized decreased penetrance. For example, the most common form of autosomal dominant dystonia (DYT1) has only a 30 to 40% penetrance. This means that many family members who have inherited the mutation never show any signs of the disease, but may pass on the abnormal gene to their children. Also, penetrance is age and test dependent. For example, by age 20 years approximately 5% of individuals who have inherited the *HD* gene will show clinical symptoms. However, by age 65 years approximately 95% of *HD* gene carriers will develop clinical symptoms. In a similar fashion, the penetrance of a gene for inherited epilepsy may be "test dependent" in that a gene carrier may never have clinical seizures but may be identified by an abnormal electroencephalogram.

Family members will also want detailed information on natural history and prognosis. This requires considerable knowledge about the disease on the part of the counselor. This information is best provided by a specialist with experience caring for a variety of patients with the disease and with knowledge of the pertinent literature. Explaining the clinical characteristics and natural history of disorders such as familial ALS, HD, hereditary ataxias, muscular dystrophies, and Charcot-Marie-Tooth disease can be very time consuming.

Further testing of family members may be recommended or optional. This testing may be required for clarifying the precise diagnosis in an affected person or may represent genetic testing to determine if an asymptomatic person carries the mutation. The indications, time, place, cost, and implications of such testing need to be explained.

Alternatives for family planning need to be discussed with couples desiring children. These include alternatives such as prenatal genetic testing during the early stages of pregnancy, abortion, adoption, artificial insemination, and preimplantation diagnosis. These alternatives often raise ethical, social, and psychological issues that need to be discussed carefully and diplomatically.

The genetic counselor may wish to refer the patient or other family members to other physicians or consultants for special diagnostic studies or long-term follow-up. Some individuals with complex emotional or behavioral issues may require specific counseling by psychologists or psychiatrists. Additional tests such as neuroimaging, electromyography (EMG), skin biopsies, or blood tests may be necessary. Additional genetic counseling may also be required.

It is often valuable to provide families with the names and addresses of local and national support groups for their particular disease. Such groups often have meetings, conferences, newsletters, and web sites that provide helpful information, guidance, and support for families. The counselor should be familiar with the strengths, weaknesses, and general qualities of such organizations.

Finally, it is important to emphasize that genetic counseling is by nature and intent a family affair that almost always involves evaluations of, and discussion with, many family members. This often requires a change of pace and orientation for physicians who are used to being focused on single patients. A genetic diagnosis is like a stone dropped in a pool of water. Health care providers must deal with the ripple effect as more and more family members learn of their risks for the disease and seek advice and evaluation.

Because direct DNA diagnostic tests are now available for a wide range of neurogenetic disorders, the remainder of this chapter provides a detailed discussion of the risks and benefits of such genetic testing.

## USE OF DIRECT DNA DIAGNOSTIC TESTS

Recent advances in molecular biology have dramatically increased the number of neurologic diseases for which causative genes have been identified. Carriers of mutations within these genes can often now be recognized by means of simple, commercially available blood tests. This phenomenon has ushered in a new era in medicine where we are able to identify carriers of mutations for untreatable, degenerative, neurologic disorders decades before the onset of symptoms. Such testing has advantages and disadvantages that need to be carefully reviewed before DNA diagnostic testing is begun.[6]

## DIAGNOSIS

Diagnosis is obviously a critical factor in the practice of neurology, and direct DNA tests are sometimes used primarily for diagnosis. The tests may be highly specific and become the gold standard of diagnostic accuracy. In fact, the identification of disease mutations is making an important contribution to the actual definition of diseases. From a practical standpoint, if a patient with unexplained chorea has an abnormal CAG trinucleotide repeat expansion in the *HD* gene, then the patient has HD (see Chapter 13 for rare exceptions). Some persons with late onset, so-called senile chorea have been found to carry the *HD* mutation.[7–9] Similarly, if a patient with unexplained myotonia has a CTG expansion in the myotonic dystrophy gene, then the patient has myotonic dystrophy. The children of such individuals are at 50% risk for inheriting the disease gene. Note that if the DNA test results are negative (normal), the physician can continue a search for other causes of the chorea or myotonia. For example, there is a form of hereditary myotonia that is clinically very similar to myotonic dystrophy, but does not involve the myotonic dystrophy gene.[10]

It is important to recognize that identification of a mutation means that an individual carries the abnormal gene, but it does not necessarily mean that the individual has developed the disease, if *disease* is defined as presence of clinical symptoms and signs. This distinction needs to be carefully explained to persons contemplating genetic testing.

Furthermore, rare patients with a disease phenotype usually associated with a trinucleotide repeat expansion may actually have a point mutation or a small deletion within the gene and may not show the expansion. Such persons are unusual but have been reported.[11] Friedreich's ataxia is a special case in which a few patients have a repeat expansion in one gene and a point mutation in the other homologous gene, producing a compound heterozygote for this autosomal recessive disease[12] (see Chapter 12). www.geneclinics.org is a website relating genetic testing to diagnosis of many neurogenetic diseases.

## PROGNOSIS

An important consequence of accurate diagnosis is a better ability to predict clinical outcome (prognosis). This has important implications for future planning by the patient, the family, the physician, and the community. Such diagnostic differences may not be trivial. For example, the following conditions can be largely distinguished by DNA testing and have markedly different prognostic implications: HD versus benign familial chorea, myotonia congenita versus myotonic dystrophy, Duchenne's muscular dystrophy versus limb-girdle muscular dystrophy, Kennedy's spinal bulbar muscular atrophy versus familial ALS, and Friedreich's ataxia versus dominant spinocerebellar ataxias. The differential diagnosis of these conditions was much more difficult in the pre-DNA testing era.

## GENETIC COUNSELING

The new DNA tests provide the high level of diagnostic accuracy necessary for specific genetic counseling. For example, limb-girdle muscular dystrophy is a heterogeneous disorder that is often autosomal recessive. From 15% to 25% of persons with a previous diagnosis of limb-girdle dystrophy, however, have been discovered to actually have mutations in the Duchenne/Becker gene.[13] Such a finding dramatically changes the genetic counseling to that of an X-linked recessive disorder. Furthermore, female carriers of Duchenne/Becker dystrophy can now be identified with much greater accuracy with important implications for potential offspring. Another similar example is the ability of DNA testing to distinguish X-linked spinal bulbar muscular (SBMA) atrophy from some forms of autosomal dominant familial ALS. In families with SBMA, females are not affected and males cannot transmit the disease to sons. Neither of these statements is true for familial ALS. Specific genetic diagnosis also allows knowledge of penetrance rates to be discussed with family members.

## THE NEED TO KNOW

Patients at risk for autosomal dominant neurologic diseases often state that a major reason for requesting DNA testing is to relieve intense, daily anxiety. They believe that the known is easier to face than the unknown. Some persons at risk for HD have stated that they would prefer learning they had inherited the HD gene rather than spend the next several decades worrying about it. The test results also enable patients to focus on specific plans for the future, including finances, career options, travel, and family planning. Of course, obtaining a negative (normal) result allows individuals to "get on with the rest of their lives." Many persons see DNA testing as a lottery or gamble and have already "decided" they will be "winners" or "losers." It is important that they be clearly reminded of the actual risk.

## RELATIVE TEST COST

The direct DNA tests listed in Table 22–2 typically cost $200 to $800 each. Compared with the costs of computed tomography (CT), magnetic resonance imaging (MRI), and EMG, such tests appear to be relatively cost effective. In some instances they may save patients an evaluation with more expensive tests that are sometimes invasive.[14] In families with myotonic dystrophy, the DNA test may replace EMG and slit-lamp examination. In families with Charcot-Marie-Tooth disease, the DNA test may replace nerve conduction studies. In children with a myopathy, the DNA tests may sometimes replace the need for a muscle biopsy. Magnetic resonance imaging studies may not be necessary for patients with chorea who prove to have HD by DNA testing.

## FUTURE TREATMENT PROTOCOLS

Most neurogenetic disorders presently have no specific treatment. In the future, DNA testing may be able to identify persons eligible for treatment or prevention therapies extremely early in the disease process. For the present, with informed consent, such testing may allow patients to enter experimental treatment trials.

## PRESYMPTOMATIC TESTING

In some cases, direct DNA tests are able to identify carriers of disease genes many years

Table 22–2. **Examples of Neurogenetic Conditions Diagnosable by Commercially Available Direct DNA Mutational Analysis***

| Condition | Pattern of Inheritance | Mutation |
|---|---|---|
| Alzheimer disease, early onset, presenilin 1 | AD | PM |
| Amyloid polyneuropathy type 1 | AD | PM |
| Amyotrophic lateral sclerosis, familial | AD | PM |
| Charcot-Marie-Tooth (CMT) type 1A | AD | Dup |
| CMT Type 1B | AD | PM |
| CMT, X-linked | XLD | PM |
| Dentato-rubral-pallido-luysian atrophy (DRPLA) | AD | TNR |
| Duchenne/Becker muscular dystrophy | XLR | PM, Del |
| Dystonia, dominant (DYT1) | AD | Del |
| Fragile X, A | XLR | TNR |
| Fragile X, E | XLR | TNR |
| Friedreich's ataxia | AR | TNR |
| Gaucher's disease | AR | PM |
| Hereditary neuropathy with pressure palsies (HNPP) | AD | Del |
| Huntington's disease | AD | TNR |
| Kallman's syndrome | XLR | PM |
| Kearns-Sayre syndrome (KS) | MT | Del |
| Kennedy's disease (X-linked spinal bulbar muscular atrophy) | XLR | TNR |
| Leber's hereditary optic neuropathy (LHON) | MT | PM |
| Lesch-Nyhan syndrome | XLR | PM |
| Medium chain acyl-CoA dehydrogenase deficiency (MCAD) | AR | PM |
| Mitochondrial encephalopathy, lactic acidosis, stroke-like episodes (MELAS) | MT | PM |
| Multiple endocrine neoplasia (MEN) IIb | AD | PM |
| Myoclonic epilepsy, ragged-red fibers (MERRF) | MT | PM |
| Myotonic dystrophy | AD | TNR |
| Neurofibromatosis type 2 | AD | PM |
| NARP (neuropathy, ataxia, retinitis pigmentosa/Leigh's syndrome) | MT | PM |
| Ornithine transcarbamylase deficiency (OTC) | XLR | PM |
| Pelizaeus-Merzbacher disease | XLR | PM |
| Spinocerebellar ataxias (types 1, 2, 3, 6, 7) | AD | TNR |
| Tay-Sach's disease | AR | PM |
| von Hippel-Lindau disease | AD | PM |

*Some disorders, such as Prader-Willi and Angelman's syndromes and Miller-Dieker lissencephaly, are associated with chromosome microdeletions that can be identified by FISH (fluorescence *in site* hydridization). AD = autosomal dominant; AR = autosomal recessive; TNR = trinucleotide repeat; XLR = X-linked recessive; XLD = X-linked dominant; MT = mitochondrial inheritance; PM = point mutation(s); Dup = duplication; Del = deletion.

before the development of clinical symptoms. For example, approximately 10% of HD patients do not develop symptoms until after the age of 60 years. A positive DNA test in such an individual at age 20 years is compatible with a 40-year latency period that could include a full and productive life. For some disorders there is a rough correlation between the length of a trinucleotide repeat expansion and age of onset, but in general these DNA tests are not useful in predicting age of onset, type of symptoms, or rate of progression.[14a]

Unfortunately, then, the test result may

exchange previous anxiety over the unknown for future anxiety regarding the dreaded onset of first symptoms with no effective treatment. Depression may be initiated or worsened. Suicide is a real but generally small risk.[15, 16, 16a] There may be subtle discrimination on the part of relatives, friends, and colleagues who learn the test results.

Surprisingly, some individuals given negative results may not be as happy as anticipated. Some suffer survivor guilt, and others are disappointed that their life is not somehow magically better. A few may lose a previously assumed explanation for their symptoms and feel at a loss to understand their persistent health problems. Initial results with DNA testing for HD show that individuals with both positive and negative results handle the information reasonably well and are able to carry on.[17] However, more longitudinal studies are required before we really understand the full, long-term psychosocial implications of this testing.[17a]

A distinction should be made between using a DNA test to establish a diagnosis in an unequivocally symptomatic patient and providing testing for an asymptomatic person at risk. The former is a diagnostic test like many others (albeit highly specific) that should be performed with the knowledge of the genetic implications. The latter "presymptomatic" situation requires careful pretest and post-test counseling that adheres to guidelines followed in experienced genetic counseling centers.[3,5,18,19]

A further important point is documentation of the presumed disease mutation in an affected family member. We have encountered individuals seeking presymptomatic DNA testing for HD and myotonic dystrophy only to discover later that affected relatives have negative DNA tests for these diseases, documenting that the families actually have some other neurogenetic disorders. Without this further information, negative DNA test results in the person initially seeking testing would have falsely suggested that they were not at risk for the family disease. This is another example of the critical importance of accurate diagnosis in genetic counseling and the role DNA testing can play in this process.

## INSURANCE AND EMPLOYMENT DISCRIMINATION

There is a legitimate concern that DNA testing may produce genetic social outcasts and that individuals testing positive for neurologic disease mutations will be denied health, life, or disability insurance and employment opportunities.[19–24] This is part of the "preexisting condition" debate regarding health insurance reform. These issues need to be faced squarely and dealt with by appropriate policies and regulations.

On the other hand, we have seen individuals whose positive DNA testing has allowed them to receive medical leave, work benefits, and pensions or job reclassification rather than being fired for "incompetence." Present regulations vary considerably on a state-to-state basis. In general, patients should be advised to obtain insurance prior to genetic testing. Many people personally pay for testing without billing insurance, but this does not necessarily prevent ultimate access to the results by third parties. Completely "anonymous" testing is also a controversial topic that seems to protect the patient, but it is fraught with potential problems, including lack of disease confirmation in the family and difficulty of follow-up.[25,26] Genetic testing is different from human immuno deficiency virus testing because DNA testing has hereditary but not infectious implications.

## PRENATAL DIAGNOSIS

Through amniocentesis and chorionic villus sampling, DNA tests can be performed on tissues from the unborn fetus. Because there are no treatments for most of the diseases that can be tested, the couple must decide whether they wish to have an abortion if the prenatal test is positive. This is clearly not a simple or easy decision for most families, and it is even more difficult if symptoms may not develop for many decades after birth. If the fetus has a positive test and the pregnancy is continued, one then faces the issues of testing a presymptomatic minor (see later). Prenatal diagnosis has been reported for HD.[27]

## TESTING OF CHILDREN

Most genetic centers will not perform DNA tests for adult-onset diseases on asymptomatic children prior to the age of 18 years, when they become legal adults. This is based on issues of autonomy and the desire for individuals to choose for themselves whether and when they want such testing.[28–31] Asymptomatic children with positive DNA tests may experience a self-fulfilling prophecy in which any physical or behavioral problem is assumed to be a result of carrying a genetic mutation. They may be treated differently by parents, siblings, other relatives, peers, or teachers. Many parents, however, feel strongly that the testing of their children is a purely parental decision. Three arguments in favor of waiting until adulthood for such testing are *(1)* no treatments are presently available for many of these disorders, *(2)* not all rational adults will choose to know their genetic status, and *(3)* children are considered entitled to an open future.[30,31]

There are legitimate reasons to test children who are *symptomatic* and in whom a genetic disease is part of the differential diagnosis. It is often appropriate to confirm the diagnosis with DNA testing, which may save considerable time, effort, and money relative to more traditional but less specific testing.[32] Our clinic has used DNA testing on many occasions to confirm the diagnosis in *symptomatic* children at risk for HD, myotonic dystrophy, Charcot-Marie-Tooth disease, Duchenne's muscular dystrophy, and mitochondrial myopathies. It is important to note that a *negative* DNA test for myotonic dystrophy has been especially useful in directing neurologists to continue further diagnostic evaluation of infants and children with unexplained myopathy. Also, in most states, any pregnant girl below age 18 years is considered an emancipated minor and is legally able to make medical decisions unencumbered by the desire of her parents. For example, we have seen a pregnant 14-year-old girl whose mother had HD. Her mother was demanding prenatal diagnosis for the unborn fetus, but the daughter disagreed and was uncertain about what course to take. Such unanticipated complexities of DNA testing are difficult challenges without easy solutions. In this case, the daughter (legally considered an adult because of her pregnancy) eventually decided to have an abortion without DNA testing.

## ADOPTION

Adoption agencies or potential adopting parents may wish to pursue DNA testing if some positive history of a genetic neurologic disorder is known in a child's family. Most medical centers decline to do such presymptomatic testing because of the issues noted earlier regarding the testing of children and the added fact that a positive test may render the child unadoptable.[28, 33] Such policies sometimes conflict with a parent's "right to know" and often need to be negotiated on an individual basis.

Another delayed aspect of this theme is becoming more common as it becomes easier for adults who were adopted as children to discover their biological parents. For example, Oregon has recently approved greater access to adoption records. Some persons are finding that they are at risk for genetic diseases for which there are DNA tests and seek genetic counseling and testing. We have been consulted by adopted adults who have recently discovered that members of their biological families have HD.

## COERCED TESTING

Prisons, courts of law, and military services may all request DNA testing for various reasons. Our clinic has experienced each of these organizations requesting evaluations of persons at risk for HD who had *(1)* committed various felonies, including murder; *(2)* requested reenlistment in the army; or *(3)* were engaged in divorce and child-custody litigation. Informed consent and appropriate legal advice are of particular importance in such situations.

It is important to determine who is asking for the genetic testing and what is the purpose of the testing. Both the autonomy and the privacy of patients must be protected within the law. It is important that attorneys, courts, and institutions understand many of the issues discussed earlier, especially the difference between a positive test and having a "disease," and the fact that most test results do not predict onset, severity, or type of symptoms. A not uncommon question is whether a person found to carry a disease gene will have symptoms or a decreased lifespan that will adversely impact the raising of children. Another issue may be whether carrying a gene for a genetic neurologic disorder influenced a criminal act involving loss of inhibition, violence, or poor judgment. Obviously, a positive DNA test is only one aspect of such complex and sometimes contentious questions.

## TWENTY-FIVE PERCENT RISK

Asymptomatic grandchildren of individuals with autosomal dominant disorders may request DNA testing. Such grandchildren are at 25% risk for inheriting the abnormal gene, that is, half the risk of their parent (who is at 50% risk). If the grandchild has a positive test, one has automatically and inadvertently also established that the child's parent is a carrier of the disease mutation.

As a general rule, such testing should not be done without the knowledge and consent of the intervening parent. Attempts should be made for a mutually agreeable family strategy toward testing. What if the whereabouts of the intervening parent are completely unknown or that person adamantly refuses involvement? What then is our obligation to the person at 25% risk requesting the test? There are sometimes no clear answers, and clinical judgment with legal and ethical advice must be used. Such questions are usually resolved in favor of the person requesting the test, based on the principle of each patient's "right to know." It should always be clarified before testing who will and who will not be informed of the test results.

## FALSE PATERNITY

Persons with an autosomal dominant disease newly diagnosed by DNA testing may sometimes have a negative family history. Occasionally, the family history is discovered to be positive on closer examination of the family. Sometimes the individual proves to be a true new mutation. New dominant mutations are being discovered for several disorders, including HD and the hereditary neuropathies. Some affected persons with a negative family history, however, are the results of false paternity and their true, but unknown, biological fathers carried the disease gene. Physicians should be aware of this possibility when DNA testing extends to additional family members.

## GENE DISCOVERY/DIAGNOSTIC TEST LAG TIME

The discovery of disease genes is advancing rapidly. (Examples of direct DNA tests for neurogenetic disorders are listed in Table 22–2.) The application of these discoveries to commercial DNA testing is occurring at a slower pace. In most cases, laboratories need many months or years of development time for confirmation of initial research results, testing of adequate controls, and refinement of techniques. Furthermore, many disorders are quite rare, and commercial testing for them is not economically justified (there are orphan tests just as there are orphan drugs). This delay in test availability can be very frustrating for families and physicians who know that the disease mutations have been found and that testing is technically possible but practically difficult. This situation can also place undue pressure on research laboratories and may blur the distinction between research and clinical testing. Examples of such orphan DNA tests presently include those for familial Alzheimer's disease with mutations in the amyloid precursor protein and presenilin 2 genes and some rare forms of hereditary neuropathies and muscular dystrophies.

In addition, many genes have a large number of slightly different mutations within them, all of which can result in clinical disease (allelic heterogeneity). It is sometimes economically and technically too burdensome to assay each individual patient for all possible mutations. Thus, direct DNA tests are not commercially available for some disorders such as neurofibromatosis type 1 and acute intermittent porphyria, even though the genes and mutations within them are known. In other instances, the established enzyme and metabolic assays are economical and accurate, and DNA tests are not required (e.g., for Tay-Sachs, $GM_2$-gangliosidosis, and phenylketonuria).

Finally, long-term banking of DNA samples is advisable for individuals affected with a genetic disorder for which there is presently no diagnostic DNA test. Such samples may prove to be highly valuable for genetic counseling of family members in the future. Local laboratories and medical school medical genetics departments can provide such information.

## SUMMARY

Genetic counseling is a complex process that involves diagnosis and education of family members regarding issues such as prognosis, recurrence risks, variable expression, and future alternatives. Genetic tests for neurologic disorders have been available for many years. The new direct DNA tests, however, are a double-edged sword with implications we have not learned to anticipate completely. On the one hand, they provide a startling degree of diagnostic accuracy with all of the associated benefits of prognosis, genetic counseling, relative economy, relief from anxiety, and ability to plan for the future. On the other hand, they raise ethical, legal, social, and procedural issues that may have no simple solutions and may increase anxiety, hardship, and depression for the patients. Thus, as with all testing in medicine, the decision to do DNA diagnostic testing must be made on an individual basis and in the full context of the patient's life. Education of the physician followed by education of and full disclosure of the issues to the patient and consultation with knowledgeable colleagues will lead to the best decisions in most cases. Hopefully, as in the past, our expertise will improve with experience.

## ADDENDUM

The current availability of DNA diagnostic tests can be obtained from *Genetests*, Children's Hospital and Medical Center, Box 5371, 4800 Sand Point Way NE, Seattle, WA 98105-0371; tel: (206)528-2689; fax: (206) 528-2687; web site: >www.genetests.org<. Portions of this chapter have appeared previously.[6]

## REFERENCES


1. Ebers GC, Sadovnick AD, Risch, et al.: A genetic basis for familial aggregation in multiple sclerosis. Nature 377: 150–151, 1995.
2. Huggins M, Block M, Kanani S, et al.: Ethical and legal dilemmas arising during predictive testing for adult-onset disease: The experience of Huntington disease. Am J Hum Genet 47: 4–12, 1990.
3. Quaid KA: Presymtomatic testing for Huntington disease: Recommendations for counseling. J Genet Counseling 1: 277–302, 1992.
4. Craufurd D, Tyler A: Predictive testing for Huntington's disease: Protocol of the UK Huntington's prediction consortium. J Med Genet 29: 915–198, 1992.
5. Bennett RK, Bird TD, Teri L: Offering predictive testing for Huntington disease in a medical genetics clinic: Practical applications. J Genet Counseling 2: 123–137, 1993.

5a. Bennett RL: The Practical Guide to the Genetic Family History, Wiley-Liss, New York, 1999.

6. Bird TD, Bennett R: Why do DNA testing? Practical and ethical implications of new neurogenetic tests. Ann Neurol 38: 141–146, 1995.
7. Davis MB, Bateman D, Quinn NP, et al.: Mutation analysis in patients with possible but apparently sporadic Huntington's disease. Lancet 344: 714–718, 1994.
8. Britton JW, Uitti RJ, Ahlskog JE, Robinson RG, Kremer B, Hayden MR: Hereditary late-onset chorea without significant dementia: Genetic evidence for substantial phenotypic variation in Huntington's disease. Neurology 45: 443–447, 1995.
9. Nance MA, Westphal B, Nugent S: Diagnosis of patients presenting to a Huntington disease (HD) clinic without a family history of HD. Neurology 47: 1578–1580, 1996.
10. Ricker K, Koch MC, Lehmann-Horn, et al.: Proximal myotonic myopathy: An new dominant disorder with myotonia, muscle weakness, and cataracts. Neurology 441: 1448–1452, 1994.
11. De Boulle K, Verkerk AJMH, Reyniers E, et al.: A point mutation in the *FMR-1* gene associated with fragile X mental retardation. Nat Genet 3: 31–35, 1993.
12. Bidichandani SI, Ashizawa T, Patel PI: Atypical Friedreich ataxia caused by compound heterozygosity for a novel missense mutation and the GAA triplet-repeat expansion. Am J Hum Genet 60: 1251–1256, 1997.
13. Norman A, Coakley J, Thomas N, Harper P: Distinction of Becker from limb-girdle muscular dystrophy by means of dystrophin cDNA probes. Lancet, March 4, pp466–488, 1989.
14. Noorani HZ, Khan HN, Gallie, Detsky AS: Cost comparison of molecular versus conventional

screening of relatives at risk for retinoblastoma. Am J Hum Genet 59: 301–307, 1996.
14a. Brinkman RR, Mezei MM, Theilmann J, et al.: The likelihood of being affected with Huntington disease by a particular age, for a specific CAG size. Am J Hum Genet 60: 1202–1210, 1997.
15. Lipe H, Schultz A, Bird TD: Risk factors for suicide in Huntington's disease: A retrospective case controlled study. Am J Med Genet 48: 231–233, 1993.
16. Wiggins S, White P, Huggins, M, et al.: The psychological consequences of predictive testing for Huntington's disease. N Engl J Med 327: 1401–1405, 1992.
16a. Almquist EW, Bloch M, Brinkman R, et al.: A worldwide assessment of the frequency of suicide, suicide attempts or psychiatric hospitalization after predictive testing for Huntington disease. Am J Hum Genet 64: 1293–1304, 1999.
17. Huggins M. Bloch M, Kanani S, et al.: Ethical and legal dilemmas arising during predictive testing for adult-onset disease: The experience of Huntington disease. Am J Hum Genet 47: 4–12, 1990.
17a. Bird TD: Outrageous Fortune: The risk of suicide in genetic testing for Huntington disease. Am J Hum Genet 64: 1289–1292, 1999.
18. Guidelines for molecular genetics predictive testing in Huntington's disease. Neurology 44: 1533–1536, 1994.
19. McKinnon WC, Baty BJ, Bennett RL, Magge M, Neufeld-Kaiser WA, Peters KF, Sawyer JC, Schneider KA: Predisposition genetic testing for late-onset disorders in adults: A position paper of the National Society of Genetic Counselors. JAMA 278: 1217–1219, 1997.
20. Natowicz MR, Alper JK, Alper JS: Genetic discrimination and the law. Am J Hum Genet 50: 465–475, 1992.
21. Billings PR, Kohn MA, de Cuevas M, et al.: Discrimination as a consequence of genetic testing. Am J Hum Genet 50: 476–482, 1992.
22. Post SG, Whitehouse PJ (eds): Genetic Testing for Alzheimer Disease: Ethical and Clinical Issues. Johns Hopkins University Press, Baltimore, 1998.
23. The Ad Hoc Committee on Genetic Testing/Insurance Issues. Background statement. Am J Hum Genet 56: 327–331, 1995.
24. Wilkie T: Genetics and insurance in Britain: Why more than just the Atlantic divides the English-speaking nations. Nat Genet 20: 119–120, 1998.
25. Mehlman MJ, Kodish ED, Whitehouse P, et al.: The need for anonymous genetic counseling and testing. Am J Hum Genet 58: 393–397, 1996.
26. Uhlmann W, Ginsburg D, Gelehrter T, et al.: Questioning the need for anonymous genetic testing. Am J Hum Genet 59: 968–970, 1996.
27. Adam S, Wiggins S, Whyte P, et al.; Five year study of prenatal testing for Huntington's disease: Demand, attitudes, and psychological assessment. J Med Genet 30: 549–556, 1993.
28. ASHG/ACMG: Report, points to consider: Ethical, legal and psychosocial implications of genetic testing in children and adolescents. Am J Hum Genet 57: 1233–1241, 1995.
29. Wertz DC, Fanos JH, Reilly PR: Genetic testing for children and adolescents. Who decides? JAMA 272: 875–881, 1994.
30. Hoffman DE, EA Wulfberg: Testing children for genetic predispositions; is it in their best interest? J Law Med Ethics 23(4): 331–344, 1995.
31. Berry AC: Predictive genetic testing in children. J Med Genet 33(9): 806–807, 1996.
32. Nance MA, and the Huntington Disease Genetic Testing Group. Genetic testing of children at risk for Huntington's disease. Neurology 49: 1048–1053, 1997.
33. Bennett RL: The challenge of family history and adoption. In Bennett RL (ed): The Practical Guide to the Genetic Family History. Wiley-Liss, New York, 1999, pp.154–159.

# INDEX

Page references in italics are for figures.
Page references followed by the letter 't' are for tables.